Ryan's

OCCUPATIONAL
THERAPY
ASSISTANT

*Principles,
Practice Issues,
and Techniques*

Third Edition

Ryan's

OCCUPATIONAL THERAPY ASSISTANT

Principles, Practice Issues, and Techniques

Third Edition

Edited by

Karen Sladyk, PhD, OTR/L, FAOTA
Bay Path College
Longmeadow, MA

Sally E. Ryan, COTA, ROH, Retired
Mounds View, MN

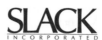

SLACK
INCORPORATED

an innovative information, education, and management company

6900 Grove Road • Thorofare, NJ 08086

Ryan's Occupational Therapy Assistant: Principles, Practice Issues, and Techniques, Third Edition is a complete revision of the classic works by Sally Ryan published by SLACK Incorporated. It includes the complete revisions of both Ryan's *The Certified Occupational Therapy Assistant: Principles, Concepts, and Techniques, Second Edition* and also *Practice Issues in Occupational Therapy: Intraprofessional Team Building*. The books were also available as *The Combined Volume: COTA Second Edition and Practice Issues in Occupational Therapy*. Now, in 2001, all of Ryan's work is completely revised and updated as *Ryan's Occupational Therapy Assistant: Principles, Practice Issues, and Techniques, Third Edition*.

Ryan's occupational therapy assistant: principles, practice issues, and techniques/edited by Sally E. Ryan, Karen Sladyk.

     p. cm.

   Includes bibliographical references and index.

   ISBN 1-55642-407-8 (alk. paper)

     1. Occupational therapy assistants. I. Title: Occupational therapy assistant. II. Ryan, Sally E. III. Sladyk, Karen.

RM735.4 .R95 2000

615.8'515--dc21

00-059568

Published by: SLACK Incorporated
                6900 Grove Road
                Thorofare, NJ 08086 USA
                Telephone: 856-848-1000
                Fax: 856-853-5991
                www.slackbooks.com

Printed in the United States of America

DEDICATION

To our family and loved ones,
past, present, and future

Contents

About the Editors

Sally E. Ryan, COTA, ROH, Retired is a graduate of the first occupational therapy assistant (OTA) program at Duluth, Minnesota in 1964. She has taken extensive coursework at the University of Minnesota as a James Wright Hunt Scholar, and at the College of St. Catherine, St. Paul. Her background includes experience in practice, clinical education supervision, and management in long-term care; consultation; and teaching in the professional occupational therapy (OT) program at the College of St. Catherine. In the past, Sally has served in a variety of leadership positions at the local, state, and national levels. She has served as representative to the American Occupational Therapy Association (AOTA) Representative Assembly from Minnesota; chair of the Representative Assembly Nominating Committee; a member-at-large of the AOTA Executive Board; member and on-site evaluator of the AOTA Accreditation Committee; and member and secretary of the AOTA Standards and Ethics Commission. She has also served as a member of the Philosophical Base Task Force, the 1981 Role Delineation Steering Committee, and as a consultant to the certified occupational therapy assistant (COTA) Task Force. She served as vice-president, secretary, and treasurer of the American Occupational Therapy Certification Board, as well as a member of the Disciplinary Action Committee. Sally is the recipient of numerous state and national awards. She was the first COTA to receive the AOTA Award of Excellence, has been recognized as an Outstanding Young Woman of America, and was among the first recipients of the AOTA Roster of Honor. The Minnesota Occupational Therapy Association has bestowed its Communication Award and Certificate of Appreciation Award on Sally. She has been invited to present numerous keynote addresses, presentations, and workshops, both nationally and internationally. Frequently her topics focus on COTA roles and relationships and intraprofessional team building. Sally has recently retired and is enjoying interior decorating, photography, needlework, and gardening.

Karen Sladyk, PhD, OTR/L, FAOTA is professor and chair of OT at Bay Path College in Longmeadow, Massachusetts. Bay Path College offers both OTA and OT programs. Karen received her bachelor's degree in OT from Eastern Michigan University and a master's degree in community health education from Southern Connecticut State University. Her practice interests in mental health and cognitive rehabilitation led to her pursuit of a doctorate in adult and vocational education at the University of Connecticut. An educator for 10 years, Karen is very interested in how students learn to become clinical reasoners. She has edited several OT texts with a focus on helping OT and OTA students master the content of OT education. In her free time she quilts, antiques for vintage jewelry, and volunteers for the local animal shelter, taking in too many strays.

Contributing Authors

Lori T. Andersen, EdD, OTR/L, received her bachelor's degree from Springfield College, her master's degree in OT from the Medical College of Virginia, and her doctorate from Nova Southeastern University. In 1994, she joined Nova Southeastern University and is an associate professor, serving as vice president of the Florida Occupational Therapy Association. Prior to entering academia, she worked in a variety of settings including acute care, home health, and rehabilitation. In her spare time she enjoys traveling, antiquing, and furniture refinishing.

Ben Atchison, PhD, OTR, FAOTA. Wife Marcia, daughters Katie and Heidi, their families, and OT students are the top priorities for Ben. He has worked in community-based OT practice for 25 years and has developed various programs and services for children and adults in family-centered venues. In addition to credentials as an OTR, he is an instructional designer/technologist and enjoys the work and play associated with computer-based instructional design and delivery.

Harriet Ann Backhaus, MA, COTA/L, ROH graduated from the OTA program at Westminster-William Woods College in Fulton, Missouri. She also began her career in rehabilitation as a part-time instructor in the OTA program at St. Louis Community College. She went on to work as a COTA and lab instructor in the Washington University Program in OT in St. Louis. She received a master's degree in gerontology and Roster of Honor (ROH) in 1992, and has served on AOTCB for 6 years. She is currently the fieldwork coordinator and an assistant professor at St. Louis Community College, and enjoys antiquing and traveling in her spare time.

Carolyn M. Baum, PhD, OTR/C, FAOTA is the Elias Michael Director and Associate Professor for OT and Neurology at Washington University School of Medicine in St Louis, MO. She served as president of both AOTA and AOTCB. She served on the National Center for Medical Rehabilitation Research and the Institute of Medicine's Committee to Assess Rehabilitation Science needs, helping to prepare a report for Congress. She heads an interdisciplinary faculty that contributes knowledge and training to understand the person and environmental factors that contribute to performance of everyday life.

Patricia K. Benham, MPH, OTR earned her undergraduate degree in OT from the College of St. Catherine in St. Paul, Minnesota, and her master of public health degree from the University of Minnesota. Her profedsional carrer has focused on pediatrics where she has held several positions in Texas and in Minnesota. She has been a faculty member in the department of OT at the College of St. Catherine and an instructor for the OTA program at the institution's St. Mary's campus. She has represented Minnesota to the AOTA's Representative Assembly. She has been employed as a lobbyist for social reform and women's issues.

Robert K. Bing, EdD, OTR, FAOTA is professor emeritus of OT at the University of Texas School of Allied Health Sciences at Galveston, Texas. He received his undergraduate degree in OT from the University of Illinois. His master of arts and doctor of education degrees were conferred by the University of Maryland. His varied clinical experiences include the United States Army, Norwich State Hospital in Connecticut, Nebraska Psychiatric Institute, Illinois Psychiatric Institute, and the University of Texas Medical Branch Hospitals, where he served as the founding dean, School of Allied Health Sciences, and professor of OT. He has also served as a member of the faculty in OT departments of six universities. Dr. Bing was elected President of the Maryland and Texas Occupational Therapy Associations and President of the AOTA. He is the recipient of the Award of Merit and the Eleanor Clarke Slagle Lectureship, and was designated as a Fellow of the AOTA. He was also named a Galveston Unsung Hero for his volunteer work and service as a liaison officer for the East Texas AIDS Project. Currently, he is retired and devoting much of his time to professional writing.

Lynda Bishop, MS, OTR/L is the assistant chair of OT and program director of the OTA program at Bay Path College. She has a bachelor's degree in OT and a master's degree in health service administration. In addition to teaching, she works part-time in home health. In her free time, she enjoys hiking, snow skiing, and taking her dogs for long walks.

Toné F. Blechert, MA, COTA, ROH is a member of the faculty and Associate Dean for 2-year degree programs at the College of St. Catherine in Minneapolis, Minnesota. She received an associate's degree from St. Mary's Junior College, a baccalaureate degree in human services from Metropolitan State University, and a master's degree in organizational leadership from the College of St. Catherine in St. Paul. Throughout her career, she has held leadership positions at the state and national level. She is a recipient of the Communication Award from the Minnesota Occupational Therapy Association and the Award of Excellence, ROH, and several Service Awards from AOTA in recognition of her leadership and exemplary contributions to the profession

Marcia Bowker, OTR, CHT is director of OT at Community Memorial Hospital in Cloquet, MN. She is certified in hand therapy, Bobath, KEY method, and Isernhagen method of functional capacity evaluation. Her focus of practice includes hand injury, industrial injury, myofascial release, neurological, and orthopedic treatment. She recently combined her work skills with her favorite hobby of quilting as a featured lecturer at the Minnesota Quilter's Annual Convention. She has acted as a consultant on ergonomics and stretching for an upcoming quilting instructional text.

Bonnie Brooks, MEd, OTR, FAOTA earned her undergraduate degree in OT at Indiana University in Indianapolis and also completed a master of science degree in Education at Loyola University in Chicago. Early in her career, she was instrumental in the development of several OTA programs and also served as a faculty member in both technical and professional education. As the assistant director of education at the AOTA, she was responsible for assisting in the development of new technical programs and for ongoing activities and initiatives in OTA education. She also served as the liaison to the COTA Task Force and the COTA Advisory Committee, and she was instrumental in providing the COTA perspective for all major AOTA committees and projects. She was also responsible for implementing the first national COTA network. She has been recognized as a Fellow by AOTA, and is now retired.

Shirley Holland Carr, MS, LOTR, FAOTA at the time of her death in 1992, was employed as an OT at the Pupil Appraisal Service for the East Baton Rouge Parish School in Louisiana, a position she held for more than eight years. She earned her undergraduate degree in education at Tufts University in Boston and received a diploma from the Boston School of OT. Later, she completed her master of science degree in psychology at Auburn University. Her many years of practice were community-oriented and included experience in child development, mental health, management, and professional and technical education. In the latter capacity, she was instrumental in planning as well as serving as the director of several OTA programs. She was a recipient of the Award of Excellence for "outstanding performance in professional development given by the Missouri Occupational Therapy Association, and she was also designated as a Fellow by AOTA.

Marianne F. Christiansen, MA, OTR is an Assistant Professor and Program Director of the OTA Program at the College of St. Catherine-Minneapolis, where she has held a faculty appointment since 1981. She entered the profession as a COTA and received her undergraduate degree in human service administration. She received a master of arts degree in health and human service administration from St. Mary's University in Winona, Minnesota. She has served on many state and national committees and boards. She is currently serving as Vice-Chair of the Accreditation Council for Occupational Therapy Education (ACOTE). In her tenure with the OTA Program, she has been an active advocate for COTA issues and concerns.

Mary Kathryn Cowan, MA, OTR, FAOTA has her bachelor's and master's degrees from the University of Minnesota. She practiced in rehabilitation and pediatrics for 14 years before teaching OT for 22 years. She worked for 2 years in a district hospital in Denmark and maintains contacts with friends there by mail and travel. She is certified in both the SCSIPT and the Bobath approach for children with cerebral palsy. She currently lives in Edinburg, TX, teaching at the University of Texas-Pan America. Her leisure interests include her Minnesota cabin, her canine companion Eliza Belle, drawing, painting, and frequent travel to Mexico.

Diane K. Direttte, PhD, OTR is an assistant professor at Western Michigan University. She earned her bachelors degree from Eastern Michigan University and her masters and doctorate degrees in OT from New York University. She worked in adult physical rehabilitation for 10 years at Kessler Institute for Rehabilitation in NJ. Her research interests include visual, visual-perceptual, and cognitive rehabilitation.

Margaret Drake, PhD, OTR/L, ATR-BC, CPAT, FAOTA has been a faculty member in four universities over 20 years. She has 12 years of mental health clinical experience and has worked overseas twice, in Saudi Arabia and Taiwan. Her research interests include history and art of healing and metaphors. Her home is in Jackson, MS with 3 cats and a dog. She has ambitions to write a series of novels about therapists.

Kathryn Melin Eberhardt, MAEd, COTA/L, ROH received her associate's degree from Southern Suburban College, and her master's degree in adult education from National Louis University. She has practiced since 1980 in mental health, physical disabilities and pediatrics and has been a full-time instructor in the OTA program at SSC since 1988. She has worked nationally and locally for the concerns of OTAs. She lives in suburban Chicago with her daughter Elizabeth.

M. Laurita (Lita) Fike, MA, OTR is an associate professor at the College of St. Catherine in St. Paul, Minnesota. She has served as director of OT at United Hospitals in St. Paul, associate director of rehabilitation services at Tucson Medical Center, director of OT at The Institute for Rehabilitation and Research in Houston, and as assistant professor of OT at the University of Texas in Galveston. After serving as assistant dean of the School of OT at Texas Women's University in Houston for 5 years, she moved back to Minnesota to be closer to her family. She is currently teaching part-time in order to devote more time to her life-long avocation of writing poetry.

Linda Florey, PhD, OTR, FAOTA has her bachelor's degree from the University of Iowa and her master's and doctoral degrees from the University of Southern California. She has worked in mental health for over 30 years and is the chief of rehabilitation services at the UCLA Neuropsychiatric Institute where she practices with children. Her academic and research interests are in play. She lives in Los Angeles, California, where she enjoys gardening in a community garden and biking on the beach.

Frank Gainer, MHS, OTR/L has his bachelor's degree from Western Michigan University and his master's degree from University of Florida. As a practitioner for 23 years he worked in a variety of settings. He is currently director of rehabilitation services for Greater Southeast Healthcare Systems of Washington, DC. He is a medical rehabilitation program surveyor for CARF, a member of the Accreditation Council for Occupational Therapy Education, and a member of the Roster of Accreditation Evaluators.

Tara J. Glennon, MS, OTR/L, BCP is an assistant professor of OT at Quinnipiac University and owner of several pediatric therapy clinics in Connecticut. She has lectured extensively on issues related to pediatric practice and has taught the SIPT certification courses for Sensory Integration International. She is hooked on audiotapes of suspense novels, and loves antique shopping and home decorating. She never misses a morning walk on the beach with Johanna and their dogs.

Dairlyn Gower, BS, COTA has been an instructor in the OTA program at Lake Superior College in Duluth, MN for 23 years. She is a graduate of that program and has her bachelor's degree in vocational-technical education from the

University of Minnesota. Over the past 15 years, she has served on a variety of committees and task forces, including the Certification Examination Development Committee and the Practice Analysis Task Force for NBCOT.

Lisa Hindbjorgen, OTS is an OT graduate student at the University of South Dakota with graduation planned for December 2000. She has a bachelor's degree in special education and psychology from Augustana College. With her love for children, Lisa plans to work in the school setting. Her hobbies include soccer, decorating, flower designing, reading, and movies.

Sue Triplett Hunt, MA, OTR received her bachelor's degree from Kansas University and her master's degree in early childhood/special education form St Joseph's College. She is an assistant professor at Quinnipiac College in Hamden, CT. Sue's professional interests include home visiting in early intervention and problem based learning. She is grateful for her son, Ian, and her friend, Michael, who provide ample support and encouragement along with quite weekends to write. Sue and her family live in Marlborough, CT where all enjoy cooking, gardening, and playing with the dog, Lucy.

Anne Birge James, MS, OTR has an advanced OT degree from Boston University and has worked full-time in a variety of clinical settings with adults with physical disabilities before becoming an educator 8 years ago. She maintains a clinical practice in home care while teaching at the University of Hartford. She lives in rural CT with her husband and daughter and never seems to find enough time for biking and cross country skiing.

Paula W. Jamison, PhD, OTR has her bachelor's degree from the University of Washington and a master's and doctorate from University of Chicago. Her master's in OT is from Western Michigan University where she returned to teach. She is currently researching effectiveness of using writing as a therapeutic tool. An avid traveler, she lives in Kalamazoo, MI with her husband and 2 cats.

Nancy Kari, MPH, OTR is Director of Program and Faculty Development for the Higher Education Consortium of Urban Affairs. She co-authored the text *Building America: the Democratic Promise of Public Work* with Harry Boyte. Her writings on public work, civic professionalism, and democracy have appeared in *The New Democrat, Policy Review, Dissent, Commonweal, The Wall Street Journal* and other publications. She is also a co-founder of the Jane Addams School for Democracy, in St. Paul, Minnesota.

Marijke Kehrhahn, MA, PhD is an assistant professor of adult and vocational education at the University of Connecticut. Her research and practice specializes in work place learning. She has worked as a staff development specialist and was Director of Volunteer Services for the 1995 Special Olympic World Games. She lives in rural CT with her husband, Ray, and daughter Jasmine. She volunteers assisting people with autism transition to adult life. She likes to use her free time to sew, read, decorate, and travel.

Barbara Kornblau, JD, OT/L, FAOTA, DAAPM, ABDA, CDSM, CCM is an OT and a practicing attorney. A graduate of the University of Wisconsin-Madison and the

University of Miami School of law, she has lectured internationally and published extensively on medicolegal issues. She has served in many volunteer roles for AOTA including President of the AOTA (2001-2003). She is a member of the faculty of Nova Southeastern University and the mother of 6 children. Her occupations include reading, quilting, genealogy and serving the community through the South Miami Rotary Club.

Barbara Larson, MA, OTR, FAOTA is an occupational health specialist with Isernhagen Work Systems in Duluth, MN. She practiced in adult rehabilitation before specializing in occupational health and industrial rehabilitation. She currently provides work injury prevention/ management services to businesses and therapists throughout America. She is adjunct faculty in OT at the College of St Catherine and the University of Minnesota.

Cheryl A. Leary, EdD is an associate professor of psychology at Bay Path College in Longmeadow, MA. Cheryl serves as senior class advisor and co-advisor to the international students at the college. She is a member of the school board for St Mary's Elementary School in Longmeadow. Prior to working at Bay Path College, Cheryl retired in 1992 from the public school system after 20 years of service as an educator and school psychologist. Her favorite hobbies are tap dancing, traveling with her husband, Chris, and shopping for goodies for her grandchildren, Meg and Robbie.

Christopher J. Leary, M.Div, MS, LPC, LADC serves as president and CEO of New Directions, Inc in Enfield, CT, an outpatient substance abuse and mental health treatment facility. In addition to holding licenses to practice counseling in CT and MA, Chris is nationally certified as an alcohol and drug counselor. His hobbies include writing, music composition, traveling, and balancing the checkbook after his wife goes shopping for the grandchildren.

Martha Logigian, MS, OTR/L has her master's degree from the State University of New York at Buffalo. She has lived in Boston, MA for 30 years where she has practiced and taught OT; 15 years as director of rehabilitation services at Brigham and Women's Hospital. She currently lives in Rochester, NY with her husband and two young daughters. Martha currently specializes in early intervention and sensory integration.

Wendy Mueller, MA, OTR/L is assistant director of Speech Pathology Services of Atlanta, GA. She supervises OT, the therapeutic preschool, and the camp programs. Wendy is a member of AOTA's Roster of Accreditation Evaluators and often a guest lecturer at local schools. Her pediatric fellowship was at University of Southern California with an internship at the prestigious Ayres' Clinic where she completed her SI certification. In addition to her professional interests, Wendy is active in the environmental organization Chattahoochee Riverkeepers, preserving local rivers and lakes. As an animal lover, she is the proud parent of 8-lb poodle, Espion.

Stanley Paul, PhD, OTR/L completed his advanced master's degree from the State University of New York at Buffalo and his doctorate at New York University. He has worked in a variety of settings and is currently assistant professor at Western Michigan University. His research interests include outcome studies, assistive technology, functional independence, adaptive design, and students with disabilities.

Deanna Proulx-Sepelak, OTR/L received her OT degree from Quinnipiac College and is currently pursuing a master's degree in health administration and a juris doctorate in law. Deanna is an adjunct faculty member at Quinnipiac College in the Department of OT and practices clinically at an acute rehabilitation hospital and a community-based setting for young adults with cognitive deficits. She and her husband Jeff reside in Middlebury, CT, and are eagerly awaiting the arrival of their first child in the early winter of 2000.

Ellen Berger Rainville, MS, OTR, FAOTA is an assistant professor of OT at Springfield College, where she teaches pediatric, clinical practice, and research courses. There she collaborates with a terrific faculty and student body. She also has a private consulting practice and is a doctoral candidate at Boston University. Her husband, Mike, and her children, Kellie, David, and Nicole, bring her great joy, as does her home is the country, her extended family, and her friends.

S. Maggie Reitz, PhD, OTR/L, FAOTA has both her bachelor's and master's degrees in OT from Towson State University in Maryland. After 10 years of clinical practice, she returned to Towson to teach, and currently serves as chairperson of the Department of OT and Occupational Science. She has completed her dissertation on coronary heart disease for a doctorate in health education. her areas of interest include occupational theory and philosophy, occupational science, ethics, and forensic issues. She resides with her husband, Fred, and their daughter, Jessica, and an unusual cat by the name of Splotch.

Denise Rotert, MA, OTR/L received her bachelor degree in OT from the University of Puget Sound and her masters degree in psychology, guidance, and counseling from the University of Northern Colorado. She spent 20 years in the US Army where she specialized in mental health treatment, substance abuse, program development and OTA education. Following retirement from the army, she joined the faculty at the University of South Dakota for 8 years and is currently self employed. Her interests include volunteer work for literacy, cooking, reading, and walking.

Angela E. Scoggin, PhD, OTR is an associate professor in the OT program at the University of Texas-Pan American. She earned her bachelor's degree in OT from the University of Florida, and master's and doctorate degrees in applied anthropology from the UNiversity of South Florida. Dr. Scoggin has over 25 years of experience as an OT, with a clinical emphasis on working with children and their families in early intervention and public school programs. She has conducted research studies related to child development and family/caregiver interactions in China, Peru, and the southern United States. In addition to teaching, her favorite occupations include traveling, family outings, and learning to play Suzuki violin with her young daughter.

Phillip D. Shannon, MA, MPA has been the coordinator of the Community Health Education and Medicaid Access Enhancement Project, co-sponsored by the Cameron County Health Department in San Benito, Texas, and by Project HOPE in Millwood, Virginia. His undergraduate degree in OT from California State University at San Jose was followed by two graduate degrees from the University of Southern California, a Master of Arts degree in OT and a Master of Public Administration degree. He has served as a program director in both technical and professional OT educational programs and is a retired officer of the United States Army. He has published extensively in professional journals, primarily on the philosophy and theory of OT, and he has published chapters in three books as well. In addition to developing and presenting numerous workshops in the United States, he developed and conducted workshops for the United States Army Seventh Medical Command in Germany from 1985-1990. He was also the principal speaker for the Sixth National Congress of the Occupational Therapy Association, Bogata, Columbia. He has been the recipient of several awards, including the Chair's Service Award from the State University of New York at Buffalo, the Service Award of the AOTA, and the Retired Educator's Award from the Association's Commission on Education. He has also been recognized as a Fellow by the AOTA. He has served as Chair of the Certification Examination Development Committee and member of the Board of Directors of the American Occupational Therapy Certification Board.

Roseanna Tufano, LMFT, OTR/L has a bachelor's degree in OT from Quinnipiac College. She has worked in a variety of mental health settings since 1980 as a practitioner and consultant with community, outpatient, and inpatient populations. At the present time, she is an assistant professor at Quinnipiac College and academic coordinator for the OT department. She teaches classes related to psychosocial functioning and clinical reasoning in both the OT and physical therapy departments. Roseanna also has her master's degree in family therapy. She is a licensed marriage and family therapist and has a small private practice. She resides with her husband, Lou, and their two children, Carisa and Brett. They are her source for love, inspiration, and fun.

Jaclyn West-Frasier, MA, OTR is an assistant professor and problem-based learning coordinator at Western Michigan University. Her past experience includes 20 years of clinical practice, including 10 years as an entrepreneur in interdisciplinary group practice. Jaclyn has been married almost as long as she has practice OT and has two children, ages 13 and 10. She and her family enjoy gardening, camping, kayaking, and mountain biking.

PREFACE

Sometimes great things happen in your life for what seems like no reason at all. That's what happened when friends Amy Drummond and John Bond approached me with what now has became known as the "Ryan Project." Sally Ryan, in my opinion a world-famous OT practitioner, was planning a new phase in her life: retirement. She was looking for someone to take over the editing of her two books, *The Certified Occupational Therapy Assistant* and *Practice Issues in Occupational Therapy*. These books had formed the educational foundation for many, many practicing OTAs. The question came, "Would I be interested?"

Needless to say, the answer was yes. I worked closely with Sally to keep the important characteristics of her books. We had several focus groups, surveys, and informal discussions with the educators who used the book. I talked with several students about their concerns. The issue of one or two books came up many times. As you can see, the decision was made for one integrated book. I'm thrilled with the results.

Four sections make up the new integrated text. The first section looks at important foundation concepts such as history, Uniform Terminology, and OT process. This was a difficult task, as our profession is experiencing such great changes now. As we await the new updated Uniform Terminology, it is helpful for students to understand our current and recent past history as well. The second section introduces students to people who are experiencing the challenges of disabilities. Some of these challenges are minor, while others are life-changing. The chapters provide general information about the disabilities, as well as important vocabulary and key concepts. The third section provides information on the "doing" of OT. Ongoing and always changing treatment techniques are introduced with the hope that students will continue to research the most current techniques. Lastly, the fourth section focuses on the management aspects of an OTA's professional life. How-to information and professional development are the main points of this section.

Six OT professionals reviewed the entire book draft independent of each other and provided us with enormous assistance with the final project. In general, the reviewers were excited about occupation-based case stories and the updated style of information. As an educator of both OTAs and OTs, I wanted the book to be easily read in order to provide current information in a student friendly manner. I'm happy to see the final results.

Editing such a large book was not an easy task. Updating 44 chapters, 4 appendices, and the front matter was a huge task. Many chapters had several authors, so the combined collaborative experience included over 150 people including authors, reviewers, and production staff. We would need another chapter just to highlight their contributions, but several people deserve special attention. I am especially thankful to Sally Ryan for her insights. All the authors clearly worked hard to provide OTA students with the best knowledge they could share. Authors that had worked with Sally on earlier editions were very tolerant of the "new kid" and were welcoming. Amy Drummond is more a friend than an editorial director. John Bond, Debra Toulson, and Kate Buczko kept me on track. Lauren Plummer made the whole project look great. My family was very tolerant of the 100 times I said, "Just a minute, I'm on the computer."

I hope this book provides you with the foundation you need to practice sound and meaningful OT. It is our hope that this book is only the beginning of a lifetime of continuing learning.

Karen Sladyk, PhD, OTR/L, FAOTA

HISTORICAL PERSPECTIVE

Work on the first edition of this text began in the spring of 1984. That year was particularly significant because it marked the 25th anniversary of certified occupational therapy assistants (COTAs) working in the field.

The project was given impetus from the fact that there was no comprehensive book written expressly for occupational therapy assistants. Discussions with technical level faculty, occupational therapists serving as clinical supervisors, and assistants emphasized the need for a text that would focus on the basic principles, concepts, and techniques of the profession; a book that would provide both an extensive and a realistic view of the roles and functions of COTAs in entry-level practice and beyond; a book that would provide examples of how to successfully build intraprofessional relationships; and, finally, a book that could be used in the clinic as well as the classroom. These objectives were adopted as a foundation for developing, organizing, and sequencing content areas in each edition.

In conclusion, it is my belief that this book will continue to serve as a model and a guidepost for occupational therapy teamwork in the delivery of services. It will serve as an incentive for the technically and professionally educated practitioners to discover the many ways in which their skills and roles complement each other. It will also serve as a catalyst for developing new skills and roles in response to the ever-changing needs of our society.

The former president of the American Occupational Therapy Association (AOTA), Carolyn Manville Baum, summed it up best in her 1980 Eleanor Clarke Slagle Address when she stated

> As a profession and as professionals, let us put our resources, intelligence, and emotional commitment together and work diligently toward the ascent of our profession. The health care system, the clients (patients) we serve, and each of us individually will benefit from our commitment.

Sally E. Ryan, COTA, ROH, Retired

FOREWORD

A mythical phoenix rising out of ashes is the international symbol of OT denoting rebuilding and recovery from adversity. This legend persists in my mind as I write the foreword for the third edition of my dear colleague's book. As the development of this edition embarked almost 4 years ago, several life and career shaping events impacted her plan to reformulate and update her pioneering book, *The Certified Occupational Therapy Assistant: Principles, Concepts and Techniques,* and incorporate it into one text with her *Practice Issues in Occupational Therapy.*

As a leader, pioneer, and visionary in the field of OT, the last decade found Sally Ryan dedicated to the complex and sometimes controversial issues of national examination and certification of OT personnel through her work on the National Board of Certification of Occupational Therapy (NBCOT). Legal disputes over several years with the leadership of the American Occupational Therapy Association (AOTA) and NBCOT tested the very core of her leadership, with her persistence, integrity, and patience prevailing. She joined with many of her colleagues to rebuild that critical corporate partnership to the benefit of the vitality of the profession.

As a loving wife and partner, she recently experienced the sudden and devastating loss of her husband. If ever there is the ultimate challenge to one's daily existence, Sally now had to reshape her career and life plan and dig deeply into all of her resources and friendships to rise as a phoenix. Part of that plan would take her into professional retirement after many amazing years as a member of the faculty at the College of St. Catherine and also cause her to embark on various business activities dealing with her husband's estate. Healing and rebuilding took her to new paths that will generate the sought-after new life.

Meanwhile, the third edition was still on the table and Sally was able to entice the talented Dr. Karen Sladyk to take the role as co-editor of the new book. Karen brings enthusiasm, a wide range of skills, and a wealth of professional experience to the challenge of updating and reshaping this longstanding, universally popular text. Over the years Karen has been dedicated to developing clinical reasoning skills in OT and OTA students and helping them learn how to become highly competent OT practitioners and effective teammates. This is a partnership made in heaven, as one can easily deduct from the quality of the third edition.

OT entered the 21st century with many of the benefits of Sally's and Karen's labors: Stronger professional OT teams; students who are prepared to meet the demands of the health care economy; and a legacy of confidence and optimism that we can tackle anything. The third edition continues Sally's and Karen's commitments to excelling at foundational skills, knowledge, and attitudes for the demands and opportunities of tomorrow's workplace. Yet they also include new horizons in inspired teamwork, wellness and prevention strategies, and a continuum of development for practice and management skill that will institute life-long learning for the team.

Karen and Sally's book not only continues to deliver a superb classroom text for the OTA student, but is also a critical text for the professional OT educational programs. Accreditation and certification requirements have increasingly asserted the importance of the professional level OT student being knowledgeable about the roles, capabilities, and responsibilities of their teammates. Sally's visionary leadership, built on by Karen's experiences, puts forth the model to emulate and demonstrates the multitude of possibilities by which the OTR's and COTA's experiences and roles complement each other. And for the practicing OTR's who want their teams to thrive and to make a difference, this book will inform and inspire you to improve your professional practice in this fast-changing marketplace.

What impresses me, is that this pioneering woman—this leader who has led the field in the accumulation and publication of the material necessary to fully prepare and develop generations of COTA's and OTR's in America—has gracefully and persistently demonstrated the characteristics we attribute to our inspirational professional symbol. Karen's expertise continues that symbol, and carries this book forward into the next generation of OTs. Lessons from the phoenix support us as we shift paradigms, question and seek best practices through research, push our search for excellence to the limit, and receive inspiration to work successfully with empathy, elegance, and grace.

Mary M. Evert, ScD(hon.), MBA, OTR, FAOTA

Historical, Philosophical, and Theoretical Principles

Looking Back, Living Forward: Occupational Therapy History

Chapter 1

Robert K. Bing, EdD, OTR, FAOTA

INTRODUCTION

Today, occupational therapy (OT) personnel face numerous predicaments. Educational preparation for practice is based predominantly on knowledge and skills that are marketable in a very competitive health care environment. The *what* of our art, science, and technology is emphasized, often at the expense of the *why*. What is missing is the sense of what has come before, of those recurring patterns that offer legitimacy and uniqueness in the health care profession.

History is an invaluable tool to assess the present and determine future courses of action. The recording of an occupational life or medical history is a testament to the past's influence on current conditions and its ability to offer approaches to alleviate problems. Fundamentally, history is experience, rather than the mere telling of quaint stories or reminiscing about past feats or failures. It is knowing enough about what has come before to know what to consider or what to rule out in evaluating the present on our way to the future. As Neustadt and May (1986) point out, we must learn how to use experience, whether remote or recent, in the process of deciding what to do today about the opportunities for tomorrow.

In the late 1700s, Western Europe was astir with a new view of life. Social, political, economic, and religious theories promoted a general sense of human progress and perfectibility (DeGrazia, 1962). Notions about intolerance, censorship, and economic and social restraints were being abandoned and replaced by a strong faith in rational behavior. Universally valid principles governing humanity, nature, and society directed people's lives and interpersonal relationships.

The changing ethic of work added a rich ingredient to this new, heady brew. Fundamental was Martin Luther's viewpoint, which declared that everyone who could work should do so. Illness and begging were unnatural. Charity should be extended only to those who could not work because of mental or physical infirmities or old age.

MORAL TREATMENT

Near the center of all of this invigorating change was the treatment of sick peo-

ESSENTIAL VOCABULARY

Habit training: Developed by Slagle to provide routine and occupation to severely ill patients.

Invalid occupations: Coined by Tracy as activities for the disabled.

Moral treatment: Change from jail-like conditions to treatment focus for people with mental illness.

National Society for the Promotion of Occupational Therapy: The forerunner of the American Occupational Therapy Association (AOTA).

Occupational nurse: First training of nurses in the use of occupation in treatment.

ple, particularly the mentally ill. Whereas long-term survivors of physical disease with physical disabilities were still rare because treatment was so inadequate, the mentally ill were a significant portion of the population.

Up to this time, the insane had been housed and handled no differently than criminals and paupers, and were often chained in dungeons. Moral treatment of the insane was one product of the Age of Enlightenment. It sprang from the fundamental attitudes of the day:

- A set of principles that govern humanity and society
- Faith in the ability of the human to reason
- Purposeful work as a moral obligation
- The supreme belief in the individual

Fast disappearing were the centuries-old notions that the insane were possessed of demons, that they were no better than paupers or criminals, and that crime, sin, vice, and inactivity were the core of insanity.

Two men of the 18th century working in different countries, and unknown to each other, initiated the moral treatment movement. These two could not have been more dissimilar. Phillippe Pinel was of the French Revolution, a physician, a scholar, and a natural philosopher. William Tuke was an English merchant, wealthy, a deeply religious Quaker, and a philanthropist.

Father of Moral Treatment— Phillippe Pinel

According to Pinel, moral treatment meant treating the emotions. He believed the emotionally disturbed individual was out of balance and the patient's own emotions could be used to restore equilibrium. The compassionate Pinel believed the loss of reason was the most calamitous of all human afflictions. The ability to reason, he claimed, principally separates the human from other living forms. As Pinel wrote in his famous treatise in 1806, because of mental illness, the human character is always perverted. His thoughts and actions are diverted, his personal liberty is at length taken from him (Pinel, 1806).

Occupation figured prominently in Pinel's scheme, primarily to take patients' minds away from emotional distress and to develop their abilities. Music and various forms of literature were used. Physical exercise and work were a part of institutional living. Pinel advocated patient farms on the hospital grounds. This period was largely an agricultural era, where one's life revolved around producing products necessary for survival and one's emotional content was elaborately interwoven. The care of animals and the necessary routines of growing crops provided patients with a respect for the authority of nature as well as the most liberty that could be tolerated. The unvarying routine to maintain farming as part of the institution

made a strong appeal to moral concepts, such as respect, self-esteem, and dignity for the patient.

The York Retreat—William Tuke

Part of this new humane concern was influenced by the beliefs and work of the Society of Friends, derisively known as the Quakers. They emerged in 17th century England and became one of the most distinctive movements of Puritanism. In the last decades of the 18th century, William Tuke and various members of his family established The York Retreat, primarily because of their religious-based concerns about the deplorable conditions in public insane asylums. Until this time, the term *retreat* had never been applied to an asylum. Tuke's daughter-in-law suggested the term to convey the Quaker belief that such an institution may be a quiet haven, a place in which the unhappy might obtain refuge (Tuke, 1813).

Several fundamental principles became evident within a short time. The approach was primarily one of kindness and consideration. The patients were not thought to be devoid of reason or feelings or honor. The social environment was to be as nearly like that of a family with an atmosphere of religious sentiment and moral feeling. Tuke and Thomas Fowler, the visiting physician, believed that most insane people retain a considerable amount of self-command. The staff endeavored to gain the patient's confidence, to reinforce self-esteem, and to arrest the attention and fix it on objects that are opposite to the illusions the patient might possess. Employment in various occupations was expected as a way for the patient to maintain control over his or her disorder (Tuke, 1813).

Pinel's major work on moral treatment was published in 1801, and Tuke's description of The Retreat appeared in 1813. These brought on a rush of reforms in institutions in Europe and, ultimately, the United States.

Sir William and Lady Ellis

Sir William Charles Ellis and his wife were in charge of newly founded county asylums in England during the first half of the 19th century. They regarded the hospital as a community—"a family"—as Sir Ellis called it. He paid little attention to medical remedies and concentrated on moral treatment principles, which he believed to be difficult but most likely to result in the gradual return to reason and happiness.

A remarkable innovation of Sir and Lady Ellis was the establishment of aftercare houses and night hospitals. Keenly aware of environmental and social influences on insanity, they envisioned these halfway houses as steppingstones from the asylum to the world (Hunter & Macalpine, 1963).

Moral Treatment in the United States

The roots of moral care and occupation as treatment were brought to the United States by the Quakers. They established asylums and immediately implemented Tuke's programs. The programs were popular because they helped maintain relatively low costs by having patients perform most of the necessary work of the asylum: growing crops and vegetables, maintaining herds, and manufacturing clothing and other goods. The typical institution was a beehive of activity largely designed to help it remain as self-sufficient as possible.

Reformers were in abundance. Borrowing heavily from The York Retreat, Thomas Eddy, a member of the board of governors of the Society of the New York Hospital, proposed in 1815 the construction of a building for exclusive use by mental patients. He envisioned a balanced program of exercise, entertainment, and occupations (Hass, 1924).

In the mid 1800s, just when it seemed that the moral movement was expected to be fully realized, unanticipated trouble came from all directions. A reform-minded humanitarian, Dorthea Lynde Dix, had been campaigning vigorously for better care of the mentally ill, including moral principles. State legislatures were responding positively by establishing public mental hospitals. By 1848, Dix decided to approach the federal government. Her vision was the establishment of a federal system of hospitals. After 6 years of wearying work, Dix was rewarded when Congress passed her bill. President Franklin Pierce, however, vetoed it, claiming states' rights would be endangered if the federal government took on the care of mentally ill patients.

State hospitals were experiencing great difficulties with a new type of patients: immigrants from Europe who were unable to adjust to the new conditions. They became public wards, often unable to use the language, and were considered unemployable. Several hospitals attempted to introduce moral principles, even establishing English instruction. The Bloomingdale, a New York Asylum made such an attempt in 1845. Classes were also held in chemistry, geometry, and the physical sciences. These classes were coupled with manual labor suitable for men and women. This approach eventually failed for many reasons. Patients often were unaccustomed to the American forms of labor. Bilingual instructors could not be found. Foreign-born mechanics and artisans could not find familiar labor. Finally, large numbers of patients were too ill to participate in the available occupations (Hass, 1924).

By the mid 1800s, the American agenda largely consisted of expansionism and slavery issues. These did not bode well for improving or increasing public care of the insane. Moral treatment, including occupations, rapidly began to disappear. By the onset of the Civil War, virtual-ly none existed in state or public-supported institutions. Custodial care continued well into the 20th century (Bockhoven, 1972).

20TH CENTURY PROGRESSIVISM

The 20th century brought with it unparalleled exuberance. The United States had largely recovered from the Civil War and acquired considerable overseas possessions as a result of the Spanish-American War. For a few years before 1900 and for some years after, nearly all Americans had become ardent believers in progress, although they did not always agree about what the word meant. Prosperity was fueled by science and technology and with a flurry of industrial inventions. Cities grew rapidly, particularly in the East and Midwest. Railroads punched their way through all kinds of barriers and in all directions, linking the country's population. The newly invented automobile served important economic purposes and became useful in leisure pursuits (Bates, 1976).

There was more than a modest amount of zaniness during this era. Many physicians regarded increased female education as the primary cause of decreased women's health. These men felt the woman's brain simply could not assimilate a great deal of academic instruction beyond high school. Some physicians went further and claimed that women who worked were in danger of acquiring predominantly male afflictions—alcoholism, paralysis, and insanity. Women were thought to have an inborn immunity to such ills.

Drug therapy was also unusual by today's standards. The pharmaceutical firm that helped to usher in the aspirin craze introduced a new medication for bad coughs—heroin. Other over-the-counter products included cocaine tablets for the throat and general nervousness. Baby syrups were spiked with morphine, and miscarriage-producing pills were, according to the ads, a sure and great remedy for women.

The Progressive Era was not always progressive. Poverty, racial injustice, ethnic unrest, sterilization of mental defectives (as they were known) and possible sterilization of social misfits, repression of women's rights because of leftover Victorian ideals, a marked increase in industrial accidents resulting in chronic disabilities, and a continued lack of concern about the institutionalized insane were all part of the times.

Chicago's Hull House

Social experiments abounded during this period, particularly in urban areas. One such experiment was Hull House, opened by Jane Addams in 1889. Hull House was intended to serve the immigrants and the poor through a variety of educational, social, and investigative programs. Along with Julia Lathrop and Florence Kelley,

Addams created an environment that helped bring OT to the forefront, as part of the restorative process of individual freedom. Eleanor Clarke Slagle, a pioneer in OT, spent two years as a staff member at Hull House and established the first training program for occupation workers (the forerunner of OT personnel).

Invalid Occupations—Susan Tracy

The first individual in the 20th century to use occupations with acutely ill patients was Susan Tracy, a nurse. She initiated instruction in activities to student nurses as early as 1902. She coined the term *occupational nurse* to signify a specialization. By 1912, she was working full-time to apply moral treatment principles to acute medical conditions. She was convinced that remedial activities should be classified by their physiological effects as stimulants or sedatives (Tracy, 1914). Tracy was also interested in experimentation and observation to enhance her practice. In 1918, she published a research paper on 25 mental tests derived from occupations (Tracy, 1918a), for example, instructing a patient in using a piece of leather and a pencil, and asking him or her to make a line of dots at equal distances around the margin and at uniform distances from the edge. This constitutes a test of judgment in estimating distances (Tracy, 1918a). Continuing with the same piece of leather, the patient is instructed to punch a hole at each dot. To do this, the patient must consider the two sides of leather and the two parts of the tool and must bring these together, thus making a simple construction test (Tracy, 1918a).

Tracy (1923) determined that high-quality work was therapeutic, worth doing well, and that practical, well-made articles have a greater therapeutic value than useless, poorly made articles. Tracy's major work, *Studies in Invalid Occupations*, published in 1918, is a revealing compendium of her observations and experiences with different kinds of patients (Tracy, 1918b). Among her many lasting principles, one stands out: the patient is the product, not the article he [or she] makes.

Re-Education of Convalescents— George Barton

The Progressive Era spawned a number of reformers who, although dissimilar in background, character, and temperament, strove to work together on common goals. Two individuals significant to OT were George Edward Barton and William Rush Dunton, Jr. Barton, by profession an architect, contracted tuberculosis during adulthood. His constant struggle led him into a life of service to physically disabled persons.

Barton founded Consolation House in Clifton Springs, NY, in 1914, an early prototype of a rehabilitation center. Today he would be considered an entrepreneur. He was an effective speaker and writer, although often given to exaggeration. Barton's main themes were hospitals and their responsibilities to the discharged patient, the conditions the discharged patient faces, the need to return to employment after an illness, and occupations and education of convalescents.

Barton's first published article in 1914 was based on a speech given to a group of nurses, in which he described a weakness in hospitals—hospitals discharge not efficients, but inefficients. An individual leaves almost any of our institutions only to become a burden upon his family, his friends, the associated charities, or upon another institution. Later in the article he warns to his subject, discharge a patient from the hospital with his fracture healed, to be sure, but to a devastated home, to an empty desk, and to no obvious sustaining employment is to send him out to a world cold. His solution was occupation to shorten convalescence and improve the condition of many patients. He ended his oration with a rallying cry: "... It is time for humanity to cease regarding the hospital as a door closing upon a life which is past and to regard it henceforth as a door opening upon a life which is to come" (Barton, 1914, p. 336).

At Consolation House, physically impaired individuals underwent a thorough review, including a social and medical history, and a consideration of their education, training, experience, successes, and failures. Barton (1922) believed that by "considering these in relation to the condition [the patient] must presumably or inevitably be in for the remainder of his life, we can find some form of occupation for which he will be fitted" (p. 320). Barton's major contribution to the re-emergence of moral treatment principles was an awakening of physical reconstruction and re-education through employment. Convalescence, to him, was a critical time for the inclusion of something to do.

Judicious Regimen of Activity— William Dunton

A medical school graduate of the University of Pennsylvania and a psychiatrist, William Rush Dunton, Jr., devoted his entire life to OT. A prolific writer, he published in excess of 120 books and articles related to OT and rehabilitation. He also served as treasurer and president of the National Society for the Promotion of Occupational Therapy (the forerunner of the American Occupational Therapy Association), and for 21 years he was editor of their official journal. As a physician, he spent his professional career treating psychiatric patients in an institutional setting. Key to his treatment methods was what he called a judicious regimen of activity. He read the works of Tuke and Pinel, as well as the efforts of significant alienists (an early term for psychiatrists) of the 19th century.

In 1895, Dunton joined the medical staff at Sheppard and Enoch Pratt Asylum in Towson, MD. From his readings and observations of patients there he concluded that acutely ill patients generally were not amenable to occupations because their weakened attention span would make involvement in activity fatiguing and harmful. Later, activities might be prescribed that use energies not needed for physical restoration. Stimulating attention and directing the thoughts of the patient in regular and healthful paths would ensure an early discharge from the hospital. Dunton developed a wide variety of activities from knitting and crocheting to printing, the repair of dynamos, and farm work to gain the attention and interest, as well as to meet the needs, of all patients. He stated that a patient makes more rapid progress if his attention is concentrated upon what he is making and he derives stimulating pleasure in its performance (Dunton, 1935). Interest in the activity was paramount in Dunton's thinking.

At the second annual meeting of the National Society for the Promotion of Occupational Therapy in 1918, Dunton unveiled his nine cardinal principles to guide the emerging practice of OT and to ensure that the new discipline would gain acceptance as a medical entity. These principles were the following:

1. Any activity should have as its objective a cure.
2. The activity should be interesting.
3. There should be a useful purpose other than to merely gain the patient's attention and interest.
4. The activity should preferably lead to an increase in knowledge on the patient's part.
5. Activity should be carried on with others, such as a group.
6. The OT should make a careful study of the patient and attempt to meet as many needs as possible through activity.
7. Activity should cease before the onset of fatigue.
8. Genuine encouragement should be given whenever indicated.
9. Work is much to be preferred over idleness, even when the end product of the patient's labor is of poor quality or is useless (Dunton, 1918).

The major purposes of occupation in the case of the mentally ill were outlined in Dunton's first book, *Occupation Therapy: A Manual for Nurses,* published in 1915. The primary objective is to divert attention from unpleasant subjects, as is true with the depressed patient; or from daydreaming or mental ruminations, as in the case of dementia praecox (schizophrenia), to divert the attention to one main subject.

Another purpose of occupation is to re-educate, to train the patient in developing mental processes through educating the hands, eyes, and muscles, just as is done in the developing child (Dunton, 1915). Fostering an interest in hobbies is a third purpose. Hobbies serve as both present and future safety valves and render a recurrence of mental illness less likely. A final purpose may be to instruct the patient in a craft until he or she has gained enough proficiency to take pride in the work. However, Dunton worried that specialization would limit interest in the world in general. (1915).

The Origin of the Term *Occupational Therapy*

There is a continuing controversy about who was initially responsible for the term *occupational therapy*—Dunton or Barton. At Sheppard and Enoch Pratt Asylum, Dunton directed the therapeutic occupations program. A special building was completed in 1902 and named The Casino. It was a dedicated space for a wide variety of occupations and amusements. In 1911, Dunton initiated a training program for nurses in patient occupations, and here he first used the term occupation therapy. This term appeared in his handwritten lecture notes, dated October 10, 1911. This is the earliest known record of the use of this term. In later years, Dunton indicated that Adolph Meyer, a renowned psychiatrist and personal and professional friend, was the first to use the terms *therapy* and *therapeutic* in connection with occupations, but that he was the first person to put occupation and therapy together as one phrase (AOTA, 1914-1917).

Barton's claim to the first use of the term appeared initially in March 1915, in the *Trained Nurse and Hospital Review.* The article was based on a speech given in Massachusetts on December 28, 1914. Before then, Barton had preferred the term occupation re-education, which accurately described his efforts at Consolation House. During preliminary discussions between Barton and Dunton about a national organization during 1915 to 1916, a series of squabbles took place, mostly through correspondence. Terminology figured heavily in these differences of opinion. Barton preferred his occupational re-education and Dunton held tenaciously to occupation therapy. Barton finally countered with occuaptioanl therapy, preferring the adjectival form. They did agree on the term *occupational workers,* since the word therapist was considered the sole property of the psychiatrist. Dunton did not change his mind until well into the 1920s (Barton, 1915; Bing, 1987).

Habit Training—Eleanor Clarke Slagle

Eleanor Clarke Slagle is considered the most distinguished 20th century OT. One of five founders of the national professional organization, she served in every major elective office. She was also executive secretary for 14 years. In the first decade of this century, she was partially trained as a social worker and completed one of the early special courses in curative occupations and recreation at the Chicago School of Civics and Philanthropy, which was associated with Hull House. She worked subsequently in a number of institutions, most notably the new Henry Phipps Clinic, Johns Hopkins Hospital, Baltimore, MD. There she served under the direction of the renowned psychiatrist Adolph Meyer. At this time, she became a devoted friend of William Dunton's family. Later, she moved to New York, where she pioneered in developing OT in the State Department of Mental Hygiene.

Slagle (1934) was knowledgeable about moral treatment principles and embraced them as the core of her thinking and practice. She emphasized that OT must be a purposely planned progressive program of rest, play, occupation, and exercise. She often spoke of the need for the mentally ill person to have a fairly well-balanced day.

Her most long-lasting contribution to the care of the mentally ill was what she entitled habit training. This plan was first attempted at the Rochester, New York State Hospital in 1901, but it was Slagle who developed and refined the basic principles for those patients who had been hospitalized for 5 to 20 years and whose behavior had steadily regressed. Habit training was 24 hours long and involved the entire ward staff. It was a re-education program designed to overcome disorganized habits, to modify other habits, and to construct new ones, with the goal of restoring and maintaining of health (Slagle, 1922).

A typical habit-training schedule called for patients to wake at 6:00 a.m., then wash, toilet, brush teeth, and air beds. After breakfast, they returned to the ward and made beds and swept. Classwork followed and lasted for 2 hours. It consisted of a variety of simple crafts and marching exercises. After lunch, there was a rest period, continued classwork, and outdoor exercises, folk dancing, and lawn games. After supper, there was music and dancing on the ward, followed by toileting, washing, teeth brushing, and preparing for bed (Slagle & Robeson, 1933).

After maximum benefit was achieved from habit training, the patient progressed through three phases of OT. The first was what Slagle called the kindergarten group. Occupations such as music, coloring, and games were graded from simple to complex. The next phase was ward classes in OT. When able to tolerate it, the patient joined in group activities. The third phase was the occupational center. "This promotes opportunities for more advanced projects... a complete change in environment; ...comparative freedom; ...actual responsibilities placed upon

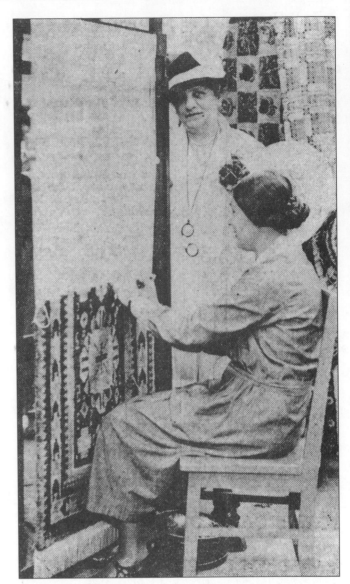

Figure 1-1. Eleanor Clarke Slagle (standing) and Margaret Kransee (1933). (Reprinted from Ryan, S. E. [1993]. *The certified occupational therapy assistant: Principles, concepts, and techniques* [2nd ed.]. Thorofare, NJ: SLACK Incorporated.)

patients; the stimulation of seeing work produced; ...all these carry forward the readjustment of patients" (Slagle & Robeson, 1933, p. 29).

Figure 1-1 shows Eleanor Clarke Slagle (standing) when she was the director of OT at the New York Department of Mental Hygiene. She is inspecting the weaving of a woolen rug by Mrs. Margaret Kransee, instructor at the Manhattan State Hospital, Wards Island, NY in 1933.

The Philosophy of Occupational Therapy—Adolph Meyer

A history of this type would not be complete without at least a brief mention of Adolph Meyer, a Swiss physician who immigrated to this country in 1892. By the end of 1910, he became professor of psychiatry at Johns Hopkins University and the first director of the Henry Phipps Clinic. Meyer "borrowed" Eleanor Clarke Slagle from Hull House for 2 years, during which time she founded the therapeutic occupations program in the clinic. Meyer's lasting contribution to psychiatry is the psychobiologic approach to mental illness and health. He coined this term to indicate that the human is an indivisible unit of study, rather than a composite of symptoms (Meyer, 1975).

Because of his friendship with Slagle and Dunton, Meyer agreed to deliver a major address at the fifth annual meeting of the National Society for the Promotion of Occupational Therapy in Baltimore, October 1921. This address has become a classic in OT literature. Meyer emphasized occupation, time, and the productive use of energy. He stated that the whole of human organization has its shape in a kind of rhythm, there are many rhythms which we must be attuned to: the larger rhythms of night, day, sleep, and waking hours; and finally the big four: work, play, rest, and sleep. The only way to attain balance in all this is actual doing, actual practice, a program of wholesome living is the basis of wholesome feeling and thinking and fancy and interests (Meyer, 1922).

In this address, Meyer successfully brought the fundamental moral treatment principles of more than a century before into contemporary OT practice and established the foundation of what now is known as *occupational behavior,* the model of human occupation and occupational performance.

Founding of the American Occupational Therapy Association

The American Occupational Therapy Association (AOTA) (1914-1917) archives hold all of the correspondence between George Barton, William Dunton, and Eleanor Clarke Slagle during the era when discussions were held about creating a national organizational to be a mechanism for exchanging views and extending information about the fledgling new line of medicine. The first letter in the series was from Dunton to Barton on October 15, 1915, wherein he suggested that Barton take the lead in organizing a central bureau for occupation workers. Barton wrote back, agreed, and suggested a title, Society for the Promotion of Occupation for Re-education. A series of false starts ensued, and Dunton became exasperated with the lack of progress. Local groups of occupation workers were forming to exchange views, and he felt they needed support and guidance from a national group. On December 7, 1916, Dunton wrote Barton again, proposing a five-member national executive committee. Disagreements between the two arose about who should be invited. They were settled on December 20, 1916, when Barton wrote Dunton with a new title, National Society for the Promotion of Occupational Therapy.

After some juggling of dates, March 15 through 17 were set for the organizational meeting and incorporation of the society. Barton invited the "big five," as he called the executive committee, to use his Consolation House for the event, as he wished to be host. The invitees, other than Dunton, included Eleanor Clarke Slagle, then the general superintendent of OT at Hull House; Susan Cox Johnson, the director of occupations, New York State Department of Public Charities; and Thomas B. Kidner, the vocational secretary, Canadian Military Hospital Commission. Susan E. Tracy, instructor in invalid occupations, Presbyterian Hospital, Chicago, was also invited but declined because of her work schedule. Isabelle Newton, Barton's secretary at Consolation House, was invited to attend in that capacity (Figure 1-2). Barton was elected president, a position he nominated himself for a few weeks before the meeting.

The next 6 months proved critical. Barton became increasingly annoyed at Dunton and Slagle, who was vice president. He suspected they were trying to overshadow his presidency. He also became involved in a heated debate about finances with Dunton, the treasurer. Subsequently, Barton refused to attend the first annual meeting on Labor Day weekend, September 1917, in New York City. He cited poor health as the reason. Dunton was elected the new president. There is no record that Barton attended any meetings of the national organization for the remainder of his life; however, he did remain a member (Licht, 1967).

The 1925 Principles

An AOTA committee, made up of physicians and chaired by William Rush Dunton, Jr., compiled an outline of lectures on OT for medical students and physicians (Adams, 1925). The members developed a definition, objectives, statements of the use of a variety of activities with different kinds of patients, therapeutic approaches, and the qualities and qualifications of practitioners. This was the first such effort since Dunton had created his principles in 1918 (Adams, 1925).

The first principle states that OT is a method of training the sick or injured by means of instruction and employment in productive occupation (Adams, 1925).

One is struck by the importance of the connection between learning by doing and purposeful activity. This was the dominant theme in several of the principles. The act of doing should be seen from the patient's point of view. For example, the treatment objectives stated that activities sought are to arouse interest, courage, and confidence; to exercise mind and body; to overcome disability; and to re-establish capacity for industrial and social usefulness (Adams, 1925).

Rules were established about the extent of activities, and attention was given to their qualities and effect on the patient. The use of crafts and work-related occupations was emphasized. Games, music, and physical exercise were not to be overlooked. A warning was offered: whereas quality, quantity, and salability may serve some objectives, these must not override the main purpose of the activity. Belief in the various properties of occupation is evident as the patient's strength and capability increase, the type and extent of occupation should be regulated and graded accordingly (Adams, 1925).

The committee made a statement about the quality of work to be expected as a therapeutic approach that inferior workmanship in an occupation which would be trivial for the healthy, may be used with the sick or injured, but standards worthy of normal persons must be maintained for proper mental stimulation (Adams, 1925).

The relationship between purposeful activity and the connections between the mind and body is found in the principle, the production of a well-made article, or the accomplishment of a useful task, requires healthy exercise of mind and body. Involvement in group activity is advised because it provides exercise in social adaptation (Adams, 1925). Evaluation rests with measuring the effect of the occupation on the patient, the extent to which objectives are being realized.

Adams (1925) believed one final principle addressed the qualifications of the practitioner as good craftsman, ability to teach, understanding, interest in the patient, and an optimistic, cheerful outlook. Elsewhere in the lecture outline, the committee recommended that therapists and aides should have a therapeutic sense, the teaching instinct, and good mental balance. Personality constitutes 50% of the value of these workers (Adams, 1925).

During this period, a number of issues were combined, including the following:
- Purposeful work and leisure
- The intricate involvement of the mind and body (interdependence of mental and physical aspects, also known as holism)
- OT as a learning process
- The therapeutic use of one's personal qualities

The literature of the next several decades, which was a period of remarkable development in the profession, gives evidence of how these principles became operational.

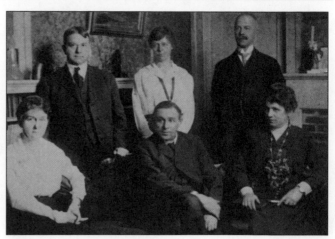

Figure 1-2. The founders of the National Society for the Promotion of Occupational Therapy. Front row, left to right: Susan Cox Johnson, George E. Barton, Eleanor Clarke Slagle. Back row, left to right: William R. Dunton, Isabel Newton, Thomas Kidner. (Reprinted from Ryan, S. E. [1993]. *The certified occupational therapy assistant: Principles, concepts, and techniques* [2nd ed.]. Thorofare, NJ: SLACK Incorporated.)

Purposeful Work and Leisure

In her early endeavors as a practitioner, Clare Spackman (1936) explored the perplexing problem of engaging the patient's interests. Her recommendation was to approach the patient through his or her interests. She noted that there are few people who have not some interest and for the therapist to make the right suggestion at the right time takes both experience and imagination.

Martha Gilbert (1936), an OT at the Choctaw-Chickasaw Sanitarium in Oklahoma, built her entire treatment program around purposeful work and leisure for children. The sanitarium was a federal institution with 75 beds for Native American children with tuberculosis and related diseases. In 1929, times were difficult, not only because of the Great Depression, but also because Native American children were not highly valued, except by those who cared for them on a daily basis. Supplies meager, she used native material to make items of interests including clay in summer and leaves in fall. The children loved to draw, garden, and march to music. Culture was a focus of activities, especially at holidays. Gilbert's approach may be seen today, as therapists and assistants carry out innovative and imaginative programs in impoverished areas of the United States and, indeed, throughout the world.

Involvement of the Mind and Body

The interaction of mind and body has remained a basic principle throughout our historical evolution. Ida Sands addresses the annual AOTA conference in 1927 with the importance of spiritual rehabilitation (1938). Beatrice Wade, a renowned clinician, educator, and administrator, spoke of the treatment of the total patient in an address in 1967. She stated that this approach is unique to OT among the health disciplines. There has always existed a strong component concerned with the ill or disabled, with the entirety of man and his functioning as a patient (Wade, 1967). This OT concept, she added, prevented an undesired separation of the psychiatric therapist from the physical disabled therapist.

Occupational Therapy as a Learning Process

Throughout the formative years, OT and education held much in common, not so much in how patients were instructed, but in the outcome of that instruction through changes in behavior and performance of a more complex nature. Harriet Robeson, a distinguished therapist, addressed a group of social workers in 1926 and affirmed some longstanding principles that OT is a re-education. She added that many think of OT as only handwork. It is far more; it is a program of work, play, and medicine to meet the mental, physical, and social needs of each patient (Robeson, 1926).

The re-education process follows the same pathway as normal education, a gradual growth through progressive development. The therapist must teach the patient to creep and to creep in the right direction (Robeson, 1926).

Irene O'Brock (1932), director of OT at the University of Oklahoma Hospitals, indicated that her program for children had an extra value, a deeper more intangible significance: the natural tendencies of life, play, and companionship. She based her treatment program on five lines of readiness:

1. To construct things
2. To communicate things
3. To find out things
4. To compete in things
5. To excel in things

Figure 1-3 shows two men engaged in activities that were typical of the times. These patients were receiving OT treatment at the Jewish Sanitarium and Hospital for Chronic Diseases in Brooklyn, NY. They were painting colorful designs on wooden plates that were sold at a bazaar. The proceeds were used to augment the hospital fund, which provided care for more than 500 disabled men, women, and children.

The Practitioner's Personal Qualities

One of the first student papers published in *Occupational Therapy and Rehabilitation*, the official journal of the AOTA, appeared in 1930. Nelda McKee (1930) of the University of Minnesota wrote *Ethics for the Occupational Therapist*. She discussed the ideals, customs, and habits that members of the profession are accumulat-

ing around the name and character of the trained therapist. Essential attributes in dealing with patients include honesty, frankness, and wisdom. She showed her insight when she stated:

> A therapist should endeavor to develop a symmetrical life. We all have a physical, mental, spiritual, and social side to our make-up which needs care and cultivation. The [therapist] is under personal obligation to keep herself from growing narrow...
>
> Above all, [she] must keep the quality of being 'teachable.' Then she will never stop developing the possibilities which she possesses. The ideal therapist never forgets that our ambitions are all directed toward one common end. We are working for the advancement of understanding and the enlargement of human life. (pp. 357, 360)

Joseph C. Doane, MD (1929), who later became president of AOTA, gave an impromptu address to conference attendees at the 1928 AOTA annual meeting. He distinguished between two kinds of workers—the occupationalist and the therapist:

> I regret to say that the occupationalists include not a few physicians and many laymen. [They believe] that OT is a very interesting and very useful plaything which begins and stops there; they see the product, rather than the patient; they comment on the beautiful colors and difficult weaves... They see nothing beyond the mere physical thing which has resulted from the activity.
>
> Then there is the other party—the therapist. The therapist looks at yarn and raffia, not as materials to be used... but as the implements or tools to be employed in the handling of much more difficult material, the disposition of the persons who are ill, a most varying and a most uncertain commodity. (pp. 13-14)

For Doane (1929), the critical importance is for the therapist to know what sick people do, think, and why they behave as they do, which is much more important than to know how to make something.

WE LIVE FORWARD

Contemporary occupational theorists and visionaries, such as Mary Reilly, Phillip Shannon, Gary Kielhofner, Janice Burke, and Elizabeth Yerxa, find ample support for their concepts in the founding, time-honored principles. For nearly two decades, between 1958 and 1977, Reilly wrote extensively about OT principles and the profession's changing role in medicine and health care. As Madigan and Parent (1985) point out:

> Reilly stated that the medical model is designed to prevent and reduce illness and does not address the reduction of incapacity that results from illness.

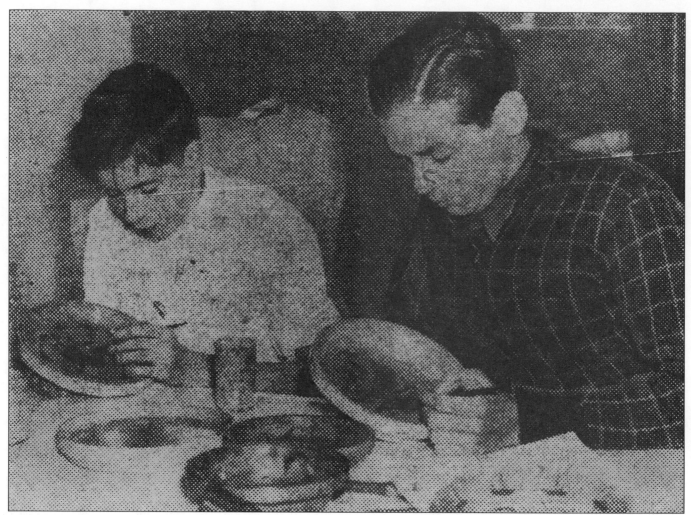

Figure 1-3. Patients in the OT Department at the Jewish Sanitarium and Hospital for Chronic Diseases, Brooklyn, NY. (Reprinted from Ryan, S. E. [1993]. *The certified occupational therapy assistant: Principles, concepts, and techniques* [2nd ed.]. Thorofare, NJ: SLACK Incorporated.)

It is the OT's [and assistant's] responsibility to activate residual adaptation of patients and to help deficit humans achieve life satisfaction through work and social involvement. (pp. 25-26)

Reilly (1962) repeatedly called for a renewed conceptualization of OT as reflected in the ideals of Dunton, Slagle, and Tracy. In addition, Reilly argued that OT needed to be concerned about the difficulties people have with their occupations all along the developmental continuum, including play and work. This she called occupational behavior.

By 1977, much of OT practice had markedly shifted away from its foundation in the original principles. Shannon (1977) viewed with alarm what was taking place. He called it a derailment:

...A new hypothesis has emerged that views man not as a creative being capable of making choices and directing his own future, but as a mechanistic creature susceptible to manipulation and control via the application of techniques... is a derailment from those... values and beliefs that legitimized the practice of OT. If OT persists in this direction, what was once and still is one of the great ideas of 20th century medicine will be swept away by the tide of technique philosophy. Should this happen the legitimacy of OT may be revoked and... its services absorbed by other health care professions. (p. 233)

Shannon was one of many graduate students under Reilly who advanced occupational behavior theory.

Six years later, Kielhofner and Burke (1983) completed an exhaustive review of the early literature and were left with a deep respect for the ideas and accomplishments of the first generation of therapists. Both a science of occupation and the art of using occupation as a medical therapy were conceived, clearly articulated, and applied. Yet, our confidence and willingness to embrace clinical problems was missing, something had been dropped out in the intervening years between the development of the principles and the time of their review.

Kielhofner (1985) and his associates proceeded with the development of what they term a *model of human occupation,* using the concepts of occupational behavior theory. The latest addition to this evolution, starting with the original principles, is called occupational science and is viewed by many as a foundation for OT well into the 21st century. Occupational science is believed to be an emerging basic science that supports occupational practice (Yerxa, 1989).

SUMMARY

OT beginnings reach back more than 200 years, to the Age of Enlightenment when human beings were emerging with a new, expanded view of "why on earth they were on Earth." There was a sense of economic, political, social, and religious progress. Ideas were forming about the importance of each human being, about the human ability to think and learn, about labor as the central focus of life, and about human existence being governed by a prevailing set of principles directed toward everyday living. These same ideals became significant in caring about and for the mentally ill.

In Europe, the birthplace of this new age, men and women, such as Phillippe Pinel, William Tuke, and Sir William and Lady Ellis, engaged their mental patients in a variety of occupations and amusements for a number of purposes:

- To restore reason
- To provide feelings of security and self-worth
- To allow as much freedom of choice and movement as possible, regardless of mental conditions
- To arrest delusional attention and fix it on objects that would help restore reason

From their experience, the caregivers established certain principles that were handed down to the present day. For more than 50 years, during the latter decades of the 19th century and the early 20th century, these principles all but disappeared because of social, economic, and political upheavals. They re-emerged in the second decade of the 20th century as OT.

In the United States during the Progressive Era, a diverse collection of men and women restated and added to the inherited principles. Among these people were William Rush Dunton, Jr., a psychiatrist; Eleanor Clarke Slagle, a partially trained social worker; Susan Tracy, a nurse; George Edward Barton, a disabled architect; and Adolph Meyer, a psychiatrist. Their contributions remain today as the cornerstone of OT principles:

1. Activity contains ingredients by which an ill or disabled individual may gain understanding of and control over one's own feelings, thoughts, and actions; habits of attention and interest; usefulness of occupation; creative expression; the process of learning by doing; skill; and concrete evidence of personal accomplishment.

2. Variations of activity provide opportunities to balance the larger rhythms of life: work, play, rest, and sleep, which must remain balanced if health is to be regained, maintained, or attained.

3. Purposeful occupation involves the intricate interplay of the mind and body, which cannot be separated if the human being is to engage in activity.

4. Involvement in remedial activity has as a major purpose the acquiring or restoring of usefulness to oneself and others as a happy, productive human being.

5. The patient is the product of his or her own efforts, not the article made nor the activity accomplished.

6. One's approach to the patient is as significant to treatment and rehabilitation as is the selection and use of an activity.

7. A knowledge of the patient's needs, an appreciation of the pain that accompanies an illness or disability, a strong desire to reduce or remove it, and a gentle firmness are among the major characteristics of the provider of therapeutic occupations.

These principles remain intact, although often restated and reworded. There is considerable evidence they will remain a part of our practice through the efforts of such individuals as Mary Reilly, Phillip Shannon, Gary Kielhofner, Janice Burke, and Elizabeth Yerxa and her associates. Occupational behavior, the model of human occupation, and occupational science offer assurances that these principles will still be with us well into the next century.

ACKNOWLEDGMENTS

The author wishes to express his profound gratitude to those people who so generously assisted in the search for materials and in the preparation of this chapter: Lillian Hoyle Parent, OTR, FAOTA; James L. Cantwell, OTR; Gary A. Wade, OTR; Florence S. Cromwell, OTR, FAOTA; and Inci Bowman, PhD, director, Truman Blocker History of Medicine Collection (AOTA Archives), Moody Medical Library, The University of Texas Medical Branch at Galveston.

Thanks also to the staff of the *American Journal of Occupational Therapy* for permission to use excerpts from previously published articles: *Occupational Therapy Revisited: A Paraphratic Journey* [1981, Vol. 35(6)] and *Living Forward, Understanding Backwards, Part 1 and 2* [1984, Vol. 38(6 and 7)].

REFERENCES

Adams, I. D. (1925). An outline of lectures on OT to medical students and physicians. *OT Rehabilitation, 4,* 277-292.

AOTA. (1914-1917). Unpublished correspondence in *AOTA Archives 1914-1917, Series 1.* Truman Blocker History of Medicine Collection, Moody Medical Library, The University of Texas Medical Branch at Galveston.

Barton, G. E. (1914). A view of invalid occupation. *Trained Nurse and Hospital Review, 52,* 328-330.

Barton, G. E. (1915). Occupational nursing. *Trained Nurse and Hospital Review, 54,* 328-336.

Barton, G. E. (1922). The existing hospital system and reconstruction. *Trained Nurse and Hospital Review, 69,* 309,320.

Bates, J. L. (1976). *The United States, 1898-1928: Progressivism and a society in transition.* New York, NY: McGraw-Hill.

Bing, R. R. (1987). Who originated the term OT? *Am J Occup Ther, 3.* Letter to the editor.

Bockhoven, I. S. (1972). *Moral treatment in community mental health.* New York, NY: Springer Publishing.

DeGrazia, S. (1962). *Of time, work, and leisure.* New York, NY: Twentieth Century Fund.

Doane, J. C. (1929). OT. *OT Rehabilitation, 8*(1), 13-14.

Dunton, W. R. (1915). *Occupation therapy: A manual for nurses.* Philadelphia, PA: W. B. Saunders.

Dunton, W. R. (1918). The principles of OT. In *Proceedings of the National Society for the Promotion of OT, Second Annual Meeting.* Catonsville, MD: Spring Grove State Hospital Press.

Dunton, W. R. (1935). The relationship of OT and physical therapy. *Archives of Physical Therapy, 16*(1), 19.

Gilbert, M. E. (1936). OT program at Choctaw-Chickasaw Sanitarium. *OT Rehabilitation, 11,* 113.

Hass, L. J. (1924). One hundred years of OT. *Archives of OT, 3*(2), 83-100.

Hunter, R., & Macalpine, I. (1963). *Three hundred years of psychiatry: 1535-1860* (pp. 871-872). London: Oxford University Press.

Kielhofner, G. (Ed.). (1985). *A model of human occupation: Theory and application.* Baltimore, MD: Williams & Wilkins.

Kielhofner G., & Burke, J. P. (1983). The evolution of knowledge and practice in OT: Past, present, and future. In G. Kielhofner (Ed.), *Health through occupation: Theory and practice in OT.* Philadelphia, PA: F. A. Davis.

Licht, S. (1967). The founding and founders of the AOTA. *Am J Occup Ther, 21,* 269-271.

Madigan, M. J., & Parent, L. H. (1985). Preface. In G. Kielhofner (Ed.), *A model of human occupation: Theory and application.* Baltimore, MD: Williams & Wilkins.

McKee, N. (1930). Ethics for the OT. *OT Rehabilitation, 9*(6), 357-360.

Meyer, A. (1922). The philosophy of OT. *Archives in OT, 1*(6). Reprinted in *Am J Occup Ther* in 1977, 31(10).

Meyer, A. (1975). The psychobiological point of view. In J. B. Brady (Ed.), *Classics in American Psychiatry.* St. Louis, MO: Warren H. Green.

Neustadt, R. E., & May, E. R. (1986). *Thinking in time: The uses of history for decision-makers.* New York, NY: The Free Press.

O'Brock, I. (1932). Occupational treatment for crippled children. *OT Rehabilitation, 11*(3), 204-205.

Pinel, P. (1806). *A treatise on insanity in which are contained the principles of a new and more practical nosology of maniacal disorders.* Translated by D. D. Davis. London: Cadell and Davis.

Reilly, M. (1962). OT can be one of the great ideas of 20th century medicine. *Am J Occup Ther, 26,* 1-2.

Robeson, H. A. (1926). How can occupational therapists help the social service worker? *OT Rehabilitation, 5,* 379-381.

Sands, I. F. (1938). When is occupation curative? *OT Rehabilitation, 17,* 117-119.

Shannon, P. D. (1977). The derailment of OT. *Am J Occup Ther, 31,* 233.

Slagle, E. C. (1922). Training aides for mental patients. *Archives of OT, 1,* 13-14.

Slagle, E. C. (1934). OT: Recent methods and advances in the United States. *OT Rehabilitation, 13,* 289.

Slagle, E. C., & Robeson, H. A. (1933). *Syllabus for training nurses in occupational therapy.* Utica, NY: State Hospital Press.

Spackman, C. S. (1936). *The approach to the patient in a general hospital.* Unpublished paper delivered at Tri-Stab Institute on OT, Farnhurst, NJ, March 9, 3-5.

Tracy, S. E. (1914). The place of invalid occupations in the general hospital. *Modern Hospital, 2*(5), 386.

Tracy, S. E. (1918a). Twenty-five suggested mental tests derived from invalid occupations. *Maryland Psychiatric Quarterly, 8,* 15-16.

Tracy, S. E. (1918b). *Studies in invalid occupations.* Boston, MA: Witcomb and Barrows.

Tracy, S. E. (1923). Treatment of disease by employment at St. Elizabeth's Hospital. *Modern Hospital, 20*(2), 198.

Tuke, W. (1813). *Description of the retreat: An institution near York for insane persons of the Society of Friends.* London: Dawson of Pall Mall.

Wade, B. D. (1967). *OT: A history of its practice in the psychiatric field.* Unpublished paper delivered at the AOTA 51st annual conference, October 1967.

Yerxa, E. (1989). An introduction to occupational science, a foundation for OT in the 21st century. *OT Health Care, 6*(4), 3.

The COTA Heritage: Proud and Dynamic

Chapter 2

Shirley Holland Carr, MS, LOTR, FAOTA

INTRODUCTION

This chapter is a story about the birth of the certified occupational therapy assistant (COTA). The story begins in the post-World War II era with Ruth Robinson and Marion Crampton, and later Ruth Brunyate Wiemer and Mildred Schwagmeyer. Described here are the circumstances that led to the creation of the COTA, the roles of some individuals who were instrumental in the development of the concept, educational training, and practice of the occupational therapy assistant (OTA), and OTA accomplishments.

You are carried from the "beginnings" to your own entry into our profession, with emphasis on the early years. If you discern more anecdotes than usual, consider that while you are reading contemporary history the writer was reminiscing.

USE OF PERSONNEL BEFORE 1960

Before World War II, many registered occupational therapists (OTRs) worked in psychiatric institutions. After 1945 and influenced by military experience, increasing numbers of therapists practiced in medical and rehabilitation settings (see Chapter One). This added to the already severe shortage of OTs in psychiatric settings during and after World War II. Psychiatric hospitals often had patient populations of between 1,000 and 6,000. With a shortage of therapists, OT services were provided by a number of aides, assistants, or technicians who were supervised by one or two OTs.

Supportive personnel (OT aides and technicians) working in psychiatric facilities were valuable and valued employees, having learned the "tricks of the trade" by modeling therapist behaviors or by trial and error. In contrast to the mobility of OTs, the employment stability of aides and technicians often made them the most knowledgeable personnel about individual patient behavior and the availability of activities and equipment in a given setting. Supportive personnel knew how to do things, but lacked goal-oriented intervention methods necessary to work without immediate supervision. This deficit

KEY CONCEPTS

- Early leaders in COTA history: Ruth Robinson, Marion Crampton, Ruth Brunyate Wiemer, Mildred Schwagmeyer.
- Roster of Honor (ROH): AOTA national award for COTAs for leadership in OT.

ESSENTIAL VOCABULARY

Grandfather clause: Ruling or law that allows OTAs not formally trained to earn credentials once formal training began for all OTAs.

Supportive personnel: Aides and technicians other than OTAs.

motivated supervisory personnel to organize courses for OTAs (Crampton, 1989).

EARLY TRAINING NEEDS AND SHORT COURSES

Several states and the military recognized the need for in-service training (on-the-job educational opportunities) for OT personnel and developed courses of varying lengths. As early as 1944, the U.S. Army developed a 1-month course. Crampton, employed by the state of Massachusetts, developed and conducted 4- and 6-week courses before approval by the AOTA. Other states with early short courses were New York, Wisconsin, and Pennsylvania (for activity aides) (Crampton, 1989).

AOTA's ROLE IN THE DEVELOPMENT OF THE COTA

The overlapping employment and association roles of Marion Crampton, Col. Ruth Robinson, Mildred Schwagmeyer, and Ruth Brunyate Wiemer were fortuitous to the development of the COTA. Each of these women had a long-standing interest in the use of supportive OT personnel, and all but Wiemer were members of the Committee on Occupational Therapy Assistants (AOTA, 1964). This committee was delegated responsibility for all developmental aspects of the OTA, including needs assessment, educational program standards, new program proposal and on-site review, and program approval (Schwagmeyer, 1989).

In addition, members of the Committee on Occupational Therapy Assistants reviewed applications for certification under the grandfather clauses. Of 460 applications, 336 individuals became COTAs. The committee also undertook the continuing education of OTs by preparing documents and acquiring grant funds to sponsor national workshops (Schwagmeyer, 1989). The focus was two-fold: appropriate supervision and use of OTAs.

Ruth A. Robinson

Col. Ruth A. Robinson was president of AOTA from 1955 to 1958 (Figure 2-1). About the same time, she became Chief of the Occupational Therapy Section of the Women's (later Army) Medical Specialist Corps, and then the first Chief of the Women's (later Army) Medical Specialist Corps. Both her military and association roles involved advocacy for the training of supportive OT personnel. She served on the Committee on Occupational Therapy Assistants from its inception as a member, chair, and consultant (AOTA, 1967).

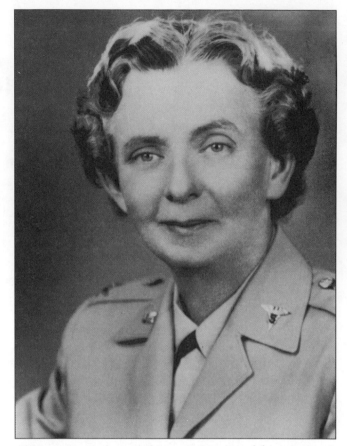

Figure 2-1. Ruth A. Robinson. (Reprinted from Ryan, S. E. [1993]. *The certified occupational therapy assistant: Principles, concepts, and techniques* [2nd ed.]. Thorofare, NJ: SLACK Incorporated.)

In an taped video interview (Cox, 1977) a few years before her death in 1989, Robinson stated that she thought her greatest contribution to the OT profession was the development of the program and curriculum to train OTAs. She also stated:

We may not realize how far advanced the OT profession was. We set a standard for other professions to follow. At first our program concentrated on the care of the psychiatric patient, just as in the early days of OT. It was frightening to some of us who felt we were not far enough advanced ourselves or secure in our own identities to be able to accept the responsibility of supervising others. We still have a long way to go. I thought the COTA ultimately would be what we thought of then as the OT, and that the COTA would be the best job in OT, leaving the OTR to do the intake work and program planning for individual patients. Recognition of the COTA through certification made me the proudest. (Cox, 1977)

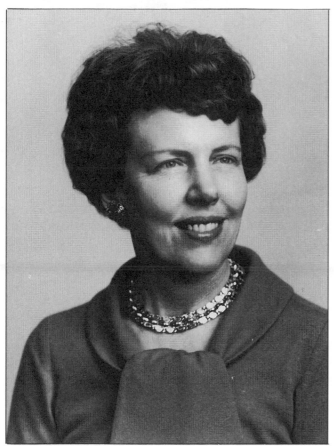

Figure 2-2. Marion W. Crampton, OTR. (Reprinted from Ryan, S. E. [1993]. *The certified occupational therapy assistant: Principles, concepts, and techniques* [2nd ed.]. Thorofare, NJ: SLACK Incorporated.)

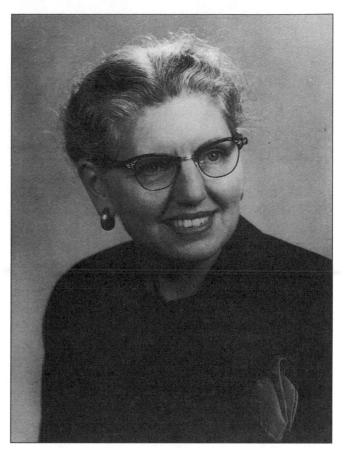

Figure 2-3. Mildred Schwagmeyer, OTR. (Reprinted from Ryan, S. E. [1993]. *The certified occupational therapy assistant: Principles, concepts, and techniques* [2nd ed.]. Thorofare, NJ: SLACK Incorporated.)

Marion W. Crampton

Marion W. Crampton was a member of the House of Delegates, a delegate member of AOTA's Board of Management, and finally a member of the board itself (Figure 2-2). She was employed by the Massachusetts Department of Mental Health to work with the state psychiatric facilities as well as the state schools under the Division of Mental Retardation. Crampton's employment involved meeting the need for OT services in her state's institutions at a time of OTR shortages. She understood the problems and needs of personnel with less than optimal preparation because that was her daily work. The OTA education program in Massachusetts was an in-service program for employed individuals with experience in OT. Crampton noted:

> The first group of students thought long and hard before applying to the course, which required leaving families for a month and returning to school after many years. Exams were especially threatening, since some students had only a 10th grade education, and had school-aged children who questioned their grades. (Crampton, 1989)

She was already involved in Massachusetts when the Committee on Occupational Therapy Assistants was formed and she was appointed chair. Crampton included "members of the loyal opposition" as she made appointments to the committee, so all sides were heard (Crampton, 1989).

As noted earlier, implementation of the OTA program brought a deluge of applications from OT personnel seeking credentialing under the grandfather clause. She recalled, "During the 2-year period, applications were reviewed in a 'round robin' composed of all committee members, who worked evenings, weekends, holidays, and even vacations to process these forms" (Crampton, 1989).

Mildred Schwagmeyer

Mildred Schwagmeyer worked in tuberculosis hospitals until recruited as assistant director of education at the AOTA national office in 1958 (Figure 2-3). Nine years later, she became director of technical education, remaining in this position until 1974 (Schwagmeyer, 1990). She became the most knowledgeable person on the subject of

OTAs at the national office and in the United States. She continued to work in OTA educational services through several title changes until her retirement.

In recalling those years, Schwagmeyer commented:

I knew in a general way about what was going on, but not that the COTA would have a real impact on my working life. After only 4 months as assistant director of the education, the division became responsible for OTA education. I became liaison to the Committee on Occupational Therapy Assistants, which reported directly to the Board of Management. At first, OTAs were only part of my job, but the work became increasingly time-consuming, demanding, and absorbing. By the 1960s, being technical education director and working with the Committee on Occupational Therapy Assistants was a full-time position. (Schwagmeyer, 1989)

She went on to recount:

As educational programs moved from hospital-based to academic-based training, concern and discussion increased on topics such as career mobility, entry-level skills, laddering, behavioral objectives, lack of appropriate textbooks and teaching aids, shortage of faculty, and overeducation by some programs leading to disappointment in graduates' work experience. (Schwagmeyer, 1989)

Five federally funded invitational workshops were held at yearly intervals between 1963 and 1968. Four were attended primarily by academic and clinical faculty, and the last included an equal mix of OTRs and COTAs. Topics included role and function, COTA/OTR relationships, and supervisions. Excellent teaching materials developed from these workshops, including the present *Guide for Supervision* (AOTA, 1994).

Schwagmeyer brought a precise use of language to her work. Among other things, she taught us that the term *COTA program* was a non sequitur. Programs are approved, but students cannot seek certification until they graduate. Even today you may sometimes hear the incorrect terminology.

After the 1964 restructuring of AOTA (1964), the functions of the Committee on Occupational Therapy Assistants were slowly integrated into the council structure (Schwagmeyer, 1989), and the committee was dissolved. Seldom have so few accomplished so much.

Ruth Brunyate Wiemer

Ruth Brunyate Wiemer was employed as an OT consultant for the Maryland Department of Health and in 1964 became president of the AOTA (Figure 2-4) (AOTA, 1967). Wiemer guided the association through the difficult period of reorganization (Wiemer, 1966). Of that period she said:

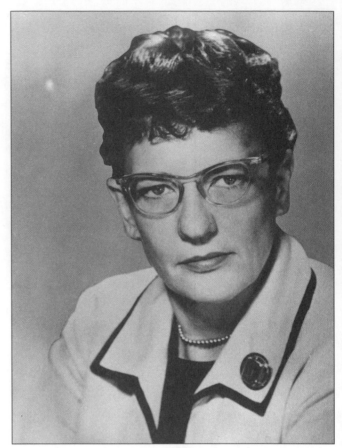

Figure 2-4. Ruth Brunyate Wiemer, OTR. (Reprinted from Ryan, S. E. [1993]. *The certified occupational therapy assistant: Principles, concepts, and techniques* [2nd ed.]. Thorofare, NJ: SLACK Incorporated.)

Communication was slow and labored, with few secretaries in the national office or in OT departments. Flying was not common; one usually traveled by car or train. Expense accounts were unheard of, either at AOTA or on the job. Little money was available for phone calls, retreats, or any type of face-to-face confrontation. (Wiemer, 1989)

She continued:

Our world changed rapidly in the 1960s after Medicare, with an explosion in the number of proprietary nursing homes and home health agencies. OT was a small, unrecognized profession without precedent for adopting such a concept [as the COTA]. Nursing had supportive personnel, but were protected by licensure; we were not. (Wiemer, 1989)

For professional OTs, COTAs became an added issue because of the following:

1. OTRs feared the unknown, especially those with no experience working with or supervising supportive personnel.

2. OTRs feared the AOTA was imposing the COTA on the profession.

3. OTRs feared giving representation to the COTA and the consequences of COTAs voting.

4. Abilities of the COTA highlighted weaknesses in OTR skills such as deficits in supervisory techniques and current clinical practice, contentment in their own comfortable niche, naively, and insufficient business acumen.

5. There was a lack of country-wide consensus on the appropriate role of OT itself (Wiemer, 1989).

In such an environment, how then were COTAs nurtured? My belief is that the leadership came from those therapists used to hierarchical order, chain of command, and discipline, such as in the military, veterans administration, or health departments. Therapists from psychiatric settings were also familiar with working with supportive personnel (Wiemer, 1989).

While others argued, Wiemer often seemed to be collecting her thoughts. Her responses were graceful, direct, organized, and reasoned, and they did not hide her advocacy for COTAs. She used a convincing metaphor in referring to the OTR/COTA problem: "Able seamen far outnumber captains and commodores, yet ships do not sink, and new ship forms, from sail to nuclear power, evolved to meet man's need. So too the varied levels of our profession can be coordinated to achieve efficiency and growth" (Wiemer, 1964).

Therapists who had not stayed abreast of current clinical practice had reason to be concerned about the role of the COTA (AOTA, 1982a). According to a 1967 "Nationally Speaking" column in the *American Journal of Occupational Therapy,* therapists must know that what was taught 15 years ago as functional treatment is taught to OTAs today as maintenance and supportive therapy (Carr, 1971). This writer's attempt to motivate other therapists may sound harsh, but the basic premise about current practice was true.

According to Wiemer:

Change eventually came about in the profession, brought about by the advent of the COTA; these included the sharpening of the roles and functions which opened up part-time positions, increased legislative efforts, and increased state licensure. A physician once asked how the OT profession had the vision to establish a subprofessional group. The profession did not; a few within it did and urged that we follow, and we did. (Wiemer, 1989)

FEELINGS OF DISTRUST

Feelings of distrust among some OTRs periodically ran high for a number of years, reigning each time new OTA rights and privileges were initiated. The following anecdote is an example of such an emotional response in the early 1970s, when the AOTA Delegate Assembly considered career mobility to allow COTAs to become OTRs by fulfilling certain fieldwork requirements and passing the national certification examination for OTs (AOTA, 1982a).

One evening, two AOTA national office staff members spoke on the subject at a district OT meeting. Heated discussion followed the presentations as a few vocal therapists expressed concern that such legislation would directly threaten their jobs. Others disagreed, and still others sat quietly, because the hour was late and the response had become familiar. A stenotypist took notes throughout the meeting so the proceedings could be distributed to therapists statewide. Apparently to prevent such dissemination, the stenotypist's tapes were "lost," but later were retrieved from a lavatory trash can. The proceedings were published (Texas Occupational Therapy Association [TOTA], 1973), the Delegate Assembly voted COTA's career mobility rights terminated in 1982 (AOTA, 1982a), and OTRs' employment was unaffected as a consequence of this or any other action pertaining to OTA rights.

As the first COTAs practiced and practiced well at the technical level (Wiemer, 1989), OTRs and COTAs began building on each other's strengths, learning to identify and complement each other's skills to the betterment of the profession. As you read further in this and in subsequent chapters, you will see how the OT/OTA relationship continues to mature.

OCCUPATIONAL THERAPY ASSISTANT EDUCATION

The initial short-term courses, such as those conducted under the auspices of the state hospital systems in Massachusetts, Wisconsin, and New York, were in-service programs (Crampton, 1989). In 1961, a program in Montgomery County, MD, was approved in general practice to train students to practice in nursing homes (Caskey, 1961). The first approved program combining psychiatric and general practice was at the Duluth Vocational-Technical School in Minnesota; it also targeted student training for nursing homes. Another Minnesota program at St. Mary's Junior College became the first approved 2-year college program (AOTA, 1965). By 1966, the original single-concept programs were being eliminated (AOTA, 1966), and soon all students were enrolled in programs that prepared them to work in general areas of OT practice, rather than in a specialized setting.

Within the parameters set by AOTA guidelines for the number of program hours, program length remained variable depending on the academic setting, length of school day, length of fieldwork, and student backgrounds. One interesting program consolidated all of the academic work into a summer. The program used the college campus and employed faculty members when the campus would otherwise be closed. All students had prior experience in OT or associated departments, or at least 2 years of college and experience working in a health facility. Such students had fewer professional socialization needs than typical junior college students but received the same OT education in an 8-hour classroom day. Fieldwork was arranged when the other college students returned to campus.

PRACTICE SETTINGS

As we have seen, COTAs were trained initially to work in psychiatric hospital practice settings and then in nursing homes and other general medical settings. Many still work in those facilities. The dispersion of OTAs into nontraditional settings came about not because of training, but because of federal legislation (Carr, 1971). Initially, Titles XVIII and XIX of P. L.89-97 (1965), more commonly known as Medicare and Medicaid, opened employment in nursing homes, related facilities, and home health agencies. Other funding opened opportunities in community health and mental health centers, day care centers, and centers for the well aging. Numbers of OTAs increased at the same time some OTs began moving from hospitals to less traditional community practice settings (Carr, 1971). OTAs joined the move to community settings, sometimes in larger numbers than OTs. Carr commented, "It may be either COTA or OTR who meanders away from traditional to new settings, but whichever goes first the other will accompany or soon follow" (TOTA, 1973). The AOTA no longer keeps yearly figures on employment settings for COTAs, but estimates (AOTA, 1987) from voluntary information on applications or surveys are the following:

- Nursing homes and related rehabilitation facilities—30%
- General hospitals—15%
- Public school systems—15%
- Psychiatric facilities/programs—8%
- Residential care facilities—8%
- Day care centers—4%
- Community mental health centers—4%
- Others—16%

With the passage of P. L. 94-142, the Education for All Handicapped Children Act of 1975, OT personnel were recruited as a related service by public schools to assist children 3 through 21 years old in learning skills necessary to participate in their individualized special education programs. P. L. 99-457, the Handicapped Amendments of 1986, gave a direct OT role in early intervention with children from birth through 2 years, and OTAs and OTs again modified their roles as they moved into schools.

As you read later in this chapter about some individual OTAs who have been singled out for honors, be aware how many have moved to nontraditional roles, some requiring OT supervision and some not. Even in roles requiring no OT supervision, it is observed that OTAs continue their relationships informally with their counterparts.

PRIDE IN RIGHTS AND PRIVILEGES HARD WON

The chronology of OTA developmental milestones, shown in Figure 2-5, chronicles hard-won rights and privileges, as well as a few not yet won. In 1980, the AOTA Executive Board formed the COTA Task Force to identify COTA concerns and formulate suggestions (AOTA, 1980, 1981). A year later, the Task Force reported the following recommendations (AOTA, 1981; Barnett, 1981):

1. Submit a resolution to the Representative Assembly to establish COTA representation. This was to include a proposal for a nationwide communication network.
2. Increase COTAs' participation on key committees and commissions and national office advisory committees.
3. Maintain a roster of COTAs qualified and interested in serving on committees at state, regional, and national levels.
4. Establish "COTA Share" column in the OT newspaper.
5. Design COTA workshops to improve technical skills.
6. Encourage utilization of COTAs as educators in professional and technical education programs.
7. Appoint a COTA liaison in the national office.

The COTA Task Force was funded for several years (AOTA, 1983) and then replaced by a COTA Advisory Committee in 1986 (Brittell, 1986). All of the original objectives were accomplished, along with many others identified by the networking of the COTA Advisory Committee. Although a proposal to elect a COTA member-at-large in the Representative Assembly was defeated in 1982 (AOTA, 1982b), a similar measure in 1983 (AOTA, 1983) created a COTA representative with voice and vote elected by the membership. It is anticipated that

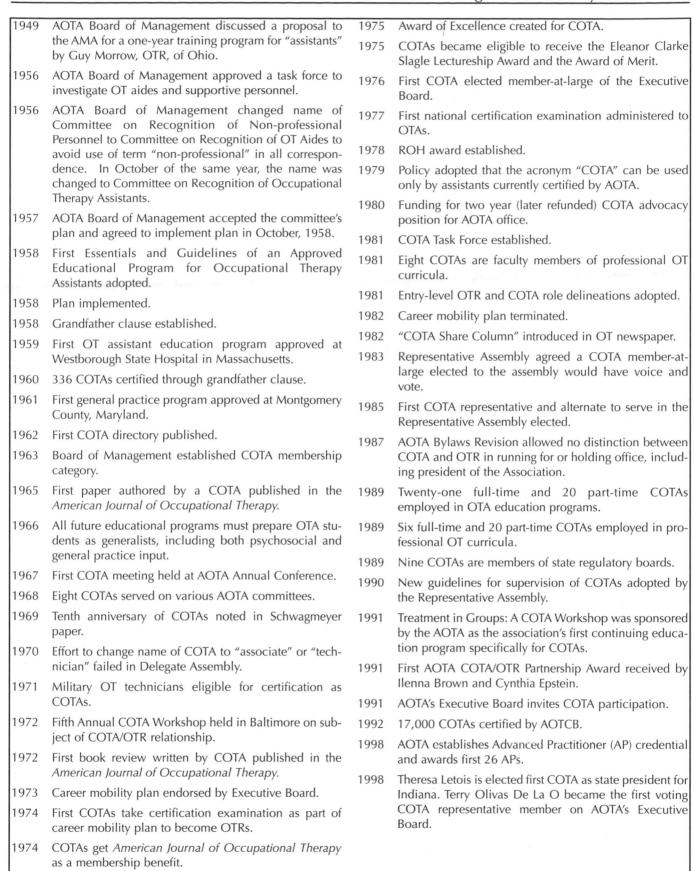

1949	AOTA Board of Management discussed a proposal to the AMA for a one-year training program for "assistants" by Guy Morrow, OTR, of Ohio.	1975	Award of Excellence created for COTA.
1956	AOTA Board of Management approved a task force to investigate OT aides and supportive personnel.	1975	COTAs became eligible to receive the Eleanor Clarke Slagle Lectureship Award and the Award of Merit.
1956	AOTA Board of Management changed name of Committee on Recognition of Non-professional Personnel to Committee on Recognition of OT Aides to avoid use of term "non-professional" in all correspondence. In October of the same year, the name was changed to Committee on Recognition of Occupational Therapy Assistants.	1976	First COTA elected member-at-large of the Executive Board.
		1977	First national certification examination administered to OTAs.
		1978	ROH award established.
		1979	Policy adopted that the acronym "COTA" can be used only by assistants currently certified by AOTA.
1957	AOTA Board of Management accepted the committee's plan and agreed to implement plan in October, 1958.	1980	Funding for two year (later refunded) COTA advocacy position for AOTA office.
1958	First Essentials and Guidelines of an Approved Educational Program for Occupational Therapy Assistants adopted.	1981	COTA Task Force established.
		1981	Eight COTAs are faculty members of professional OT curricula.
1958	Plan implemented.	1981	Entry-level OTR and COTA role delineations adopted.
1958	Grandfather clause established.	1982	Career mobility plan terminated.
1959	First OT assistant education program approved at Westborough State Hospital in Massachusetts.	1982	"COTA Share Column" introduced in OT newspaper.
1960	336 COTAs certified through grandfather clause.	1983	Representative Assembly agreed a COTA member-at-large elected to the assembly would have voice and vote.
1961	First general practice program approved at Montgomery County, Maryland.		
1962	First COTA directory published.	1985	First COTA representative and alternate to serve in the Representative Assembly elected.
1963	Board of Management established COTA membership category.	1987	AOTA Bylaws Revision allowed no distinction between COTA and OTR in running for or holding office, including president of the Association.
1965	First paper authored by a COTA published in the *American Journal of Occupational Therapy*.	1989	Twenty-one full-time and 20 part-time COTAs employed in OTA education programs.
1966	All future educational programs must prepare OTA students as generalists, including both psychosocial and general practice input.	1989	Six full-time and 20 part-time COTAs employed in professional OT curricula.
		1989	Nine COTAs are members of state regulatory boards.
1967	First COTA meeting held at AOTA Annual Conference.	1990	New guidelines for supervision of COTAs adopted by the Representative Assembly.
1968	Eight COTAs served on various AOTA committees.	1991	Treatment in Groups: A COTA Workshop was sponsored by the AOTA as the association's first continuing education program specifically for COTAs.
1969	Tenth anniversary of COTAs noted in Schwagmeyer paper.		
1970	Effort to change name of COTA to "associate" or "technician" failed in Delegate Assembly.	1991	First AOTA COTA/OTR Partnership Award received by Ilenna Brown and Cynthia Epstein.
1971	Military OT technicians eligible for certification as COTAs.	1991	AOTA's Executive Board invites COTA participation.
1972	Fifth Annual COTA Workshop held in Baltimore on subject of COTA/OTR relationship.	1992	17,000 COTAs certified by AOTCB.
		1998	AOTA establishes Advanced Practitioner (AP) credential and awards first 26 APs.
1972	First book review written by COTA published in the *American Journal of Occupational Therapy*.	1998	Theresa Letois is elected first COTA as state president for Indiana. Terry Olivas De La O became the first voting COTA representative member on AOTA's Executive Board.
1973	Career mobility plan endorsed by Executive Board.		
1974	First COTAs take certification examination as part of career mobility plan to become OTRs.		
1974	COTAs get *American Journal of Occupational Therapy* as a membership benefit.		

Figure 2-5. Chronology of COTA developmental milestones. Information complied from author and *OT Practice*, July/August 1999b, p. 21. (Adapted from Ryan, S. E. (1993). *The certified occupational therapy assistant: Principles, concepts, and techniques.* 2nd ed. Thorofare, NJ: SLACK Incorporated.)

when OTAs are routinely elected to the Representative Assembly from their states, such a special at-large position will be unnecessary. Two OTAs have been elected to the Representative Assembly from their states in the past. Theresa Letois is currently the president of her state association and Terry Olivas De La O is the first elected representative to the Executive Board (AOTA, 1999b).

OTAs describe the 1980s as having had two phases. In the early part, they expended their energy claiming a fair share of responsibility in the Association. Their effort paid off, and in the latter part of the decade increasing numbers of OTAs were involved in local, state, and national professional activities. The maturity of the OTA group was especially obvious when the COTA Advisory Committee voluntarily withdrew the proposal to change the title of OTAs and discouraged any further action on that long-held dream because the legal and economic implications outweighed the benefits (AOTA, 1980).

In 1989, 21 full-time and 20 part-time OTAs were employed as faculty in technical education programs, and 6 full-time and 20 part-time OTAs were on faculties of professional curricula. Nine OTAs were members of state regulatory (licensure or registration) boards. Can the day be far off when OTAs are directors of educational programs (Jones, 1989)? Ten years ago, only the visionaries among us would even have dreamed that in 1987 the AOTA would change its bylaws (AOTA, 1987), allowing no distinction between OTAs and OTs running for elected national office, including the office of president. Jones commented that with the labor shortage (where this chapter began), OTAs are becoming administrators, hiring OTs as consultants and clinicians (1989).

MULTIPLYING SLOWLY

The fears of some OTs, as outlined by Wiemer (1989), that COTAs would become more numerous than OTRs, has not yet happened. The number of OTAs has increased, but their impact on the profession is far greater than numbers indicate. As you read the information on outstanding OTAs, compare it with the membership statistics shown in Figure 2-6 and see if you agree.

The decrease in membership from 1986 to 1988 was expected, due to a change in the method of counting after the separation of certification and membership in 1986 (AOTA, 1987).

ROSTER OF HONOR

The ROH recognizes OTAs with at least 5 years of experience who, with their knowledge and expertise, have made a significant contribution to the continuing education and professional development of members of the association and provide an incentive to contribute to the advancement of the profession (AOTA, 1999a). Become familiar with their names so you will recognize them when you meet them (and you will). Many of the recipients also received the Award of Excellence (AOTA, 1999b), which recognizes the contributions of OTAs to the advancement of OT and provides an incentive to contribute to the development and growth of the profession.

The following people are a select group of early recipients of these honors, which the AOTA bestows on OTAs. Each year other distinguished OTAs join the ranks of these leaders, presented here with our pride in their accomplishments.

Sally E. Ryan of Mounds View, MN, received the ROH (1979) and the Award of Excellence (1976) for outstanding achievements and contributions in education, committee work in professional organizations at affiliate and national levels, and for identifying the needs of the OTA as a membership group. She is a retired member of a professional OT curriculum faculty and is both an editor and author of textbooks for OTA students.

Betty Cox of Baltimore, MD, received the ROH (1979) and the Award of Excellence (1977) for leadership in increasing the involvement of OTAs both in the practice arena and in the Association. Her own business offers professional seminars in health-related subjects, both nationally and internationally. She is president of a publishing company that produces books on OT.

Terry Brittell of New Hartford, NY, received the ROH and the Award of Excellence (1979) for outstanding contributions to OT in the areas of practice and clinical education and for service to the profession and for services to the community. At the same psychiatric facility where he was a traditional OTA, he was the coordinator of a stress management program for employees, and of the Mental Health Players, a community prevention program based on role playing.

Charlotte Gale Seltser of Chevy Chase, MD, received the ROH (1981) in recognition of her program development for the visually handicapped. Once retired, Seltser enjoyed volunteering at the National Eye Institute of the National Institutes of Health teaching patients appropriate independence and coping skills and referring them to community agencies.

Toné Frank Blechert of Excelsior, MN, received the ROH and the Award of Excellence (1981) in recognition of her outstanding contributions to OT in the area of OT technical education. As a master degree faculty member of a junior college, she taught mental health concepts and group dynamics to OTA students and coordinated academic advisement for all students.

Ilenna Brown of Plainfield, NJ, received the ROH (1984) for fostering pride and pursuit of excellence for COTA practitioners. In a 550-bed nursing facility, Brown

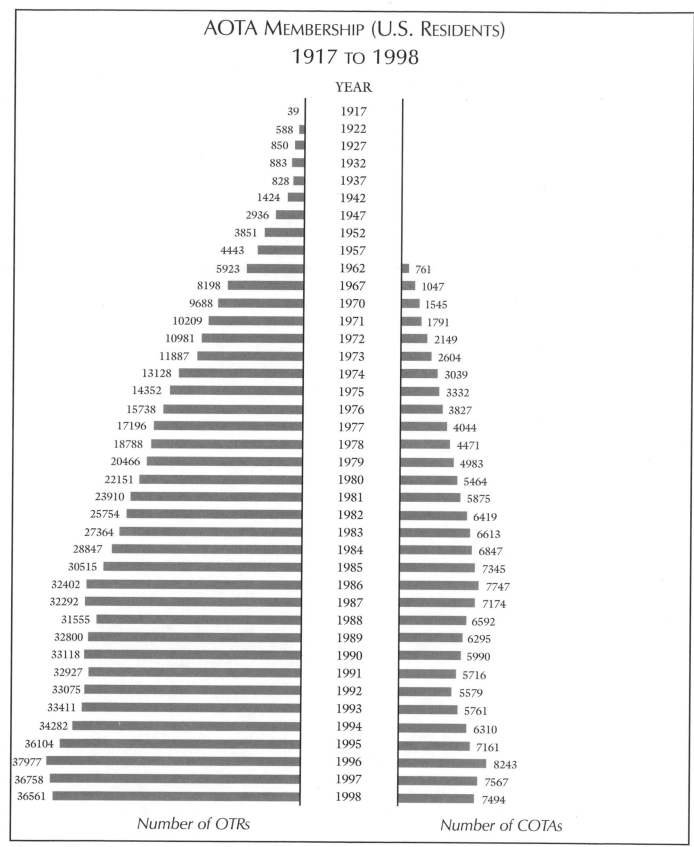

AOTA MEMBERSHIP (U.S. RESIDENTS)
1917 TO 1998

Number of OTRs	YEAR	Number of COTAs
39	1917	
588	1922	
850	1927	
883	1932	
828	1937	
1424	1942	
2936	1947	
3851	1952	
4443	1957	
5923	1962	761
8198	1967	1047
9688	1970	1545
10209	1971	1791
10981	1972	2149
11887	1973	2604
13128	1974	3039
14352	1975	3332
15738	1976	3827
17196	1977	4044
18788	1978	4471
20466	1979	4983
22151	1980	5464
23910	1981	5875
25754	1982	6419
27364	1983	6613
28847	1984	6847
30515	1985	7345
32402	1986	7747
32292	1987	7174
31555	1988	6592
32800	1989	6295
33118	1990	5990
32927	1991	5716
33075	1992	5579
33411	1993	5761
34282	1994	6310
36104	1995	7161
37977	1996	8243
36758	1997	7567
36561	1998	7494

Figure 2-6. AOTA membership statistics for OTRs and COTAs (AOTA, 2000). (Reprinted in part from Ryan, S. E. (1993). *The certified occupational therapy assistant: Principles, concepts, and techniques.* 2nd ed. Thorofare, NJ: SLACK Incorporated.)

was the supervising OTA and rehabilitation coordinator for programs carried on cooperatively by OT, physical therapy, and rehabilitation nursing.

Barbara Larson of Mahtomedi, MN, received the ROH (1985) for exemplary leadership and promotion of the profession. Larson returned to school to become an OTR and now has a master's degree. She was the coordinator of an industrial rehabilitation clinic and currently consults in occupational health and industrial rehabilitation. She was the past president of her state association at the time of her award.

Patty Lynn Barnett of Birmingham, AL, received the ROH (1986) for dynamic leadership in the promotion of OTAs. At the time, Barnett was a faculty member of a university OT curriculum where she taught activity classes and coordinated clinical education for assistant students.

Margaret S. Coffey of Russiaville, IN, received the ROH and Award of Excellence (1986) for excellence in role expansion and commitment to COTAs. With a master's degree, she enjoys a diverse life with the care for two children, a weaver's group, and co-authored *Activity Analysis & Application: Building Blocks of Treatment* (3rd ed.) with two OTs.

Barbara Forte of Palm Springs, CA, received the ROH and the Award of Excellence (1986) because through exemplary qualities of dedication and commitment, she provides outstanding leadership in local, state, and national organizations. She articulates the emerging role of OTAs and serves as a role model. Forte has broad experience in delivering community-based clinical services and private mental health programs.

Robin Jones of Chicago, IL, received the ROH and the Award of Excellence (1987) because she exemplifies excellence and professionalism and is recognized as a strong OTA role model by her peers. She is recognized as an outstanding practitioner, teacher, and advocate for OT. Jones has experience as the director of an independent living center, master's degree student, and vice chair of her state's licensure board.

Teri Black of Madison, WI, received the ROH and Award of Excellence (1989) for leadership modeling for OTA/OT professional development. She has experience teaching in an area technical college and practices in a nursing home. Black served two terms as chair of her state's licensure board.

Sue Byers of Gresham, OR, received the ROH (1989) for exemplary role modeling for OTAs and students. As a member of the faculty of an OTA education program, Byers taught and practiced in home health.

Diane S. Hawkins of Baltimore, MD, received the ROH (1991) in recognition of her significant contributions in staff development and communications. Diane was a faculty consultant for the AOTA workshop "Treatment in Groups: A Workshop for COTAs" and an associate faculty member for the Sheppard and Enoch Pratt National Center for Human Development.

Eleanor Clarke Slagle Award

As of yet, no OTA has received the Eleanor Clarke Slagle Award, the highest honor given by the AOTA to any OTA or OT. This honor may be waiting for you or one of your peers.

Summary

To summarize in allegory, picture a young fruit tree growing well, but having the potential of producing a limited amount of fruit. On advice of well-experienced practitioners, a graft of another tree is applied to increase productivity and quality of fruit. Although traumatic to the tree and to the graft bud at first, the surgery is successful. The graft takes well, and the whole tree develops and becomes stronger than before, even stronger than it could have been if left alone to grow naturally. Now after more than 30 years, the subtle difference in a part of the tree is indistinguishable, unless you are up close or know fruit trees very well.

Editor's Note

At the request of the author, the writing style has not been modified to third person, to conform with other chapters. Rather, the terms *you* and *your* have been retained where appropriate to assist in engaging the reader in the story as it unfolds.

Acknowledgments

Marion Crampton, Mildred Schwagmeyer, and Ruth Wiemer shared their early COTA stories and allowed me to use their materials; I avow my appreciation. I also thank those who helped me document memories and flesh out the intervening years. These individuals include Patty Barnett and Sally Ryan, Robert Bing, Bonnie Brooks, Marie Moore, Dottie Renoe, Lauren Rivet, Ira Silvergleit, and the ROH award winners. Lisa Dickey was a patient co-proofreader, and Joel G. Swetnam has generously shared his computer graphic skills.

References

AOTA. (1964). Annual report, committee on OTAs. *Am J Occup Ther, 18,* 45-46.

AOTA. (1965). Board of management report. *Am J Occup Ther, 19,* 100.

AOTA. (1966). AOTA: Delegate assembly minutes. *Am J Occup Ther, 20,* 49-53.

AOTA. (1967). Presidents of the AOTA (1917-1967). *Am J Occup Ther, 21,* 290-298.

AOTA. (1980). Representative assembly minutes. *Am J Occup Ther, 43,* 844-870.

AOTA. (1981). COTA task force chart of concerns. *OT News, 35*(8).

AOTA. (1982a). Representative assembly report. *Am J Occup Ther, 36,* 808-826.

AOTA. (1982b). 52nd annual conference, annual business meeting. *Am J Occup Ther, 36,* 808-826.

AOTA. (1983). Representative assembly minutes. *Am J Occup Ther, 37,* s92.

AOTA. (1987). Member data survey. *OT News,* September.

AOTA. (1994). Guide for supervision of OT personnel. *Am J Occup Ther, 48,* 1054-1056.

AOTA. (1999a). *Award nomination form, ROH.* Bethesda, MD: Author.

AOTA. (1999b). Fortieth anniversary timeline: OTA history. *OT Practice, 21,* July/August.

AOTA. (2000). *AOTA membership statistics.* Bethesda, MD: Author.

Barnett, P. (1981). COTA task force report. *OT News, 35,* August.

Brittell, T. (1986). *AOTA COTA advisory committee final report.* Bethesda, MD: Author.

Carr, S. H. (1971). Models of manpower utilization. *Am J Occup Ther, 25,* 259-262.

Caskey, V. (1961). A training program for OTAs. *Am J Occup Ther, 15,* 157-159.

Cox, B. (1977). *AOTA's visual taped history: Ruth A. Robinson.* AOTA Archives, Moody Medical Library, University of Texas Medical Branch, Galveston, Texas.

Crampton, M. (1989). *Presentation at 30th anniversary COTA forum.* Baltimore, MD.

Jones, R. (1989). *Presentation at 30th anniversary COTA forum.* Baltimore, MD.

Schwagmeyer, M. (1989). *Presentation at 30th anniversary COTA forum.* Baltimore, MD.

Schwagmeyer, M. (1990). *Personal correspondence to S. Carr.* January 4.

TOTA, Southeast District (1973). *Proceedings of meeting.* October 15.

Wiemer, R. (1964). Unpublished report of workshop summary: *Workshop on the training of the OTA.* Detroit, MI.

Wiemer, R. (1966). AOTA conference keynote address. *Am J Occup Ther, 20,* 9-11.

Wiemer, R. (1989). *Presentation at 30th anniversary COTA forum.* Baltimore, MD.

Philosophy and Core Values of Occupational Therapy

Chapter 3

Phillip D. Shannon, MA, MPA

INTRODUCTION

A vital aspect of the educational preparation of the OTA is an appreciation of the philosophy on which the practice of OT is based. Why is this so vital? There are at least four reasons that provide a rationale.

First, the philosophy of any profession represents the profession's views on the nature of existence. These views reflect the reasons for its own existence in responding to the needs of the population served. For example, a somewhat complex question addressed in philosophy is: "What is man?" Is man a physical being, a psychological being, a social being, or all of these? If man is perceived by a profession as a physical being only, then in responding to the needs of "man the patient" the action is quite clear: the practitioner deals only with the body, not with the mind. As inconceivable as this particular belief might appear, the practices of some professions reflect a narrow perspective of man. Sometimes, as it will be discussed later, a profession does not practice what it believes.

Guided by its philosophical beliefs, a grand design evolves to specify the purposes or goals of the profession. Lacking an understanding of the philosophical basis for this grand design, the practitioner cannot be sure that the goals he or she is pursuing are worth pursuing or that the services provided are worth providing.

A second reason for understanding the philosophy of the profession is that philosophy guides action. Indeed, it is only within the context of a profession's philosophy that actions have meaning. Attending to the leisure needs of the patient, for instance, is one of the major concerns of OT, because its practitioners believe that man seeks a sense of quality to life. One aspect of a quality life, like a satisfying work life, is a satisfying leisure life. Consequently, using arts and crafts to promote the leisure interests and skills of the patient and, therefore, the quality of life of the patient, is an action that makes sense because the action has philosophical meaning.

One of the primary reasons for studying philosophy, according to Thomas (1983), is to clarify beliefs so that the action that comes from those beliefs is sound and consistent. Clarifying the beliefs of the profes-

KEY CONCEPTS

- Importance of philosophy: Profession's views, guide action, explain practice, appreciation.
- Metaphysics: The ultimate nature of man and life.
- Epistemology: The study of truth.
- Axiology: The study of values.
- Philosophy of Adolph Meyers: Founding beliefs of OT.

ESSENTIAL VOCABULARY

Philosophy of life: Personalized view of oneself and the world.

Quality of life: Satisfaction in the occupations of living.

sion should be regarded as a critical component of the OTA's education to ensure that his or her actions are sound and consistent; that is, that the OTA's entry-level behaviors are based on and consistent with a set of guiding philosophical beliefs.

A third rationale for understanding the philosophy of OT is the direct relationship between the growth of the profession and the ability of its practitioners to explain their reasons for existence. In the present era of accountability, where the justification for programs and the competition for resources to support these programs is greater than in previous years, one cannot assume that those external to the profession, such as physicians, will perceive OT as an intrinsically good or essential service. Claims of goodness must be substantiated with evidence. That evidence must be supported philosophically, otherwise it will lack a context for its interpretation. For example, documented evidence that a patient's range of motion in the left elbow was increased by 5 degrees as a result of OT's intervention is important. What strengthens this evidence, however, are the reasons for intervening in the first place. These reasons are linked to the philosophical beliefs of the profession.

Finally, it is not sufficient for the OTA to be skilled in applying the techniques of the profession. On the contrary, he or she must have some appreciation, philosophical and theoretical, of the reasons why these techniques are applied. Lacking this appreciation, the OTA will apply these techniques without being able to communicate their value to the patient, thereby failing to motivate the patient's active involvement in treatment.

Certainly from the initial stage of patient referral to the last stage of discontinuing the patient's treatment, the philosophical beliefs of the profession must remain in the foreground. For the OTA, who has major responsibilities along the entire continuum of health care, these beliefs and the actions that stem from them must be understood and practiced. Indeed, this is the first duty of the OTA.

WHAT IS PHILOSOPHY?

To appreciate fully the philosophy of OT, one must appreciate and understand philosophy in general. Basically, philosophy is concerned with the "meaning of human life, and the significance of the world in which man finds himself" (Randall & Buchler, 1960, p. 5). Man is, by nature, a philosophical creature. Questions such as "Who am I?", "What is my destiny?", and "What do I want from life?" are questions of meaning and purpose that concern all human beings. Each individual, in responding to questions such as these, develops a personalized view of oneself and the world, commonly referred to as a philosophy of life. This philosophy represents a fundamental set of values, beliefs, truths, and principles that guide the person's behavior from day to day and from year to year.

The philosophy of a profession also represents a set of values, beliefs, truths, and principles that guides the actions of the profession's practitioners. Typically, as with individuals, the philosophy evolves over time and sometimes changes as a profession matures. Each profession, in shaping and reshaping its philosophy, has choices to make in three philosophical dimensions. These include metaphysics, epistemology, and axiology.

Metaphysics

Metaphysics is concerned with questions about the ultimate nature of things, including the nature of man. With regard to the nature of man in particular, the mind/body relationship is of special interest to the philosopher. Are mind and body two separate entities, one superior to the other, or are mind and body a single entity representative of the "whole"—the whole person? The first position, that of mind/body separation, is the dualistic position. The second position, that of mind/body as one entity, is the position of holism.

While most (if not all) professions claim to be holistic, the truth in this claim is seen to the extent to which the actions of the profession are consistent with its beliefs. Assume, for example, that the actions of "profession X" are directed toward exercise as the means for promoting a healthy body (e.g., a healthy "physical" body). Assume also that profession X claims to be holistic, asserting a concern for the whole person. In actuality, it is dualistic because the body is viewed as superior to the mind; the goal of exercise, in this case, is a healthy body, not a healthy body and a healthy mind. There is a contradiction, therefore, in what profession X believes and what it does. Its actions do not follow from its beliefs, and the claim of holism is illegitimate. When exercise is seen as promoting the health of the "whole," a more holistic approach is demonstrated.

Epistemology

The second dimension pertinent to shaping and reshaping the philosophy of a profession is the dimension of epistemology, which is concerned with questions of truth. What is truth? How do we come to know things? How do we know that we know? One way of knowing is by experience. One knows, for example, that the flame of a fire brings pleasure in terms of the warmth it provides, but also that it produces pain if it is touched by the bare hand. Usually, one only needs to experience this pain once to "know that he or she knows." Is experience the only route to truth or knowing? From a holistic perspective, there are many routes to truth and knowing. Intuition, for instance, is considered to be as truthful as experiential learning or the logic reasoned by the powers of the intellect. For the dualist, on the other hand, the subjective realities of intuition and experience cannot be accepted as truths. On the contrary, only the objective reality of rational thought can be admitted as truth; truth is logic.

Axiology

The third dimension of philosophy is axiology, which is concerned with the study of values. Two types of questions are addressed by axiology: questions of value with regard to what is desirable or beautiful in the world (aesthetics) and questions of value with regard to the standards or rules for right conduct, or ethics. Most people would agree that a long life is a desirable thing—something that is valued. Some people might argue that a long life without a sense of quality to one's life is a life that is not worth living. Almost everyone would maintain that it is wrong to take a life, yet there are those who believe that "a life for a life" might be justified in some instances.

Conflicting values and standards often produce dilemmas that are difficult to resolve. If life is valued, for example, is it right or moral to disconnect the support systems maintaining the life of the person who has been certified as "brain dead?" Is it right or moral to prolong a life that may not be a life worth living? These are difficult questions of value about what is desirable or beautiful in the world and about the standards that will be applied in pursuing that which is valued.

Each profession has choices to make about what it considers beautiful and desirable in the world and the ethical principles that it will follow in achieving its goals. For medicine, the preservation of life is the first priority, and perhaps this is as it should be, for medicine. But, is this the highest priority of the other health care professions? Should it be the highest priority? A profession that claims to be holistic cannot be satisfied with saving lives. Instead, a holistic profession would maintain that a life worth saving must be a life worth living.

Given this brief glimpse of metaphysics, epistemology, and axiology, dimension can be discussed as it relates to the philosophy of OT. Specifically, four questions will be addressed:

1. The metaphysical question of "What is man?"
2. The epistemologic question of "How does man know that he knows?"
3. The aesthetic question of "What is beautiful or desirable in the world?"
4. The ethical question of "What are the rules of right conduct?"

Two approaches will be taken in responding to these questions. First, the philosophy of Adolph Meyer (1977), who was primarily responsible for providing OT with a philosophical foundation for practice, will be examined. Second, the extent to which this philosophical base has survived the test of time will be explored.

THE EVOLUTION OF OCCUPATIONAL THERAPY

OT evolved from the moral treatment movement that began in the early 19th century (Bockhoven, 1971). If there was a single purpose to which the champions of this movement were committed, it was to humanize and to provide more humane forms of treatment for the mentally ill incarcerated in the large asylums in this country and abroad. Marching under the banner of humanism, the leaders of this movement sought to defend and preserve the dignity of all human beings, particularly the sick and the disabled.

Among these humanists who carried the movement into the 20th century was the psychiatrist Adolph Meyer (Figure 3-1), whose paper on "The Philosophy of Occupation Therapy" (1977) laid the foundation for the practice and promotion of OT. Meyer's philosophy was on his observations of everyday living. From his beliefs about the nature of man, about life, and about a life worth living, the pioneers of the profession emerged to chart its course. Although Meyer has been quoted frequently in the literature of recent years, a more extensive discussion of his philosophy is provided here because, to date, his thoughts have not been examined within the context of metaphysics, epistemology, and axiology.

A Retrospective Glance at the Philosophy of Adolph Meyer

What Is Man?

Meyer's perspective of man was holistic: Our body is not merely so many pounds of flesh and bone figuring as a machine, with an abstract mind or soul added to it. (Rather it is a live organism acting) in harmony with its own nature and the nature about it.

For Meyer, three characteristics distinguished man from all other organisms: sense of time, capacity for imagination, and need for occupation.

A sense of time, past, present, and future, was the central theme of Meyer's philosophy. He believed that a sense of time, and particularly time past (experience), provides man with an advantage over other living organisms in terms of adapting in the present and manipulating the future. This capacity to learn from experience, when blended with the capacity for imagination or creativity, allows man to alter his environment. The squirrel, for example, is totally dependent on its environment for food and shelter during the winter months. Man, on the other hand, through experience and imagination, has been able to alter his environment to ensure survival from hunger through food preservation techniques and protection from the cold via heat-producing systems.

The need for occupation was regarded by Meyer (1977) as a distinctly human characteristic. He defined occupation as a form of helpful enjoyment, which clearly transcends the notion of occupation as being limited to work. On the contrary, the meaning of occupation was extended by Meyer to include all of those activities that comprise a normal day, particularly work and play. He considered occupation important to all, the sick as well as the healthy. Each individual must achieve a balance among his occupations, a balanced life of not only work and play, but also of rest and sleep (Meyer, 1977).

How Does Man Know That He Knows?

Man learns not only by experience, but also by "doing": engaging mind and body in occupation. By doing, man is able to achieve. Fidler and Fidler (1978), in reiterating this theme in the 1970s, maintained that doing is linked to becoming, to realizing one's potential. Fundamental to achieving and becoming is doing. In doing, man comes to know about himself and the world. In doing, man knows that he knows.

What Is Desirable or Beautiful in the World?

For Meyer (1977), man is not content simply existing in the world. Instead, man seeks a sense of quality to life that comes from the pleasure in achievement. It is in engaging the total self that man comes to experience the pleasure in achievement, which Reilly (1962), in her Eleanor Clarke Slagle lectureship, articulated so beautifully: "That man, through the use of his hands as they are energized by mind and will, can influence the state of his own health." Again, it is in doing that man achieves and is able to acquire a sense of quality in his life.

What Are the Rules of Right Conduct?

Meyer (1977), in outlining the guiding principles for the practice of OT, maintained that the occupation worker should provide opportunities, not prescriptions. Prescriptions tend to constrain the development of one's potential, whereas opportunities nourish it. To apply prescriptions is to treat the patient as an object; to offer opportunities is to regard the patient as a person. Inherent in this principle of right conduct is a belief in the type of relationship that the occupation worker should maintain with the patient—a helping relationship, a caring relationship, a relationship where patients are indeed treated as persons and not as objects.

To summarize, Meyer's perspective of man was holis-

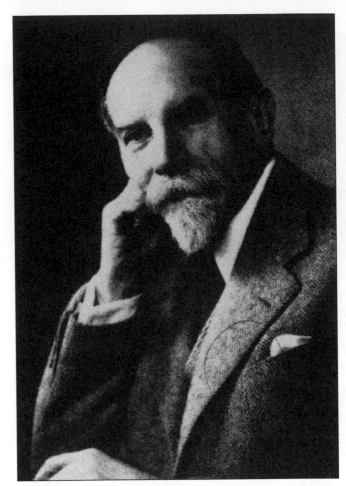

Figure 3-1. Dr. Adolph Meyer, psychiatrist and early occupational therapy proponent and philosopher (Fabian Bachrach photo). (Reprinted from Ryan, S. E. [1993]. *The certified occupational therapy assistant: Principles, concepts, and techniques* [2nd ed.]. Thorofare, NJ: SLACK Incorporated.)

tic. He emphasized doing as the primary route to truth and to achieving a sense of quality in one's life. Prerequisite to doing, however, is opportunity. Lacking the opportunity to do, man, like the squirrel, cannot control his own destiny. On the contrary, man becomes the squirrel, controlled and manipulated by his environment.

The Test of Time

Has the philosophy of Adolph Meyer, which provided the direction for the practice and promotion of OT, survived the test of time, or has the profession, as it matured, changed its direction, based on a different set of values, beliefs, truths, and principles? The answer is reflected in the report to the AOTA on the Project to Identify the Philosophical Base of Occupational Therapy (Shannon, 1983), which was submitted to the Executive Board of the representative assembly. This report did not represent "an official position" of the AOTA with regard to the philosophy of OT, but it is the documentation of a 6 1/2-year project designed to trace the philosophical beliefs of the profession historically and to interpret those beliefs within the context of more modern times. In reviewing the degree to which the beliefs of Adolph Meyer have withstood the test of time, the four philosophical questions addressed earlier are once again discussed in the following sections.

What Is Man?

The belief in holism has persisted in the profession (Shannon, 1983). Indeed, one of the unique aspects of OT is its integrating function, where mind and body are activated to promote the patient's total involvement in the treatment process. To lose sight of this function is to lose sight of one of the major contributions of OT—attending to the "whole person."

One might speculate that it is the profession's commitment to holism that has attracted people to OT rather than to some of the other health professions that appear less holistic. Even in OT, however, the concept of holism, although universally professed, is not uniformly applied in practice. Action is not always consistent with belief. When practice takes the form of dealing only with the mind, only with the body, or worse yet, with only parts of the body, the commitment to holism has been compromised, and there is a contradiction between what one believes and what one does.

For example, hand rehabilitation has become a highly specialized area of practice. Unquestionably, there is a significant contribution to be made to health care in this area. However, when some of the practitioners in rehabilitation begin to refer to themselves as "hand therapists" vs. "OTs," there is an implicit shift away from holism. The belief in holism may remain, but the explicit actions that follow are sometimes not holistic. Only when hand rehabilitation focuses on the whole person does it retain its holistic function.

Another contradiction between belief and action is in mental health practice. Probably one of the first signs indicating the shift away from holism in mental health is when the practitioner uses the title "psychiatric occupational therapist" or "psychiatric occupational therapy assistant." "Psychiatric occupational therapy" personnel tend to focus only on the mind of the patient to the exclusion of the patient's body. Furthermore, when the practitioner's actions are directed primarily toward the unconscious mind, as in providing activities for the sublimation of innate drives, attention is not even focused on the whole mind, much less the mind and body. Again, the belief in holism may be contradicted by the practitioner's actions.

Surely these examples are not characteristic of most practitioners in mental health; nor is "hand therapy" necessarily limited to the treatment of the hand. However, when the broad concerns of OT are narrowed, the patient is somehow cheated in the process.

Also surviving the test of time is the belief in Meyer's distinguishing characteristics of man. Indeed, in responding to the needs of "man the patient," OT has placed a high priority on time as a continuum in the life of a patient, designing programs of treatment within the context of the patient's past, present, and future. In implementing these programs, the patient's capacity for imagination or creativity is challenged in the interest of serving the need for occupation.

Occupation, as defined in the report from the AOTA Project to Identify the Philosophical Base of Occupational Therapy, is goal-directed behavior aimed at the development of play, work, and life skills (Shannon, 1983). If, as Reilly (1962) proposed, man's need for occupation is that vital need of man served by OT, then to reduce the concept of occupation to the level of exercising bodily parts with weights and pulleys or to the level of occupying the patient's mind with activities that bear little or no relationship to the nature of his or her occupation, is to deny this vital need. In addition, another unique aspect of the profession is somehow lost in the transformation of belief into action.

In contrast, by drawing on the patient's past experiences in work and play and in exploring the patient's values, capacities, and interests, the therapist should provide experiences that will serve the patient's need for occupation. In addition, in tapping the creative potential of the patient in areas such as problem-solving and decision-making, the therapist can expand the patient's capacities for altering the environment, thereby, expanding the potential for adapting in the present and for controlling his or her own destiny into the future.

How Does Man Know That He Knows?

From the beginning, OT has believed in the active vs. the passive involvement of the patient in treatment, that is, in doing. As Meyer believed, however, doing is but one way of knowing. There are multiple routes to truth—experience, thinking, feeling, and doing—which the modern day practitioner also accepts as reality (Shannon, 1983). One knows, for example, what happiness means because it has been experienced and because it can be felt. Happiness cannot be measured, but this does not make it any less real.

Among the many ways of knowing, doing is emphasized in the profession as the means for acquiring the skills for daily living and knowing one's capabilities in the present and one's potential for the future. Here again, the opportunities for doing must be framed within the context of the whole person. Consider, for example, the active engagement of the patient in sensory integration activities. One of the major reasons for involving a patient in this type of activity is that the ability to receive and process sensory information is one way of knowing. For example, one knows that it is cold, and, therefore, that the body should be protected with warm clothing because one is able to feel cold, process this input, and take the appropriate steps to protect oneself.

Lacking the ability to process sensory information, the person is denied an important, if not critical, source of information. In this case, doing, in the form of involving the individual in sensory integration activities, is an important step in the process of knowing. On the other hand, if the patient benefits from involvement in OT are limited to those derived by applying the techniques of sensory integration, then OT has not served its holistic function, nor has it served the patient's need for occupation.

The practitioner takes a step away from this belief in doing when the action of "having the patient do" is replaced with the action of "doing to the patient." Another unique aspect of OT is obscured when the patient is denied the opportunity for doing.

What Is Desirable or Beautiful in the World?

To subsist, according to Meyer, is not enough for man. Man seeks something beyond subsistence or survival: the "good life," a life of quality. In maintaining this position over the years, OT has focused its attention in two directions: minimizing the deficits and maximizing the strengths of the patient (Shannon, 1983). Attending to one without attending to the other is incomplete and insufficient if the goals go beyond mere survival.

Traditionally, OT has minimized its contribution to the survival aspects of care and maximized its role in promoting a life of quality for its patients. Perhaps this is as it should be, perhaps not. Perhaps it is a matter of interpretation, that is, how one defines survival in terms of whether or not this position is legitimate. Consider, for example, the patient who has not learned the techniques of wheelchair mobility. This individual will not survive, at least not as a self-sufficient being. Consider also the patient who cannot dress him- or herself and is unable to organize time to meet the demands of daily living. This patient will not survive with any degree of autonomy or self-respect. Furthermore, as Shannon (1983) summarized, bodies and minds not active will die. Also, people who lack quality in their lives sometimes engage in self-destructive behaviors, such as alcoholism, that lead to deterioration and death (Shannon, 1985). Does OT contribute to the preservation of life? Surely, as these examples suggest, OT contributes to the survival of the patient directly, if survival is interpreted to mean the ability to care for self, and indirectly, by adding a sense of quality to the lives of those served by the profession.

Reilly (1962) stated that the first duty of an organism is to be alive; the second duty is to grow and be productive. If survival is the first priority of the organism, then perhaps the position of the profession can be strengthened by developing an argument for the practice and promotion of OT that includes a commitment to the survival of the patient, as well as to the quality of his or her life (Shannon, 1985). In developing this argument, it must be made clear that the first priority of the profession is to teach the patient skills that will ensure survival. The second priority is to guide the patient toward the realization of his or her potential and social worth as a member of society, as evidenced, according to Heard (1977), by the ability to perform an occupational role. Indeed, it is for these reasons that man engages in occupation; it is also for these reasons that OT exists.

OT has expressed its commitment to the second priority, but its actions are often directed to the first. As Heard maintained, it is in addressing the second priority, and particularly the social worth of the patient, that OT has been most negligent (Heard, 1977). Yet, in attending to the social worth of the patient, the profession is making a major contribution to a more healthy society. Certainly, in making this contribution, as Yerxa (1979) argued that it must, the profession's value is increased and its survival guaranteed.

What Are the Rules of Right Conduct?

Meyer's principle of providing opportunities, not prescriptions, for patients has been one of the distinguishing characteristics of the profession. In applying the rule of nonprescription, the patient becomes an active partner in treatment. Why is this important?

First, the skills and habits necessary for the performance of occupational roles cannot be administered to the patient, but must be acquired by the patient. Second, prescriptions tend to foster externally controlled behaviors (pawn), whereas opportunities encourage internally controlled behaviors (origin) as defined by Burke (1977). In applying prescriptions, the patient is treated as a pawn, externally controlled by those responsible for his or her care; in offering opportunities, the patient is treated as origin, drawing upon the strengths within him or her to assume control for his or her own life. If taking charge of one's own life is important and assuming control for one's own destiny is valued, providing opportunities and not prescriptions is a necessary first step.

In offering opportunities for patients to take charge of their own lives, two major ethical principles guide the actions of the practitioner (Beauchamp & Childress, 1983). The first of these is the principle of nonmaleficence, which states that not only should one do no harm, but also that one should promote the good. The second is the principle of beneficence, or the rule that one should show kindness and caring. Perhaps no profession can lay greater claim to applying these principles than OT. The principle of showing kindness and caring, however, raises the issue of patient vs. client. Which is more legitimate: a therapist/patient relationship or a therapist/consumer relationship?

In a therapist/patient relationship, the client is perceived as an object, an "it," because only one aspect of the client becomes the focus of attention. The therapist/patient relationship is similar to that of a used car salesperson who has only one goal: to sell the client a used car regardless of whether the client can afford gasoline to operate the car or whether the client has the financial resources to insure and maintain it.

In a therapist/consumer relationship, the patient is perceived not as an object, but as a person. Patients expect that their total well-being will be improved when seeking health care (Reilly, 1984).

Over the years, OT has prided itself on the fact that it cares. In caring about its patients, clients, or consumers, the profession has demonstrated that it is holistic and humanistic. If a different type of caring evolves, then any future claim of being a holistic, humanistic enterprise will have to be denied.

SUMMARY

The philosophical beliefs guiding the contemporary practice of OT can be traced to Adolph Meyer, whose philosophy of occupation therapy was framed within the context of metaphysics, epistemology, and axiology. Meyer's philosophy was both holistic and humanistic. As it persists in the present to guide the actions of the OT practitioner, so will it persist in the future to provide direction for the profession as it continues to mature.

The philosophical beliefs identified in this chapter and the principles for practice that evolved from these philosophical beliefs are summarized in Table 3-1, which also contains descriptions of situations when these beliefs and principles are compromised. The COTA owes allegiance to these beliefs and principles when responding to the needs of those served by the profession.

EDITOR'S NOTE

In the context of this chapter, the term "man," in the philosophical sense, refers to the generic term "mankind," which is considered standard and gender inclusive.

REFERENCES

Beauchamp, T. L., & Childress, J. F. (1983). *Principles of biomedical ethics*. New York, NY: Oxford University Press.

Bockhoven, J. S. (1971). Legacy of moral treatment 1800s to 1910. *Am J Occup Ther, 25,* 223-225.

Burke, J. P. (1977). A clinical perspective on motivation: Pawn versus origin. *Am J Occup Ther, 31,* 254-258.

Fidler, G. S., & Fidler, J. W. (1978). Doing and becoming: Purposeful action and self-actualization. *Am J Occup Ther, 32,* 305-310.

Heard, C. (1977). Occupational role acquisition: A perspective on the chronically disabled. *Am J Occup Ther, 31,* 243-247.

Meyer, A. (1977). The philosophy of occupation therapy. *Am J Occup Ther, 31,* 639-642.

Randall, J. H., & Buchler, J. (1960). *Philosophy: An introduction*. New York, NY: Barnes and Noble, Inc.

Reilly, M. (1962). OT can be one of the great ideas of 20th century medicine. *Am J Occup Ther, 16,* 1-9.

Reilly, M. (1984). The importance of the patient versus client issue for OT. *Am J Occup Ther, 6,* 404-406.

Shannon, P. D. (1983). Report on the AOTA project to identify the philosophical base of OT. January, 1983. Condensed under the title: *Toward a Philosophy of OT*. August, 1983.

Shannon, P. D. (1985). From another perspective: An overview of the issue on the roles of OTs in continuity of care. *OT Health Care, 2,* 3-11.

Thomas, C. E. (1983). *Sport in a philosophic context*. Philadelphia, PA: Lea and Febiger.

Yerxa, E. (1979). The philosophical base of OT. *In OT: 2001 AD*. Rockville, MD: AOTA.

Table 3-1
Summary of Philosophical Beliefs, Principles, and Contradictory Practices

Philosophical Beliefs	Principles for Practice	Beliefs/Principles Compromised
Metaphysical Position		
The belief in holism, in mind and body as one entity	Attending to the whole person	Attending only to the mind or only to the body or parts of the body
The belief in the uniqueness of or in man's distinctly human qualities, that include an appreciation of time, past, present, and future	Designing intervention programs within the context of the patient's past, present, and future	Attending to the present needs of the patient without considering the patient's past experiences and goals for the future
The capacity for imagination	Challenging the patient's capacity for imagination or creativity	Providing prescriptions versus opportunities
The need for occupation	Promoting a balanced life of work, play, rest, and sleep	Placing an emphasis on the treatment of pathology to the extent that the acquisition of skills that will support occupational role is minimized or ignored
Epistemologic Position		
The belief that there is not just one, but many routes to knowing or learning	Valuing experience, thinking, and feeling in the process of doing en route to knowing or learning	Treating the patient as a passive versus active participant during the process of intervention
Axiologic Position— **The Aesthetic Component**		
The belief that man seeks a life beyond subsistence, a life of quality	The first principle: teaching survival skills by minimizing deficits and maximizing strengths	Teaching survival skills without attending to the patient's potential beyond survival or his or her social worth
	The second principle: providing opportunities for achievement, for the realization of one's potential and one's social worth	
Axiologic Position— **The Ethical Component**		
The humanistic belief that patients should be treated as persons, not objects	Protecting the patient from harm; promoting good	Neglecting the patient's safety or security needs and/or failing to protect the patient's rights as a patient and as a human being
	Demonstrating kindness and caring	Promoting a therapist-client versus therapist-patient relationship
	Providing opportunities versus prescriptions	Applying remedies that discourage individual initiative

(Reprinted from Ryan, S. E. [1993]. The certified occupational therapy assistant: Principles, concepts, and techniques [2nd ed.]. Thorofare, NJ: SLACK Incorporated.)

Human Development

Cheryl A. Leary, EdD

INTRODUCTION

Welcome to the world of understanding human development. As an OT practitioner, you will encounter many people in the course of your work who will need your help. In order for you to be helpful and successful in your work, you will need to know about human development. What you may not realize is that you already know a great deal about human development. The purpose of this chapter is to introduce you to specific information that will help you understand some of the cognitive, behavioral, social, psychological, and emotional issues that directly affect human development and have an impact on everyday life experience.

Each developmental period will be discussed by presenting the milestones that occur throughout normal human development. (A summary can be found in Appendix A.) The science of human development has its own vocabulary. Terminology will be presented throughout this chapter that is specific to the various developmental periods. Also, terminology will vary according to the unique perspective of the different theorists around human development. In fact, each theorist in this discussion proposes his or her own "stages" of human development. There are many theorists and many different models for us to use in considering the topic of human development. The advanced student of human developmental theory will certainly want to look into the role of culture and its impact on development within a family system. For the sake of brevity and clarity, we will limit our focus in this chapter to a select few who have had a dramatic impact on human developmental theory.

THE THEORISTS

Jean Piaget (1896-1980)

With the birth of a newborn, there come many changes for the entire family. The entire family becomes focused on the well-known developmental milestones. Is she crawling, walking, or is she eating solid food? Did she talk yet? We are all

KEY CONCEPTS

- Piaget's stages of cognitive development: Asserts that our ability to think and solve problems develops in defined stages from birth through adulthood. We have certain innate abilities that are refined as we mature and experience life.

- Erikson's stages of psychosocial development: These eight stages are most often presented as psychosocial "crises." These crises are resolved in the context of genetic history, personal circumstances, and the environment.

- Maslow's hierarchy of needs: Provides an organized framework in which we can understand our needs as human beings. Needs range from basic survival to self-understanding and actualization.

Table 4-1
Erikson's Eight Stages of Psychosocial Development

1. Basic trust vs. mistrust	(birth to 1 year)
2. Autonomy vs. shame and doubt	(1 to 3 years)
3. Initiative vs. guilt	(3 to 6 years)
4. Industry vs. inferiority	(6 to 12 years)
5. Identity vs. role confusion	(12 to 19 years)
6. Intimacy vs. isolation	(19 to 25 years)
7. Generativity vs. stagnation	(25 to 50 years)
8. Ego integrity vs. despair	(50 and older)

captivated by the developmental progress of our loved ones.

One scientist who was also captivated by the development of his own children is considered one of the pioneers in understanding human development. Jean Piaget was born in Switzerland and began his early career as a biologist. He was a scientist who was able to allow his scientific mind to venture into the part of him that was a parent and a father. In observing his own children develop, he formulated his theories around cognitive development and established four distinct stages for cognitive development.

The first stage, the sensorimotor stage, starts at birth and continues for approximately the first 2 years of life. During this period, "the infant gradually becomes able to organize activities in relation to the environment through sensory and motor activity" (Papalia & Olds, 1998, p. 23). Piaget's second stage of cognitive development is the preoperational stage (2 to 7 years). In this stage, the child develops a representational system and uses symbols such as words to represent people, places, and events. The third stage in the paradigm of Piaget is the concrete operations stage (7 to 12 years). In this stage, we witness the onset of the use of logic by the child. The child can solve problems logically when they are focused on the here and now. The fourth and final stage for Piaget is the formal operations stage (12 years through adulthood). In the formal operations stage, the person can think abstractly, deal with hypothetical situations, and think about possibilities (Papalia & Olds, 1998).

Erik Erikson (1902-1994)

Another theorist whose name is recognized and remembered by most students of human developmental theory is Erik Erikson. Erikson, who was a follower of Freud, proposed a theory of psychosocial development that covers eight stages across the life of an individual. In each of these stages, a crisis in personality arises and needs to be resolved in order to effect healthy ego development. For some, there is little resolution to the psy-

chosocial crises, and, as a result, they go through life with a certain amount of imbalance. For example, in Erikson's first developmental stage, the psychosocial crisis is trust vs. mistrust. If an appropriate balance is not the resolution of this first-stage psychosocial crisis, then the person will be subject to either trusting too much or not trusting enough as he or she develops. Virtus in medio stat. Virtue stands in the middle and balance is the key. Always keep in mind that balance is essential to effecting appropriate resolution of the psychosocial crisis in each of Erikson's stages of development. Also, the psychosocial crisis in each stage of Erikson's model need not be a single event but could also be a cluster of events that occur over a period of time in the maturational process. See Table 4-1 for a detailed breakdown of each of the stages of development as proposed by Erikson (Seifert, Hoffnung, & Hoffnung, 1997).

Keep in mind that Erikson's theories were criticized for not adequately addressing issues of both male and female human development. Jean Baker Miller asserted that personality grows within relationships. She believes that "during toddlerhood and early childhood, rather than striving for autonomy and individuation, both boys and girls continue to place the highest importance on intimate connections" (Papalia & Olds, 1998 p. 25).

Abraham Maslow (1954)

Maslow offers another unique approach to understanding our quest for knowledge of human development. The Freudian and neo-Freudian schools of psychology would assert that all behavior is a manifestation of need. Maslow utilized this assertion in formulating his model of human development and growth. His well-known model is called Maslow's Hierarchy of Needs and is almost always pictured as a triangle with basic physiological needs at the bottom and self-actualization at the top (Figure 4-1).

Maslow's assertion is that these basic needs are the prime motivators of human behavior. In fact, only when

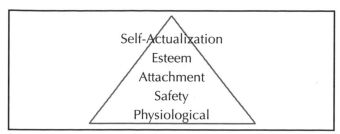

Figure 4-1. Maslow's Hierarchy of Needs.

people have satisfied the basic needs can they move on to satisfy the higher needs. In Maslow's hierarchy, the most basic need is physiological. Food and water are necessary to sustain physical life. Shelter is needed to sustain safety from the elements. Because of our need to belong, the shelter now becomes a home with a family, a family that is part of a community, a community that is part of a larger system. Within that family and community, there is a need to have esteem. The highest need is to be self-actualized and find self-fulfillment; that is, the person finds his or her real place in the community and in the world and is comfortable with it.

THE DEVELOPMENTAL PERIODS

Each developmental theorist has established his or her own specifically defined periods of time over the lifespan in which developmental milestones are achieved. For the sake of our discussion here, the developmental periods are broken down as follows:

- Infancy and toddlerhood—birth to 2 years of age
- Childhood—2 to 12 years of age
- Adolescence—12 to 21 years of age
- Young adulthood—21 to 35 years of age
- Middle adulthood—35 to 60 years of age
- Senior adulthood—60 years of age onward

Infancy and Toddlerhood

The infancy and toddlerhood period runs from birth to about 2 years of age or the onset of language skills. It is a period of time marked by intense care for the infant on the part of caregivers, usually parents.

For Piaget, this is the sensorimotor period in which the child will begin to exhibit reflex behaviors such as visual acuity skills, palm reflex, and sucking. We also see the onset of the preoperational period in which the child is not able to distinguish between reality and fantasy.

In the Erikson paradigm, we see the child caught up in the balancing act of trust vs. mistrust. The child is completely dependent upon others for his or her care. The child learns to trust that when hunger arises and the child cries, a caregiver will bring food. If there is significant inconsistency in this pattern, the child will begin to devel-

op a sense of mistrust. Also, during this period of time, the child will begin the second stage of attaining autonomy vs. shame and doubt. The child begins to move more freely on her own by crawling, standing, or walking. The child begins to establish a better sense of self in relation to the environment. Shame and doubt arise in response to the reaction of the caregivers to the child's new sense of independence.

Maslow would assert that basic physiological and safety needs are predominant during this period, that is, the child is caught up in getting nourishment and feeling safe. We all know that babies are not afraid to let us know when they are hungry or need changing. Loud noises and overly reactive adults can easily frighten babies.

Physically, the infant/toddler is growing rapidly. During these years, the infant/toddler learns to walk, talk, and eat solid foods. Toilet training is also accomplished. Freud would frame these times as the oral and anal phases of development.

Childhood

The period of childhood runs from about 2 years of age to 12 years of age. We see tremendous growth and learning occurring during this developmental period. In considering the thinking of Jean Piaget, this stage of life is a combination of his preoperational and the concrete operations periods. In the preoperational stage, children begin using symbols to represent what was for them a reality at the sensorimotor stage. Make-believe play is helpful for the child to develop the ability to distinguish reality from the appearance of reality (Berk, 1998). In essence, a doll could be a representation of the mother, the father, or anyone in the family system that the child opts to have the doll represent. The concrete operations stage spans from 7 to 11 years of age. During concrete operations, thought is more logical, flexible, and organized than it was during early childhood (Berk, 1998). The child is able to apply logic and organizational skills in concrete situations. Abstract thought comes later. For Erikson, this is the time of initiative vs. guilt, industry vs. inferiority, and the beginning of identity vs. role confusion. Remember that healthy ego development seeks a balance between initiative and guilt, industry and inferiority, and identity and role confusion. The child who is seeking to resolve the conflict of initiative vs. guilt exhibits wonderful spontaneity in his or her behaviors. If the behaviors meet the approval of the social structure in which the child is being reared, then the child feels affirmed. If approval is not given, then the child will feel guilt. For example, a child uses crayons to do some coloring in a coloring book. If she stays in the lines of the picture, she is given approval. If the same child took the crayons and applied the various colors to the living room walls to create some modern art, disapproval of the caregivers would soon follow, and the child would begin to feel guilt. These types of patterns consistently arise in early childhood to help the child achieve the proper balance between initiative vs. guilt. OT focuses on developmentally appropriate and rewarding activities to encourage healthy growth in early childhood.

With the psychosocial crisis of industry vs. inferiority, the child continues to negotiate his or her role among a wider social structure (i.e., peers and school). In meeting the challenges of this stage, the child will sustain healthy ego development by becoming more industrious in problem-solving and skillful at play. However, the child does these things in relationship to peers. If the child does not achieve the appropriate balance in this stage, he or she may be subject to feelings of inferiority. By age 12, the child should have established an optimal balance of trust vs. mistrust, autonomy vs. doubt and shame, initiative vs. guilt, and industry vs. inferiority. The child now enters into the turbulent years of adolescence with a fairly healthy ego.

Now, how many people do you really believe enter into adolescence with a fairly healthy ego? We now encounter Erikson's fifth stage of development, identity vs. role confusion, and our developing person is only 12 years old. This stage will be discussed in more detail in the section on adolescence.

In the Maslow paradigm, we now see the child seeking to belong and to be loved within the context of the family system. The child becomes aware of his or her full name (i.e., the first name followed by the family name). The child's needs for belonging and loving are met within the context of the family. School and peers also play a significant role in helping to meet the need to belong and to be loved.

Physically, the child is still growing rapidly during this period. Emotional and psychological changes are directly related to the physical maturation process. Children are becoming aware of sex differences and gender roles. They also learn to relate to other members of the family and to distinguish right from wrong. Throwing, catching, and utilizing simple tools are critical to maturation during this period. Children learn to get along with their peers, and they progress in the skills of reading, writing, and math. Children begin formulating attachments outside of the home toward peers and other social groups.

Adolescence

The period of adolescence runs from 12 years of age to 21 years of age. It is a time of great change for a young person. During this period, the child grows into an adult body, which grows at a rapid rate. Freud would say that along with any significant change in the body comes a significant change in behavior and psychological makeup.

During this time, the child becomes more acutely aware of sexual feelings and drives.

For Piaget, the child reaches the final stage of cognitive development during the adolescent years. This is the formal-operational stage. Abstract thinking and syllogistic reasoning should be flourishing in the child during this period. Syllogistic reasoning is basic deductive reasoning. An example of syllogistic reasoning is as follows: All OT students learn to practice OT skills. Mary is an OT student. Therefore, Mary will learn to practice OT skills.

In the Erikson paradigm, the primary psychosocial crisis of adolescence is identity vs. role confusion. This is the time that young people move their sense of identity away from their families toward their peers and heroes among their peers. For many kids, the heroes are sports figures, rock stars, or actors. These young people have become an economic reality for big business and are readily targeted by these companies for sales. In the quest for a solid identity, teens will attach to a certain style of clothing, jewelry, or fad that each adolescent will purchase in order to identify the self with the larger community of adolescents. Not to belong to the accepted grouping is to suffer role confusion and risk becoming a "geek" among your peers. Rules for belonging and identification vary from group to group. What qualifies an adolescent for belonging to a youth group at church varies from what qualifies an adolescent for belonging to a gang or scouting organization.

The crisis of identity vs. role confusion is probably most obvious during the adolescent years. The struggle with role confusion is most obvious in the teen who strives to assume the identity of an adult but shirks the responsibilities of adulthood. Consider this scenario: A teenager borrows dad's car with the strict admonition from dad that traffic violations will result in loss of car privileges. The teen accepts a challenge from a peer to engage in a drag race down Longmeadow Street and gets stopped by the police, who issue the teen a traffic citation. He may have won the race, but he also probably lost the privilege of using his father's car.

For Maslow, these years continue the process of seeking to belong. However, now the adolescent needs to belong to his or her peer group more than to the family. Esteem needs also must be achieved during this time of life. Healthy ego development is contingent upon peer recognition of the competence of the adolescent. In the car scenario above, the teen may have lost his car privilege, but he gained status among his peers because he proved his competence when challenged. This example also gives evidence to the fact that the previous Eriksonian psychosocial crisis of initiative vs. guilt is still being played out even in adolescence. OT for adolescents understands the importance of peers in helping teens gain functional skills.

Physically, the adolescent is usually very fit. The growing adolescent body should be able handle any tasks as it progresses toward the adult body. However, emotionally and psychologically, the adolescent is in turmoil. Any discussion of adolescent psychology and emotions cannot be had without reference to the changing physical body. The body is evolving into an adult body, and the adolescent struggles with acceptance of the body that nature has given. Acne can be a very sensitive issue for the adolescent. For girls, body size and physical attractiveness directly affects the level of acceptance by peers. This is the time when many young women develop an eating disorder. Independence is a valued prize to be won in adolescence. The typical rite of passage for new independence is the highly valued driving license. It is during adolescence that one begins to develop a sense of moral purpose and subscribes to a given ethical system of values.

Young Adulthood

Young adulthood is the time in which many parents breathe a sigh of relief if they and their children have survived the turbulent period of adolescence with minimal harm to themselves and the family. Young adulthood spans the years from age 21 to age 35. During this time, the young adult typically has completed his or her education or training to become economically independent from the parents. This is a time when many young adults seek out intimacy and marriage.

Erikson's intimacy vs. isolation is the psychosocial crisis to be resolved during young adulthood. Just when you thought that you had it all together from your adolescence and you established a strong sense of self, a real identity uniquely your own, you go and fall in love. What does falling in love mean? It means that you begin to sacrifice little parts of your individual identity in favor of the "we." Of course, Erikson would say that the identity must be firmly established before true intimacy can take place. However, Jean Baker Miller of the Stone Center would disagree. She asserts that "identity and intimacy can develop simultaneously. Autonomy, creativity, and assertion can all grow within the context of relationships" (Seifert, Hoffnung, & Hoffnung, 1997, p. 463). In either case, intimacy brings about significant changes for both parties who seek an intimate relationship with each other.

Intimacy in young adulthood brings the young adult into stronger alliances and dependencies on friends and lovers vs. ongoing attachment to the family. The young adult is usually on his or her own and living in a residence away from the family.

In the Maslow paradigm, young adults are still struggling to achieve those goals that meet their need for esteem, competence, and recognition in their families and among their peers. There is really too much to be done during this time to consider self-actualization needs. In fact, many young adults will grow old without attaining true self-actualization. The demands of economic survival become the mandated primary focus for the next 45 years. Usually, entrepreneurs who work hard in their young adulthood and achieve a high degree of economic success by age 45 claim a lot of self-satisfaction and report that they are self-actualized. However, true self-actualization is not tied to economic success. True self-actualization is realized in gut-level acceptance of one's self in relationship to family, significant others, friends, community, and the world.

Physically, the young adult is capable of achieving peak performance. There is less of a chance that the body will be significantly harmed from years of poor nutrition and lack of exercise. However, poor nutrition, lack of exercise, and accidents will always take a toll on the wellness of the body regardless of age. Emotionally, the young adult is in search of intimacy and relationships. These are exciting years for attachment and partnership. If this thrust toward intimacy is compromised, the result could be isolation, withdrawal, and depression. Psychologically, the young adult has begun a career and is working to improve his or her place on the economic strata. As part of their integration into the adult social network, many young adults take on civic responsibilities. Strong attachments are formed with peer groups. OT for young adults usually addresses the need for independence and supports the attainment of normal development at this stage.

Middle Adulthood

The middle adulthood years span from 35 to 60 years of age. Middle adults are, for the most part, well established in their careers. For many middle adults, the children have moved out and are on their own. There is a new freedom from child-rearing responsibilities. This stage of life becomes even more exciting as middle adults become grandparents.

A growing trend over the past 20 years is the significant number of grandparents who are taking on the responsibility of raising their grandchildren because their own children have become inadequate parents. In such situations, the parents do not accept the responsibility of parenting their own children. The grandparents step in to provide the needed nurturing and guidance for their grandchildren. This brings to light many developmental issues for both grandparents and grandchildren who are now relating to each other as if in a parent/child relationship. Grandparents should be slowing down and enjoying retirement but are now caught up in running after little ones and changing diapers. Children can feel some sense of embarrassment when their legal guardians show up at the PTA and are, frequently, 20 years or so older than the parents of their peers.

Erikson's psychosocial crisis for middle adulthood is generativity vs. stagnation. This stage does not necessarily focus on biological generativity. In fact, middle adults focus on being very productive in their jobs and hobbies.

They desire to leave something of themselves to benefit not only their children, but also all humanity. The balance between generativity and stagnation is accomplished by not allowing oneself to waste time. Middle adults become very conscious of time and its importance. Mortality becomes more and more a reality for middle adults.

Physically, the body of the middle adult is getting older and more inclined to sedentary ways. Middle adults tend to be productive at the expense of their bodies. They just forget to take care of the body through good nutrition and exercise. They are focused on economics and planning for retirement. Their incomes are hopefully better than when they first started working in their adolescent years. Their familial responsibilities are minimal, and they have a new freedom to engage in personal hobbies and interests. Psychologically, middle adults are independent, capable, and viewed as leaders in most family systems.

Senior Years

In the final discussion of developmental stages, we turn our focus to people age 60 and over. During this time period, the senior adult is doing the final balancing act of Erikson's paradigm, ego integrity vs. despair. The whole idea behind integrity is wholeness. Having lived a long and fruitful life, the senior adult can begin to rest comfortably in the conviction that his or her life was meaningful on this planet. If imbalance has carried through the entire life of the senior adult, then the senior adult faces feelings of meaninglessness in life and tends to despair. Death becomes the final insult to a life of frustration and toil. On the other hand, for the senior adult who has successfully integrated his or her entire life, death is understood as a necessary part of a life well lived. OT can play an important role in helping the senior find meaningful activities in life.

The senior adult faces an increasing incapacity to function independently as the years progress. Dignity and honor should be the hallmarks of the senior years. Unfortunately, dignity and honor for the elderly exist only in certain cultures and not in all. Historically, in Asian cultures, for example, people hold a deep respect and honor for ancestors and for their elderly family members. This trend in more modern Asian cultures is changing. In cultures that foster a highly developed economy, multiple income earners are necessary to maintain a certain standard of living. This forces many families to turn the care of their dependents over to a paid caregiver. Many modern families need day care, not only for their children, but also for their elderly parents. Nursing homes, senior day care facilities, and assisted living communities are becoming more common as a resolution for elder care.

Many senior adults are physically fit. However, for seniors, there is a loss of bone mass, muscle mass, poor eyesight, and wrinkled skin. Senior adults have significantly more involvement in medical services as their bodies give evidence to either years of care or years of neglect and/or abuse. Emotionally, the senior adult may be grieving the death of a lifelong partner or the deaths of friends and peers. These are years of loss for the senior adult. Loneliness and depression are directly related to the isolation that may result when senior adults do not adjust adequately to their multiple losses during this time. Social involvement with peers is a must. Psychologically, the senior adult has integrated a lifetime of experience, relationships, and emotions. The senior adult needs to feel that these experiences are valued. On a more practical side, living arrangements must be made and the ability to care for self must be monitored by family or professionals. Memory tends to fail and the level of care is increased in direct proportion to the inability of the senior adult to care for self.

SUMMARY

In this chapter, we have looked at human development from the perspective of Piaget, Erikson, and Maslow. An additional consideration was given to Jean Miller Baker, who stresses the importance of relationships in personality development. The major developmental periods were examined with some emphasis on physical, emotional, and psychological expectations of people in those developmental periods. Any advanced study of human development should consider looking at the work of Carol Gilligan and Lawrence Kohlberg around issues of moral development.

REFERENCES

Berk, L. A. (1998). *Development through the lifespan*. Needham Heights, MA: Allyn & Bacon.

Papalia, D. E., & Olds, S. W. (1998). *Human development* (7th ed.). Boston, MA: McGraw-Hill.

Seifert, K. L, Hoffnung, R. J., & Hoffnung, M. (1997). *Lifespan development*. Boston, MA: Houghton Mifflin.

Uniform Terminology: Our Language

Chapter 5

Ben Atchison, PhD, OTR, FAOTA

INTRODUCTION

It was an interesting tour for the students in the OTA program as they observed several individuals involved in a variety of activities in a community-based program for persons with developmental disabilities. The OTA who was conducting the tour noted that one of the clients demonstrated dyspraxia and was involved in a therapeutic program to enhance motor planning skills. "So," asked the normally inquisitive student, "does his program involve dexterity activities?" "No," replied the tour guide, "his fine motor coordination is fine. As I said, it is more of a motor planning problem." The student was confused and a little embarrassed, but she remembered that her supervisor on her last fieldwork experience had explained that dyspraxia was the same thing as poor dexterity. "Why," she asked herself, "is this person using this term so differently than what I was taught?"

This student's experience is not uncommon. The language used to describe the many components of OT practice is not always consistent. Try this experiment: Ask a few OTAs to define activities of daily living (ADLs). Undoubtedly, several variations will be offered. The reason for this lack of consistency is that each of those persons you asked probably learned the definition from another person without the benefit of a standard glossary. It presents a problem, however, when the terms that describe the practice of OT are not consistent because it causes confusion among those who are not OTs, including clients, families, other health care team members, and third party payers. For example, if one therapist states that intervention was aimed at improving "self-care" and another uses the term "ADLs" to define self-care, there is a lack of certainty as to the activities included in each term used. However, if all OTs describe "ADLs" in the same way, there is better assurance that others will better appreciate the full spectrum of ADLs and that the term encompasses more activities other than self-care.

KEY CONCEPTS

- Uniform Terminology: Meaning of language in OT.
- Rationale of OT: To provide structure and definition of OT.

ESSENTIAL VOCABULARY

Occupational Performance Areas: Describes the occupational role of an individual in terms of three major categories: ADLs, work and productive activities, and play or leisure activities.

Occupational Performance Components: Provides one with a format for a complete activity analysis. These components are identified in UT3 as: sensorimotor components, cognitive integration and cognitive components, and psychosocial skills and psychological components.

Occupational Performance Contexts: Situations or factors that influence an individual's engagement in desired and/or required performance areas (AOTA, 1994, p. 1047).

Uniform Terminology: Published by AOTA, ensures that health professions use common language when completing required documents.

DEVELOPMENT OF THE UNIFORM TERMINOLOGY SYSTEM

The lack of consistency in the use of terminology is not unique to OT. In fact, a law was passed (P. L. 95-142) in 1977 that, in part, required health care facilities to establish a uniform reporting system to ensure that health professions used common language when completing required documents (Dohli & Leibold, 1998). In part, this law was passed in response to significant billing fraud and abuse in both the Medicare and Medicaid programs by all health-related disciplines. In response to this law, the AOTA created a task force to develop the *Uniform Terminology System for Reporting Occupational Therapy Services* (1979). The Uniform Terminology system has been revised twice since its initial development in 1979. Each revision reflected changes in OT practice and provided more precision in the definitions of terms. The most recent document was published in 1994 and is often referred to as UT3, which stands for *Uniform Terminology (3rd ed.)* (AOTA, 1994). Within this document are three major categories:

1. Performance areas
2. Performance components
3. Performance contexts

PRACTICAL APPLICATION OF *UNIFORM TERMINOLOGY (3RD ED.)*

There are several ways that the UT3 benefits OTs in their everyday practice. First, it provides a reference for the evaluation and intervention process. When the system is used in its entirety, a complete or holistic approach is ensured. For example, when an evaluation is conducted to determine the effects of chronic obstructive pulmonary disease on the ability to perform home management tasks, the impact of this condition on physical-motor components is emphasized. Yet, when using the UT3 grid, which is illustrated in Table 5-1, the therapist will equally consider the effects of this condition on the psychological well-being of the client. Second, a uniform understanding and articulation of terms promotes a common use of language among OT clinicians, educators, researchers, and students. For example, a research article on "The Effects of Compensatory Devices on Perceptual Processing for Children with ADHD" should define "perceptual processing" in the same way that clinicians use the term. Students should learn the term in the same way, no matter what school they receive their education. Third, a consistent use of terms prevents confusion among the consumers of OT, including clients, families, payers, and other professionals, when terms are used to describe evaluation and intervention (Dohli & Leibold, 1998). The OT and OTA collaborate on both evaluation and intervention goals and, in doing so, discuss with the client and family members the approach they are using to meet those goals. The terms used to describe the approach must be consistent to provide a clear understanding of what they are doing.

UNIFORM TERMINOLOGY: PERFORMANCE AREAS

The performance areas describe the occupational role of an individual in terms of three major categories:

A. Activities of daily living
B. Work and productive activities
C. Play or leisure activities

Each of these areas are addressed with an individual during the OT evaluation and intervention process, and it is most important that the therapist considers the dynamic nature of occupational performance. The roles that a person plays change not only over a period of time, but also on a daily basis. As an OT student, consider the emphasis on performance in the work and productive area and specifically in educational activities. At times, it is a dominant role, even to the exclusion of some ADLs and perhaps many desired play or leisure activities. Of course, this emphasis shifts when classes are finished for the term. A break in the academic calendar shifts the major activity from academic work to the pursuit of leisure interests. However, some individuals do not have the benefit of being able to focus on one major role. Consider the student who is a single parent, holds down a full-time job, and attends school full-time as well. His or her roles obviously shift rapidly during a given day, often resulting in negative effects on well-being.

In order to determine the relative importance of occupational performance areas to an individual, the therapeutic relationship with a client begins with a "person-centered" approach. That is, the OT considers with the client the perceived needs, interests, and expectations for resuming each of the occupational performance areas. This process continues into the intervention program as the emphasis in each area changes as events occur in the client's daily life.

CASE EXAMPLE

Dorothy, a 55-year-old woman, was diagnosed in 1996 with diabetic neuropathy, which is a complication of diabetes that results in loss of sensation and motor function and further compromises circulatory function. In Dorothy's case, her diabetic condition was very severe and led to multiple amputations over the next 2 years. At the

Table 5-1
UT3 Grid

I. Performance Areas

A. Activities of Daily Living
  1. Grooming
  2. Oral Hygiene
  3. Bathing/Showering
  4. Toilet Hygiene
  5. Personal Device Care
  6. Dressing
  7. Feeding and Eating
  8. Medication Routine
  9. Health Maintenance
  10. Socialization
  11. Functional Communication
  12. Functional Mobility
  13. Community Mobility
  14. Emergency Response
  15. Sexual Expression
B. Work and Productive Activities
  1. Home Management
    a. Clothing Care
    b. Cleaning
    c. Meal Preparation/Cleanup
    d. Shopping
    e. Money Management
    f. Household Maintenance
    g. Safety Procedures
  2. Care of Others
  3. Educational Activities
  4. Vocational Activities
    a. Vocational Exploration
    b. Job Acquisition
    c. Work or Job Performance
    d. Retirement Planning
    e. Volunteer Participation
C. Play or Leisure Activities
  1. Play or Leisure Exploration
  2. Play or Leisure Performance

II. Performance Components

A. Sensorimotor Component
  1. Sensory
    a. Sensory Awareness
    b. Sensory Processing
      (1) Tactile
      (2) Proprioceptive
      (3) Vestibular
      (4) Visual
      (5) Auditory
      (6) Gustatory
      (7) Olfactory
    c. Perceptual Processing
      (1) Stereognosis
      (2) Kinesthesia
      (3) Pain Response
      (4) Body Scheme
      (5) Right-Left Discrimination
      (6) Form Constancy
      (7) Position in Space
      (8) Visual-Closure
      (9) Figure Ground
      (10) Depth Perception
      (11) Spatial Relations
      (12) Topographical Orientation
  2. Neuromusculoskeletal
    a. Reflex
    b. Range of Motion
    c. Muscle Tone
    d. Strength
    e. Endurance
    f. Postural Control
    g. Postural Alignment
    h. Soft Tissue Integrity
  3. Motor
    a. Gross Coordination
    b. Crossing the Midline
    c. Laterality
    d. Bilateral Integration
    e. Motor Control
    f. Praxis
    g. Fine Coordination/Dexterity
    h. Visual-Motor Control
    i. Oral-Motor Control
B. Cognitive Integration and Components
  1. Level of Arousal
  2. Orientation
  3. Recognition
  4. Attention Span
  5. Initiation of Activity
  6. Termination of Activity
  7. Memory
  8. Sequencing
  9. Categorization
  10. Concept Formation
  11. Spatial Operations
  12. Problem Solving
  13. Learning
  14. Generalization
C. Psychosocial Skills and Components
  1. Psychological
    a. Values
    b. Interests
    c. Self-Concept
  2. Social
    a. Role performance
    b. Social Conduct
    c. Interpersonal Skills
    d. Self-Expression
  3. Self-Management
    a. Coping Skills
    b. Time Management
    c. Self-Control

III. Performance Contexts

A. Temporal Aspects
  1. Chronological
  2. Developmental
  3. Life Cycle
  4. Disability Status
B. Environment
  1. Physical
  2. Social
  3. Cultural

time the home-care-based OT and OTA made their first visit to Dorothy's home in 1998, she was a quadrilateral amputee. She had bilateral above knee amputations in addition to a left below elbow and right below MCP amputation, leaving her metacarpals and thumb intact. She had received extensive rehabilitation as an in- and out-patient during the past year but was not able to continue outpatient services due to transportation difficulties.

In the course of the initial interview, it was determined that Dorothy had received a master's degree in social work and was working with Children and Family Services until she could no longer tolerate the demands of the job. She lived in a neat, well-kept, and accessible apartment and had assistance of a certified nursing assistant (CNA) who came to her home daily. She was able to meet all of her ADL needs with the assistance of the CNA and felt that any attempt to do these things independently would be too time-consuming and difficult. Her perceived needs were quite different from the therapist's, who wanted to focus on her personal care and began suggesting adaptive devices that would enable her to do some tasks without as much assistance. However, she did not have an interest in this. Her major concerns included functional communication, functional and community mobility, and emergency response. Once this was understood, the therapist developed a plan that included a program to provide needed adaptations and instruction in the use of a personal computer, which she had purchased and wanted to be able to use. She enjoyed writing and wanted to pursue development of a book about her life experiences. Functional mobility issues centered about her ability to transfer from her wheelchair to bed and back, and a program was initiated to determine the feasibility of developing independent transfer skills. She was referred to a local service that sold specialized vans that would enable her family to provide transportation and thus allow her to resume some of her previous interests and limit her homebound status. Finally, it was suggested that she enroll in a program that provided her with a direct telephone link to a 24-hour emergency rescue service.

OCCUPATIONAL PERFORMANCE AREAS

When learning about occupational performance areas, keep in mind that the activities listed in each area are not necessarily those that individuals do themselves without help from anyone. It is important to note the concept of "independence" is defined in OT as the "ability to self-determine activity performance, regardless of who actually performs the activity" (Hinojosa & Kramer, 1998, p. 252.)

The performance areas include three major categories:
A. ADLs
B. Work and productive activities
C. Play or leisure activities

ADLs include specific activities that are referred to in UT3 as self-maintenance tasks. Each are listed and defined below.

1. *Grooming*—Obtaining and using supplies; removing body hair (use of razors, tweezers, lotions, etc.); applying and removing cosmetics; washing, drying, combing, styling, and brushing hair; caring for nails (hands and feet); caring for skin, ears, and eyes; and applying deodorant.

2. *Oral Hygiene*—Obtaining and using supplies; cleaning mouth; brushing and flossing teeth or removing, cleaning, and reinserting dental orthotics and prosthetics.

3. *Bathing/Showering*—Obtaining and using supplies; soaping, rinsing, and drying body parts; maintaining bathing position; and transferring to and from bathing positions.

4. *Toilet Hygiene*—Obtaining and using supplies; clothing management; maintaining toileting position; transferring to and from toileting position; cleaning body; and caring for menstrual and continence needs (including catheters, colostomies, and suppository management).

5. *Personal Device Care*—Cleaning and maintaining personal care items, such as hearing aids, contact lenses, glasses, orthotics, prosthetics, adaptive equipment, and contraceptive and sexual devices.

6. *Dressing*—Selecting clothing and accessories appropriate to time of day, weather, and occasion; obtaining clothing from storage area; dressing and undressing in a sequential fashion; fastening and adjusting clothing and shoes; and applying and removing personal devices, prostheses, or orthoses.

7. *Feeding and Eating*—Setting up food; selecting and using appropriate utensils and tableware; bringing food or drink to mouth; cleaning face, hands, and clothing; sucking, masticating, coughing, and swallowing; and management of alternative methods of nourishment.

8. *Medication Routine*—Obtaining medication, opening and closing containers, following prescribed schedules, taking correct quantities, reporting problems and adverse effects, and administering correct quantities by using prescribed methods.

9. *Health Maintenance*—Developing and maintaining routine for illness prevention and wellness promotion, such as physical fitness, nutrition, and decreasing health risk behaviors.

10. *Socialization*—Accessing opportunities and interacting with other people in appropriate contextual and cultural ways to meet emotional and physical needs.

11. *Functional Communication*—Using equipment or systems to send and receive information, such as writing equipment, telephones, typewriters, computers, communication boards, call lights, emergency systems, Braille writers, telecommunication devices for the deaf, and augmentative communication systems.

12. *Functional Mobility*—Moving from one position or place to another, such as in-bed mobility, wheelchair mobility, transfers (wheelchair, bed, car, tub, toilet, tub/shower, chair, floor). Performing functional ambulation and transporting objects.

13. *Community Mobility*—Moving self in the community and using public transportation, such as driving or accessing buses, taxi cabs, or other public transportation systems.

14. *Emergency Response*—Recognizing sudden, unexpected hazardous situations, and initiating action to reduce the threat to health and safety.

15. *Sexual Expression*—Engaging in desired sexual and intimate activities.

Work and productive activities are purposeful activities for self-development, social contribution, and livelihood. Each are listed and defined below.

1. *Home Management*—Obtaining and maintaining personal and household possessions and environment.

   a. *Clothing Care*—Obtaining and using supplies; sorting; laundering (hand, machine, and dry clean); folding; ironing; storing; and mending.

   b. *Cleaning*—Obtaining and using supplies; picking up; putting away; vacuuming; sweeping and mopping floors; dusting; polishing; scrubbing; washing windows; cleaning mirrors; making beds; and removing trash and recyclables.

   c. *Meal Preparation and Cleanup*—Planning nutritious meals; preparing and serving food; opening and closing containers, cabinets, and drawers; using kitchen utensils and appliances; cleaning up and storing food safely.

   d. *Shopping*—Preparing shopping lists (grocery and other); selecting and purchasing items; selecting method of payment; and completing money transactions.

   e. *Money Management*—Budgeting, paying bills, and using bank systems.

   f. *Household Maintenance*—Maintaining home, yard, garden, appliances, vehicles, and household items.

   g. *Safety Procedures*—Knowing and performing preventive and emergency procedures to maintain a safe environment and to prevent injuries.

2. *Care of Others*—Providing for children, spouse, parents, pets, or others, such as giving physical care, nurturing, communicating, and using age-appropriate activities.

3. *Educational Activities*—Participating in a learning environment through school, community, or work-sponsored activities, such as exploring educational interests, attending to instruction, managing assignments, and contributing to group experiences.

4. *Vocational Activities*—Participating in work-related activities.

   a. *Vocational Exploration*—Determining aptitudes; developing interests and skills; and selecting appropriate vocational pursuits.

   b. *Job Acquisition*—Identifying and selecting work opportunities and completing application and interview processes.

   c. *Work or Job Performance*—Performing job tasks in a timely and effective manner; incorporating necessary work behaviors.

   d. *Retirement Planning*—Determining aptitudes; developing interests and skills; and selecting appropriate avocational pursuits.

   e. *Volunteer Participation*—Performing unpaid activities for the benefit of selected individuals, groups, or causes.

Play or leisure activities are listed and defined below.

1. *Play or Leisure Exploration*—Identifying interests, skills, opportunities, and appropriate play or leisure activities.

2. *Play or Leisure Performance*—Planning and participating in play or leisure activities. Maintaining a balance of play or leisure activities with work and productive activities and ADLs. Obtaining, utilizing, and maintaining equipment and supplies.

OCCUPATIONAL PERFORMANCE COMPONENTS

Imagine you are watching someone prepare a meal and you are recording the activity on a video camera. As you watch the playback, you have been asked to observe the skills and knowledge that are needed for this activity. There are many and you are not quite sure where to begin so you focus on the movements required for this activity. However, you are aware that meal preparation requires more abilities than those related to motor function, such as sequencing for following a recipe, attention to boiling water and baking bread, and perhaps emotionally coping with a burned meal. Another valuable aspect of the UT3 is the breakdown of the component skills needed to perform a particular activity. It provides one with a format for a complete activity analysis. These components are identified in UT3 as:

A. Sensorimotor components

B. Cognitive integration and cognitive components

C. Psychosocial skills and psychological components

They collectively are labeled occupational performance components. The specific terms and definitions within the components are listed below.

The sensorimotor component is the ability to receive input, process information, and produce output. These components are listed and defined below.

1. *Sensory*

   a. *Sensory Awareness*—Receiving and differentiating sensory stimuli.

   b. *Sensory Processing*—Interpreting sensory stimuli.

      (1) *Tactile*—Interpreting light touch, pressure, temperature, pain, and vibration through skin contact/receptors.

      (2) *Proprioceptive*—Interpreting stimuli originating in muscles, joints, and other internal tissues that give information about the position of one body part in relation to another.

      (3) *Vestibular*—Interpreting stimuli from the inner ear receptors regarding head position and movement.

      (4) *Visual*—Interpreting stimuli through the eyes, including peripheral vision and acuity, awareness of color and pattern.

      (5) *Auditory*—Interpreting and localizing sounds, and discriminating background sounds.

      (6) *Gustatory*—Interpreting tastes.

      (7) *Olfactory*—Interpreting odors.

   c. *Perceptual Processing*—Organizing sensory input into meaningful patterns.

      (1) *Stereognosis*—Identifying objects through proprioception, cognition, and the sense of touch.

      (2) *Kinesthesia*—Identifying the excursion and direction of joint movement.

      (3) *Pain Response*—Interpreting noxious stimuli.

      (4) *Body Scheme*—Acquiring an internal awareness of the body and the relationship of body parts to each other.

      (5) *Right-Left Discrimination*—Differentiating one side from another.

      (6) *Form Constancy*—Recognizing forms and objects as the same in various environments, positions, and sizes.

      (7) *Position in Space*—Determining the spatial relationship of figures and objects to self or other forms and objects.

      (8) *Visual-Closure*—Identifying forms or objects from incomplete presentations.

      (9) *Figure Ground*—Differentiating between foreground and background forms and objects.

      (10) *Depth Perception*—Determining the relative distance between objects, figures, or landmarks and the observer, and changes in planes of surfaces.

      (11) *Spatial Relations*—Determining the position of objects relative to each other.

      (12) *Topographical Orientation*—Determining the location of objects and settings and the route to the location.

2. *Neuromusculoskeletal*

   a. *Reflex*—Eliciting an involuntary muscle response by sensory input.

   b. *Range of Motion*—Moving body parts through an arc.

   c. *Muscle Tone*—Demonstrating a degree of tension or resistance in a muscle at rest and in response to stretch.

   d. *Strength*—Demonstrating a degree of muscle power when movement is resisted, as with objects or gravity.

   e. *Endurance*—Sustaining cardiac, pulmonary, and musculoskeletal exertion over time.

   f. *Postural Control*—Using righting and equilibrium adjustments to maintain balance during functional movements.

   g. *Postural Alignment*—Maintaining biomechanical integrity among body parts.

   h. *Soft Tissue Integrity*—Maintaining anatomical and physiological condition of interstitial tissue and skin.

3. *Motor*

   a. *Gross Coordination*—Using large muscle groups for controlled, goal-directed movements.

   b. *Crossing the Midline*—Moving limbs and eyes across the midsagittal plane of the body.

   c. *Laterality*—Using a preferred unilateral body part for activities requiring a high level of skill.

   d. *Bilateral Integration*—Coordinating both body sides during activity.

   e. *Motor Control*—Using the body in functional and versatile movement patterns.

   f. *Praxis*—Conceiving and planning a new motor act in response to an environmental demand.

g. *Fine Coordination/Dexterity*—Using small muscle groups for controlled movements, particularly in object manipulation.

h. *Visual-Motor Integration*—Coordinating the interaction of information from the eyes with body movement during activity.

i. *Oral-Motor Control*—Coordinating oropharyngeal musculature for controlled movements.

Cognitive integration and cognitive components concern the ability to use higher brain functions. They are listed and defined below.

1. *Level of Arousal*—Demonstrating alertness and responsiveness to environmental stimuli.
2. *Orientation*—Identifying person, place, time, and situation.
3. *Recognition*—Identifying familiar faces, objects, and other previously presented materials.
4. *Attention Span*—Focusing on a task over time.
5. *Initiation of Activity*—Starting a physical or mental activity.
6. *Termination of Activity*—Stopping an activity at an appropriate time.
7. *Memory*—Recalling information after brief or long periods of time.
8. *Sequencing*—Placing information, concepts, and actions in order.
9. *Categorization*—Identifying similarities of and differences among pieces of environmental information.
10. *Concept Formation*—Organizing a variety of information to form thoughts and ideas.
11. *Spatial Operations*—Mentally manipulating the position of objects in various relationships.
12. *Problem-Solving*—Recognizing a problem, defining a problem, identifying alternative plans, selecting a plan, organizing steps in a plan, implementing a plan, and evaluating the outcome.
13. *Learning*—Acquiring new concepts and behaviors.
14. *Generalization*—Applying previously learned concepts and behaviors to a variety of new situations.

Psychosocial skills and psychological components concern the ability to interact in society and to process emotions. They are listed and defined below.

1. *Psychological*
   a. *Values*—Identifying ideas or beliefs that are important to self and others.
   b. *Interests*—Identifying mental or physical activities that create pleasure and maintain attention.
   c. *Self-Concept*—Developing the value of the physical, emotional, and sexual self.

2. *Social*
   a. *Role Performance*—Identifying, maintaining, and balancing functions one assumes or acquires in society (e.g., worker, student, parent, friend, religious participant).
   b. *Social Conduct*—Interacting by using manners, personal space, eye contact, gestures, active listening, and self-expression appropriate to one's environment.
   c. *Self-Expression*—Using a variety of styles and skills to express thoughts, feelings, and needs.

3. *Self-Management*
   a. *Coping Skills*—Identifying and managing stress and related factors.
   b. *Time Management*—Planning and participating in a balance of self-care, work, leisure, and rest activities to promote satisfaction and health.
   c. *Self-Control*—Modifying one's own behavior in response to environmental needs, demands, constraints, personal aspirations, and feedback from others.

In Dorothy's situation, performance component areas were identified that she needed to develop to enable her to pursue the performance areas that she felt were most important. The two areas that would require the most direct intervention were functional communication and functional mobility. For functional communication goals, the motor components needed to enable her to use a computer included development of physical endurance, postural control and alignment, motor control, and visual-motor integration. The cognitive components required to learn computer use include attention span, problem-solving, learning new concepts, and sequencing. Because Dorothy was focused on developing a book about her life experiences, the ability to clearly express her thoughts and feelings and share those were central to her success.

In terms of functional mobility, her desire to be less dependent for transfers from her wheelchair to her bed required a plan that incorporated an analysis of neuromusculoskeletal abilities and requirements including ROM, strength, endurance, postural control, and postural alignment. For each component, a further analysis was conducted to determine the particular mobility, strength, etc., needed to perform the transfers.

The nature of Dorothy's disability would easily lead to the assumption by others, as the team did initially, that she needed to first develop basic self-care skills. Additional concerns would be raised about lack of self-concept, coping skills, role performance, and self-control. Yet, these were her strengths. She knew her physical limitations and had worked through her loss. She had been active in her efforts to "reclaim" her occupational roles and she now knew what her priorities were.

Occupational Performance Contexts

In the study of disabling conditions, OT students learn about the occupational performance areas and components that are commonly affected by a particular condition. When the OT and OTA work together to develop a therapeutic plan that is appropriate for a client, decisions about what is appropriate and meaningful for this person begin with an understanding of the condition and the common problems associated with that condition. From here, a treatment protocol is developed. Superimposed on this protocol is the consideration of the context in which this person will perform occupational roles and tasks. This is referred to as performance contexts.

Performance contexts are defined in the *Uniform Terminology for OT* as "situations or factors that influence an individual's engagement in desired and/or required performance areas" (AOTA, 1994, p. 1047). There are two major categories of performance context. The first category is referred to as the temporal aspects, which are related to the chronological, developmental, and life cycle phases and disability status of the individual. Consider the impact of a C-6 spinal cord injury for a person who is 25 years old. The developmental maturation of this person, the phase of his or her life, and the acuteness of the injury are uniquely different for this person than they are for a 78-year-old person who experiences the same traumatic event. Even if two people are the same age, a condition has a unique impact depending on the developmental status and life phase of each person. The developmental tasks expected for each person are clearly different. Therefore, their treatment needs are unique.

The second category of performance context is environmental aspects. This includes physical, social, and cultural factors that impact on occupational performance. Physical context includes accessibility to and interaction with the objects within a particular environment. A person may be able to access his or her home safely and perform necessary occupations, however, it is necessary to determine if he or she is able to do what is needed beyond the context of home. How different is his or her ability to perform similar tasks when in church, synagogue, school, the mall, or theater? Considering the variation in physical environment and the challenges that each subsequently pose is necessary to ensure reclamation of occupational performance.

In addition to the challenges that the physical environment poses, social context has a significant impact on occupational performance. Consider the ways in which your family, friends, teachers, and other significant people influenced you in the establishment of your values, customs, roles, and routines. One grows dependent on the availability of these individuals, especially when stressful events occur. The success of the OT intervention process is dependent, in large part, on understanding the social matrix that exists for the client and enabling effective interaction with these resources.

The third aspect of environmental considerations is the cultural context. This includes customs, beliefs, activity patterns, behavior standards, and expectations of the society in which the person lives (AOTA, 1994). It is essential that the cultural mores of an individual be considered and respected. So often the routines of OT programs are based on standards for white, middle class people. Recognizing that there are many variations to how people perform occupation among different cultures is essential to effective intervention. For example, it is expected in some cultures that a large group of family members keep continuous vigil at a patient's bedside when ill. Rather than see this behavior as an interruption to the routine of caregivers, it would be necessary to adapt the routine to facilitate the return to health.

Cultural context can also be viewed in terms of society as a whole. The policies of a state or a nation result in laws that affect access to resources and either affirm or deny personal rights such as health care, education, employment, and economics. These policies are based on beliefs, values, customs, expectations, and behavior standards that a particular society holds for its members. A chasm often exists between OT beliefs and values and the reality of health care economics. Clearly, this has an effect on the ability to provide individual clients with ideal OT intervention. Nevertheless, it behooves the OT profession to continually monitor the impact of service delivery in the larger context of political policy and legislation.

In summary, the integration of contextual considerations with specific occupational performance areas and components affected by a particular condition culminates in the holistic view that occupational therapists strive to achieve in practice. The word "context" comes from the Latin word "contexere," which means "to weave together" and suggests a holistic view of the "whole situation, background, or environment relevant to some happening or personality" (*Webster's New World Dictionary,* 1957, p. 319). In a time in which standardized treatments are felt to be effective for economic productivity, practitioners are confronted with the challenge of infusing the temporal and physical aspects of context in the therapeutic event.

Summary

The UT3 is more than a list of terms; it is a basis of explaining what it is OT concerns itself with. It helps to define the "domains" of the profession in a consistent, clearly descriptive approach. It is a dynamic system as the terms will change as theory in OT changes to develop new ways of thinking about "occupation" and as research continues to provide the practitioner with new ways of applying theory.

EDITOR'S NOTE

With a practice as exciting and always changing as OT, readers will have to update their knowledge when Uniform Terminology, 4th edition is available. Plans are to have the new document reflective of terminology contained in the second version of the International Classification of Impairments, Disabilities, and Handicaps code (ICIDH-2).

REFERENCES

AOTA. (1979). *OT output reporting system and uniform terminology system for reporting OT services.* Bethesda, MD: Author.

AOTA. (1994). Uniform terminology for occupational therapy (3rd ed.). *Am J Occup Ther, 48,* 1047-1054.

Dohli, C., & Leibold, M. (1998). Uniform terminology and its application to OT evaluation. In J. Hinojosa & P. Kramer (Eds.), *Evaluation: Obtaining and interpreting data.* Bethesda, MD: AOTA.

Hinojosa, J., & Kramer, P. (1998). Appendix B: Uniform terminology for OT. In J. Hinojosa & P. Kramer (Eds.), *Evaluation: Obtaining and interpreting data.* Bethesda, MD: AOTA.

Webster's new world dictionary. (1957). Cleveland, OH: World Publishing Co.

Activity Analysis: Our Tool

Chapter 6

Sally E. Ryan, COTA, ROH, Retired

Karen Sladyk, PhD, OTR/L, FAOTA

INTRODUCTION

The meanings of activity, purposeful activity, and occupation are currently debated by OT educators and scholars. However, the role of activity analysis remains extremely important in OT. This process involves the "breaking down" of an activity into detailed subparts and steps, which is a necessary foundation for all activities of daily living, play/leisure, and work tasks used in intervention. Activity analysis is an examination of the therapeutic characteristics and value of activities that fulfill the patient's many needs, interests, abilities, roles, and occupations. Without such analysis, it may be impossible to use the proper application of activity or to obtain the best treatment results to meet the patient's occupation needs. Skill in activity analysis is critical to determine the validity of the use of activities in OT assessment and treatment.

The type of activity analysis used will be determined, at least in part, by the individual therapist's or assistant's frame of reference (Crepeau, 1998). Such analysis will also be influenced by the use of particular techniques and variations in the use of equipment. While there is no universally accepted method of activity analysis, it is useful to consider the general categories of Uniform Terminology: sensorimotor, cognitive, and psychosocial (AOTA, 1994). Other considerations should include factors such as the supplies and equipment needed, cost, the number of steps required for completion, time involved, supervision required, space needed, precautions, and contraindications. It is also helpful to think of functional requirements of the activity and then analyze them in terms of gradability. Functional requirements may be defined as components of an activity that require motor performance and behaviors for adequate completion. Gradability refers to a process whereby performance of an activity is viewed step by step on a continuum from simple to complex or slow to rapid (Holm, Rogers, & James, 1998).

The activity analysis yields the kind of data needed for determining therapeutic potential of a particular activity in relation to established patient goals, interests, and needs. Therapeutic potential is the degree of likelihood that therapeutic goals will be

KEY CONCEPT

- Activity analysis: Study of a task's subparts and process.

ESSENTIAL VOCABULARY

Adaptation: Modifying a task to make it easier for a person to complete.

Grading: Viewing an activity on a continuum from simple to complex, typically grading an activity more challenging as a person has gained skill.

Therapeutic potential: The degree of likelihood that a therapeutic goal can be achieved.

achieved. As specific techniques and equipment vary considerably for many activities, so will the results of an activity analysis. Once an activity is thoroughly analyzed, it can be adapted for therapeutic purposes.

HISTORICAL PERSPECTIVES

The profession of OT was founded on the notion that being engaged in activities promotes mental and physical well-being and, conversely, that the absence of activity leads to dysfunction (AOTA, 1980). Through their activities, human beings show their concern with how to survive, be comfortable, have pleasure, solve problems, express themselves, and relate to others. They come to know their strengths and they fulfill their roles in life. Thus the term occupation, as used in OT, is in the context of the individual's directed use of time, energy, interest, and attention (AOTA, 1980).

Activities being the foundation of the profession, historical definitions and other accounts place a strong emphasis on occupations or purposeful activities.

When William Tuke established the York Retreat in England in the late 1800s, employment in various occupations was a cornerstone of treatment in this facility for mental patients. Review of historical accounts of Tuke's work show that he had spent some time analyzing activities. For example, activities and occupations were selected to elicit emotions that were opposite of the condition; a melancholy patient would be given activities that had elements of excitement and were active, whereas a manic patient would be engaged in tasks of a sedentary nature. The habit of attention was a key element in using activities for treatment (Tuke, 1913).

Among the early pioneers of our profession, history records the work of Susan Tracy in relation to the process of analyzing activity. Tracy's work with mentally ill patients led her to believe that remedial activities "...are classified according to their physiological effects as stimulants, sedatives, anesthetics..." (Tracy, 1914). Over time, she analyzed the use of leather projects with patients and identified various components of a specific activity that would measure abilities in areas such as judgment, visual discrimination, spatial relationships, and making choices (Tracy, 1914). In 1918, she published a research paper, "Twenty-Five Suggested Mental Tests Derived From Invalid Occupations" (Tracy, 1918).

Eleanor Clarke Slagle's work in developing the principles of habit training certainly reflects her knowledge of activity analysis, as she placed particular emphasis on the gradation of activities and a balance among them (Slagle, 1922). The 1918 principles, established by the founders of our profession, also address aspects of activity that imply an ability to analyze the activity's properties. Emphasis was placed on the qualities of particular activities, with crafts and work-related activities being prominent; games, music, and physical exercise were also used (Dunton, 1918).

The terms employment, labor, moral treatment, recreation, amusement, occupation, exercise, and diversion among others, have been used by different writers at various times to describe the forms of treatment used by OT personnel. The philosophy of the profession also places a strong emphasis on activities. Throughout our history, particular properties of activities were also addressed, giving strong roots to our basic belief in the activity analysis process. Activity properties are those characteristics of activities (e.g., being goal-directed, having significance to the individual, requiring involvement, gradability, adaptability, etc.) that contribute to their therapeutic potential.

Contemporary definitions of OT are summarized in the 1981 definition of the profession, developed for licensure purposes, which describes OT as the therapeutic use of self-care (ADLs), work, and play/leisure activities to maximize independent function, enhance development, prevent disability, and maintain health. It may include adaptations of the task or the environment to achieve maximum independence and to enhance the quality of one's life (AOTA, 1981). Implicit in the latter statement is the ability to analyze activities. One must indeed know the particular properties and possibilities of a variety of activities to adapt the task to help the patient attain his or her goals. A related point, emphasized by Mosey (1986), is that activities used by OT personnel include both an intrinsic and a therapeutic purpose. This point is important to consider during activity analysis. Further, the reader should understand the OT process outlined by Moyer (1999).

ACTIVITY ENGAGEMENT PRINCIPLES

OT personnel must know various types of activities. Some of the categories of activities used in evaluation and treatment are the following:

- Crafts—Beading, ceramics, gifts
- Sensory awareness—Music, dance, hiking
- Movement awareness—Dance, drama
- Fine arts—Sculpting, painting, music
- Construction—Woodworking, electronics, computers
- Games—Bingo, checkers, parachute games
- Self-care—Dressing, feeding, hygiene
- IADLs—Cooking, homemaking, community mobility
- Communication—Social activities, Internet
- Vocational—Collecting, reading
- Recreational—Sports, leisure interests
- Educational—Mathematics, writing, publishing

For activities to be considered purposeful and therapeutic, they must possess certain characteristics (Hopkins & Smith, 1983), which include the following:

- Be goal-directed.
- Have significance to the patient at some level.
- Require patient involvement at some level (mental, physical, or both).
- Be geared toward prevention of malfunction and/or maintenance or improvement of function and quality of life.
- Reflect patient involvement in life task situations (ADLs, work, and play/leisure).
- Relate to the interests of the patient.
- Be adaptable and gradable.

The selection of appropriate activities for evaluation and treatment of patients must be based on sound professional judgment that is well grounded in knowledge and skill. As activity specialists, OTs and OTAs must have strong skills in this area (Punwar, 1994). A thorough knowledge of and experience in analyzing a wide variety of activities is an essential element of this process. The *Standards for an Accredited Educational Program for the OTA* stats that analysis and adaptation of activities is a requirement for entry-level personnel (AOTA, 1998). Mosey (1986) stresses that purposeful activities cannot be designed for evaluation and intervention without analysis. Dunn (1989) states that if activities are to be the core of OT, they must be delineated, classified, and analyzed in terms of therapeutic value.

PURPOSE AND PROCESS OF ACTIVITY ANALYSIS

The purpose of activity analysis is to determine if the activity will be appropriate in meeting the treatment goals established for the patient. To analyze an activity with knowledge and skill, it is necessary to know how to perform the processes involved. It is also relevant to know the extent to which the activity fosters or impedes various types of human performance and interaction.

The patient must be receptive to the activity selected, in other words, it must be meaningful to the patient. Patients will be more motivated and participate if their interests, life tasks, and roles are considered. In addition, the patient's functional level should be considered. The individual may be interested in the activity and it may relate directly to his or her life tasks and roles, but due to performance deficits, it cannot be accomplished.

The process of analyzing an activity involves breaking it down to illustrate each step in detail that leads to the expected outcome. Consideration must be given to numerous factors that are used to achieve activity completion, as shown in examples later in this chapter.

An activity analysis can be helpful when determining the use of an activity for an evaluation or for treatment. When analyzing an activity intended for evaluative purposes, it must be broken down into separate components to determine what opportunities exist to objectively measure what is to be evaluated. For example, as Early (1993) points out, when the purpose of engagement in an activity is to measure decision-making skills, the activity selected must provide choices, as well as decision points, to allow it to be useful. She also stresses that OT personnel must know the exact responses and outcomes that might potentially occur and how they relate to the patient's ability to make decisions. An interpretation of observations of the individual's engagement in the activity (performance) would follow. When the activity is intended to be used for treatment, it again must be broken down into small units to determine which components (constituent parts) of the activity will help to achieve the treatment goals, such as to increase ROM, to improve attention span, or to decrease isolative behavior.

The environment is also important to consider during analysis of an activity. As many OTAs treat patients in their home, activity analysis in a home environment is likely to be more true and meaningful to the patient. The context section of Uniform Terminology will be more accurately analyzed in a home environment.

An accurate analysis of an activity allows OT personnel to select activities that will address the needs and goals of the patient therapeutically. This process also aids in determining the therapeutic potential of specific activities and their purposeful use. The absence of a thorough activity analysis is likely to prevent achievement of the best treatment results.

DEVELOPING SKILLS

Skill in activity analysis is critical to determine the validity of the use of activities in OT intervention programs. Prerequisite to achieving skill is the ability to understand the basic components of the activity, that is, the fundamental processes, tools, and materials required for task completion. Self-analysis of a simple, frequently engaged in activity, such as bathing, is useful as an initial step. Asking questions, such as the following, is recommended.

- Why is the activity important to a person?
- What supplies and equipment are needed?
- What is the step-by-step procedure needed to complete this task?
- What other factors should be considered?

Once these questions have been answered, look at the information critically to determine if precise information was recorded. Recheck to be sure that no important factors were omitted. Ask a family member or peer to also answer these questions. In comparing results, differences in answers emphasize the uniqueness of the individual. Other questions can then be considered, such as how to adapt the activity for persons with various disabilities.

Experience in engaging in a wide variety of activities is also important in building skill, as it allows the OTA to make comparisons and formulate potential applications based on several possibilities. Practice in using several forms of activity analysis and receiving objective feedback is also way to develop skill. Once skill is achieved, the OTA can more easily select the most appropriate activity, which is of interest to the patient, relates to his or her life tasks and roles, is within the individual's functional capacity to perform, and provides opportunities for goal achievement (Trombly & Scott, 1995). Goal achievement is the accomplishment of tasks and objectives that one has set out to do.

RELATED CONSIDERATIONS

Frame of Reference

OT personnel use many approaches to analyze activities. The type of activity analysis is determined, at least in part, by the individual therapist's or assistant's frame of reference. For example, if a developmental frame of reference is used, activities are analyzed to determine the extent to which they might contribute to the age-specific development and related areas of occupational performance. If gratification of oral needs was a goal of treatment, it would be important to analyze the activity in teens for opportunities for eating, sucking, blowing, and encouraging independence, among other factors (Mosey, 1986).

Activity analysis is also influenced by the use of particular techniques and variations in the use of equipment recommended, such as in sensory integration and in the theoretical approaches of Rood, Bobath, or Brunnstrom. Additional information on theoretical frameworks and approaches may be found in Chapter 7.

Adaptation

To adapt an activity means to modify it (Early, 1993). It involves changing the components that are required to complete the task. Adaptations are made to allow the patient to experience success in task accomplishment at his or her level of functioning. For example, an individual who has had a stroke, resulting in paralysis of one side of the body, will need to use a holding device such as a lacing "pony" or a vice to stabilize a leather-lacing project. A change in positioning of the project, due to loss of peripheral vision and neglect of the involved side, is another important adaptation. Although few adaptations

are required in this example, all of the components of the specific activity must be considered for potential changes to increase their therapeutic potential.

Grading

Grading of an activity refers to the process of performance being viewed step by step on a continuum that progresses from simple to complex. For example, a patient might begin by lacing two precut layers of leather together, using large prepunched holes and a simple whip stitch, to make a comb case. Once this is satisfactorily completed, additional challenges, such as the following, could be introduced over several treatment sessions:

- Use of saddle stitching, followed by single cordovan and double cordovan lacing, on other short-term leather projects.
- Use of simple stamping, followed by tooling and carving to decorate the project.
- Application of basic finishes, or more advanced techniques, such as antiquing and dyeing with several colors.

Activities may also be graded according to rate of time, varying from slow to rapid (e.g., a musician who wants to increase finger speed after hand surgery). An important concept is that the grading of activities builds on what has already been accomplished in progressive stages.

FORMS AND EXAMPLES

Although no universally accepted method of activity analysis exists, the following outline, checklist, and examples are provided to assist the reader in understanding the many diverse and complex factors inherent in the process of activity analysis. Study and use of these materials provides the OTA with opportunities to gain new skills or improve existing ones. Although every effort has been made to make these examples as complete as possible, other relevant aspects could undoubtedly be included. Some of the examples are formatted in such a way that they could be filled out and used as protocols for an OT clinic, thus ensuring that all personnel had information about a particular activity and its potential therapeutic uses. Those with limited experience in activity analysis should focus first on the general outline shown in Figure 6-1. From time to time, unfamiliar terminology may be introduced. Definitions may be found by consulting a dictionary or reviewing Uniform Terminology (AOTA, 1994).

An example of the narrative format of activity analysis shown in Figure 6-1 is presented in Figure 6-2. (Note: Each of the Uniform Terminology sections could easily be expanded with further justification of the practitioner's clinical thinking. The reader may want to further expand the format presented in the following figures.)

Name of activity:	Sensorimotor components: Use Uniform Terminology to consider sensory awareness, processing, neuromusculoskeletal, and motor issues.
Number of individuals involved:	Cognitive components: Use Uniform Terminology to consider integrative and cognitive skills.
Supplies and equipment: List all materials needed.	Psychosocial components: Use Uniform Terminology to consider psychosocial and psychological skills.
Procedure: List all steps required.	ADL performance areas: How can this activity assist in ADLs?
Cost: List costs and source for all materials. Separate consumable from nonconsumable.	Work/productive performance areas: How can this activity assist in this area?
Preparation: List any processes needed to be complete before session.	Leisure/play performance areas: How can this activity assist in leisure/play?
Time: List time needed for each step in procedure, include setup and cleanup.	Adaptation: List the ways in which this activity can be made easier.
Space needs or setting required: List space requirements including setting.	Grading: List the ways in which this activity can be made more challenging.
Activity qualities: To whom is this activity likely meaningful?	Disabilities: List the disabilities for which this activity could be recommended.
Occupation: What occupational roles would use this activity?	Goal: Write a primary goal that involves this activity.
Supervision: List supervision requirements and degree.	Temporal aspects: Describe how chronological, developmental, life cycle, and disability status influence this activity.
Precautions: List safety issues.	Environmental aspects: Describe how physical, social, and cultural status influence this activity.
Contraindications: List issues that indicate a person should not do this activity because it would be harmful.	Other issues:

Figure 6-1. General outline to structure an activity analysis in a narrative format. (Adapted from AOTA. (1994). *Uniform terminology in OT* [3rd. ed.]. Bethesda, MD: Author.)

Name of activity: Volleyball.

Number of individuals involved: 8 to 15.

Supplies and equipment: Volleyball, net, poles, score pad, and pen. Optional: Refreshments and prizes.

Procedure: Stand in designated space. Reach (shoulder flexed, elbow extended, forearm supinated, wrist in neutral, fingers flexed) to hit the ball over the net when it approaches you. Move side to side and front to back within your designated space to hit the ball. Rotate to the space on your right after score is made. Optional: Start a new game after the established score is reached.

Cost: None if equipment is available; otherwise about $60 (see *Supplies and equipment*).

Preparation: 5 to 10 minutes to obtain equipment and set up.

Time: 1 hour, 5 minutes—5 minutes to set up equipment, 5 minutes to instruct group (process, rules, scoring), 45 minutes for actual activity participation, and 10 minutes to clean up, pack, and store equipment.

Space needs or setting required: Outdoor area or large room free of obstacles and furnishings.

Activity qualities: Teens and young adults may find this meaningful. High potential for noise due to excitement and competitive behavior.

Figure 6-2. An example of a narrative format activity analysis.

Occupation: Leisure interests such as exerciser. Social interests such as peer supporter.

Supervision: Direct to ensure proper follow-through and safety.

Precautions: Participants with low tolerance may need frequent breaks; participants with short attention span or memory deficits may need frequent cueing. Aggressive players may need limit setting. Thoroughly instruct in proper serving and other motions required to reduce potential for injury.

Contraindications: Avoid use with individuals with serious cardiopulmonary and respiratory problems. Not appropriate for the very young or those having pronounced perceptual and motor deficits.

Sensorimotor components: Sensory awareness required. Sensory processing including tactile, proprioceptive, vestibular, visual, and auditory. Perceptual processing needed includes kinesthesia, pain response, body scheme, right-left discrimination, position in space, figure ground, depth perception, and spatial relations. Neuromuscular needs include reflex, range of motion, muscle tone, strength, and endurance. In addition, postural control and alignment are needed. Motor needs are gross, crossing the midline, laterality, bilateral integration, praxis, and visual-motor integration.

Cognitive components: Attention span, initiation, termination, memory for rules, sequencing, problem solving, and learning (if new to game).

Psychosocial components: Interests, self-concept, role performance, social contact, interpersonal skills, self-expression, coping skills, and self-control are needed.

ADL performance areas: Gross motor skills of volleyball can be helpful in dressing and functional mobility.

Work/productive performance areas: If teen, volleyball may be helpful in physical education classes in school. If adult, volleyball has rules and structure helpful to adults working in gross motor jobs such as assembly line work of large items.

Leisure/play performance areas: Volleyball is an activity that can be continued as a leisure pursuit in most communities through local recreation programs.

Adaptation: Potential for adaptation or modification is very good. May use a foam ball, balloon, punching balloon, or a beach ball. May be played while seated. Instead of a net, two people can hold up a piece of crepe paper. Playing for points and rotations may be omitted (also see *Grading*). Use more people on one or both teams to reduce the area covered. Decrease emphasis on time; allow game to proceed as tolerated; add breaks.

Grading: Decrease time allocated and encourage increased participation. Decrease the number of people on the floor at any given time. Have players add wrist weights to hands or ankles.

Disabilities: People with gross motor issues that can tolerate resistive weight from hitting the ball. Teens with sensory integrative issues or conduct disorders. Adults with mental health issues such as schizophrenia or depression.

Goal: Within one OT treatment session, the patient will raise her hands over her head and hit a balloon 50% of the time the balloon is sent to her from the opposite team.

Temporal aspects: Volleyball is typically a game played by teens and young adults; however, the game can be adapted for chronological, developmental, life cycle, and disability status issues.

Environmental aspects: Volleyball is typically played outdoors or in a large gym area. The game can be adapted to smaller rooms with chairs and balloons. The social aspects can be increased by having players call out names or socialize at each step of the game. Cultural aspects would have to be addressed on an individual basis as some cultures may not encourage people playing games.

Other issues: Prizes may be awarded for best serve, most points scored by a single person, good sportsmanship, etc.

Figure 6-2 continued. An example of a narrative format activity analysis.

ACTIVITY ANALYSIS CHECKLIST

The Activity Analysis Checklist, shown in Figure 6-3, is a faster method of determining the particular components of an activity, as it requires less writing than the narrative general activity analysis outline (see Figure 6-1). The Activity Analysis Checklist has an area to justify your thinking in a comment area. Students using the form for assignments may find it helpful to scan the form into a computer for future assignments. Figure 6-4 shows the same form used to analyze the specific activity of brushing teeth.

SUMMARY

Activities are universal and historically have remained a primary foundation for the profession. Activity analysis is a deeply rooted concept, which has withstood the test of time and continues to be an important cornerstone for accurate assessment and effective intervention by OT personnel. The basic concepts and processes have been described to provide a fundamental understanding of the knowledge base and skills necessary for activities analysis. These skills include activity engagement principles, methods for developing skills, and concepts of grading and adapting activities. Forms and examples of the analysis of specific activities were also presented.

Emphasis was placed on the need for the activity analysis process and the information that may be gained through exploration of activity properties and possibilities. Skill in activity analysis is essential to determine the validity of the activities used for assessment and treatment. A thorough and accurate activity analysis allows the practitioner to select the most appropriate activity, which is of interest to the patient, relates to his or her life tasks and roles, and provides opportunities for goal achievement.

REFERENCES

AOTA. (1980). *Reference manual of official documents of the AOTA*. Rockville, MD: Author.

AOTA. (1981). Resolution Q: Definition of OT for licensure. Minutes of the 1981 AOTA Representative Assembly. *Am J Occup Ther, 35*, 798-799.

AOTA. (1994). Uniform terminology in OT (3rd ed.). *Am J Occup Ther, 48*, 1047-1054.

AOTA. (1998). *Standards for an accredited educational program for the OTA*. Bethesda, MD: Author.

Crepeau, E. B. (1998). Activity analysis: A way of thinking about occupational performance. In M. E. Neistadt & E. B. Crepeau (Eds.), *Willard & Spackman's OT*. Philadelphia, PA: Lippincott.

Dunn, W. (1989). Application of uniform terminology in practice. *Am J Occup Ther, 43*, 817-831.

Dunton, W. R. (1918). The principles of OT. In *Proceedings of the National Society for the Promotion of OT, second annual meeting*. Catonsville, MD: Spring Grove State Hospital Press.

Early, M. B. (1993). *Mental health concepts and techniques for the OTA*. New York, NY: Raven Press.

Holm, M. B., Rogers, J. C., & James, A. B. (1998). Treatment of occupational performance areas. In M. E. Neistadt & E. B. Crepeau (Eds.), *Willard & Spackman's OT*. Philadelphia, PA: Lippincott.

Hopkins, H. D., & Smith, H. L. (Eds.). (1983). *Willard & Spackman's OT* (6th ed.). Philadelphia, PA: Lippincott.

Mosey, A. C. (1986). *Psychosocial components of OT*. New York, NY: Raven Press.

Moyer, P. (1999). *Guide to OT practice*. Bethesda, MD: AOTA.

Punwar, A. J. (1994). *OT principles and practice*. Baltimore, MD: Williams & Wilkins.

Slagle, E. C. (1922). Training aides for mental patients. *Archives of OT, 1*, 13-14.

Tracy, S. E. (1914). The place of invalid occupations in the general hospital. *Modern Hospital, 2*(5), 386.

Tracy, S. E. (1918). Twenty-five suggested mental tests derived from invalid occupations. *Maryland Psychiatric Quarterly, 8*, 15-16.

Trombly, C., & Scott, A. D. (1995). *OT for physical dysfunction*. Baltimore, MD: Williams & Wilkins.

Tuke, S. (1913). *A description of the retreat: An institution near York for insane persons of the Society of Friends*. London, England: Dawson of Pall Mall.

Name of activity:					
Check the appropriate box:					
Uniform Terminology (AOTA, 1994)	*None*	*Minimal*	*Moderate*	*Maximal*	*Clinical Thinking Comment*
Sensory Awareness					
Tactile					
Proprioceptive					
Vestibular					
Visual					
Auditory					
Gustatory					
Olfactory					
Stereognosis					
Kinesthesia					
Pain Response					
Right-Left Discrimination					
Form Constancy					
Position in Space					
Topographical Orientation					
Reflex					
Range of Motion					
Muscle Tone					
Strength					
Endurance					
Postural Control					
Postural Alignment					
Soft Tissue Integrity					
Gross Coordination					
Crossing the Midline					
Laterality					
Bilateral Integration					
Motor Control					
Praxis					
Fine Coordination/Dexterity					
Visual-Motor Integration					
Oral-Motor Control					
Level of Arousal					
Orientation					
Recognition					
Attention Span					
Initiation of Activity					
Termination of Activity					
Memory					
Sequencing					
Categorization					
Concept Formation					
Spatial Operations					

Figure 6-3. A checklist outline to structure an activity analysis.

Uniform Terminology (AOTA, 1994)	None	Minimal	Moderate	Maximal	Clinical Thinking Comment
Problem-Solving					
Learning					
Generalization					
Values					
Interests					
Self-Concept					
Role Performance					
Social Conduct					
Interpersonal Skills					
Self-Expression					
Coping Skills					
Time Management					
Self-Control					
Chronological Context					
Developmental Context					
Life Cycle Context					
Disability Status Context					
Physical Context					
Social Context					
Cultural Context					
Grooming					
Oral Hygiene					
Bathing/Showering					
Toilet Hygiene					
Personal Device Care					
Dressing					
Feeding and Eating					
Medication Routine					
Health Maintenance					
Socialization					
Functional Communication					
Functional Mobility					
Community Mobility					
Emergency Response					
Sexual Expression					
Home Management					
Care of Others					
Educational Activities					
Vocational Activities					
Play/Leisure Exploration					
Play/Leisure Performance					

NARRATIVE INFORMATION OF ACTIVITY:

Figure 6-3 continued. A checklist outline to structure an activity analysis.

Name of activity: **Brushing teeth**
Check the appropriate box:

Uniform Terminology (AOTA, 1994)	None	Minimal	Moderate	Maximal	Clinical Thinking Comment
Sensory Awareness			X		Receive/be aware of sensory info
Tactile			X		Feel toothbrush in hand
Proprioceptive			X		Be aware of movement
Vestibular		X			Less impact unless dizzy
Visual			X		See toothbrush, water, sink
Auditory	X				Less impact to hear water
Gustatory			X		Taste of toothpaste
Olfactory	X				Less impact of smell
Stereognosis			X		Find brush not comb, razor
Kinesthesia		X			Movements of brushing
Pain Response	X				Less unless brush slips
Right-Left Discrimination	X				Not needed
Form Constancy			X		Distractions might affect
Position in Space				X	Relationship of body to sink
Topographical Orientation	X				Not needed
Reflex	X				Only if water too hot/gag
Range of Motion			X		For brushing movement
Muscle Tone			X		For brushing movement
Strength			X		For brushing movement
Endurance			X		For brushing movement
Postural Control			X		To stand or sit at sink
Postural Alignment			X		To stand/sit at sink, balance
Soft Tissue Integrity		X			Only if hand/mouth sores
Gross Coordination		X			More fine motor
Crossing the Midline				X	Get both sides of teeth
Laterality			X		Can be done one-handed
Bilateral Integration			X		Opening toothpaste
Motor Control			X		To control toothpaste
Praxis				X	To motor plan to mouth
Fine Coordination/Dexterity				X	Manage supplies, brushing
Visual-Motor Integration				X	Put paste on, brush teeth
Oral-Motor Control				X	Rinse paste
Level of Arousal				X	Must be alert
Orientation	X				Not needed
Recognition			X		Of supplies needed
Attention Span			X		At least 3 to 5 minutes
Initiation of Activity			X		To begin brushing
Termination of Activity			X		To end brushing/rinse
Memory			X		Remember all teeth
Sequencing			X		Order of steps
Categorization	X				Not needed
Concept Formation	X				Not needed
Spatial Operations	X				Not needed

Figure 6-4. A completed activity analysis using a checklist outline.

Uniform Terminology (AOTA, 1994)	None	Minimal	Moderate	Maximal	Clinical Thinking Comment
Problem-Solving			X		If drop cap/paste/brush
Learning		X			Likely learned early
Generalization		X			To other activities/eat
Values			X		All the psychosocial area
Interests			X		must include some level
Self-Concept			X		of motivation for the
Role Performance			X		person to be interested
Social Conduct			X		in engaging in task of
Interpersonal Skills			X		brushing teeth.
Self-Expression			X		
Coping Skills			X		
Time Management			X		
Self-Control			X		
Chronological Context					This activity is usually
Developmental Context					done by a parent until
Life Cycle Context					independent in skill.
Disability Status Context					Brushing teeth typically
Physical Context					valued by most people.
Social Context					
Cultural Context					
Grooming				X	Importance of grooming
Oral Hygiene				X	Brush teeth
Bathing/Showering				X	Importance of grooming
Toilet Hygiene	X				Not needed
Personal Device Care				X	Denture care, braces
Dressing	X				Not needed
Feeding and Eating				X	Similar skills to brushing
Medication Routine	X				Not needed
Health Maintenance				X	Prevent tooth decay
Socialization				X	Fresh breath
Functional Communication				X	Others will participate
Functional Mobility	X				Not needed
Community Mobility	X				Not needed
Emergency Response	X				Not needed
Sexual Expression				X	Others will have interest
Home Management	X				Not needed
Care of Others				X	Brush children's teeth
Educational Activities			X		Others will participate
Vocational Activities			X		Others will participate
Play/Leisure Exploration	X				Not needed
Play/Leisure Performance	X				Not needed

Figure 6-4 continued. A completed activity analysis using a checklist outline.

NARRATIVE INFORMATION OF ACTIVITY:

Supplies: Toothpaste, toothbrush, water, sink.

Procedure: Open toothpaste, squeeze paste, close toothpaste, turn on water, brush all teeth, rinse mouth, rinse brush/sink, turn off water. Generally, the task can be completed in 5 minutes and for under $5, not including sink. This activity is likely meaningful to most people and often a prerequisite to many occupational roles such as spouse, worker, peer.

Precautions: Skin may be burned with hot water, child may gag on brush, paste may be too minty hot for sensitive mouth.

Contraindications: Severe oral problems.

Adaptation for ease: Limited distractions, use of mirror, verbal cueing, adaptive equipment.

Gradation for challenge: Can include finding supplies in medicine cabinet, making choices on supplies, using weights on wrists.

Figure 6-4 continued. A completed activity analysis using a checklist outline.

Frames of Reference and Models in Practice

Chapter 7

Diane K. Dirette, PhD, OTR

The terms explored in this chapter include theory, frame of reference, and model. A simplified definition of a theory is a description of a set of phenomena and the relationships among the concepts in those phenomena (Mosey, 1996). A *frame of reference* is a guideline for practice that provides direction for evaluation and treatment of particular deficits in the OT domain of concern. A frame of reference is not written to address a particular diagnosis such as spinal cord injury, but is designed to address deficits that may occur in a variety of diagnoses. Frames of reference link theoretical concepts to treatment.

INTRODUCTION

The parts of a frame of reference include the theoretical base, the function/dysfunction continua, the behaviors and signs indicative of function/dysfunction, and the postulates regarding change (Mosey, 1996). The theoretical base is the concepts drawn from various theories that support the use of the guidelines. The function/dysfunction continua are the deficits addressed by the frame of reference. The behaviors and signs indicative of function/dysfunction guide the therapist in the evaluation phase of the intervention. The postulates regarding change guide the intervention used to ameliorate the deficits.

Theories are used as the foundation for developing frames of reference. The theoretical foundation of OT comes from the biological sciences (e.g., anatomy and physiology), psychology, sociology, and medicine. For example, the biomechanical frame of reference, discussed later in this chapter, is based on anatomy, physiology, and kinesiology.

The term *model* is used in different ways in the OT literature. Some authors use the term interchangeably with the term frame of reference (Katz, 1998; Tufano, 1999). Other authors use the term model to mean overarching concepts that guide the general approach to clinical practice (Christiansen & Baum, 1997; Kielhofner, 1997). Mosey (1996) concluded that it is not a necessary and is a sometimes confusing term in an applied profession. For the purposes of this chapter, the term model is used as defined by the authors who present their work in the format of models or overarching concepts. These authors do not

KEY CONCEPTS

- Theory: A set of phenomena and relationships.
- Frame of reference: Guideline of practice based on theory.
- Model: Theoretical concepts used to guide practice in a specific arena.

ESSENTIAL
VOCABULARY

Function/dysfunction: How a frame of reference views wellness and non-wellness.

Postulates of change: how change occurs within a frame of reference.

Theoretical base: The theory that supports a frame of reference.

present specific guidelines for evaluation and treatment as done in frames of reference.

THE USE OF FRAMES OF REFERENCE IN OCCUPATIONAL THERAPY

The following discussion of frames of reference is separated into different practice areas. However, many individuals with whom the OT practitioner works will have deficits in many areas. For example, a person with a cerebrovascular accident may have deficits in physical function, which lead the therapist to use the rehabilitation or neurodevelopmental treatment frame of reference. That same person may have deficits in social role functioning which would lead the therapist to also use the role acquisition frame of reference. If the theoretical concepts of the frame of reference are not in conflict with one another, the frames of reference may be used in combination for a thorough treatment plan to address the deficits faced by the person.

If the theoretical concepts are not compatible, the therapist would not be using these frames of reference in treatment with the person. For example, the theoretical base of the psychoanalytical frame of reference focuses on exploring underlying issues that lead to behaviors. The behavior modification frame of reference is based on the concepts of addressing only outward behaviors without the need for exploration of underlying processes. Therefore, these frames of reference would not be used when treating one individual.

FRAMES OF REFERENCE FOR PHYSICAL FUNCTION

Biomechanical

Originated by Bolderin, Taylor, and Licht. Adapted from Dutton (1995).

Theoretical Basis

Anatomy, physiology, and kinesiology.

Assumptions

1. Purposeful activity can be prescribed to remediate loss of range of motion (ROM), strength, and endurance.
2. If ROM, strength, and endurance are regained, the person will automatically use these prerequisite skills to regain functional skills.
3. The body must be rested, then stressed.
4. The person must have an intact brain that can produce isolated, coordinated movements.

Function/Dysfunction Continua

1. Structural stability, endurance, edema, ROM, and strength.

Behaviors Indicative of Function/Dysfunction

1. Structural stability (measured by observation of positioning and control).
2. Passive ROM (PROM) and active ROM (AROM) (measured by observation and goniometry).
3. Muscle strength (measured by manual muscle testing).
4. Peripheral edema (measured by observation, volumetery, and circumfrential measures).
5. Endurance (measured by observation of the duration and/or intensity of activities performed).

Postulates Regarding Change

1. If the therapist uses orthoses and positioning, structural damage will be prevented.
2. If the therapist uses orthoses, positioning, and rest followed by stress, structural stability will be regained.
3. If the therapist prescribes increased duration and/or intensity of activities, then endurance will be gained.
4. If the therapist uses elevation, pressure, temperature control, and ROM, then peripheral edema will be reduced.
5. If the therapist uses PROM, active assisted ROM (AAROM), AROM, scar prevention, orthoses, and positioning, then PROM will be maintained.
6. If the therapist uses heat, scar remodeling, passive stretch, active stretch, orthoses, positioning, and activities, then ROM will be increased.
7. If the therapist uses AROM and activities, then strength will be maintained.
8. If the therapist uses isometric, active assistive, active, and progressive or regressive resistive exercises, then strength will be increased.

Neurodevelopmental Treatment

Originated by Berta and Karl Bobath. Adapted from Dutton (1995).

Theoretical Basis

Neurology and developmental theories.

Assumptions

1. It is important to remediate foundation skills that make normal skill acquisition possible.

2. Normal movement is learned by experiencing what normal movement feels like.

3. Postural control is essential for limb movement.

4. Normal movement cannot be imposed on abnormal muscle tone.

5. The brain has plasticity.

Function/Dysfunction Continua

1. Axial control (control of neck and trunk).

2. Automatic reactions (righting reactions, equilibrium reactions, protective limb extensions).

3. Limb control with specific focus on the scapula and pelvic mobility and stability.

Behaviors Indicative of Function/Dysfunction

1. Reflex development (evaluated through observation).

2. Automatic reactions (evaluated using observation of the quality of movement).

3. Synergies (evaluated using clinical observation of positioning and movement patterns).

4. Muscle tone (evaluated using manual and visual observation of resistance to passive and active movements).

Postulates Regarding Change

1. If the therapist uses passive elongation, reflex inhibiting patterns, positioning, and weight shifts, then hypertonia can be inhibited.

2. If the therapist uses joint compression, joint traction, manual resistance, and weight shifts, then increased tone for hypotonia can be facilitated.

3. If the therapist uses passive elongation, active weight shifts, passive pelvic tilts, and active axial rotation, then axial control can be facilitated.

4. If the therapist uses reflex inhibiting patterns and desired combinations of movement patterns, then automatic reactions can be facilitated.

5. If the therapist uses dissociation of synergy patterns, reflex inhibiting patterns, limb weight shifts, place and hold, and postures and movements with rotational and reciprocal limb movements, then limb control can be facilitated.

Rehabilitation

Originated by Dunton. Adapted from Dutton (1995).

Theoretical Basis

Systems theories and learning theories.

Assumptions

1. A person can regain independence using compensation when underlying deficits cannot be remediated.

2. Motivation for independence cannot be separated from volitional and habitual subsystems.

3. Motivation for independence cannot be separated from environmental contexts.

4. A minimum level of emotional and cognitive prerequisite skill must be present to make independence possible.

5. Clinical reasoning should take a top-down approach. Focus should first be on environmental demands and resources. Then, volitional and habitual subsystems should be considered followed by functional capabilities and then prerequisite skills/deficits.

Function/Dysfunction Continua

1. This frame of reference addresses activities of daily living, work, and leisure activities.

Behaviors Indicative of Function/Dysfunction

1. Ability to safely perform activities of daily living in a timely manner.

2. Ability to safely perform home management tasks in a timely manner.

3. Work behaviors, work tolerance, general work traits, and/or specific work skills.

4. Ability to participate in meaningful leisure activities.

5. Clinical observations and interviews are used to evaluate these performance areas.

Postulates Regarding Change

1. If the therapist uses adaptive devices, orthotics, environmental modifications, wheelchair modifications, ambulatory aids, adapted procedures, and/or safety education, then independence in ADLs, home management, work, and leisure will be maximized.

Proprioceptive Neuromuscular Facilitation

Originated by Kabat. Adapted from Voss, Ionta, and Myers (1985).

Theoretical Basis

Neurophysiology, anatomy, and kinesiology.

Assumptions

1. Normal movement and posture are dependent upon a balanced interaction of antagonists.

2. The growth of motor behavior has cyclic trends as evidenced by shifts between flexor and extensor dominance.

3. Early motor behavior is dominated by reflex activity. Mature motor behavior is reinforced or supported by postural reflex mechanisms.

4. Normal motor development proceeds in a cephalo-caudal and proximo-distal direction.

5. Developing motor behavior is expressed in an orderly sequence of total patterns of movement and posture.

6. Normal motor behavior has an orderly quality with overlapping occurring.

7. Improvement of motor ability is dependent on motor learning.

Function/Dysfunction Continua

1. This frame of reference addresses movement patterns and postures.

Behaviors Indicative of Function/Dysfunction

1. Smooth, controlled functional movement patterns of the head, neck, trunk, and extremities.

Postulates Regarding Change

1. If the therapist prevents or corrects imbalances between antagonists, then normal movement and posture are possible.

2. If the therapist assists the person through reversing movements, then there is interaction of the antagonists.

3. If the therapist uses reflex support, then voluntary movements are reinforced.

4. If the therapist has the person perform movement patterns in diagonal and spiral as well as forward, backward, sideward, and circular directions, then total patterns of movement and posture are achieved.

5. If the therapist uses appropriate sensory cues and demands, then learning of motor acts is enhanced.

FRAMES OF REFERENCE FOR PSYCHOSOCIAL FUNCTION

Role Acquisition

Originated by Anne C. Mosey. Adapted from Mosey (1986).

Theoretical Basis

Sociology, psychology, and behavioral learning theories.

Assumptions

1. The individual has an inherent need to explore the environment.

2. What an individual must learn (roles) is specified by the society and cultural group in which he or she lives.

3. Learning basic skills, social roles, and temporal adaptation includes a socialization process and a learning process.

4. In the typical developmental process, the individual interacts in an environment where he or she is relatively free to explore and to acquire interests, goals, and competencies. Atypical development occurs when the environment is not conducive to learning, either in the past or at the present time.

5. Emphasis should be placed on purposeful activities, including both individual and group activities.

Function/Dysfunction Continua

1. The areas of concern can be viewed as hierarchical in nature, with task skills and interpersonal skills forming the base; family interactions, activities of daily living, school/work, and play/leisure/recreation forming the middle; and temporal adaptation making up the top portion of the pyramid.

Behaviors Indicative of Function/Dysfunction

1. Adequate participation in the physical, cognitive, and psychological aspects of tasks. Evaluation of task skills is usually accomplished through data gathered from a general interview and the Survey of Task Skills.

2. Initiation and participation in interpersonal interactions. Evaluation of interpersonal skills is typically accomplished through use of an interview, an evaluation group, and the Interpersonal Skill Survey.

3. Adequate family interactions including the child role, the adolescent role, the parent role, and general family interactions. Evaluation tools include observation and general interview.

4. Participation in activities of daily living. Evaluation includes observation and the Activities of Daily Living Survey.

5. Adequate participation in school or work roles. Evaluation is accomplished through interview, observation, and the School Survey or Work Survey.

6. Appropriate play/leisure/recreation participation. Evaluation includes interview, observation, and the Leisure/Recreation Survey.

7. Temporal adaptation for adequate participation in activities of daily living and roles. Evaluation is accomplished through a general interview and the Activity Configuration.

Postulates Regarding Change

1. Long-term goals are set based on the client's expected environment.
2. The sequence of the change process is generally task skills, interpersonal skills, social roles beginning with activities of daily living and temporal adaptation.
3. The sequence, however, need not be rigidly adhered to and is often best determined by the client.
4. Task and interpersonal skills can be taught separately initially or they can be taught within the context of the learning of social roles.
5. An adequate repertoire of behavior is acquired through selected application of the principles of learning during activities that a) elicit the relevant behavior, b) are interesting to the client and allow for exploration and movement toward mastery, and c) include socialization.
6. Emphasis is on designing activities that will change the behavior and thus alleviate the problem rather than delving into intrapsychic reasons for the problem.
7. The therapist must know very specifically what kind of behavior he or she wishes to promote or enhance and can thus be accomplished through activity analysis and synthesis.

Behavioral

Adapted from Bruce and Borg (1993).

Theoretical Basis

The behavioral frame of reference is based on concepts drawn from experimental psychology, classical conditioning (Pavlov), operant conditioning (Skinner), and social learning theories (Bandura).

Assumptions

1. Behavior is predictable, measurable, and objective.
2. A person's verbalization and self-descriptions are behaviors.
3. The patient has a repertoire of behaviors (adaptive and maladaptive) that have been learned through selective reinforcement from the environment.
4. The patient's repertoire of behavior determines his or her ability to function in activities of daily living, work, and leisure.
5. Through positive and differential reinforcement and the systematic application of learning techniques, the patient can learn to modify and control his or her behavior.
6. Only behavior that is demonstrated can be reinforced.

7. New behavior may be established through the use of continuous or frequent and predictable reinforcement; however, the most stable behavior is that maintained by intermittent reinforcement.
8. If maladaptive behavior is only occasionally reinforced, it is strengthened.
9. The strength of the patient's response is influenced by bodily conditions such as those related to emotions, drives, and the use of drugs.
10. The skills for adaptive functioning in the natural environment are independent and not stage-specific.

Function/Dysfunction Continua

1. The focus of this frame of reference is on the behaviors that elicit or inhibit functioning in the areas of activities of daily living, work, and play/leisure. There is an emphasis on the stimuli that act as cues to the behavior and the reinforcers for specific behaviors.

Behaviors Indicative of Function/Dysfunction

1. Age-appropriate, culturally acceptable behaviors that contribute to or interfere with adaptive function.
2. Behaviors necessary for adequate function in the person's natural environment.
3. The frequency of specific adaptive and maladaptive behavior.
4. The ability of the person to discriminate among stimuli and to generalize learning effectively.
5. Evaluation is completed through a combination of observation and rating of task performance and interview using questionnaires or behavior checklists. Some examples of assessment tools include the Kohlman Evaluation of Living Skills (KELS), the Bay Area Functional Performance Evaluation (BaFPE), the Comprehensive Occupational Therapy Evaluation (COTE), and the Scorable Self-Care Evaluation (SSCE).

Postulates Regarding Change

1. Activities are used to teach specific skills and to provide simulated learning experiences.
2. Pleasurable activities are used as reinforcement of adaptive behaviors.
3. Maladaptive behaviors are decreased through negative reinforcement or ignoring those behaviors.
4. Activities are graded to provide progressively more difficult learning challenges to shape adaptive behaviors needed to function in the community environment.
5. Group and individual activities are used to increase the person's ability to generalize the behaviors

learned during treatment to a broad range of situations.

6. Clear, concrete goals increase the person's understanding of the focus of treatment, which in turn expedites the treatment process.

7. Some appropriate treatment tools include shaping, forward and backward chaining, scheduled reinforcement, modeling, and token economies.

Object Relations

Adapted from Mosey (1986) and Bruce and Borg (1987).

Theoretical Basis

The basis is an eclectic integration of principles from Freudian, Jungian, neo-Freudian, existential-humanistic, social, and ego psychologies.

Assumptions

1. The behaviors of man are defined in terms of a dynamic balance between needs, drives, affect, cognitive processes, and the will.

2. Through the interrelationship of these inherent elements, man relates to objects in such a way as to realize his unique potential.

3. This relationship, however, is rarely perfectly tuned, and imbalance leads to inattention to aspects of the self and the environment. Some of these aspects are unconscious and interfere with self-actualization.

4. Through the use of cognitive processes, man is able to correct the imbalance between that which is conscious and that which is unconscious, and thus continue toward self-actualization.

Function/Dysfunction Continua

1. Feelings of inferiority.
2. Differentiation from the non-human environment.
3. Trust in one's fellow man.
4. Control of sexual impulses.
5. Emotional separation from one's parents.
6. Establishing mature love relationships.
7. Finding one's place as a contributing member of a social system.
8. Selecting a guiding system of values.
9. Perception of the self as an unacceptable object.
10. Investment of aggressive energy in the self.
11. Free-floating libidinal energy.
12. Free-floating aggressive energy.
13. Threatened emergence of unconscious content.
14. Acceptance of the unacceptable aspects of the self.
15. Acceptance of the opposite sex characteristics of the self.
16. Relatedness to the non-human environment.

Behaviors Indicative of Function/Dysfunction

1. A well-established sense of self.
2. An ability to trust.
3. Appropriate communication skills.
4. Behavior that is consistent and congruent with verbalizations.
5. Ability to establish and maintain relationships.
6. Ability to identify and meet needs, including safety, physical, love, belonging, self-esteem, and self-actualization.
7. Ability to respond to change.
8. Appropriate investment and use of energy.
9. Ability to cope with the anxiety of self-discovery and change.
10. Tools for evaluation may include a general interview, activities, and the Fidler Battery.

Postulates Regarding Change

According to Bruce and Borg (1993), activities and the discussions around them are used for one or more of the following:

1. To provide an avenue for appropriate expression of feeling.
2. To provide an opportunity to improve ego function.
3. To provide a means to establish or re-establish a sense of self and control.
4. To provide a vehicle for learning new skills, improving skills, or gaining confidence in skills already held.
5. To provide an opportunity for trying out new roles or gaining confidence with already established roles.
6. To provide a vehicle for learning more about one's self and one's relationship to others.
7. To provide a means toward increased self-acceptance.
8. To facilitate movement toward flexibility in approaching life tasks.
9. The treatment process occurs in individual and group situations with persons who are reality oriented and capable of logical thinking. To facilitate a dynamic understanding of behavior and problems, the OT uses creative media or semi-structured experiences to help the patient project his [or her] thoughts, feelings, needs, fantasies,

desires, and frustrations onto the end product (activity), or [he or] she uses structured activities to assist the patient in increasing organizational and problem-solving skills."

Cognitive Behavioral

Adapted from Bruce and Borg (1993).

Theoretical Basis

Based on principles from social learning, cognitive, and behavioral theories.

Assumptions

1. The person's emotions and behavior reflect his or her cognitive function.
2. The person develops as a result of the interaction of the cognitive system, behaviors learned, and the social and physical environment.
3. The person can learn skills and strategies that he or she can use independently to face problems and find solutions.
4. When the person masters the use of his or her body and objects, he or she has a resource for problem-solving.
5. When a person learns new cognitive strategies to respond to the present, he or she is preparing to confront and solve future problems.
6. When a person changes his or her present knowledge and skill level, he or she changes his or her past knowledge and self-image.
7. The self-monitoring process can be learned.
8. Self-regulation is a balance in which present knowledge and cognitive functioning and new learning and challenges complement each other to facilitate growth, optimal function, and the quality of life.

Function/Dysfunction Continua

1. Self-knowledge.
2. Dependence and independence.
3. Self-interest and interest in others.
4. Personal views of reality and the ability to be empathetic.
5. Identity with others and an autonomous identity.
6. Ability to express and control feelings.

Behaviors Indicative of Function/Dysfunction

1. Optimum function reflects a balance of the two extremes for each of the continua and is associated with feelings of competence.
2. Self-regulation is evidenced by the person's ability to monitor relevant data that come from the self and the environment, to use these data to choose and implement new behaviors, and to practice these behaviors until they become automatic.
3. Dysfunction is usually seen when the predominant behaviors are at the extremes of the continuum or when cognitive function does not meet developmental expectations and is associated with feelings of incompetence. This may include one or more of the following behaviors:
    *   Insufficient, inflexible, or distorted self-knowledge.
    *   Reasoning that may be illogical, not coinciding with reality, or involve inferences that do not have a basis.
    *   Limited exploration of one's environment.
    *   Failure to establish an autonomous identity.
    *   Limited problem-solving skills.
4. Evaluation is viewed as an ongoing process and can include the use of observation, tests, and interviews. Some assessment instruments include the Task Check List, the Allen's Cognitive Level Test, and the Lower Cognitive Level Test.

Postulates Regarding Change

1. Treatment does not eliminate the disorder but provides cognitive, affective, and behavioral learning experiences to teach skills, strategies, and methods of coping.
2. Treatment is more effective when specific techniques and skills (activities) are learned than when only verbal methods are utilized.
3. Treatment activities can help the person to act upon the environment as well as help with self-monitoring of thoughts, feelings, and behaviors.
4. The arrangement of the learning environment influences cognitive function and can facilitate cognitive development and stimulate problem-solving.
5. The person can benefit from a structured treatment setting that controls distractions and provides repeated opportunities for skill practice and problem-solving.
6. The complexity of tasks can be modified to promote successful learning.
7. The therapeutic tasks used should consider the person's cognitive knowledge, level of function, and interests.
8. Tasks with a high probability of success can stimulate cognitive development.
9. Therapy should stress the highest degree of self-regulation, not the highest cognitive developmental level.

PEDIATRIC-FOCUSED FRAMES OF REFERENCE

Several of the physical dysfunction and psychosocial frames of reference listed previously are used in pediatric practice. The following was developed for use with pediatrics, but is also used in some settings for treatment of adults.

Sensory Integration

Originated by Ayres. Adapted from Kimball (1999).

Theoretical Basis

Neuroscience and developmental theories.

Assumptions

1. The central nervous system is hierarchically organized. Cortical processing relies on adequate organization of inputs supplied by the lower brain centers.
2. Meaningful registration of stimuli must occur before the central nervous system can make a response to in and, therefore, allow for higher functioning to occur.
3. The brain is innately organized to program a person to seek out stimulation that is organizing or beneficial in itself.
4. Input from one sensory system can facilitate or inhibit the state of the entire organism. Input from each system influences every other system and the whole organism.
5. There is plasticity within the central nervous system.
6. Normal human development occurs sequentially.

Function/Dysfunction Continua

1. Sensory modulation.
2. Functional support capabilities.
3. End-product abilities.

Behaviors Indicative of Function/Dysfunction

1. Indicators of function in the sensory system modulation are noted by normal responses in the following areas: tactile system, auditory system, relationship to gravity, movement level, oral arousal, olfactory arousal, visual system, attention level, post-rotary nystagmus, sensitivity to movement, proprioceptive sensitivity, and emotional arousal. Under- or over-registration, as noted by the level of response, would be indicators of dysfunction.
2. Indicators of function in the functional support capabilities would include normal responses in the following areas: suck-swallow-breathe, tactile discrimination, sensory discrimination, movement level, oral discrimination, olfactory discrimination, visual discrimination, proprioceptive discrimination, attention level, emotional discrimination, cocontraction, muscle tone, balance and equilibrium, developmental reflexes, lateralization, and bilateral integration. Dysfunction would be noted by poorly developed capabilities in the areas listed above.
3. Indicators of function in the end-product abilities would include adequate praxis, form and space perception, behavior, academics, language and articulation, emotional tone, activity level, and environmental mastery. Dysfunction would be noted by poorly developed skills in the areas listed above.
4. Evaluation is completed using clinical observations, parent and teacher and child interviews, and several assessment tools including one or more of the following: the Sensory Integration and Praxis Test, Touch Inventory for Elementary School-Aged Children, Tactile Defensiveness Checklist, Sensory Profile, and the Bruininks-Oseretsky Test of Motor Proficiency.

Postulates Regarding Change

1. If intervention involves several sensory systems and requires intersensory integration, then it will be more powerful and more likely to bring about an adaptive response.
2. If the therapist provides a situation in which the child can act on his or her environment, then the child will be more likely to produce adaptive responses. The child's self-initiated actions also use the more efficient feed-forward neurological mechanisms that build motor patterns rather than only the neurologically less efficient feedback.
3. If the child moves his or her own body volitionally during therapy rather than being moved by someone else, then effective motor patterns are more likely to develop.
4. If the therapist provides a situation that requires an adaptive response that is developmentally appropriate, then the adaptive response is more likely to occur and more likely to promote growth.
5. If the activity presented to the child is challenging yet achievable, then it will facilitate an improved adaptive response.
6. If the therapist provides the child with a sense of emotional safety, then the child will be more likely to actively engage in the therapy process.
7. If the therapist provides the child with constant feedback during the therapy session, then the child

will gain a greater understanding of what he or she is doing and what he or she has done.

8. If the therapist provides activities that involve controlled change and variety, then the child is more likely to make an adaptive response rather than develop a learned behavior.

9. There are also specific postulates regarding change that address each of the three levels of continua. They are not listed here. The postulates address function/dysfunction continua using the above guidelines. They are considered to be hierarchical. This means each of the levels should be addressed in order. For example, if there are deficits in sensory system modulation, they should be addressed before addressing functional support capabilities.

COGNITIVE/PERCEPTUAL FRAMES OF REFERENCE

Cognitive Rehabilitation

Developed by OTs at Loewenstein Rehabilitation Hospital. Adapted from Averbuch and Katz (1998).

Theoretical Basis

Neuropsychological and cognitive theories (developmental and information processing).

Assumptions

1. Each brain region is involved in various functions and interacts with other regions in completing a specific task.

2. Every normal act is a result of a dynamic balance between all brain structures.

3. Higher mental processes in the human cortex constantly change during child development and are influenced by the environment (learning and training process).

4. The functional system as a whole can be disturbed by a lesion in one area.

5. It can be disturbed differently by lesions in different localizations.

6. The normal intellect involves processing information from the environment, the memory, and the feedback received after an action.

7. The normal individual actively seeks and assimilates information in relation to his or her ability to understand and then remember it.

8. Perception, thinking, and memory are constantly interacting.

9. Impaired intellectual processes can be improved through cognitive retaining.

Function/Dysfunction Continua

1. This frame of reference addresses cognition (the acquisition, organization, and use of knowledge), perception, visual-motor organization, thinking operations (executive functions), memory, attention, and concentration.

Behaviors Indicative of Function/Dysfunction

1. Basic cognitive task performance in the various cognitive subcomponents.

2. Comparison of current cognitive performance to premorbid information.

3. Sensorimotor function.

4. Functional performance of daily activities.

5. Assessment of cognition may be completed using various cognitive batteries, including the Loewenstein Occupational Therapy Cognitive Assessment, the Rivermead Behavioral Memory Test, the Behavioral Inattention Test, and/or the Neurobehavioral Cognitive Status Examination.

Postulates Regarding Change

1. In the first phase, component specific (perception, visuomotor organization, thinking operation, and memory) training is completed using specific tools in a "laboratory environment."

2. In this environment, the therapist instructs the person to complete tasks that are at the level of the person's capabilities for that specific component.

3. The level of difficulty for each task is increased when the person masters the task.

4. The person is trained to develop specific strategies for each specific component.

5. Once the person has internalized the given cognitive strategies and can manipulate them on different tasks, the person is trained to adjust and adapt them to activities of real life.

Dynamic Interactional

Originated by Toglia. Adapted from Toglia (1998).

Theoretical Basis

Concepts are drawn from neuropsychology and learning theories.

Assumptions

1. Cognition is the individual's capacity to acquire and use information in order to adapt to environmental demands. Cognitive abilities are not conceptualized as specific components, but as the underlying strategies and potential for all learning.

2. Cognitive function, the ability to receive, elaborate, and monitor incoming information, is influenced by the dynamic interaction between the individual (strategies, metacognition, the learner characteristics), the task, and the environment.

3. Cognitive abilities are modifiable and vary with the characteristics of the task, the environment, and the individual.

Function/Dysfunction Continua

1. Processing strategies.
2. Metacognition.
3. Learning capabilities.
4. Transfer of learning to varied tasks and environments.

Behaviors Indicative of Function/Dysfunction

1. The ability to select and use efficient processing strategies to organize and structure incoming information.

2. The ability to anticipate, monitor, and verify the accuracy of performance.

3. The ability to link new information with previous experience.

4. Flexible application of knowledge and skills to a variety of situations.

5. Assessment methods include the use of the Dynamic Interactional Assessment, which includes awareness questioning, response to cueing and task grading, and strategy investigation; the Dynamic Visual Processing Assessment; and the Toglia Category Assessment.

Postulates Regarding Change

1. Task and environmental variables are systematically changed to enhance the person's ability to process, monitor, and use information across new tasks and situations.

2. The person is taught to use processing strategies for varied tasks.

3. The processing strategies are practiced in a variety of different situations to increase the person's understanding of the conditions in which the strategies are useful.

4. Strategies such as self-prediction, role reversal, self-questioning, self-evaluation, structured error monitoring systems, and videotape feedback are used to increase metacognitive function.

5. When the person has internalized the ability to estimate and self-monitor performance, he or she is moved from a cued to an uncued condition.

6. Motivation and individual personality characteristics are considered when selecting treatment activities.

7. Individual treatments need to be combined with group treatments to reinforce self-monitoring or task strategies.

Neurofunctional Approach

Developed by Giles, Clark-Wilson, and Yuen. Adapted from Giles (1998).

Theoretical Basis

Neuroscience and learning theories.

Assumptions

1. Deficits in memory, attention, processing, and frontal lobe functions interfere with a person's ability to perform daily functional skills.

2. The person's cognitive abilities and learning characteristics impact the manner in which daily functional skills can be retrained.

3. Damage to the cerebral cortex often results in deficits in adaptive behavior and the ability to reacquire adaptive patterns of behavior.

4. The extent and location of injury to the cerebral cortex places constraints on human learning, but the ability to acquire new behaviors is retained in all but the most profoundly impaired persons.

Function/Dysfunction Continua

1. This frame of reference focuses on performance areas, including activities of daily living, work and productive activities, and play or leisure activities.

Behaviors Indicative of Function/Dysfunction

1. Function is defined as adequate completion of performance areas in a naturalistic environment in which cues are not provided and demands are not specifically manipulated.

2. Assessment methods include observation, standardized assessments, questionnaires, checklists, and rating scales. If the person is not able to perform tasks in a naturalistic environment, structure and cues are provided to obtain baseline information. If, despite careful observation, the origin of some functional skills deficits remain unclear, the OT may use standardized testing to attempt to elicit the true cause of the problem and develop an adequate treatment plan.

Postulates Regarding Change

1. Practice of functional skills leads to modification of the person's previous responses and replaces them with new and more adaptive ones.

2. New metacognitive control strategies can be formed through the development of a new and

more accurate model of basic cognitive functioning.

3. Cognitive overlearning is used to focus the person's attention on the behavior or area of skills deficit and to develop a verbal label for the behavior.

4. Learning of functional skills is increased through reinforcements, task analysis (to determine the steps of the activity that need cueing), chaining, prompts, practice, shaping, antecedents, and overlearning (practicing a skill well beyond the point where the person is able to produce the behavior).

5. When the focus of therapy is on the person being able to set and pursue his or her own goals, the person can learn about his or her own cognitive abilities and develop effective metacognitive control strategies.

MODELS USED IN OCCUPATIONAL THERAPY

Client-Centered Models

Originated by Law, Christiansen, and Baum. Adapted from Tufano (1999).

Two models for practice in OT that focus on the client as the center of treatment include the Canadian Model of Occupational Performance (CMOP) and the Person-Environment Occupational (PEO) performance model. The CMOP is an open system based model that focuses on the interaction of the environment, occupational roles, and the person. The environment includes social, cultural, institutional, and physical components. Occupation includes self-care, leisure, and productivity. The person is viewed holistically and not just as the components of the disability.

The PEO performance model is also an open system based-model that focuses on activities of daily living, motivation, and the personal characteristics that influence the person's ability to manage the environment. Performance is the result of complex relationships between the person and the environment, and occupation facilitates adaptation. Stages of development influence motivation, skills, and roles.

According to both of these models, the client should be the focus of treatment. The client identifies meaningful occupations that are then used by the therapist to promote health. Occupation is addressed from an intrinsic and environmental perspective.

Model of Human Occupation

Originated by Reilly and Kielhofner. Adapted from Tufano (1999).

The Model of Human Occupation (MOHO) is based on general systems theory, existential/humanism, ego psychology, cognitive theory, sociology, and biology (Kielhofner, 1997). Man is viewed as an open system with input, throughput (comprised of volitional, habitual, and performance subsystems), output, and feedback. Information enters the human system as input, is processed as throughput, and results in output from the person. Occupation is viewed as behavior that is internally gratifying and used to fulfill a variety of culturally and socially accepted roles. Occupation is subject to feedback from the environment and is instrumental to one's self-development.

The focus of treatment from this model is on the promotion of health through a balance of self-care, work, and play activities. The person's use of objects and tasks, participation in social organizations, and cultural influence should all be considered when selecting occupations. Goals should be mutually set by the therapist and the client to restore age-appropriate occupations and improve role functioning.

Occupational Science

Originated by Yerxa. Adapted from Tufano (1999).

Occupational science is based on biological and social sciences, the humanities and open systems theory. Human beings are viewed as complex multilevel systems who participate in their environment. Illness, disease, or other life experiences limit the person's ability to adapt to the environment and participate in occupation. Emphasis is placed on the human as a holistic being and not as the parts of the human.

The focus of treatment from this model is on the use of meaningful occupations to enable humans to achieve competency and a sense of efficacy. The therapist needs to be aware of each person's unique qualities in language, culture, experience, and spiritual meaning.

REFERENCES

Averbuch, S., & Katz, N. (1998). Cognitive rehabilitation: A retraining model for clients following brain injuries. In N. Katz (Ed.), *Cognition and occupation in rehabilitation: Cognitive models for intervention in OT.* Bethesda, MD: AOTA.

Bruce, M. A., & Borg, B. (1987). *Frames of reference in psychosocial OT.* Thorofare, NJ: SLACK Incorporated.

Bruce, M. A., & Borg, B. (1993). *Psychosocial OT: Frames of reference for intervention* (2nd ed.). Thorofare, NJ: SLACK Incorporated.

Christiansen, C., & Baum, C. (1997). *OT: Enabling function and well-being* (2nd ed.). Thorofare, NJ: SLACK Incorporated.

Dutton, R. (1995). *Clinical reasoning in physical disabilities.* Baltimore, MD: Williams & Wilkins.

Giles, G. M. (1998). A neurofunctional approach to rehabilitation following severe brain injury. In N. Katz (Ed.), *Cognition and occupation in rehabilitation: Cognitive models for intervention in OT.* Bethesda, MD: AOTA.

Katz, N. (1998). *Cognition and occupation in rehabilitation: Cognitive models for intervention in OT.* Bethesda, MD: AOTA.

Kielhofner, G. (1997). *Conceptual foundations of OT.* Philadelphia, PA: F. A. Davis.

Kimball, J. G. (1999). Sensory integration frame of reference: Theoretical base, function/dysfunction continua and guide to evaluation. In P. Kramer & J. Hinojosa (Eds.), *Frames of reference for pediatric OT* (2nd ed.). Baltimore, MD: Lippincott, Williams & Wilkins.

Mosey, A. C. (1986). *Psychosocial components of OT.* New York, NY: Raven Press.

Mosey, A. C. (1996). *Applied scientific inquiry in the health professions: An epistemological orientation* (2nd ed.). Bethesda, MD: AOTA.

Toglia, J. P. (1998). A dynamic interactional model to cognitive rehabilitation. In N. Katz (Ed.), *Cognition and occupation in rehabilitation: Cognitive models for intervention in OT.* Bethesda, MD: AOTA.

Tufano, R. (1999). Frames of reference in OT. In K. Sladyk (Ed.), *OT Study Cards in a Box.* Thorofare, NJ: SLACK Incorporated.

Voss, D. E., Ionta, M. K., & Myers, B. J. (1985). *Proprioceptive neuromuscular facilitation: Patterns and techniques* (3rd ed.). Philadelphia, PA: Harper & Row.

Therapeutic Intervention Process

Chapter 8

Sally E. Ryan, COTA, ROH, Retired

INTRODUCTION

The profession of OT has developed a specific plan for therapeutic intervention known as the OT process (AOTA, 1994c; Moyers, 1999). It is made up of five distinct procedural categories that should be carried out in a particular order. (Exceptions are noted in the discussion of each category.) Service management is considered a sixth category. These sections are as follows:

1. Referral
2. Evaluation, including screening and assessment (AOTA, 1994a)
3. Treatment planning
4. Treatment implementation (including periodic re-evaluation)
5. Program discontinuation (including discharge planning and follow-up)
6. Service management

The AOTA has established general standards of practice for OT service programs and OT practitioners providing direct service. These standards were developed as guidelines to assist members of the profession. They have been reprinted in Appendix B because they detail important aspects of the OT process in which the OTA serves an important role. In recent times, more specific standards of practice have been adopted in the areas of physical disabilities, developmental disabilities, mental health, home health, and school settings, and other areas. These are published in the *Reference Manual of the Official Documents of the AOTA*, which is available from the products division of AOTA. Further detail of occupational practice can be found in AOTA's *Guide to OT Practice* by Moyers (1999).

REFERRAL

Requests for OT services may come from many sources, including physicians, physical therapists, teachers, social workers, and other health professionals, as well as parents and patients themselves. Referrals may be initiated and/or received by the OT either before or after the patient's initial screening. All referrals must be documented in writing and become a part of each patient's permanent record. The OTA may initiate patient referrals in

ESSENTIAL VOCABULARY

Activity analysis: Study of a task's subparts and process.

Performance areas: Uniform terminology sections of ADL, work, and play/leisure that are occupation based.

Performance components: Uniform terminology sections related to sensorimotor, cognitive, and psychosocial aspects of occupation that support the performance areas.

Performance contexts: Uniform terminology sections that describe the factors that influence the performance areas such as temporal and environmental concerns.

KEY CONCEPTS

- Referral: Request for occupational therapy services.
- Evaluation: Screening and assessment of an occupational therapy consumer.
- Intervention planning: Identifying problems, goals, and treatments.
- Treatment implementation: Putting the treatment plan in action and re-evaluating as needed.
- Program discontinuation: Ending services when goals are reached or consumer is unable to make further progress.
- Service management: Process of delivery of the therapeutic intervention.

the area of ADLs. When an OTA receives a referral, whether initiated or not, it must be given to the supervising OT who is ultimately responsible for any action taken regarding the referral (AOTA, 1994c).

The AOTA does not require that a referral be received before services can be provided. When there is no referral, the OT must assume all responsibility for the delivery of services. In some instances, state laws or the requirements established by health care facilities mandate the receipt of a referral. For example, the Commission on Accreditation of Rehabilitation Facilities (CARP), the Joint Commission on Accreditation of Healthcare Organizations (JCAHO), and Medicare regulations require that a physician's referral must be obtained if OT services are to be provided (Punwar, 2000). Figure 8-1 shows an example of a referral form used in a major hospital.

EVALUATION

The process of evaluation includes both screening and assessment (AOTA, 1994a) and must take place before individual program planning. Evaluation is used to describe the process of collecting and interpreting data. Assessment refers to specific tools (AOTA, 1994a). A thorough assessment provides a comprehensive "picture" of the patient based on a complete analysis of all of the screening and evaluation data. It is a predictor of the need for OT or other services and the estimated duration of treatment.

SCREENING

Screening of individuals who may benefit from OT services can be carried out by various health care providers. For example, a physical therapist may believe that a young man has stress management problems that are contributing to his diminished physical condition. A recreational therapist may note that a child has difficulty maintaining balance when participating in some play activities. Both of these individuals would be advised to seek an OT screening to determine the extent to which evaluation and treatment might alleviate or mediate the presenting problem.

The process of screening patients is necessary to determine whether a patient needs OT services. Screening involves the collection and analysis of specific data and facts. Information is obtained by observing the patient while he or she is performing tasks or engaging in social interactions; through interviews with the patient and family or significant others, such as a roommate or a close friend; or through a review of the patient's general history from sources that may include the medical chart, a psychologist's report, or a teacher's appraisal. The OTA collaborates with the supervising OT in the screening

process by collecting and reporting selected information as requested. For example, he or she may use a structured interview form to gather information about the patient's educational background, employment history, hobbies, and ADL skills. If the OT's analysis of the screening information indicates that OT treatment would be beneficial, a comprehensive evaluation is performed.

ASSESSMENT

The purpose of evaluation is to determine the patient's current level of functional performance and to identify performance deficits. The OT is responsible for all aspects of the assessment; however, the OTA may carry out some evaluative tasks under supervision. These tasks may include administering an interest checklist or an activity configuration and summarizing the information in a written report. In addition, the OTA can observe the patient in a specific situation and report on interpersonal skills, coordination, strength, and endurance as they relate to ADL skills and tasks.

The profession of OT is concerned with function and uses specific procedures and activities to:
- Develop, maintain, improve, and/or restore the performance of necessary functions
- Compensate for dysfunction
- Minimize or prevent debilitation
- Promote health and wellness (Punwar, 2000)

The occupational performance areas, performance components, and performance contexts delineated in the document *Uniform Terminology for OT* (3rd ed.) (AOTA, 1994d), provide the framework for a comprehensive evaluation. Examples are as follows:

Performance Areas

1. ADLs—Grooming, dressing, feeding and eating, socialization, functional communication, sexual expression
2. Work activities—Home management, care of others, educational and vocational activities
3. Play or leisure activities—Exploration and performance

Performance Components

1. Sensorimotor components—Sensory awareness, muscle tone, reflexes, perception, position in space, proprioception
2. Cognitive integration and cognitive components—Level of arousal, orientation, recognition, attention span, memory
3. Psychosocial skills and psychological components—Coping skills, self-expression, values, self-management

Patient _____   Date Referral Received _____
          Last   First   M. Initial

Address _____   Zip_____
Medicare # _____   Medicare # _____
Contact Person _____   Physician _____
Phone # _____   Phone # _____
Relationship:_____

Primary Diagnosis: _____
Date of Onset: _____
Secondary Diagnosis:_____
Restrictions and Precautions: ❏ None   ❏ Specify: _____
Medical Prognosis: ❏ Excellent   ❏ Good   ❏ Fair   ❏ Poor   ❏ Guarded
❏ Patient   ❏ Family   is aware of Diagnosis and Prognosis

Physician's Plan of Treatment

❏ Physical Therapy: ❏ Evaluation and Treatment   ❏ Other_____
Specify Rx/Modalities: _____
Rehabilitation Goals: _____
Frequency: _____   Duration: _____ Wk/Mos   Equipment: ❏ Yes   ❏ No

❏ Occupational Therapy: ❏ Evaluation and Treatment   ❏ Other_____
Specify Rx/Modalities: _____
Rehabilitation Goals: _____
Frequency: _____   Duration: _____ Wk/Mos   Equipment: ❏ Yes   ❏ No

❏ Speech Pathology: ❏ Evaluation and Treatment   ❏ Other_____
Specify Rx/Modalities: _____
Rehabilitation Goals: _____
Frequency: _____   Duration: _____ Wk/Mos   Equipment: ❏ Yes   ❏ No

❏ Social Work: ❏ Evaluation and Treatment   ❏ Other_____
Rehabilitation Goals: _____

Physician Certification: I ❏ certify   ❏ recertify that the above Skilled Rehabilitation Services are required and authorized by me.

Physician's Signature _____   Date _____

Figure 8-1. Outpatient, referral, and treatment care plan. Adapted from Irene Walter Johnson Rehabilitation Institute, St. Louis, MO. (Reprinted from Ryan, S. E. [1993]. *Practice issues in OT: Intraprofessional team building.* Thorofare, NJ: SLACK Incorporated.)

Evaluation is necessary to determine the patient's strengths and weaknesses, needs, and the degree of change possible through OT intervention. OTs and OTAs use a variety of specific evaluations. Many are discussed in the individual case studies presented in Section II and the techniques of practice described in Section III.

The OT analyzes and interprets screening and evaluation data to determine the total assessment results. Recommendations for continuance or dismissal from OT are made. Services other than OT that may assist the patient are identified and referral may be made.

Information obtained through a comprehensive evaluation also assists OT practitioners in determining the activities that will be most beneficial in assisting the patient in performance deficit areas.

TREATMENT PLANNING

Treatment planning involves identifying the patient's problems and selecting goals that are reasonable to achieve and developing the methods to achieve them (Early, 1994). Hopkins and Tiffany (1981) stressed the need to use a problem-solving process in setting treatment objectives and carrying them out. This process is summarized as follows:

1. Problem identification
2. Solution development
3. Development of a plan of action
4. Implementation of the plan
5. Assessment of results

In the treatment planning process, both long- and short-term objectives and time lines are established. Specific activities related to the patient's occupations are analyzed, selected, and sequenced to assist the patient in meeting the goals. Specific frames of reference, methods, and approaches are also determined, and adaptations are planned. The patient's goals, values, cultural identification, stage of biological and mental development, and interests and abilities are all carefully considered as an integral part of the process. The active involvement of the patient, as well as family members and significant others, in all phases of treatment planning is important and influences the overall effectiveness of the plan. Motivation and cooperation often increase when the patient has a thorough understanding of the treatment process and feels that he or she has had an integral part in the planning.

Failure to include the patient in planning may result in ineffective or unnecessary intervention strategies. For example, if the patient is a woman who has had a stroke needs to perform ADL tasks with one hand, it is often a common practice in OT to include goals related to meal preparation. This may be stereotypical planning in some cases, as evidenced by the report of one OTA. The woman was placed in a cooking group and later told the

OTA that her husband did all of the cooking and related tasks and she "never set foot in the kitchen nor did she plan to!" Another area where stereotypical planning might occur is housework. Setting goals related to tasks such as cleaning and doing the laundry would be inappropriate for a person who always hires outside help to do them and has the necessary financial resources to continue to do so. These brief examples illustrate the importance of including the patient in the treatment planning process. Outcomes of intervention must relate to the needs and priorities of the individual.

A strong background in a variety of different activities, together with knowledge and skill in activity analysis, is a critical factor in effective treatment planning. The therapeutic potential of age-appropriate activities and their various properties, components, and potential for adaptation must be related to the specific treatment goals.

The OTA contributes to many aspects of the program plan; however, the OT is responsible for the final plan that will best meet the patient's needs and objectives and is acceptable to the patient (Early, 1994).

The long-term objectives of such a plan are to develop, improve, restore, or maintain the patient's abilities that allow for a more productive and meaningful life. They may be quite broad in focus and are written to reflect the expected outcome of treatment. The short-term objectives relate to the long-term objectives and contribute to their achievement. They must be stated in achievable, measurable outcomes and be met in a short enough time span to serve as a record of improvement. Short-term objectives address more immediate, specific goals. They may be viewed as "mini-steps" that will lead to the desired result (Punwar, 2000).

Treatment planning is a critical component of the OT process. It involves setting the problem and identifying the steps necessary in solving the problem (Parham, 1987). The former is the role of the OT, and the latter is a collaborative OT and OTA process, with the OT having the ultimate responsibility.

TREATMENT IMPLEMENTATION

All OT treatment is based on the treatment plan. Treatment implementation is putting the plan into action. Effective treatment requires the patient to participate in selected purposeful activities designed to achieve the established goals. The OTA, working under close supervision, may implement a program for acutely ill individuals, such as a patient who has had a recent stroke or someone who is depressed and suicidal. Close supervision is essential because of the complex problems and degree of change frequently seen that may require a modified treatment approach or re-evaluation by the OT (AOTA, 1994b). If the patients are in a more stable, non-acute, or controlled condition, the assistant may carry out treatment procedures with greater independence, as directed by the supervising OT. The OTA may also be responsible for monitoring the patient's performance and providing a summary report. It is the OTA's responsibility to keep the supervising therapist informed of all changes in patient performance and any other pertinent facts. As treatment progresses and changes are noted, the assistant may contribute suggestions for program modifications and additions that will help the patient reach the established goals.

In the event that the patient is not making satisfactory progress, the OT will conduct a reevaluation to determine necessary changes in the program plan and the treatment procedures. Reevaluation refers to repeating certain assessments and analyzing the findings. Results may indicate that objectives have been set at too high a level or are unrealistic (Punwar, 2000). Perhaps methods, activities, and/or time frames need to be modified. Specific aspects of the re-evaluation may be delegated to the assistant. Re-evaluation also takes place before discharge to determine discontinuation and discharge planning. Comparison of re-evaluation data with that obtained in the initial evaluation provides an objective means of measuring change.

Program Discontinuation

Program discontinuation takes place when the patient has reached all of the established goals or it is determined that the patient can no longer benefit from OT services. Among other tasks, the OTA may assist in this process by providing specific information on progress or lack of progress to be included in a summary report. The OTA may also provide instructions for a home-based program, identify community resources and personnel, or recommend environmental adaptations that may assist the patient after discharge.

Although the Standards of Practice adopted by AOTA (1994c) do not specify that patient follow-up must occur, it is desirable to gather such information to determine the effectiveness of treatment, general adjustment outcomes, and the degree to which the patient is able to resume social, family, work, and leisure roles. This task could be performed collaboratively by an OT and OTA, with the OT determining the final conclusions. Follow-up also provides additional support to the patient in the transition from illness to wellness.

Service Management

Service management is a process that involves planning, structuring, developing, coordinating, documenting, and evaluating the delivery of all OT services to ensure quality, efficiency, and effectiveness. It is the organizational framework and system that supports the OT process in therapeutic intervention. Service management is essential in the delivery of OT services. Because this area has so many specific components, it will be discussed in depth later in this book. Specific information relative to documentation may be found in Chapter 38.

Summary

Therapeutic intervention follows a specific plan called the OT process. This process includes sets of tasks that should be carried out in a particular order. Referral, evaluation (including screening and assessment), treatment planning, treatment implementation (including re-evaluation), and program discontinuation (including discharge planning and follow-up) are presented. Service management is a system that allows the OT process to be carried out. The OTA may participate in all aspects of the process as directed by the supervising OT.

References

AOTA. (1994a). Clarification of the use of the terms assessment and evaluation. *Am J Occup Ther, 48,* 1072-1073.

AOTA. (1994b). Guide for supervision of OT personnel. *Am J Occup Ther, 48,* 1045-1046.

AOTA. (1994c). Standards of practice for OT. *Am J Occup Ther, 48,* 1039-1043.

AOTA. (1994d). Uniform terminology for OT (3rd ed.). *Am J Occup Ther, 48,* 1047-1054.

Early, M. B. (1994). *Mental health concepts and techniques for the OTA.* New York: Raven Press.

Hopkins, H. L., & Tiffany, K. G. (1981). OT—A problem solving process. In H. Hopkins & H. Smith (Eds.), *Willard & Spackman's OT* (77th ed.). Philadelphia, PA: Lippincott.

Moyers, P. (1999). *Guide to OT practice.* Bethesda, MD: AOTA.

Parham, D. (1987). Toward professionalism: The reflective therapist. *Am J Occup Ther, 41,* 555-561.

Punwar, A. J. (2000). *OT principles and practice.* Baltimore, MD: Williams & Wilkins.

Occupation: An Individual Choice

Chapter 9

Bonnie Brooks, MEd, OTR, FAOTA

INTRODUCTION

One of the foundations of OT theory is that humans have a need to be active and participate in various occupations. Occupation is essential for basic survival and optimal mental and physical health. Occupation is also an integral part of survival and a basic drive of every person. Within this individual frame of reference, a person's activities and occupations enable him or her to function as a central part of a larger whole. It is the difference between existing and actively participating. Participation and optimal functioning within a person's environment provide an individual with feelings of purpose and self-esteem throughout his or her life span (Moyers, 1999).

What does the word occupation mean? To those in OT, it means engaging in purposeful activity. Occupations are effective in preventing or reducing disability and in promoting independence through the acquisition of skills, as the following examples illustrate.

- The occupation of a preschool child with a disability is learning the motor skills necessary to enter school.
- The primary occupation for a young adult may be planning for a career or vocation.
- Occupation for others may be providing for financial security through employment, which may require a variety of activities.
- Occupation for an individual with serious cardiac problems may include learning to conserve energy while doing daily activities.
- An occupation for the elderly may be prolonging participation in rewarding activities and maintaining personal independence.

An occupation may require a variety of activities and skills. For example, the occupation of self-care includes the activities of bathing, shaving, dressing, and feeding, each of which requires varying degrees of skill in gross and fine motor coordination and judgment.

OT is the art and science of directing an individual's participation in selected tasks to restore, reinforce, and enhance performance. OT facilitates teaming of skills and functions essential for adaptation and productivity, for diminishing or correcting

KEY CONCEPTS

- Occupation: The roles and tasks that give meaning and purpose to one's life.
- Disruptions in occupation: Environmental, community, culture, or tradition changes.

ESSENTIAL VOCABULARY

External environment: Contexts such as climate, community, and economics.

Internal environment: Aspects such as motivation, wellness, and emotional state.

Occupational performance areas: ADLS, work, and play/leisure.

pathology, and for promoting and maintaining health. The word occupation in the professional title refers to goal-directed use of time, energy, interest, and attention. OT's fundamental concern is developing and maintaining the capacity to perform, with satisfaction to self and others, the tasks and roles essential to productive living and mastering self and the environment throughout the life span (AOTA, 1979).

Three main types of occupation are necessary for the achievement of optimal performance and quality of life: ADLs, work, and leisure. These areas are discussed in greater depth later in this book. Acquiring and maintaining skills in these areas enable a person to interact successfully with the environment. Activities and skills also enable a person to engage in a variety of occupations that result in the establishment of the individual's lifestyle.

OT provides service to those individuals whose abilities to cope with tasks of living are threatened or impaired by developmental deficits, the aging process, physical injury or illness, or psychological and social disability (Reed & Saunderson, 1999).

Intervention programs in OT are designed to enable the patient to become adequate or proficient in basic life skills, work, and leisure, and thereby competent to resume his or her place in life and interact with the environment effectively. As each patient is unique, each treatment approach must be individualized. With these goals in mind, this chapter focuses on case studies and examples of how OT intervention can be individualized in relation to the environment, society, change, and prevention.

CASE STUDIES IN OCCUPATION

The profession of OT recognizes that the level of optimal function to which a patient may aspire is highly individual and determined by all of the circumstances of the individual's life (AOTA Council on Standards, 1972). No two patients are alike, even if they are the same age and have identical problems or disabilities. Intervention programs should be individualized and focus on the uniqueness of the individual. To understand the multitude of factors that create an individual lifestyle, a description of John and Darlene follows. They will be referred to later in this chapter to illustrate various content areas.

Case Study 1

John is a 24-year-old obese man. He smoked two packs of cigarettes a day for 4 years and recently quit. He appears in good health.

Family Information

John is the oldest of three children. His sisters, aged 19 and 21, are away at college. His mother is 53 years old and in good health. His father is 57 years old and has high blood pressure. Three years ago the father experienced two severe heart attacks and was hospitalized both times. The following year the father had three minor attacks. He had generalized weakness and has been very depressed; however, he exhibited significant improvement recently.

Vocational Information

John graduated from college 2 years ago. He returned home to manage the farm because of his father's illness. The crop farm is located 25 miles outside a rural town in southern Minnesota. Employment opportunities were very limited for John in that particular region of the state, and he had just accepted a job to work as an accountant in Duluth. He plans to move there in 4 months.

Leisure and Socialization

During the winter, John watches television a great deal and plays cards. Recently, he decided to take half-hour walks twice a day to lose weight. In the summer, John plays softball on a local team, goes swimming, and meets socially with friends.

Case Study 2

Darlene is a 35-year-old woman in good health. She is slightly underweight because of constant dieting.

Family Information

Darlene is an only child. She lived in California and was married for 5 years, but divorced 2 years ago. She has no children. Her mother is 62 years old, her father is 65 years old, and both are retired. They are healthy and travel extensively, spending most of their time in Florida. Darlene currently lives in her parent's home located in a wealthy suburb of New York City.

Vocational Information

Darlene worked for a short time prior to her marriage at age 27. Before that time she took classes at a local college periodically and worked in her father's office part-time. Darlene completed a computer course 3 years ago and now works as a full-time programmer for a moderate salary. She pays no expenses while living in her parents' home; however, she does buy groceries and presents for her parents periodically. Her parents recently decided to sell their home and move to a condominium in Florida.

Leisure Information

Darlene is very active. She goes out every evening and frequently takes weekend trips. She is very fashion conscious, often attending fashion shows, and identifies shopping as a major interest. After shopping sprees, she and her friends frequently go to art galleries or the theater. Darlene belongs to a health spa, racquetball club, and country club. She enjoys golf and swimming.

John and Darlene have been introduced to provide a context to examine some of the factors that have impact on the development of their present lifestyles. These include the effect of the environment, sociocultural aspects, local customs, and economic implications. All of these factors must be considered to gain an understanding of individuals' current lifestyle, who they are, what roles they have, what they want and expect, and what they need.

ENVIRONMENTAL CONSIDERATIONS

A person's environment is comprised of all of the factors that provide input to the individual. The environment includes all conditions that influence and modify a person's lifestyle and activity level. Environmental considerations vary significantly in complexity. They can be as simple as climate, geographic location, or economic status or as complex as considering the sociocultural aspects of traditions, local customs, superstitions, values, beliefs, and habits.

Every individual has two environments that constantly provide input: internal and external. These environments are so closely integrated in an individual's life that it is often difficult to consider them separately. Both internal and external environments must be considered in designing treatment intervention that will allow a person to function at maximum capacity. This coordinated approach is the essence of total patient treatment in OT.

External Environment

The external environment is comprised of a number of factors, including climate, community, and economic status. One of the most obvious external environmental factors is the climate. Some climates are warm or cold for most of the year and offer extremes in temperatures and weather hazards during several months. Many regions experience four seasons. In general, spring and fall are periods of transition. Whereas winter and summer exhibit extremes in weather, such as floods, hurricanes, tornadoes, or blizzards. Individual responses to climates and weather conditions vary. Many people dislike the winter months and restrict their activities. It is very common for some people to gain weight during these months and then lose the added pounds when the weather permits them to resume their outdoor activities.

The Effects of Climate on John and Darlene

The impact of winter weather is greater for John than for Darlene. Darlene's work and leisure activities occur within a much smaller geographic area than those of John. Her suburban environment offers a variety of transportation options. The winter months impose more restrictions on John. This period of snow storms and icy conditions usually limits his transportation, which in turn restricts his opportunities for socialization. During severe weather, John restricts his leisure activities to watching television and playing cards, and he frequently gains weight during this period. Summer also affects John more than Darlene. Although Darlene experiences some changes, these have minimal impact on her activity level. John's farm work requires heavy labor as soon as the soil is workable, beginning with the first sign of spring and continuing well into the fall. He completely changes his leisure, recreation, and social activities, which include playing on a softball team, swimming, and meeting with friends.

External environment can affect a patient through secondary issues, such as the splinting problems seen in Case Study 3.

Case Study 3

A patient living in Georgia was required to wear a basic cock-up splint. During his monthly visits to the clinic, his splint always needed significant adjustments. It was discovered that he would frequently leave the splint on the back shelf of the car. The internal temperature of the closed car in a hot climate was excessive. The splint had been fabricated from a low temperature material, which tended to change shape in the high heat. A new splint was made from a heavier material that would withstand high temperatures, thus solving the problem.

Severe cold can also affect the selection of splinting materials. Some are made of plastic, which can become brittle and shatter on impact in extreme cold. Metal braces and splints can also be very uncomfortable in extreme temperatures. Special attention should be given to lining the splint to protect the skin that comes into contact with the device.

Community

Another important environmental consideration is the type of community in which the person lives. There are three basic types of communities: rural, urban, and suburban. Each type has different characteristics that can affect an individual's occupations, activities, and lifestyle.

The Effects of Community on John and Darlene

John is well-known in his small farming community. His neighbors know that he completed college and returned home to help his father. John knows the grocer, auto mechanic, drug store clerk, dentist, and physician personally.

Darlene shops and receives necessary services in a variety of places and therefore does not know many of these people personally. She knows the names of two women who work in her favorite boutiques. Personalized service and recognition can be status symbols if deliberately developed.

Internal Environment

One method of separating the internal and external environments is by considering the physiologic feedback provided by the various body systems. This feedback is the body's way of informing a person of his or her ability to respond to the daily requirements of the external environment. Moods and emotional states can be considered parts of an internal environment that influence the way a person responds to the external environment. Depressed persons frequently respond more slowly to their environment and may decrease social activities. Some may further restrict the environment by remaining at home. Self-image is another example of previous feedback from the external environment that creates an internal set or environment. These internal environments can exist long after the external environment has changed. Phobias are yet another example of adverse internal environments. They are defined as abnormal fears or dreads and are as illustrated in the following case.

Case Study 4

Mrs. Anderson is 45 years old, married, and the mother of two children, aged 13 and 17. Her husband's job as an industrial consultant requires periodic travel for up to 4 consecutive weeks at a time. He is generally at home one week at a time between trips.

Approximately 8 years ago, Mrs. Anderson began to decline social invitations from friends when her husband was at home. She would excuse herself for some minor or nonexistent complaint or say that their time together was so limited that they needed to be alone as a family. Eventually, she reached the stage where she encouraged her husband to attend events without her because of headaches.

Mrs. Anderson no longer liked driving the car. She complained about heavy traffic, crowded grocery stores, and rude clerks in department stores. She located a small grocery store that would deliver orders, and she began buying mail-order clothing. Cosmetics and other items were ordered through door-to-door distributors. Her family became concerned and began encouraging her to go for rides or have an occasional dinner out. Mrs. Anderson was very uncomfortable and obviously in a state of anxiety. Finally she simply refused to leave her home.

Mrs. Anderson was exhibiting symptoms of agoraphobia, a Greek term meaning fear of the marketplace, which, in current usage, refers to a fear of open or public places. In all probability, her agoraphobia had occurred as a result of previous environmental feedback; however, once the condition developed, it then became an internal environment affecting her occupation and effectiveness as a member of her family unit.

Economic Environment

The economic environment of the community and the economic status of individuals must also be considered. Values and standards vary greatly and affect OT treatment, as shown in the two case examples to follow.

Case Study 5

Susan was 16 years old when she was diagnosed as having juvenile arthritis, affecting her right hand. The rheumatologist referred her to OT to have a splint fabricated, which would block metacarpophalangeal (MCP) flexion of all four fingers. A variety of splints were presented to the patient and her family. All were visually unacceptable. The patient agreed to wear the "ugly" splint when she was at home, but adamantly refused to wear it in public. Her family supported her in this decision, even though they understood the medical benefits that could be achieved by a regular wearing schedule. The parents requested that the occupational therapist work in collaboration with their local jeweler to design something more attractive.

Working with the jeweler, the OTR designed rings for each finger, which were connected by chains to a large medallion on the back of the hand. The medallion was then connected by chains to a snug, wide bracelet. The design proved to be highly workable, although not ideal medically. The final product was made of 14-carat gold and studded with rubies and pearls. The patient wore it constantly and several of her friends requested similar jewelry. It seemed that the "splint" had become a status symbol in her social group.

Case Study 6

A diagnosis of rheumatoid arthritis had far reaching implications for Mrs. Kennedy, a 36-year-old woman employed as a bank clerk in a small community. Weight bearing had become very painful, and a total hip replacement and bilateral knee surgery had been recommended.

Several months before the diagnosis was made, persistent pain and stiffness had forced Mrs. Kennedy to give up her job in the bank, even though her salary was important to maintain the family's modest standard of living. She had allowed her health insurance coverage to lapse and was in the process of applying for coverage under her husband's policy when her condition was diagnosed. As a result, she was denied coverage.

Mrs. Kennedy was referred to OT for homemaking training and self-care activities before surgery. The evaluation revealed the need for a variety of adaptive equipment, including a wheelchair and a ramp to access her home. She also needed a commode, as the only bathroom was upstairs. A utility cart would be needed for basic kitchen activities.

When these recommendations were presented, Mrs. Kennedy began to cry. She explained that the family had already remortgaged their home to pay for her medical bills and the planned surgery. There was no money for the necessary equipment. She felt that in less than a year she had gone from being a contributing member of society to becoming a burden on her family. She was worried about the effects of financial stress on her husband and her inability to care for their two small children. The mere mention of possible sources of community assistance brought a fresh flood of tears.

The OTA working with Mrs. Kennedy had grown up in a small community and knew how important it was for people to maintain their pride and sense of self-worth. She also knew that friends and neighbors would welcome the opportunity to help Mrs. Kennedy and others like her who might need assistance. She suggested to the OT that they contact the local Kiwanis and Lions Clubs to propose the development of a community adaptive equipment bank. She also recommended that Mrs. Kennedy be asked to serve as coordinator of the equipment bank, receiving requests from physicians and family members, arranging for purchase and delivery of equipment, and mainlining records and inventory. The occupational therapist approved the plan, which was put into action within 2 weeks. Mrs. Kennedy was pleased to have an opportunity to use her office and managerial skills and to have the use of the equipment until she recovered from her surgery.

SOCIOCULTURAL CONSIDERATIONS

Many communities contain diverse ethnic groups. People from the same cultural background have common traditions, interests, beliefs, and behavior patterns that give them a common identity. Frequently, these individuals tend to cluster in geographic areas to preserve their customs, values, traditions, and at times their native language. The ethnic neighborhood can be viewed as a society within a society. These clusters or environs provide individuals with opportunities for perpetuation of their culture and lifestyles.

Some cultures are matriarchal, or female controlled, whereas others are patriarchal, or male controlled. The roles and performance expectations of the oldest, middle, or youngest child can also vary among cultural groups. In some societies, the number of male children may determine the financial security of the parents in later life.

Customs

A custom is a pattern of behavior or a practice that is common to many members of a particular class or ethnic group. Although rules are unwritten, the practice is repeated and handed down from generation to generation. Cultural implications can have a significant impact on designing OT intervention techniques that enable a person to function at his or her maximum in the specific environment, as shown in Case Study 7.

Case Study 7

Mrs. Franko is a 61-year-old Italian woman who recently had a stroke. Her primary residual deficit was mild, right-sided hemiparesis. Mrs. Franko was also slightly disarthric and difficult to understand, as her native language was Italian.

When she returned home from the hospital, Mrs. Franko was depressed, unmotivated, and not interested in beginning any ADLs. When cooking activities were suggested, she became very upset and burst into tears. This behavior was discussed with one of her sons, and it was discovered that the entire family routinely gathered at the parents' home for Sunday dinner. Mrs. Franko greatly enjoyed this custom. She made all of her own pasta and canned homegrown tomatoes for sauce. She did not want her daughters-in-law to bring food or assist too much in meal preparation. Convenience foods and ready-made pastas had never been used, and the suggestion was totally unacceptable to the family.

In home care OT, Mrs. Franko was encouraged to regain her cooking skills, which required some minor adaptations. Her family bought her an electric pasta machine since she was no longer able to knead and roll her own pasta. Her heavy cooking pots were replaced with new, lightweight styles.

Once Mrs. Franko regained her cooking skills and resumed a role that was very important to her, she became receptive to relearning other aspects of ADL skills.

Traditions

Traditions are inherited patterns of thought or action that can be handed down through generations or can be developed in singular family units; they also may be perpetuated through subsequent generations. Many families develop their own special traditions during holidays, birthdays, vacations, and other occasions.

Customs and traditions may also occur on a daily basis and can be highly individualized. Their origin may be unknown and not related to any particular sociocultural custom or event, as illustrated by the following case.

Case Study 8

Mr. Wisneski is 50 years of age and was admitted to the Veterans Hospital with a diagnosis of multiple sclerosis. He was confined to a wheelchair and exhibited severe weakness of the upper extremities. His wife was 45 years old and they had six children all living at home who ranged in age from 4 to 16 years.

In OT, Mr. Wisneski participated in dressing activities, bathing, and transfer techniques and was actively experimenting with a variety of adaptive equipment that would assist him in resuming to his previous employment. Although he was a very quiet, nonverbal person, he seemed highly motivated and always carried through on any requests made as a part of his treatment.

When the OTA suggested that he begin shaving techniques, Mr. Wisneski said that it simply was not necessary and told the assistant not to worry about it. The OTA reminded him of the accomplishments he was making in independent living skills and pointed out that this was one more activity in which he could achieve independence. He acquiesced and went along with the program to please the OTA. One day, when Mr. Wisneski had successfully shaved himself, the OTA asked him if he did not feel better shaving independently. Mr. Wisneski replied that "it felt okay"; however, in his family it was a tradition for the wives to shave their husbands. Mr. and Mrs. Wisneski felt that this daily activity reaffirmed their commitment to each other and was a daily declaration of their devotion.

Superstitions

Superstitions can be difficult to identify and define. They can be customs, traditions, and beliefs of a very small population that may be geographically localized. They can also be highly individualized and border on mental or emotional pathologic states. Webster's dictionary defines them as "beliefs and practices resulting from ignorance and fear of the unknown" (Guralnik, 1982). They are also viewed as a statement of trust in magic. Superstitions are further defined as irrational attitudes of the mind toward supernatural forces.

It can be very difficult for OT personnel to deal with superstitions. It may be easy for a therapist or an assistant to point out how "ridiculous" superstitions are and to present facts that disprove such "ignorant" notions. The personal environment, standards, values, traditions, and beliefs of the OTA and OT can, at times, be in direct conflict with those of the patient. OT personnel must realize that the ultimate goal of OT is to return the individual to his or her lifestyle with all of its implications. The following case illustrates this point.

Case Study 9

Mrs. King is an 82-year-old woman who was admitted to the hospital with severe circulatory disturbances in her left leg. This condition resulted in surgical amputation of the lower left extremity.

The patient was referred to OT for generalized strengthening activities, cognitive stimulation, and reality reorientation. Although she frequently did not know where she was, past memory appeared to be intact. Mrs. King presented herself as a very pleasant person with a warm, personable manner.

During one of her initial treatment sessions, it was noted that she wore a small bag of coins tied tightly around her right thigh with several strips of gauze. When the occupational therapist questioned her about this, she explained that the bag of coins "kept evil spirits away" and made a person happy. She elaborated further, saying that she had always worn the bag on her left leg, but since the doctors had to remove that leg, she would now have to tie it to the right one. This situation had not been noted during prior medical examinations, as Mrs. King always removed the bag when she disrobed.

OT intervention consisted of introducing a 6-inch wide cohesive, light woven, elastic bandage, applied lightly on the thigh, with the small bag of coins attached with a safety pin. This solution was acceptable to Mrs. King. She also reported that all of the other family members also observed this practice. Therefore, all 12 family members were also instructed in this new method.

Values, Standards, and Attitudes

Values, standards, and attitudes are other aspects of an individual that develop through environmental transaction and influence lifestyle. These facets of a person's life usually result from feedback received from other people within one's work and leisure environments, as well as from the individual's sociocultural status, economic status, and self-image. They are very personal and become an important part of a person's internal environment. The presence of disease or injury can be very disruptive and require reassessment of all aspects of an individual's life and lifestyle, requiring some temporary or permanent adaptations. It is important for OT personnel to use intervention techniques that can be adapted to minimize the stresses that occur when the patient's values, standards, and attitudes are in jeopardy or must be compromised to some extent. Two case examples are presented to elaborate on these points.

Case Study 10

Mr. Hanson, a 50-year-old farmer living in a rural community in Indiana, had sustained a nerve injury to his left wrist. When his wrist was maintained in 50 degrees hyperextension, he could perform most precision patterns and his hand was functional.

All standard splints were unacceptable to Mr. Hanson, who stated that he would "feel like a sissy" and would not wear any of them in front of his friends. The solution was to fabricate a splint from a tablespoon, which was bent and angled to the correct medical alignment. The spoon was then riveted to a wide leather wrist band. Mr. Hanson wore the splint daily and enjoyed joking with his friends that he was "always looking for a meal." This adaptation was the change that convinced the patient to wear the appliance.

Case Study 11

Mrs. Nadeau was 60 years old when she had a stroke, which resulted in left hemiparesis. She had slight subluxation of the left shoulder. Shoulder subluxations are common, as the pull of gravity on the paralyzed or weakened limb frequently causes the ligaments surrounding a joint to stretch and the head of the humerus to pull out of the socket. Hemiplegic arm slings are sometimes recommended during ambulation to prevent this condition. These slings are very noticeable and not very attractive.

The patient was a very well-dressed, fashion-conscious woman of financial means. She frequently met with friends for luncheons and other social gatherings at her country club. Wearing the sling was an embarrassment for her. The solution involved adapting a leather shoulder bag to wear on these occasions. The bag was strong and large enough to support her forearm, and the strap was adjusted to a length that would support the humeral head in the shoulder joint. A wooden handle was attached to the bag, which maintained Mrs. Nadeau's wrist in hyperextension and held her thumb in opposition.

Consideration of these individual values and self-images enabled the occupational therapist to use everyday objects to fabricate necessary medical appliances in a form that was acceptable to both of the patients and compatible with their lifestyles.

Each occupational therapist and assistant has values, standards, and attitudes that may be in direct conflict with those of the patient, thus making it difficult to work with some individuals as noted in the example that follows.

Case Study 12

An occupational therapist was working one half day per week in a very small, rural general hospital. When she reported for work, she found four treatment requests for one patient, Mr. Smithe. Two were referrals from physicians requesting immediate initiation of feeding and toileting activities. There were also memoranda from the director of nursing and the hospital administrator requesting the same services. Mr. Smithe had been admitted for prostate surgery. He refused to use the toilet in his room, preferring instead a small, rectangular, plastic-lined wastepaper basket.

The patient was seen for an initial evaluation during the lunch hour. The meal consisted of cube steak with gravy, mashed potatoes, carrots, and a dish of sherbet. Mr. Smithe used no utensils; he ate with his fingers and licked up some foods. This behavior, together with his lip smacking and belching noises, was in total violation of the therapist's standards and values, as well as those of two female aides who cleaned up the food scatterings on the bed.

Limited information was available in Mr. Smithe's medical record. In addition to the problems discussed previously, nursing notes indicated that his behavior was that of a very hostile and angry person. It was difficult to determine whether Mr. Smithe was experiencing mental changes that required psychiatric intervention, whether his behavior was a reflected form of his personal lifestyle, or whether a combination of both was involved. Intake records revealed that Mr. Smithe refused to state his age or financial status.

Since there was no social worker available, the occupational therapist was requested to gather additional information from neighbors and the community. Mr. Smithe was described by his neighbors as an antisocial recluse. He had lived for at least 40 years in a large old toolshed on the back acres of a farm, which was a long distance from town. There had been windows in the building; however, he had covered them with roofing material many years ago. His home had no electricity or running water. He was always piling up wood and rubbish, so the neighbors felt certain that he had some sort of stove for cooking and heating.

The therapist visited a small grocery store nearby to see if Mr. Smithe bought food there. It was reported that he had indeed shopped there as long as the elderly owners remember. Mr. Smithe would slip a grocery list under the door and specify when he would pick up the items. He always paid in cash and requested that no females be present when he came to the store. He would talk with the male owner and periodically try new products that he recommended. If the owner's wife or other females were present, Mr. Smithe would slip in the back entrance, grab his groceries, pay, and leave hurriedly. With this information, the therapist made the following changes when she returned to the hospital:

- A male orderly was assigned to the patient.
- Mr. Smithe was informed that he could eat in any manner he chose; however, he would have to change his own linen. He began to cover himself with a large towel when eating and folded it neatly when finished.
- A portable commode was placed in his room. He liked it and stated that he had disliked the coldness

of the toilet seat and the loud rushing of water. He also disliked two females taking him to the bathroom.

If Mr. Smithe had recently developed this lifestyle, intervention techniques may have been different. When an OT or OTA encounters a lifestyle that has existed for over 40 years, it requires different consideration. At times it can be difficult to understand how persons living in the same general environment respond in such highly individualized manners.

CHANGE AND ITS IMPACT

Changes in lifestyles, roles, and activity levels occur throughout the life cycle. Normal changes are expected at various ages. For example, a child is expected to walk and talk at a certain age, and a young adult is expected to begin a career when he or she has completed the necessary education.

Changes can be self-imposed or superimposed on an individual. Self-imposed and superimposed changes and their resulting influence on the individual can occur over a prolonged period or they can be very sudden. The length of time and timing of such change have an impact to varying degrees on lifestyles, roles, self-image, and activity levels.

Retirement, whether self-imposed or superimposed, is a change that affects most aspects of a person's life. Many professionals are becoming involved in pre-retirement planning. These programs are designed to help people consider the various aspects of their life and plan ahead. The emphasis is on all important areas, not just financial planning.

Stress

The potential for stress is inherent with any change. Individuals react very differently to what appears to be the same stress situation. People who have explored different environments and adapted to change may have some sense of mastery over their environment. They can recall and apply previous actions and thoughts that either worked successfully or were ineffective. This provides them with more resources and information to plan an action and respond appropriately.

John and Darlene: Follow-Up

Both John and Darlene will be experiencing significant changes in their environment. These changes will affect their activities, roles, and lifestyles. John's decision to relocate in Duluth is a self-imposed change. He has given a lot of thought to this decision to move and start a new career. This cognitive planning has prepared him for the changes in his environment, new roles, and a markedly different lifestyle from the one he has established on the farm.

Darlene's future change had been superimposed on her by her parent's decision to move. She must now identify and evaluate alternatives and make a decision. She could locate a place of her own or move to Florida with her parents. These two alternatives offer very different considerations in terms of finances, employment, social status, and activities, as well as the total physical environment.

As these changes occur, they will create stress for both John and Darlene. Individuals who have made significant changes in the past often find that they can draw on these past events in terms of future decision-making and adjustment.

Severe Disruptions

Disruptions are sudden changes in a person's environment that require immediate attention and response. They are usually superimposed on an individual. Disruptions can be as simple and temporary as a common cold or loss of a job, or as complex and permanent as a stroke or death of a loved one. Most disruptions are high stress situations for the individual directly affected. Disruptions can also directly affect and cause stress for other persons in the client's environment.

Case Study 13

Michael, a mentally retarded young man functioning at about a 5-year-old level, had a severe disruption when his parents were in an automobile accident. Due to multiple injuries they both sustained and the length of time needed for rehabilitation, it was necessary to move Michael from his home to an institution. Michael's reaction to this abrupt change was evidenced by withdrawal and frequent tantrums. The OTR at the facility visited the parents in the hospital to gain information that might assist in helping Michael to adjust to his new environment. She learned that Michael had particular food preferences, had favorite television programs, and enjoyed hearing bedtime stories. Other details of his daily routine were discussed. The therapist then made the appropriate changes in Michael's daily regimen, and Michael discontinued his tantrums and began relating to others.

SUMMARY

It is much easier for health care personnel to treat arthritis, a hand injury, a personality disorder, a suicide attempt, or an amputee than to treat the whole person. The latter requires knowledge and insight about the individual's development, values, lifestyles, environments, self-images, roles, and activities in planning and implementing purposeful and meaningful therapeutic programs.

The goal of OT is to return the person to his or her environment with the skills necessary to resume previous occupations and roles. OT is concerned with the quality of life, which is determined by the individual and his or her environment. The relationship between humans and their environs goes far beyond the simple stimulus and response theory. A total transaction occurs between the individual and the external and internal circumstances that make up the person's unique environment.

To effectively treat a person and not a disability, all members of the profession must know the sociocultural, economic, psychological, and physical aspects and view them in relation to the standards, values, and attitudes of the patient's total environment. Occupational therapists and assistants are performance specialists who design and implement highly individualized developmental, remediation, and prevention programs.

REFERENCES

AOTA. (1979). *The philosophical base of occupational therapy, Resolution #531*. Bethesda, MD: Author.

AOTA Council on Standards. (1972). OT: Its definition and functions. *Am J Occup Ther, 26,* 204-205.

Guralnik, D. B. (1982). *Webster's new world dictionary*. New York, NY: Simon and Schuster.

Moyers, P. (1999). *Guide to OT practice*. Bethesda, MD: AOTA.

Reed, K., & Saunderson, S. (1999). *Concepts of OT*. Baltimore, MD: Williams & Wilkins.

Teaching and Learning

Chapter 10

Karen Sladyk, PhD, OTR/L, FAOTA

INTRODUCTION

Everyone thinks they understand teaching and learning. After all, if you have a high school diploma, you have had at least 13 years of teaching and learning experience. If you have any additional schooling, you have had even more experience with the topic. But teaching and learning is much more than learning in school. Even for the healthy adult, who may never need rehabilitation services, most of what he or she "knows" did not come from school. In fact, when adults are asked to list everything they have learned and where they learned it, only about 25% of the list was learned in school (Sheckley, 1984). All the rest (75%) was learned experientially in life. This experiential learning fits nicely with OT because experiential learning is life bound and the occupation of OT is life bound as well.

Just because we learn through our life experiences does not mean that scholars have not tried to capture the educational experience. Just as there are many frames of reference in OT, there are many educational theories in learning. This chapter will briefly look at educational theories,

Mosey's concepts on teaching and learning, Allen's view of cognitive disabilities, and applications in OT.

THEORIES IN ADULT LEARNING

Vast and numerous books have been written about educational theories. This section will look at theories specific to adults, commonly called andragogy. The educational foundations of your schooling through high school were based on pediatric theories, often called pedagogy. If you remember your medical terminology classes, you can see the word root focuses on the child or the adult.

Adults like to learn in different ways than do children. You may still use some of the skills learned in grade school in adulthood, such as making flashcards or lists for reminders, but you do not likely use every skill learned earlier now that you are an adult. Sometimes, teachers that use pedagogy techniques on adults actually insult the adult learner. An example of this is an experience I had recently.

Feeling that I was isolating myself in my work, I signed up for a holiday cookie class

KEY CONCEPTS

- Learning: Acquiring of knowledge or skill.
- Experiential learning: Learning through life experiences.
- Teaching and learning principles: Developed by Mosey to address learning in OT treatment.

at the local adult education program. On the first night, I learned that we would be baking cookies in "teams of three" and that there would be no cookies to take home because the class always ate them all. I was disappointed but I went along. My baking partners were significantly older than I was and they already had ideas of what we should make for the next week, so again I went along. After planning all the ingredients, I was sent to our assigned kitchen to find the 9x13-inch pan for next week. When I returned to the table with the pan, the teacher asked, "How do you know the size?" I started to explain how I estimated a 1-foot measurement then added an inch. I was handed a ruler to double check. I started to measure the bottom of the pan when one of my partners insisted I turn the pan over to measure the top. The pan was a half-inch short. I thought to myself, I'm here to relax, not worry over small details like this. I left the class and promptly withdrew. This educational experience had not met my needs.

I told this story to everyone at work the next day and besides all the ribbing I took from my peers, one physical therapist offered to show me how she makes her famous biscotti cookies. That was a perfect match for me. She showed me what I wanted and needed to know, not drilling me as I learned. Because of how I learned these skills, I was able to "transfer my training" to other tasks. The experience was positive.

The important lesson here is that adults learn differently. Some even like to learn the way they did in primary or secondary school, however, others want different approaches. The key to teaching adults is flexibility and continual assessment of meeting their learning needs.

Adult learners are a widely diverse group that encompasses many different styles, goals, and experiences (Cross, 1988). Understanding some of the major characteristics of this group can lead to more effective application of knowledge and transfer of learning to life situations. When interpreting major characteristics of adult learning, caution should be made to avoid labeling a diverse group with limited characteristics.

We live in a complex society were continual learning is no longer a luxury, but a necessity (Cross, 1988; Wlodkowski, 1990). Adults are independent thinkers with a variety of thought and experiences that come with them when they embark on new learning. Addressing this diversity of experience and needs will help the educator or therapist succeed.

Adults come to each learning experience with an integration of all prior learning experience (Kolb, 1984). For example, if a teenager had negative experiences in high school, he is likely to come to a vocational training program with negative feelings. If a patient has had positive experiences all during her rehabilitation program, she is likely to be open to new experiences in an outpatient clinic. Formal and informal experiences (Bandura, 1978) are included in this integration of experiences, so academic success in the past is more than just good grades. It includes interactions with teachers, parents, and peers. As the adult gets older, work experiences are added to this integration. Have you ever been "forced" to go to a work inservice that was way over your head or so simple it was a waste of time?

Brookfield (1990) points out that adults learn best in situations of mutual respect. Fostering the growth of the learner along a path to an ideal goal is the job of the teacher. He advocates that teachers help students identify and challenge assumptions and context, imagine and explore alternatives, and view knowledge with reflective skepticism.

Simply providing the learner with information does not foster the transfer of knowledge. This learning situation does not foster mutual respect and clearly makes the teacher the powerful partner with "all the knowledge."

Chaffee (1998) says that the key to successful adult thinking consists of eight steps:

1. Think critically
2. Live creatively
3. Choose freely
4. Solve problems effectively
5. Communicate effectively
6. Analyze complex issues
7. Develop enlightened values
8. Think through relationships

He encourages adults to transform themselves through thinking and to create a life philosophy to follow. This requires a strong commitment to self-analysis that many adults cannot call upon because of other factors.

Adult behavior is an interaction of person and environment (Bandura, 1978). Although most people believe that the learner's responsibility is to learn, the learner will act on his or her learning within the structure of his or her environment. In some cultures, women are not expected to be learners. Teaching a person from this environment may be extremely difficult.

When addressing the unique learning needs of adults, several themes emerge. Adults have an educational history that may be positive or not. Adults learn through their experiences (experiential learning). Motivation can support learning, however, adults typically learn within their own environments. Mutual respect plays an important role in adult learning. All of these factors can influence the transfer of training to life situations. All of these factors, if negative, can cause a negative loop that is recursive and self-fulfilling. The goal of the teacher is to manage these factors in a way that is positive to the adult learner.

MOSEY'S TEACHING-LEARNING PROCESS

Although teaching and learning have been a part of OT from the beginning, Mosey's (1986) book on psychosocial OT was one of the first to link educational theory and psychological theory with OT treatment. She details 16 principles to guide therapist/patient interaction in learning. She reminds practitioners that learning principles do not provide firm rules, but provide a base to begin to facilitate learning. A principle may carry more importance with one person than another. The therapist's judgment is the key to patient success. The following guidelines are adapted from Mosey's (1986) work.

When teaching in OT treatment, the practitioner will:

- Use good communication skills—Collaboration is a valued aspect of the therapeutic relationship that begins with the practitioner using good communication skills. The therapist should sit squarely toward the patient without crossing arms or legs. Good, comfortable eye contact and a relaxed approach will make the patient comfortable. Use open-ended questions in patient conversations. Open-ended questions are questions that require more than a one-word answer. This type of question should comprise the majority of the therapist's questions. Use open-ended questions to probe for details about a patient's life. For example, "What about that activity makes you tired, Seth?" Use closed-ended questions carefully and only when you need a specific answer. For example, "Where does the splint cause you pain, Annie?"

- Accept the client for who he or she is—All human beings have the right to good health. The practitioner should keep biases in check and be reflective of any behavior that appears judgmental. Remain the professional in the relationship and avoid behaviors that reflect friendship on a nonprofessional level.

- Begin treatment at the consumer's current level—This allows the person initial success before moving onto the next level. When the person is ready for the next level, provide what Allen, Earhart, and Blue (1992) call the "just-right challenge." Remember everyone learns at different rates.

- Acknowledge the patient's current culture and environment—This can include heritage, country of origin, age, gender, and memberships. The person's assets and limitations are important to address in light of his or her culture and environment. All of these factors can have a positive and/or negative influence on returning to health. For example, membership in a street gang or social club can hinder a person remaining alcohol free, but membership in a church or fitness club can help.

- Communicate effectively in volume and pace—Consider how you are saying something as well as what you are saying. Patients with hearing problems usually hear better with their eyeglasses on because they pick up on the visual clues of speech. Confused patients perform better with simple, clear cues, such as "open the toothpaste."

- Encourage the learner to be an active learner—Empower the client to be the leader of his or her treatment. Encourage learning with all the sensorimotor components to reinforce the task.

- Control the consequences of learning—Pleasurable experiences reinforce the consumer to want to learn again. Always process the experience whether in a group or individually after the learning experience. Provide opportunities to make errors and then discuss how things could go better next time. If need be, stop an experience if safety is an issue because safety is always addressed first in treatment.

- Provide an opportunity for trial and error—This is empowering for the patient when consequences are controlled. Use first and last experiences to demonstrate how far the patient has improved. Stay open-minded to ways the patient wants to "try something out." The patient may know better than the practitioner.

- Provide opportunity for practice and repetition—No one likes to learn something by rote memory, but opportunities to practice skills provide mastery. Just like trial and error, use the first and last experiences to show the client his or her progress.

- Encourage the consumer to set his or her own goals—Too often practitioners write treatment goals in patient's records and the patients participated very little in the planning process. A practitioner should never solely develop goals for a patient even when goals may be influenced by insurance reviewers. The patient should always work with the therapist in developing goals for him- or herself because of motivation and responsibility. The practitioner's expertise is making sure the patient's goals are not too high or too low.

- Practice skills in different situations—Learning is often specific to an experience but practice in different situations allows the client to generalize the skill or transfer the training. For example, the electric dryer in the ADL kitchen is different from the electric dryer in the client's home or the gas dryer in the local laundromat.

- The learner should understand what is being learned—Too often the consumer does not understand what is being learned. This is especially true for head injured or confused patients. Too many times this leads to the patient making negative statements about OT, including to the media, who repeat the story without knowing the details of the situation. The practitioner must repeat the purpose of the task until he or she is sure the patient understands. Check for understanding during the processing stage of treatment to see the patient's understanding. Educate staff, family, and friends at every available opportunity.

- Learning moves from simple to complex—This integrates earlier discussions of helping clients succeed throughout their treatment process. The idea of learning moving from simple to complex is nicely illustrated by the rating system for ski slopes—bunny trail to black diamond.

- Encourage creative problem-solving—Often times traditional approaches to a problem may not be the right answer for clients with nontraditional issues. The practitioner should role model and encourage his or her consumer to "think outside of the box."

- Acknowledge that everyone handles stress and anxiety differently—Learning is frustrating, stressful, and anxiety-producing. Remember anatomy exams? Learners deal with this stress in different ways. Some "shut down" and become very quiet. Some get loud and angry. Some get the giggles and laugh at everything. The practitioner needs to watch for signs that learning is causing stress or anxiety and process this information with the client.

LEARNING WITH A COGNITIVE DISABILITY

The cognitive disabilities frame of reference was developed on the belief that some patients have cognitive disabilities due to a biological or chemical defect in the brain. Because of this disability, cognitive functioning is impaired (Allen et al., 1992). These cognitive disabilities result in a decrease in the person's ability to learn. OT can assist with adaptation to maximize functioning but cannot improve cognitive functioning unless the patient has demonstrated a prior higher level. Medication can sometimes help improve functioning.

Allen's Cognitive Level Test (Allen et al., 1992) is a task-based assessment that provides information on a patient's cognitive functioning. Cognitive functioning is measured on a scale from 1 to 6, with 1 indicating severe impairment and 6 indicating normal cognitive functioning. In addition, each level is subdivided into smaller units to allow for scoring between levels. For example, a patient may score 4.6.

Each level indicates a higher level of cognitive functioning and are briefly summarized here.

- Level 1—Conscious but profoundly disabled. Stares, may sit, walk, or chew with simple commands. Needs 24-hour nursing care.

- Level 2—Actions related to comfort or discomfort. Short attention span of less than 10 minutes. May wander or resistant to caregiver assistance. Needs 24-hour nursing care.

- Level 3—Manual actions. Pointless or destructive manipulation of objects. Behavior may be inappropriate or not goal-directed. Needs cues to groom.

- Level 4—Goal-directed with cues. Pace is slow and person pays little attention to environment. Needs support in community, as plans are often unrealistic.

- Level 5—Trial and error problem-solving. Often impulsive or careless. Fails to see consequences of behaviors, especially long-term.

- Level 6—Plans ahead. Thinks ahead before acting and can predict consequences of behavior. Independent and organized (Allen et al., 1992).

The cognitive level of a patient can help guide the practitioner in developing treatment goals (Allen et al., 1992). Patients with lower cognitive levels benefit most from changes to the environment to keep them safe. Patients with fluctuating cognitive functioning benefit from further evaluation and tasks that provide the just-right challenge. Patients with higher level scores benefit from learning activities within their cognitive functioning (Allen et al., 1992).

APPLICATION OF LEARNING THEORIES

Teaching and learning have been a foundation for OT from its early history. There are as many different theories on learning as there are different types of OT consumers. Choosing the right approach to each consumer requires clinical reasoning skills (Mattingly & Fleming, 1994). The practitioner must consider the procedures he or she is using, his or her interaction with the patient, and his or her understanding of the patient's world all at the same time. Learning theories can assist the therapist in his or her clinical reasoning.

Case 1

You are the OT personnel for a vocational program for young men leaving prison. This program accepts men 19 to 21 years old who have had one incarceration and a good behavior record while in prison. The vocational program trains these young men in cable TV installation and has an excellent record of job placement and work history. Your job is to evaluate basic skills in ADLs and pre-work skills. You often find that your clients hold a high school diploma but lack skills in reading and social skills needed on the job. They are often resistive to "learning."

Discussion

Understand how the principles of adult learning can be applied here. Your clients are likely bringing with them negative learning experiences that have reinforced a negative attitude about new learning. What motivating factors might you use? What principles of Mosey's work might be useful?

Case 2

You are the primary practitioner for a home-based Alzheimer's program. This community-based program aims to keep cognitively impaired clients at home as long as possible. You work closely with an OT who comes in for periodic patient evaluation and provides collaborative supervision as you need it. Other members of the team include nursing, home health aides, and a physical therapist assistant. The team is concerned that a patient is no longer safe at home. He has wandered out of the home several times and locked his wife outside in the cold when she went to get the mail. His vision appears to be decreasing because he has had two recent falls. You ask the OT to come in for an evaluation and she uses the ACL test, modified with large holes. The patient scores a 2.4. Other professionals evaluate the client and agree that 24-hour nursing care is required. The problem is that his wife does not believe this and wants to keep him home because of their wedding vows. "I can teach him what he needs to stay safe, he trusts me," she says. She is clearly showing the strain of his care on her health.

Discussion

This is an interesting case because it involves learning on many levels. Allen, Earhart, and Blue (1992) show us that a person functioning at 2.4 is not capable of learning even from someone he trusts. The 2.4 score is slightly higher than a 2.0 but can still require 24-hour nursing care. However, at this time, the patient's wife cannot see or understand his functioning.

Let's look specifically at the wife's learning. What reasons could be interfering with a clearer, objective view of her husband's functioning? First reaction might say guilt, but this does not explain everything. She may have negative attitudes from earlier experiences about nursing

homes that she brings to this experience. Similar to the young men in the case above, this appears in a "resistive" attitude. She may not understand the cognitive decline of her husband. The OT and OTA can work together to explain the process using Mosey's principles of learning. What other resources could the OTA call upon to assist the wife in objectively evaluating the home situation? How would the OTA use learning theories to prepare these other resources to address issues with the wife?

SUMMARY

Teaching and learning is a complex process of mutual respect, sharing information, guiding progress, and understanding adults. Educational theories help OT practitioners understand and practice teaching in treatment. OTs, including Mosey and Allen, help explain teaching and learning from the perspective of patient needs.

REFERENCES

Allen, C. K., Earhart, C. A., & Blue, T. (1992). *OT treatment goals for the physically and cognitively disabled.* Bethesda, MD: AOTA.

Bandura, A. (1978, April). The self system in reciprocal determinism. *American Psychologist,* 344-357.

Brookfield, S. D. (1990). *Understanding and facilitating adult learning.* San Francisco, CA: Jossey-Bass Publishers.

Chaffee, J. (1998). *The thinker's way: 8 steps to a richer life.* Boston, MA: Little, Brown and Co.

Cross, K. P. (1988). *Adults as learners.* San Francisco, CA: Jossey-Bass Publishers.

Kolb, D. A. (1984). *Experiential learning.* Englewood Cliffs, NJ: Prentice-Hall.

Mattingly, C., & Fleming, M. H. (1994). *Clinical reasoning: Forms of inquiry in therapeutic practice.* Philadelphia, PA: F. A. Davis Co.

Mosey, A. C. (1986). *Psychosocial components of OT.* New York, NY: Raven Press.

Sheckley, B. G. (1984). The adult as learner: A case for making higher education more responsive to the individual learner. Two part series, *CAEL News, 7*(8) and *8*(1).

Wlodkowski, R. J. (1990). *Enhancing adult motivation to learn.* San Francisco, CA: Jossey-Bass Publishers.

Occupations and Disabilities

A Baby with Visual Deficits

Chapter 11

Mary Kathryn Cowan, MA, OTR, FAOTA
Angela E. Scoggin, PhD, OTR
Patricia K. Benham, MPH, OTR

INTRODUCTION

This chapter discusses a case study of a young child with a visual impairment within the context of early intervention services based on a family-centered model of care. Federal legislation that impacts services provided to children ages birth to 2 years and their families will be reviewed.

Concisely stated, "Visual impairments can result from problems with any part of the visual system, including the eyes, eye muscles, optic nerve, or the area of the cerebral cortex that processes visual information" (Gersh, 1991, p. 69). In order to be classified as legally blind in the United States, an individual must have 20/200 or poorer corrected visual acuity in the best eye or a visual field of 20 degrees or less. While a child with normal vision can clearly see a particular object that is 200 feet away, the legally blind child, with glasses or other correction, must be only 20 feet away to see the object with the same clarity. The definition of legal blindness is also met if the child's peripheral vision is limited to 20 degrees or less rather than the over 180 degrees in a normal visual field (Snow, 1996). A child classified as having low vision has acuity, or visual clarity, of 20/70 or poorer. It is important to note that these criteria for measuring vision were developed with adults, and that measuring vision in infants and young children cannot be as precise and will also require observation of functional vision used during daily activities (Senitz et al., 1990).

Although there are numerous factors that may be associated with visual deficits in infants and young children, hereditary disorders and the effects of prematurity are the most common causes (Senitz et al., 1990). Some of the most common conditions in children treated by OT practitioners include retinopathy of prematurity (ROP) (a term synonymous with retrolental fibroplasia [RLF]), cataracts, and cortical blindness/visual impairment. ROP may occur in extremely premature infants, especially those with medical complications and those exposed to excessive oxygen. Children with healed ROP are also more likely to have myopia, strabismus, and amblyopia. In myopia, also referred to as nearsightedness, the child has much better

KEY CONCEPTS

- Early intervention laws: Laws providing services for newborns to 3-year-olds.
- Family-centered approach: The family is the consumer, not just the child.
- Cultural implications: Performance context is specific to each family.
- Developmental evaluation: Children with blindness often have developmental delays.
- Program goals and objectives: Specific behavioral goals for treatment.
- Play and feeding activities: Encourage development skills.
- School adaptations: Providing learning in the most supportive environment.
- Transition planning: Promoting skills to transition to other areas in life.

vision at close range than farther away. The child with strabismus demonstrates an inability of the eyes to converge on the same image. The term amblyopia refers to decreased vision most often resulting from the brain suppressing the visual image to one eye in order to prevent double vision (Berkow, 1992).

Chromosomal abnormalities and maternal diseases, such as rubella during pregnancy, are the most common causes of congenital cataracts. Congenital cataracts result in a cloudy or opaque, rather than clear, lens of the eye and require early surgical removal, followed by the use of visual correction such as glasses for the infant (Berkow, 1992). In cortical blindness/cortical visual impairment, the child's vision is functionally impaired because the visual cortex of the brain cannot process the visual information received from the eyes. This condition results from extensive neurological damage, as seen in children with severe cerebral palsy or victims of near drowning (Snow, 1996).

The Impact of Visual Impairment on Occupational Performance of Children

The effect of early visual impairment on a child's performance of occupational roles and activities varies greatly according to the extent of the visual impairment itself, as well as the number and extent of accompanying disabilities. However, considering visual impairment alone, it is known that developmental motor delays are common when infants with blindness are compared to sighted children (Adelson & Fraiberg, 1977). Touch and sound must provide the stimuli for reaching and movement behaviors in children with visual impairment, which will lead to normal play in infancy, and these do not stimulate the child to reach or move as early as visual stimuli will with sighted children (Senitz et al., 1990). Many social behaviors are learned through the visual experience, and then imitation of that experience occurs as the child evaluates his or her social world and develops his or her own repertoire of social behavior. Early visual impairment in and of itself is not a cause of any occupational performance problems, but rather an obstacle to overcome so that a child's true performance abilities may be developed and utilized and further disability prevented.

Occupational Performance Areas Affected by Visual Impairment

- Self-care—The development of independence in eating and drinking as well as independence in dressing may be delayed because children with blindness from birth may not have developed the necessary motor skills required for each task, or they have been unable to imitate the performance from other children or adults due to the lack of vision. Other areas of self-care that may be affected as the child gets older are the social aspects of grooming, eating in social situations, selecting food in cafeterias and stores, and mobility in the community.

- Play—Children with visual impairment may have underdeveloped play skills due to delays in motor/mobility skills, lack of exploratory behavior, or stimulation from the environment.

- School—As the child develops and attends primary and elementary school, mobility in the new environment can be limited by visual impairment, and all school skills that usually require vision will need to be monitored. These activities include reading and all material presented in a visual manner (worksheets, instruction on a blackboard, teacher demonstration, etc.) and developing a method of communication through written format. Additionally, potential areas of limitation may also include the visual and social aspects of lunch and recess activities.

Occupational Performance Components Affected by Visual Impairment

Although the performance components of sensorimotor, cognitive, and personal/social are not part of the disability of blindness, a lack of development in these components can occur if a child does not receive adequate environmental and interpersonal stimulation during infancy and early childhood. When other disabilities, such as neurological impairment, exist along with a diagnosis of early blindness, there can be significant impairment in sensorimotor, cognitive, and personal/social abilities from birth.

Frames of Reference

Frames of reference that appear to be most appropriate for children born with severe visual impairment include the developmental and occupational behavior frames. The developmental frame of reference, as developed by Lela Llorens, views OT as the facilitator of development, which will help the child master each developmental life task and the ability to cope with life expectations. The occupational behavior frame, as developed by Mary Reilly, emphasizes play as the occupation of children, and within the world of play the child develops basic mastery and competence of all skills needed during the child's lifetime (Hinojosa, Kramer, & Pratt, 1996). If other disabilities are present, neurodevelopmental, sensory integrative, and biomechanical frames of reference must be considered.

AOTA Policy, Public Law, and Early Intervention Services

AOTA supports the provision of early intervention services using a family-centered approach that incorporates professional collaboration, as outlined in the AOTA Position Paper, *OT Services in Early Intervention and Preschool Services* (AOTA, 1996). Children make the most progress when their needs are constantly viewed within the context of the family. Purposeful, self-initiated activity continues to be the cornerstone of OT treatment, but parents are encouraged to actively participate in their child's treatment plan and to take satisfaction in their occupational roles as parents. OT practitioners strive for "best practice" by providing state-of-the-art treatment approaches while developing new and innovative strategies to better meet the needs of infants and their families. Prevention as well as intervention are stressed, and OT practitioners collaborate with community agencies to assist families in the many transitions that they face at this stage in their children's lives.

The position of AOTA is in agreement with the federal mandates regarding early intervention services. The U. S. Congress first enacted the Education of the Handicapped Act (EHA), also called P. L. 94-142, in 1975. This act mandated that public schools provide educational services for children with disabilities ages 5 through 21. P. L. 99-457 amended EHA in 1986 by mandating services for preschoolers with disabilities (Part B) and giving the states options for developing early intervention systems for infants, toddlers, and their families (Part H). Congress amended EHA in 1990, changing the name to the Individuals with Disabilities Education Act (IDEA) (Maruyama et al., 1997). The most recent amendments of IDEA, authorized in 1997, place increased emphasis on transition planning for school to work, team collaboration, and justification for instances when the child is placed in settings that do not include peers without disabilities (Muhlenhaupt et al., 1998). Mandates for early intervention are now included in Part C of IDEA. Other changes include the use of the terms "service coordinator" instead of "case manager" and "adaptive behavior" instead of "self-care."

The purpose of IDEA is to ensure that children with disabilities ages 3 through 21 receive a free appropriate public education in the least restrictive environment. Part B addresses the needs of children with disabilities ages 3 through 21. Part H (now included in Part C) is the Early Intervention Program for Infants and Toddlers with Disabilities. It provides states with financial assistance to:

Develop and implement a statewide, comprehensive, coordinated, multidisciplinary, interagency program of early intervention services for infants and toddlers with disabilities and their families;

facilitate the coordination of payment for early intervention services from federal, state, local, and private sources. (34 C.F.R. 3 03. 1 [a][b], as cited in Maruyama et al., 1997, p. 14)

Since each state develops its own early intervention system, OT practitioners must be aware of the regulations and guidelines for the states in which they practice.

OT is a primary service in early intervention programs and a related service for children 3 through 21 years, who are served through the public school system. As a primary service, OT can be provided either alone or in combination with other early intervention services to eligible children ages birth through 2 years. The goal of services is to enhance the child's functional ability and prevent or minimize future impairment by meeting the needs of the child and family as they relate to the child's development. Early intervention mandates require a multidisciplinary team model and a family-centered approach. Services should be provided in the child's natural environments and are based on a collaboratively developed Individualized Family Service Plan (IFSP). Eligible children include those who are developmentally delayed or who have a diagnosed condition that places them at risk of developmental delay (Maruyama et al., 1997).

In contrast, OT, as a related service under Part B of IDEA, is provided to children with identified disabilities who need OT in order to benefit from special education. A multidisciplinary, student-focused team model addresses the child's educational needs. Service delivery should be conducted in the least restrictive environment and in a regular educational setting with non-disabled peers to the maximum possible extent. Each child must have a written Individualized Education Program (IEP) that outlines how the student's educational needs will be met and how the school will ensure that needed services are provided (Maruyama et al., 1997).

Other federal legislation that may impact the OT practitioner working with infants and young children includes the Head Start Act of 1964. The Head Start program may assign at least 10% of its placements to preschoolers with disabilities. Additionally, the Early Head Start program provides family-centered services for low-income families with children ages birth through 2 years. Title XIX of the Social Security Act of 1965 (Medicaid) and the Americans with Disabilities Act of 1990 (ADA) are additional federal laws that are relevant for OT service provision (Maruyama et al., 1997).

Case Study

The following case study has been adapted from Benham (1993). Alejandro is a 15-month-old child with a diagnosis of RLF, or retrolental fibroplasia. RLF is a bilateral condition that may occur as the result of a child being placed in an incubator that has an excessive amount of oxygen. The elevated oxygen levels destroy the rapidly growing blood vessels in an infant's retina. When the child is returned to normal room air, the blood vessels grow back haphazardly, and scar tissue forms. As the scar tissue contracts, it pulls the retina away from the choroid, causing the retina to detach. It is difficult to determine the degree of functional damage for an infant affected by RLF; however, blindness usually develops within several weeks. Once blindness occurs, there is no effective treatment. Other factors that contribute to the origin and development of the condition include apnea (temporary cessation of breathing), asphyxia, sepsis (presence of pathogenic microorganisms or their toxins in the blood or other tissues), nutritional deficiencies, and a large number of blood transfusions given during a short period of time (Thomas, 1989).

Referral

Alejandro was diagnosed as developmentally delayed and visually impaired as a result of RLF. He was born prematurely at 32 weeks' gestation, weighing 3 pounds. He suffered severe respiratory distress and required oxygen, which resulted in a visual impairment diagnosed as RLF. When he was discharged from the hospital at age 3 months, no motor impairments were noted, and the extent of his visual impairment was unknown. At age 15 months, Alejandro was referred to the Early Intervention Program at the state Department of Health and Human Services by his pediatrician after an initial examination that revealed delays in several areas of development on the Denver II Revised Developmental Screening Test (Frankenberg et al., 1989). A service coordinator was assigned and the early intervention team members began their assessments. Team members included a teacher of the visually impaired, an orientation and mobility specialist, a psychologist, an ophthalmologist, an OT, and an OTA.

Assessment and Evaluation Process

The OT/OTA Team

When early visual impairment has been diagnosed by an ophthalmologist, an estimate of residual vision established, and the diagnosis of any accompanying disabilities completed, the OT/OTA team can discuss how each team member will be involved with the child. If blindness or severe visual deficit is the only disability present, the OT usually completes the evaluation with the assistance of the OTA, and program planning developed by the team may well be carried out by the OTA. If additional, increasingly complex disabilities exist (such as neurological problems), the OT may not only need to carry out the evaluation, but carry out the treatment program with the assistance of the OTA (AOTA, 1996).

Selected Evaluations

Considering the occupational performance areas which may be impacted by early visual deficits, tests of general development may be the first choice for assessment of young children since they can give a picture of a child's play, self-care, and personal social abilities, as well as motor abilities. If the child is school-aged, more detailed evaluations of school, classroom, and environmental demands on the child will be required. This information can be obtained from interview of teachers, school checklists, self-care checklists, or formal evaluations such as the School Function Assessment (SFA) (available from Therapy Skill Builders, a division of the Psychological Corp., 555 Academic Ct., San Antonio, TX 78204-2498) or the Pediatric Evaluation of Disability Inventory (PEDI) (available from PEDI Research Group c/o Stephen M. Haley, Dept. of Rehabilitation Medicine, New England Medical Center Hospital #75K/R, 750 Washington St., Boston, MA 02111-1901). If multiple handicaps are present, more extensive evaluation of self-care (especially eating), sensory integrative, and motor functions may need to be completed by the OTR for children of all ages.

At the initial team meeting for Alejandro, the Family Needs Survey (Baily & Simeonsson, 1985) was administered by the early intervention team. It was also decided by the OTR and COTA that OT evaluation needs would include assessment of:

- Fine and gross motor development
- Reflex maturation
- Self-care or adaptive behavior activities
- Sensorimotor development
- Play development

OT evaluations selected for Alejandro included:

- Developmental Programming for Infants and Young Children (Schafer & Moersch, 1981)
- The Milani-Comparetti Motor Development Screening Test (1992)
- Takata's Play History (1974)
- Sensory history

Results of Family Interview

Alejandro's family included his mother, father, and two older female siblings, ages 3 and 5 years. The family had recently moved to the United States from Honduras as a result of the father's employment opportunities. The father, who is Hispanic, and the mother, who is European-American, are professionals and employed outside of the home. The paternal grandmother takes care of Alejandro during the day and has a different view of Alejandro's condition than the mother. She believes that Alejandro's condition is a result of mal-puesto (bad luck) and that he should be accepted "as he is." The mother is aware of the possibilities for Alejandro in the future, due to volunteer experiences at a local high school for retarded children. In general, the family would like to have more information about Alejandro's development and expressed a desire to have only one or two professionals involved in their son's care. Because the OTA speaks Spanish and English, she will work closely with the OT in assessment and programming for Alejandro. Both the OT and the OTA described in this study are practicing at the advanced level as defined by the AOTA document *Guide for Supervision of OT Personnel* (AOTA, 1996).

Results of Occupational Therapy Evaluation

- Alejandro's gross motor, fine motor, self-help, and play development were delayed.
- Alejandro's gross motor development was typical of blind children; that is, the milestones achieved are those that do not require self-initiated mobility. He sits alone briefly, but usually uses his arms for support. No trunk rotation was noted, and he is not able to achieve a sitting position independently. In a prone position, he moves by belly-crawling, in an amphibian pattern. Occasionally, he will attempt to support himself on his hands and knees and rocks back and forth. He raises his head when in a prone position on extended arms, but has weak neck extensors and a lack of visual motivation to maintain the position. Rolling is achieved accidentally. If he hears his mother voice, he will try to follow the sound, resulting in spontaneous rolling.
- Primitive reflexes appear integrated, with the exception of a slight Moro reflex reaction when startled by unexpected noises or a change in position. Righting reactions are emerging in prone, supine, and sitting. Muscle tone is slightly hypotonic.
- Fine motor developement is in the 8- to 9-month range, due to resistance to tactile exploration and his visual impairment. He does not reach for objects by using sound location.
- Self-care or adaptive behavior activities are performed at the 9- to 11-month age range. He is able to chew, take food off of a spoon, and hold his bottle. He will not hold a spoon or finger feed himself. He refuses to try new foods and mealtime is often unpleasant.
- Play skills are limited primarily to solitary play. The OTA observed that his grandmother is very protective of him in regard to other children if they bump into him or try to engage him in play. He frequently engages in self-stimulating behaviors such as eye poking, waving his hands in front of his face, and rocking.
- The sensory history revealed that he does not enjoy "rough-housing" and cries when moved unexpectedly. He enjoys being rocked, but he does not like being held firmly or cuddled. Alejandro is orally defensive and does not readily mouth objects. He is resistive to tactile exploration of his parents' faces. He does not enjoy putting his hands in soft or "messy" textures.
- The teacher of the visually handicapped assessed Alejandro's remaining vision, using the Functional Vision Inventory for the Multiple and Severely Handicapped (Langley, 1980). Based on this assessment and the ophthalmologist's medical assessment of the child's eyes, Alejandro was thought to have remaining vision that he was not using optimally. The vision teacher made recommendations that were to be incorporated into the IFSP regarding optimal light conditions, distance of objects, object size, and visual field presentation.

General Goals

Child and family strengths that were identified by the team included the child's desire to participate in family interaction, the parents' desire to encourage independence, and the grandmother's interest in the child's well-being. The family identified the following areas of need:
- To have the child participate in play with siblings.
- To understand the child's condition and to have realistic expectations.
- To have the child become independent in feeding.
- To decrease the child's self-stimulation behaviors.
- To have the child walk independently.
- To have the parents and grandmother appreciate each other's point of view regarding treatment.

The family/team wrote the following treatment goals into the IFSP:
- Decrease blindisms or mannerisms.
- Stimulate remaining vision.
- Decrease tactile defensiveness.
- Increase independence in feeding.
- Encourage normal play development and interaction with siblings.
- Increase tolerance for vestibular stimulation.
- Develop adequate righting and equilibrium reactions in sitting, kneeling, and standing.
- Enhance age-appropriate gross and fine motor development.

Writing Measurable Goals and Objectives

In early intervention and school programs, annual goals are written to the general area of need, and specific measurable objectives are written under each goal. Each objective must include four components:

1. The learner (the child).
2. The behavior or performance expected.
3. The conditions or circumstances under which the behavior will occur.
4. The criteria for measuring the degree of success of this objective.

Refer to the case study presented at the end of the chapter for examples of both goals and objectives.

Samples of Alejandro's Goals and Objectives

- Goal 1—Alejandro will feed himself using a spoon or fingers as appropriate with minimal assistance and compliant behavior.

    Objective 1—Alejandro will consistently tolerate his hand on the spoon using a hand-over-hand backward chaining technique as his grandmother directs food toward his mouth at mealtimes.

    Objective 2—Alejandro will tolerate the introduction of one new food each week, as presented by his grandmother using a positive but firm approach.

- Goal 2—Alejandro will initiate a play activity by reaching for a toy given a sound or light cue, with minimal prompting.

    Objective 1—Alejandro will visually attend to toys for 45 seconds when a light is shone on them.

    Objective 2—Alejandro will demonstrate a preference for social interaction by bellycrawling toward a sibling playing nearby to increase proximity to her.

Treatment Activities/Techniques

Play is the primary therapeutic medium with infants and young children, along with the introduction of technology to aid limited vision or blindness. Through play, body scheme, movement, and fine motor development are enhanced by using all forms of sensory stimulation and guided movement as needed. Children with visual impairment need maximal stimulation from sound, touch, movement, and remaining sight in order to develop the desire to move, to reach and manipulate objects, care for themselves, and lead productive occupational lives (Snow, 1996).

Treatment Activities for Alejandro

The treatment activities, which focused on feeding and play, were carried out by the OTA, who worked well with Alejandro's grandmother. The OT would make a home visit once a week in the evening when both parents would be present. Treatment sessions would be videotaped to document progress and to ensure the accuracy of the home program instruction. Following are treatment activities developed from the sample goals and objectives previously written.

- During play time, place Alejandro's hand on a spoon and move him through the motions of banging the spoon on various surfaces. Talk about the different sounds and whether the noises were loud or soft. To direct his visual attention to the spoon or object, wrap it with fluorescent tape. Initially, place him in a supported sitting position, as he is not able to maintain unsupported sitting. This will free his hands. As sitting balance improves, encourage him to sit with one arm support and gradually move to independent sitting with hands engaged in play at midline. Gradually decrease the pressure of the "helping hand" on his hand until he is holding the spoon independently.

- During snack time, put peanut butter or honey on the spoon and encourage him to bring the spoon to his mouth. Initially, the spoon may need to be redirected 100% of the way, but the distance for which assistance is required should be gradually decreased. Visually impaired children need to have experiences that will enhance body perception, so telling him about his hand and where it is in relation to his mouth is important. Because Alejandro is also orally defensive, thus decreasing the amount of oral play in which he engages, he needs assistance in developing proprioceptive awareness of the hand-to-mouth pattern.

- Encourage finger feeding by having him finger-paint with whipped cream. Allow him to put his fingers in the mouth of his grandmother to give her a taste, and encourage him to lick his fingers. He will benefit from variety in his sensory experiences, so add puffed rice cereal and fruit-flavored gelatin cubes to the whipped cream to add tactile and oral texture.

- Make arrangements for the grandmother to visit a preschool classroom for visually impaired children during lunchtime to observe independent self-feeding. Also arrange to have a Spanish-speaking mother of one of the children talk to the grandmother about the progress her child has made with self-feeding.

- In a darkened room, shine a flashlight on a toy and direct Alejandro's face in the proper direction. Gradually increase the length of time he looks at the toy. Direct his hand toward the toy. Present toys such as Lite Brite (Hasbro Corp., Pawtucket, RI) while he is in a prone position, thereby also encouraging him to maintain neck extension for a prolonged period. This enhances visual attention and encourages use of remaining vision and to reach toward sound cues.

- Encourage sibling interaction by playing games such as "So Big" and "Patty Cake." Start out by engaging him in play with one sister initially to facilitate one-to-one interaction. Be sure that his sister is in close enough physical contact so that Alejandro can feel her presence. Gradually, increase the distance so that he will have to reach arm's length to pass a ball or tickle his sister. Be sure interactions are fun for both children.

- As Alejandro improves in his tolerance of vestibular stimulation, increase the use of activities that have physical and tactile components, such as rolling up in a blanket with his sister or riding "horsey back."

- The grandmother and the parents will need to be reminded to let the siblings comfort each other if there is an accident or hurt feelings during their play. This can be encouraged by having them hug or kiss the hurt or rub it to make it feel better as an additional tactile activity. Alejandro has been overprotected from the normal day-to-day bumps, bruises, and disagreements that occur among siblings. Efforts need to be made to allow the children to solve their own problems to empower the children and solidify Alejandro's family position.

Several examples of additional specific treatment activities are shown in Figures 11-1 through 11-5.

Discharge Planning/Transition Planning

The OT scheduled a meeting with the family in their home 2 weeks before the anticipated date of discharge from the OT program. Segments of the videotape were reviewed, demonstrating the many goals that Alejandro had achieved. The parents and the grandmother indicated their appreciation and thought that the entire family had benefited from the intervention program. The service coordinator would continue to follow Alejandro and his family, assisting them in identifying appropriate community resources and groups as necessary. He would also receive services from the teacher of the visually impaired, primarily for premobility training. Preschool services that Alejandro would be eligible for were also discussed.

CLINICAL PROBLEM-SOLVING

Alejandro demonstrated "blindisms." What activities would be appropriate to decrease these behaviors?
If "blindisms" are present, purposeful activities should be used to distract the child, especially those

activities using movement or proprioception. Blindisms such as pressing or poking the eyes can cause dark circles under the eyes, the eyes sinking into the head, and even deform the bony structures around the eyes. It is important that they do not become an established pattern (Senitz et al., 1990).

Although peanut butter and honey are used in a treatment activity with Alejandro, what precautions should be considered with these foods?
Peanuts are often a cause of allergy, and use of peanut butter should be discussed with the family before use in a feeding program. Honey is not recommended for children under 1 year of age, due to a possibility of causing infant botulism (Berkow, 1992).

Jason is 3 years old and, along with the diagnosis of cerebral palsy spastic quadriplegia, is considered to be cortically visually impaired. What additional considerations need to be made when considering the OTR/COTA team relationships for this child?
If multiple handicaps are present, the OTR will select and carry out appropriate neurodevelopmental, sensory integrative, or other specialized evaluations or treatment techniques that will treat components of the child's occupational performance problems.

John has a diagnosis of visual impairment due to ROP. He is in the third grade of a public school. What occupational performance problems do you think might exist in his case? What therapeutic interventions would you recommend for John? How would OT service be provided to John under IDEA 1997?
Self-care may need to be emphasized in terms of orientation to food and location of utensils. Social development may need to be enhanced and guided as John comes increasingly more in contact with others in the home, neighborhood, and school activities. Mobility training, Braille reading and writing techniques, as well as low vision training are provided by specialists in these areas; however, OT can prepare the child for learning these techniques by developing early perceptual/sensory sensitivity, manipulation, and mobility skills (Snow, 1996). For the child in a school-based program, the need for assistive devices or technology is usually decided by the child's IEP team, based on the recommendations of the specialists involved (usually the ophthalmologist, special education teacher, and OT). Magnification of images, increased light, reduction of glare, and increasing contrast are basic adaptation techniques used when there is visual impairment. Under public law (IDEA 1997), OT is provided as a "related service" for children with visual impairment as determined by the child's IEP team.

Melanie is 15 years old, mildly mentally handicapped, and visually impaired due to meningitis in early infancy. What occupational performance problems might you anticipate in her case? What services are required by

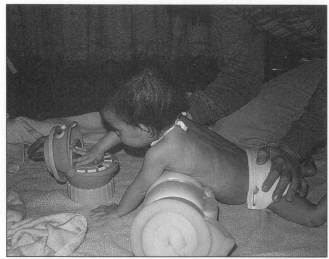

Figure 11-1. A bolster provides trunk support, allowing arms to extend to play with the Big Mouth Singer. (Reprinted from Ryan, S. E. [1993]. *Practice issues in OT: Intraprofessional team building.* Thorofare, NJ: SLACK Incorporated.)

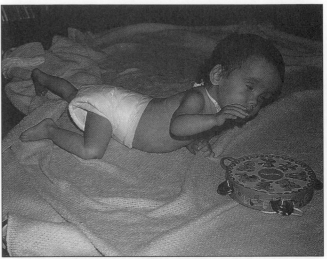

Figure 11-2. Eliciting location and reaching through the use of a tambourine. (Reprinted from Ryan, S. E. [1993]. *Practice issues in OT: Intraprofessional team building.* Thorofare, NJ: SLACK Incorporated.)

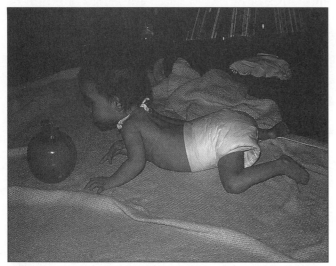

Figure 11-3. The Happy Apple provides sound as a stimulus for self-initiated belly crawling. (Reprinted from Ryan, S. E. [1993]. *Practice issues in OT: Intraprofessional team building.* Thorofare, NJ: SLACK Incorporated.)

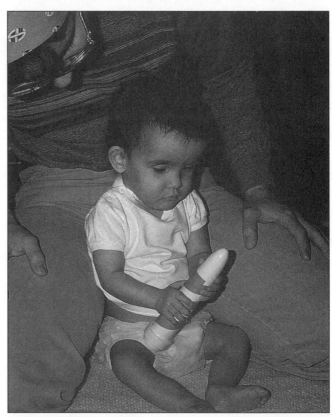

Figure 11-4. A supported sitting position allows both hands to be engaged in activity using a battery-powered vibrator wrapped with fluorescent tape. (Reprinted from Ryan, S. E. [1993]. *Practice issues in OT: Intraprofessional team building.* Thorofare, NJ: SLACK Incorporated.)

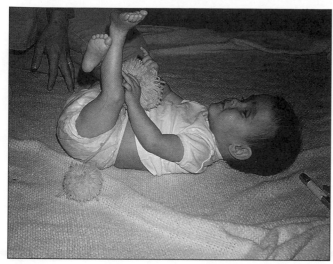

Figure 11-5. A handmade yarn pom-pom is used for tactile awareness and body stimulation. (Reprinted from Ryan, S. E. (1993). *Practice issues in OT: Intraprofessional team building.* Thorofare, NJ: SLACK Incorporated.)

IDEA 1997 at her age level? What type of an OT service plan would be appropriate for Melanie?

Some children with visual impairment, especially when combined with a mental handicap, need guidance with reading social cues and behavior, developing independence and care in self-grooming, and appropriate social etiquette in eating and work situations. According to law, an ITP must be written at age 14, and vocational planning is essential. Working in the community will need to be discussed as an option, and the vocational counselor now becomes part of the planning team. The skills for selected jobs can be developed in OT. Assistive technology that will assist in development of job skills should be considered by the ITP team. Low technology devices, for example, may include magnifiers and bold-writing pens; high technology devices may include stand-alone print enlargement systems, character enlargement systems for computers, Braille output devices, voice output systems, audio tactile devices, scanning systems, notetaking devices, and laptop computers (Mann & Lane, 1991). (For up-to-date technology, contact organizations for persons with visual impairments, such as the American Foundation for the Blind, 15 W. 16th St., New York, NY 10011 or Vision Foundation Inc., 818 Mt. Auburn St., Watertown, MA 02172.)

REFERENCES

Adelson, E., & Fraiberg, S. (1977). Gross motor development in infants from birth. In S. Chess & A. Thomas (Eds.), *Annual progress in child psychiatry and child development* (pp. 130-149). New York, NY: Brunner/Mazel Publishers.

AOTA. (1996). *Reference manual of the official documents of the AOTA.* (6th ed.). Bethesda, MD: Author.

Baily, D., & Simeonsson, R. (1985). *Family needs survey.* Chapel Hill, NC: Frank Porter Graham Child Development Center.

Benham, P. K. (1993). The child with visual deficits. In S. Ryan (Ed.), *Practice issues in OT: Intraprofessional team building* (pp. 27-34). Thorofare, NJ: SLACK Incorporated.

Berkow, R. (Ed.). (1992). *The Merck manual of diagnosis and therapy.* Rahway, NJ: Merck & Co., Inc.

Frankenberg, W. I., Dodds, J. B., Archer, P., et al. (1989). *Denver II* (3rd ed.). Denver, CO: Denver Developmental Materials, Inc.

Gersh, E. S. (1991). Medical concerns and treatments. In E. Geralis (Ed.), *Children with cerebral palsy: A parents' guide* (pp. 57-89). Bethesda, MD: Woodbine House, Inc.

Hinojosa, J., Kramer, P., & Pratt, P. N. (1996). Foundations of practice: Developmental principles, theories, and frames of reference. In J. Case-Smith, A. S. Allen, & P. N. Pratt (Eds.), *OT for children* (3rd ed.). St. Louis, MO: Mosby.

Langley, B. M. (1980). *Functional vision inventory for the multiple and severely handicapped.* Chicago, IL: Stoelting Co.

Mann, W. C., & Lane, J. P. (1991). *Assistive technology for persons with disabilities.* Rockville, MD: AOTA.

Maruyama, E., Chandler, B., Clark, G. F., Dick, R. W., Lawlor, M. C., & Jackson, L. L. (1997). *OT services for children and youth under the Individuals with Disabilities Education Act.* Bethesda, MD: AOTA.

Milani-Comparetti Motor Development Screening Test (3rd ed. Rev.). (1992). Omaha, NE: Meyer Rehabilitation Institute.

Muhlenhaupt, M., Miller, H., Sanders, J., & Swinth, Y. (1998). Implications of the 1997 reauthorization of IDEA for school-based therapy. *School System Special Interest Section Quarterly, 5*(3), 1-4.

Ryan, S. (Ed.). (1993). *Practice issues in OT: Intraprofessional team building.* Thorofare, NJ: SLACK Incorporated.

Schafer, D. S., & Moersch, M. (1981). *Developmental programming for infants and young children.* Ann Arbor, MI: University of Michigan Press.

Senitz, C., Bride, B. M., Adrian, J., & Semmler, C. J. (1990). Visually impaired children. In C. J. Semmler & J. G. Hunter (Eds.), *Early OT intervention—Neonates to 3 years* (pp. 262-274). Gaithersburg, MD: Aspen.

Snow, E. (1996). Services for children with visual or auditory impairments. In J. Case-Smith, A. S. Allen, & P. N. Pratt (Eds.), *OT for children* (3rd ed., pp. 717-742). St. Louis, MO: Mosby.

Takata, N. (1974). Play as prescription. In M. Reilly (Ed.), *Play as exploratory learning: Studies in curiosity behavior.* Beverly Hills, CA: Sage.

Thomas, C. L. (Ed.). (1989). *Taber's cyclopedic medical dictionary* (17th ed.). Philadelphia, PA: F. A. Davis.

A Toddler with Pervasive Developmental Disorder

Chapter 12

Tara J. Glennon, MS, OTR/L, BCP

INTRODUCTION

The fourth edition of the *Diagnostic and Statistical Manual of Mental Disorders* (DSM-IV) clarifies the criteria for the diagnosis of autism or pervasive developmental disorder (PDD), also referred to as autistic spectrum disorders (1994). The disorder is a behaviorally defined syndrome that has a biological base. The diagnostic criteria include qualitative impairment in reciprocal social interactions, qualitative impairment in verbal and nonverbal communications and imaginative play, restricted repertoire of activities and interests, and onset prior to age 3. In addition, experts include disturbances in developmental rates and sequences that affect motor, cognitive, and socioemotional areas; and disturbances in response to sensory stimuli as evidenced by hyperreactivity, hyporeactivity, or extreme alternating between these two states. It is also important to note that these characteristics can be observed with other developmental disorders and should be considered as additional diagnoses in order to be addressed accordingly.

Although the DSM-IV (1994) describes the symptomatology, there appears to be many subtypes. There are three categories of functioning identified in DSM-IV. In order for the diagnosis of autism to be made, at least two items from Category 1 and one item from both Categories 2 and 3 needs to be identified. However, there are many children who demonstrate several of the criteria, without meeting the number or combination required to meet the diagnosis of autism. If the child does not meet the autism criteria, the diagnosis of PDD would be made. With so many possible combinations, it has been speculated that different etiologies also exist. Therefore, there should be no "norm" for intervention. Rather, the symptomatology should be identified, specific research information should be analyzed, and various interventions should be considered.

The last point to be addressed with regard to autistic spectrum disorders is severity. Again, based on the combination of symptoms and the severity of each symptom, there is a wide range of disability. For example, one child may be intellectually

KEY CONCEPTS

- Medically based services: Paid for by insurance carrier upon medical necessity.
- School system practice: Guided by federal law for a free and appropriate education.
- Medical vs. educational services: Differences in service delivery models and team approaches.
- OT/OTA collaboration: Intricate interactions between two practitioners who each have necessary information and understanding of performance.

average, or even superior, and possess several communicative and interactional limitations. Another child may function in the mentally deficient range with no ability to participate in self-care activities. For this reason, each child who carries an autistic spectrum diagnosis needs to be treated on an individual basis with no preconceived notions of what the maximum level of independence will be.

HISTORICAL PERSPECTIVE

Henry Maudsley, the first psychiatrist to pay specific attention to very young children with severe issues in the developmental processes, considered these issues to be psychoses. This thought was commonplace until fairly recently. For it was only in 1943, a mere 50 plus years ago, that a paper titled "Autistic Disturbances of Affective Contact" was written by Dr. Leo Kanner (1943). Kanner, who first coined the term *infantile autism,* was a psychiatrist at Johns Hopkins Medical Center when he established the hallmarks of the disorder. At the time, he was working from a group of 11 patients who demonstrated similarities in their symptoms. The original concept of the disorder was described as a lack of responsiveness on the part of the child to environmental input and an inability to relate to people and situations from the beginning of life. As this original concept continued to be refined and clarified, DSM revisions reflected the changes in perspective (Sponheim, 1996), and intervention plans were modified and clarified.

At the time of original identification, intervention was minimal and inadequate, as the preliminary theories identified the mother as part of the problem. It was thought that the child ceased to interact because the mother was "cold" to the child. Unprepared and uneducated physicians cited this theory as late as 1990. In fact, before 1980, children with any PDD were classified as having a type of childhood schizophrenia (Petty et al., 1984). Physicians, pediatricians, and psychologists who are now current with the literature understand that autistic spectrum disorders are considered to be neurobiological disorders. Additionally, with more refined diagnostic information, the incidence of autistic spectrum disorders has been reported as high as 1 in every 500 births (Ritvo et al., 1990). These numbers imply than autistic spectrum disorders are more common that cystic fibrosis, which occurs 1 in every 2,500 births, and Down syndrome, which is 1 in every 1,000 births (Cohen & Volkmar, 1997).

RESEARCH CONSIDERATIONS RELATED TO OCCUPATIONAL THERAPY

Studies emerging in the 1970s have continued with full force today, secondary to the increased incidence of the disorder. Discovering the etiology or etiologies of autistic spectrum disorders, which would lead to prevention and more effective interventions, has been a challenge. Although technological advances in neuroimaging and neurochemical analysis have advanced this cause, the results have been mixed. Researchers have provided us with conflicting information and a variety of possibilities. Therefore, this section will focus on anatomical findings that would be considered to directly impact the role of OT personnel.

Researchers have identified neurological abnormalities in the limbic system, cerebellum, thalamus, and reticular formation (Bauman & Kemper, 1994; Courchesne et al., 1988). Rimland (1985), a leading researcher even today, cited that the symptomatology might be secondary to a deficit in perceptual capacities, possibly due to brainstem dysfunction, especially in the reticular formation. Rimland theorized that this results in "perceptual inaccessibility," as evidenced by a lack of preparedness to respond. Ornitz and Ritvo (1968), also authors on this topic, reflect on the possibility of faulty sensory modulation. Modulation, a term which will be discussed later in the chapter, refers to a lack of response or exaggerated response to certain environmental stimuli. Ornitz identifies a lack of orientation and attention to stimuli, inconsistent responses to sensory input, increased sensitivity to sensory input, which is termed *defensiveness*, and possible increased awareness of sensation coupled with a tendency to seek the input.

The limbic system, which is actually several structures that function together, include the hippocampus circuits and the amygdaloid complex. These structures function with the adjacent neocortices, hypothalamus, brainstem, and reticular system. As a review, the limbic system is involved in survival mechanisms, including frustration, anger-rage-violence continuum, hormonal and immune systems, and long-term memory. Bauman and Kemper (1985) identified smaller neurons and issues with cell density within the limbic system structures of individuals diagnosed as autistic.

Bauman and Kemper (1985) also identified cerebellar irregularities. The cerebellum, which has distinct regions responding to different sets of input, has been found to be 20% to 30% smaller in person's diagnosed with autism. The Purkinje cells, which typically have extensive dendrite trees whose axons go down into the white matter of the cerebellum, are the sole output of the cerebellar cortex. With the diagnosis of autism, however, Purkinje cells have been noted to be fewer in number and have immature axons. The result of these cerebellar findings is pertinent for OT, as information being processed within the cerebellum is compromised secondary to the defects in the Purkinje cells. Additionally, the two hemispheres of the cerebellum are divided by the vermis, which functions as a relay station. The sections of the vermis found to be affected in the autistic population carry information related to visual and vestibular information. Therefore, communication between the two halves of the cerebellum through the vermis regarding visual and vestibular information is compromised.

Frames of Reference

Despite the frame of reference utilized on behalf of the child with an autistic spectrum disorder, any interventionist must always consider the child's role within the environment. Occupational behavior is the basis of our profession. It is imperative that environmental adaptations be completed and opportunities presented so that the child can acquire the skills necessary to meet the demands of the environment. This concept is universal to many frames of reference, based on developmental principles, acquisitional considerations, and coping concepts, so that the child is able to take care of his or her own needs.

The most common intervention strategy for OT staff working with this diagnosis is sensory integration. This approach, developed by Dr. A. Jean Ayres, was outlined for parents in a book titled *Sensory Integration and the Child* (Ayres, 1972). Sensory integration is a clinical frame of reference based on extensive research of normal development, experimental neuroscience, studies with children diagnosed with learning disabilities, concepts on mind-brain-body, and open systems theory. Ayres was the co-founder of Sensory Integration International (SII) in Torrance, CA, a non-profit agency dedicated to research and education, and founder of the Ayres Clinic, purchased by SII after her death. It should be noted that her groundbreaking clinical insights initially met with resistance in the late 1960s. The information, however, eventually altered the way OTs work with children. Sensory integration theory emphasizes the importance of sensory processing as a foundation for learning within all developmental sequences. Ayres developed the Southern California Sensory Integration Test (SCSIT) and was instrumental in the creation and interpretation of the Sensory Integration and Praxis Tests (SIPT), an updated sensory integrative assessment tool developed in the mid 1980s. While these assessment tools are only to be administered by OTs, the results are also valuable for the OTA.

The role of the OTA can be quite extensive within home-, school-, clinic-based therapy and institutional environments. The intricacy of this frame of reference requires intense cooperation between the OT and OTA. The primary emphasis of OT staff working with autistic spectrum disorders would be to educate other team members on the utilization of sensory integrative techniques so that these strategies can be incorporated into everyday experiences (Hanschu, 1997; Wilbarger & Wilbarger, 1991).

Dr. Mary Reilly, an OT, developed a concept of play that has expanded how we value the play experience (Parham & Fazio, 1997). She believed that play gave meaning to the daily life of a child and provided opportunities to learn rules, develop interactions, and form the basis for adult competencies. As clinicians working with a child diagnosed with autism/PDD, the play experiences chosen must provide opportunities for the child to grow and develop socially and emotionally. Within this framework, capitalizing and expanding upon what the child finds intriguing is a useful technique in expanding the child's play sequences as well as motor planning opportunities. As attempts are made to provide an environment in which the play experience is meaningful and accessible for the child on the autistic spectrum, the therapist would need to incorporate sensory integrative components.

Assessment

Within the arena of pediatric practice, the evaluation process for a child on the autistic spectrum is always complex. Due to the fact that the effects are pervasive, as noted in the diagnosis, full team evaluation and intervention planning often occurs, particularly within the educational system. This interdisciplinary approach is often considered to be most appropriate for these children. This section will focus on the assessment tools utilized by OT personnel. Once this information is identified, it can be incorporated into the full team evaluation. As the OTA may in fact be the therapist assigned to this team, full understanding of what assessment tools have been utilized is essential. In addition, if the child is referred for a medically based evaluation, a full team evaluation may not be available. In that case, the OT would assess the child, and the results would be shared with the OTA for collaboration and intervention planning. Therefore, this section is offered to the OTA not only to understand his or her role within this process, but to appreciate the evaluation tools completed by the OT. Please also refer to the chapter regarding the pediatric diagnosis of cerebral palsy for additional information regarding the pediatric evaluation process and the tools utilized under medical and educational scenarios.

Despite the assessment tool identified for use, the OTA can play an integral role in the initial phase of the process. Observations of functional performance within the classroom or home environment would be important to complete. Additionally, conversations with the parent or teacher to determine their concerns regarding the child's performance cannot be emphasized enough. It is the parent and teacher who are part of the child's natural environment and are able to share pertinent information that might not be readily observed by a third party. During these observations, the assistant's knowledge of task analysis is helpful when attempting to identify areas of concern through observation of functional performance. This initial phase of the evaluation process should also include a chart review. It is quite important to review other team members' observations in order to document how areas of deficit noted within those reports impact varying domains of function. For example, if the speech pathologist identifies a language processing disorder, this would impact how the child follows through on commands related to occupational performance. Additionally, this review would also allow the OT staff to gain preliminary information as to where OT concerns might be impacting performance in other domains of functioning. For example, if the OT personnel determine sensitivities to auditory stimulation, this might relate to the teacher reporting that the child retreats to the corner during music class. This information obtained by the OTA should then be shared with the OT as the more formalized stage of the evaluation begins.

With the diagnosis of PDD, the level of severity would impact the assessment procedure chosen. When choosing an assessment tool, it should be remembered that children who are significantly impaired would not be able to complete standardized assessments. In fact, many standardized assessments should not be implemented if a known diagnosis interferes with the child's ability to complete the assessment. If the child is able to attend successfully, understand the directions, follow the commands, and plan his or her responses, a standardized tool might be implemented.

The first area to be assessed should be sensory processing. If standardized assessment tools are possible, the SIPT might be chosen. This assessment, only appropriate for children age 4 to 8 years, 11 months, requires a specialty certification to administer and interpret. The therapist certified to administer this assessment tool would be able to make an educated decision as to whether the tool is appropriate or not. If the child is not able to participate in a standardized procedure, there are several formalized, but nonstandardized, tools focusing on sensory processing. Each of the following tools is designed for a particular age group.

1. The Test of Sensory Functioning in Infants (TSFI), published by Western Psychological Services (WPS) in 1989, is for children birth through 18 months. This tool of quantified observations is helpful if there are concerns noted in the young child.

2. The DeGangi-Berk Test of Sensory Integration (TSI), also published by WPS (1983), was created by the same author as the TSFI but is used for children 3 to 5 years. There is a more formalized scoring of the identified quantified observations, which results in a score classification of normal range, at risk, or deficient. The areas addressed include postural control, bilateral integration, and the influences of residual reflexes.

3. Reisman and Hanschu (1992) created the Sensory Integration Inventory of Individuals with Developmental Disabilities (SII-DD), a formalized questionnaire to identify issues in specific areas of sensory processing. This tool, which is not age specific, is designed as a formalized questionnaire that can be completed by the family or educational staff. The SII-DD is used to identify sensory processing issues which present as behaviors that might interfere with functional participation within the environment. The results of the questionnaire need to be interpreted by the OTR secondary to the complicated and evolving theory of sensory integration.

In addition to the tests of sensory processing, traditional standardized motor assessments could be helpful. These include:
1. Test of Visual Perceptual Skills—Revised (TVPS-R), by Gardner (1996), is a non-motor test assessing seven areas of visual perceptual functioning. There are upper and lower divisions of the test depending on the child's age, 4 to 12 years for lower division and 12 to 17 years, 11 months for upper division.

2. Test of Visual Motor Skills—Revised (TVMS-R), also by Gardner (1995), has upper and lower divisions. The revised test has categories of visual motor functioning, such as intersecting lines, the ability to close or connect designs, angulation, and change of direction of the strokes.

3. The Beery Developmental Test of Visual-Motor Integration (VMI) (Beery, 1997) is another test of visual motor functioning.

4. The Bruininks-Oseretsky Test of Motor Proficiency (BOTMP) (1978) is used for children 4 1/2 years to 14 1/2 years. This tool is useful for assessing underlying skills such as speed and dexterity, upper extremity control, and response speed.

5. Miller and Roid (1994) created the Toddler and Infant Motor Evaluation (TIME), for children 4 months to 3 1/2 years. The intent of the tool is to identify motor delays and deviations in eight domains related to motor abilities. This assessment tool may be useful if the referred child is younger than 4 years and therefore ineligible for most other standardized tools.

6. Peabody Developmental Motor Scales (PDMS) (Folio & Fewell, 1983) is also appropriate for younger children who might not be able to complete other assessment tools. The PDMS is utilized for children birth to 6 years, 11 months.

With the diagnosis of autism, there are numerous occasions when a child appears to possess the motor ability to complete a task, but does not demonstrate the skill within the appropriate context. For example, a child may be noted to climb up on high furniture and balance with extreme precision. However, the child is unable to complete a prerequisite skill of standing on one foot for a specified amount of time. Again, the role of OT would be to assess occupational performance. Therefore, the certified assistant should develop competencies in and be able to implement criterion-referenced assessments. These tools are designed to gain descriptive information of functional domains of performance, outline components of skills which are present or absent, and describe the child's current functioning, while providing guidelines for future skill emergence. During these observations, the OTA should remember to clinically observe sensory processing, including defensiveness, modulation, registration, and integration. If a criterion-referenced tool is used, the OTA may in fact complete most of the data gathering and collaborate with the OT to write up a formal report. The following criterion referenced tools might be appropriate.

1. The Brigance Diagnostic Inventory of Early Childhood Development (Brigance, 1991), a tool for children birth to 6 years, is particularly appropriate for school settings as it allows for other disciplines to complete additional sections related to other domains of functioning. Domains appropriate for OT include fine motor, dressing, and feeding. The certified assistant is able to complete these portions of the evaluation and share the findings with the OTR for analysis and coordination with other assessment findings.

2. The Hawaii Early Learning Profile (HELP), published by the Vort Corp. (1995), outlines skills for two age groups: birth to 3 years and 3 to 6 years. As this evaluation tool provides an in-depth task analysis of all daily living skills (e.g., dressing, feeding, fine motor, and visual motor skills), it is an appropriate tool for the COTA to complete. Again, this tool would be helpful as the child with autism may have the necessary motor skills to complete a task but may not demonstrate active participation in functional activities.

CASE STUDY

Review of Medical Records Pertinent to Educational Intervention

Ethan is a 3-year, 2-month old boy who was referred to the Board of Education. He has received medically based OT services since being diagnosed with PDD at 2 ½ years of age. These services have focused on sensory integrative functioning as the clinic where he receives OT specializes in sensory processing disorders. At the time of the original referral, Ethan was not able to be assessed via standardized measures. The following clinical issues, which will require coordination with the educationally based services, were presented in the medically based OT report.

1. Defensive responses to tactile, vestibular, and auditory inputs. The following definition, noted within the medical report, should be shared with the educational team in order to understand how Ethan may be responding to sensory experiences within the educational environment.

    All of us have a protective system in our bodies that responds to certain sensations that are interpreted as potential danger. For example, touching a hot stove or having a spider crawl on our arm makes us react by quickly removing our arm, getting an internal response of fear or anxiety, or brushing our skin until the "annoying touch" goes away. Certain people, however, have what is termed as "tactile defensiveness," which is an overactivation of this protective sense. These people, due to a misperception of the tactile experience, respond "protectively" to certain touches that most people would not find annoying, noxious, or potentially dangerous. For example, individuals with tactile defensiveness can be described as avoiding, sometimes overactive, emotional, or responding with behavioral outbursts. It is also important to recognize that the literature supports that people who are defensive to tactile stimuli are often sensitive to sights, sounds, movements, tastes, and/or smells. If more than one sensory system is involved, it is termed "sensory defensiveness."

2. Decreased body awareness in space secondary to inefficient proprioceptive processing.

    The proprioceptive system refers to the perception of joint and body movement, as well as position of the body, or body segments, in space. It enables us to check on the spatial orientation of our bodies or body parts in space, the rate and timing of our movements, how much force our muscles are exerting, and how much and how fast a muscle is being stretched. When considering the educational implications, the OT personnel decided that fine motor functioning should be investigated due to the influence that efficient proprioceptive feedback has on the development of fine motor skills.

3. Decreased motor planning skills were identified via clinical observations and parent reports. As the educationally based OT and OTA discussed this issue, it was determined that a functionally based, criterion-referenced assessment tool should be utilized rather than standardized assessment tools.

Educational Assessment and Staff Training

Upon referral to the local school district, Ethan was assessed with the Childhood Autism Rating Scale (CARS) by the special education teacher and the speech language pathologist. This assessment tool, published by Western Psychological Services in 1988, contains several categories including relating to people, imitation, body use, object use, adaptation to change, and responses to sensory experiences. Based on the results, a referral to OT as a related service was completed. A related service is defined as that which is necessary to support the special education instruction. OT, as an educationally based related service, is not intended to be a medical service but rather must be necessary for educational performance. The law that outlined OT services as a related service was written in the early 1970s. Although the laws have been revised, expanded, and redefined since that time, OT has always remained as a related service for the child to benefit from special education.

During the assessment period, the team decided that OT staff should begin training the educational staff based on the information provided by the medically based OT, which also coordinated with the CARS results and preliminary clinical observations within the classroom setting. The following two concerns were focused upon by OT for initial staff training.

1. Sensory defensive responses to tactile, vestibular, and auditory inputs were identified in the medically based report and supported within the CARS results. With reference to intervention, literature supports that this issue needs to be addressed first. Therefore, training was implemented at the earliest opportunity. It was important to emphasize that negative responses to sensory experiences might not be readily apparent to the staff at the moment of occurrence. Defensiveness, which has cumulative effect, can be impacting the individual without being noticed by staff until a dramatic behavioral response is demonstrated. The primary procedure to address defensiveness, called the Wilbarger Protocol (Wilbarger & Wilbarger, 1991), requires strong doses of deep touch pressure followed immediately by quick joint compressions. The Wilbarger Protocol is ideally implemented every 2 hours for maximum effect. The OT staff is responsible for training and monitoring staff implementation of the protocol on a regular basis. Although every 2 hours is ideal, the constraints of a classroom routine may influence this schedule. In an attempt to follow this schedule as closely as possible, the other team members were trained in carrying out the program.

2. Sensory modulation concerns were mentioned within the medically based OT report but not emphasized. This may have been due to the fact that within a one-on-one environment, modulation concerns were not readily apparent. However, within the hustle and bustle of a classroom environment, Ethan's modulation concerns were quite evident. His sensory seeking behaviors appeared to be associated with modulation difficulties. Modulation is the ability to regulate/maintain arousal so that a person can orient, focus attention on meaningful sensory events, and maintain an alert but relaxed state. It is this optimum level of arousal that allows us to function meaningfully within our environment. It was determined by the team observations that Ethan was seeking out sensory experiences which appeared to have an organizing effect. These experiences included movement (e.g., running, rocking, and swinging), as well as proprioceptive input such as pulling, pushing, biting toys, poking his fingers into people, and hiding under the pile of pillows in the reading corner.

It was important to emphasize to the staff that the protocol for defensiveness works best within the context of a sensory program to address modulation. This program, often called a sensory "diet" to reflect the concept of many inputs provided in a well-balanced format, can occur within the natural context of the classroom (Wilbarger & Wilbarger, 1991). Components are not meant to be different from the typical classroom routine. Rather, these components are meant to augment naturally occurring situations. This diet emphasizes the exact types of inputs which Ethan was seeking on his own, but provides the experiences in a more socially appropriate manner. Frequent movement breaks, gross motor tasks, input to muscles and joints, and heavy work experiences are the main components of the sensory diet. This input should occur frequently, some say as often as every hour, to maintain the system in a calm, yet attentive state.

Although a sensory diet is individualized and must be flexible to respond to a child's fluctuating sensory needs, it was important to provide the staff with structured suggestions. The sensory diet outlined for Ethan is exhibited in Figure 12-1. Additionally, based on Ethan's auditory sensitivities, a program of Therapeutic Listening (Frick, 1998) was outlined. This program can be flexible within the educational environment. In addition, it would possibly assist with transitions, another area of concern noted within the CARS results, as it provides grounding and organization.

Child's Name: Ethan W.   Date: September 2000
Therapist: Tara G.

Please implement checked items.

Morning Routine:
☐ Push the car door closed
☐ High five to bus driver upon greeting
☐ Carry heavy object from bus to classroom (object: _____)
☐ Walk around school building (up/down the hills/stairs) while deep breathing
☐ Hold open the school door for the other children
☐ Pull open the classroom door
☐ Vigorous handshake with teacher or assistant when entering classroom
☐ Brisk rub over back by staff while coat is on (remember to ask permission)
☐ Joint compressions (as instructed by therapist) after coat is removed
☐ Shoulder squeezes after coat is removed
☐ Wall push-ups after coat is removed
☐ Remove chairs from on top of the table and put in correct location at table
☐ Errand of pushing cart or pulling the wagon while delivering a message to office
☐ Push something while delivering attendance
☐ Pull a friend in a wagon
☐ Apply wrist or ankle weights
☐ Put on weighted vest

Circle Time:
☐ Drag chairs to and from the circle area
☐ Carry containers with circle time materials to and from circle area
☐ Carry stack of carpet squares to the circle area
☐ Greet each child with a handshake or high five
☐ Play with squeezy ball (or other fidget) while at circle time
☐ Therapy band or Lycra around legs of the chair
☐ Lycra around the trunk of the child to encapsulate
☐ Provide long strokes down back while seated in chair
☐ Provide shoulder/trunk compressions (as instructed by therapist)
☐ If sitting on floor, provide own personal space
☐ If sitting on floor, provide back support
☐ Allow for movement up and down for changing the calendar, etc.
☐ Carry containers to put materials away

Figure 12-1. Sensory diet outlined for Ethan.

Documentation of Educationally Based Services

As with any federally funded program, a legal document must be designed in order to outline the necessary services. Within the school system, the Individualized Education Plan (IEP) is the legal document that addresses the child as part of his or her educational environment (Blossom, Ford, & Cruse, 1996). The IEP is designed by a group identified as the Pupil Planning and Placement Team (PPT). Members of this team include parents, special and regular educators, an administrator, special service providers such as OT personnel, the student if appropriate, and other invited members, which could include an attorney, parent or child advocate, or other parent support. The IEP serves as a tool for measuring progress, ensuring communication, and providing ongoing evaluation of the child.

The IEP, which is updated at least every year, must include the child's current level of educational performance, annual goals, short-term/behavioral objectives, the services required to meet objectives, and criteria to assess whether objectives have been met (AOTA, 1997). It is imperative that the goals and objectives be specifically related to education. Each year, at the annual IEP meeting, the previous goals are measured to determine progress, continued or additional services are decided, and new goals are developed as appropriate. At that time, the roles of the OTR and COTA are to collect data and provide information to the team to assist with discussions and the decision-making process. Throughout each of these phases, the OT staff must remember to translate technical information into educational terms so that interdisciplinary team members can utilize this information effectively.

For Ethan, the delivery of educationally based OT services by a certified assistant is appropriate. In addition to educating the team on sensory strategies, the COTA is able to address the fine motor and daily living concerns found as a result of the criterion-referenced assessment process. The goals and behavioral objectives outlined in Ethan's IEP included:

1. Following the Wilbarger Protocol, Ethan will be able to maintain a seated position for 5 minutes of circle time, for 4 out of 5 consecutive school days.

2. Through the use of a sensory diet and vestibular stimulation, Ethan will sustain eye contact with the speech pathologist during a two-turn reciprocal imitation game, in three out of four consecutive attempts.

3. Through sensory strategies and backward chaining techniques, Ethan will execute all steps of putting on his coat with assistance for zipper engagement, in 4 out of 5 consecutive school days.

4. While sitting at the table with two classmates, Ethan will cut on a line within a ½-inch deviation, in three out of four attempts.

Service Delivery

Through a team discussion, it was decided that the educationally based OT intervention would be delivered within the classroom environment. The parents agreed to this model of service delivery as they valued the idea that the OT staff would function as a role model for the implementation of sensory strategies, as well as assisting the staff with understanding the nonverbal sensory messages demonstrated by Ethan. Additionally, classroom delivery would allow the therapist to address the fine motor, visual motor, and daily living skills as they naturally occur for all of the children.

SUMMARY

The incidence of PDDs, also referred to as autistic spectrum disorders, is on the incline. As practitioners with unique knowledge of sensory processing, we are in a position to positively contribute to the intervention plans for these children. The therapist's ability to facilitate play and motor development, as well as the ability to task analyze and focus on specific skill development, is specifically useful when program planning for the child with PDD. The multiple issues involved, including sensory processing, motor planning, relating to others, and adaptation to change, emphasize the need for intense cooperation between the OT and OTA. Each professional collects specific information with respect to the individual's level of functioning, and collaboration and synthesis is necessary in order to develop a comprehensive plan of action. Several frames of reference are appropriate, some requiring more intensive training than others. For example, the use of sensory integration requires intense and consistent attention on the part of the therapist through professional development opportunities. For this approach, although extensive clinical experience is considered optimal for medically based intervention, educationally based services are more manageable for the assistant. For within the educational environment, occupational behavior predominates and is inherent in the role of the assistant and is the basis of our profession.

CLINICAL PROBLEM-SOLVING

Jenny, a 39-year-old woman, has resided in the state's institution for individuals with mental retardation since she was 25. Her diagnoses include autism, mental retardation, and receptive/expressive receptive language disorder. The institution recently received a state grant to provide augmentative communication devices for 20 clients. The OTA, who had been working with Jenny for the past 6 months utilizing sensory integrative techniques, identified Jenny to the speech language pathologist as a candidate. Based on the observations that Jenny's interactions and relatedness improved following sensory integrative interventions, the OTA felt that this would be an ideal time to require more formalized communication from Jenny. Based on collaboration between the speech pathologist and certified assistant, a simple device requiring Jenny to press a switch with a picture attached was developed. The plan was to train Jenny to press the switch when she wanted more of a desired sensory activity. This was mastered fairly quickly based on its simple cause and effect nature. At that point the device was adapted for two pictures. The intent of this step was for Jenny to identify which activity she wanted based on a choice of two activities. If this was accomplished, the device could be expanded to include more choices. Based on the fact that the sensory input was desired by Jenny, and also had a positive organizing effect, the potential for using a communicative device during these activities was optimum. The OTA would continue to provide sensory possibilities for Jenny, while the speech pathologist would continue to provide access to communication.

Questions for Discussion

- Based on the living environment, what types of sensory diet activities could be outlined for Jenny? Remember, sensory diets include frequent movement breaks and heavy work experiences, which are incorporated into the naturally occurring experiences.
- If you were able to order $500 worth of equipment from the Southpaw catalog, what would you order for Jenny?

William Z., an 8-year-old boy with Asperger's syndrome, was referred for an educationally based OT evaluation. Mrs. Z. indicated difficulties at home which included meltdowns some afternoons, decreased ability to manage family events, and difficulty following verbal instructions. The OT completed three standardized assessments that were mastered at or above age level. Based on the fact that children within the autistic spectrum often possess skills that they are unable to functionally utilize within a more distracting environment, the certified assistant was asked to observe William within his natural environments. The OTA observed William and interviewed his teachers. When discussing the outcomes with the OT, it became apparent that William functioned appropriately within his classroom, art class, physical education, and in the cafeteria, but

he did have some difficulty organizing himself on the playground. While not minimizing Mrs. Z.'s concerns, William did not qualify for educationally based OT services. Strategies to address the playground concerns included outlining the activities in which William should participate, organizing a group game prior to the children going outside, and monitoring and redirection by the playground aide should William appear to be non-productive. At the meeting to discuss the outcome of the evaluation, Mrs. Z. continued to express concerns regarding William's home performance. The school administrator outlined the laws governing educationally based OT and stated that she may wish to consult her pediatrician for a medically based referral. Additionally, although the educational system is not responsible for providing educationally based services, the administrator did agree to providing a sensory diet for use at home. The OTA met with Mrs. Z. to demonstrate the Wilbarger Protocol and emphasized implementation before leaving for school, upon his return from school, and just after dinner time. Additionally, since the fall season provides many opportunities for outdoor activities, Mrs. Z. received a list of suggested activities. These activities included raking, digging up the summer plants, pushing the wheelbarrow around to pick up the fallen twigs, and bagging the leaves. All of these tasks would provide heavy muscle work as well as a variety of head positions to activate the vestibular system.

Questions for Discussion

- What other activities could be suggested as part of an 8-year-old boy's typical afternoon or weekend?
- It was suggested to William's parents that he be enrolled in body oriented, extracurricular activities. The possibilities included swimming, karate, horseback riding, yoga, and gymnastics. What are the sensory experiences in each of these activities that support the sensory diet concepts?

Carlos was 25 years old when he was referred for a medically based OT consultation by the state. The intent of the referral was to determine if OT could diminish Carlos' self-abusive behaviors. The assistant working within the state system had gone to a conference regarding the topic and thought that this might be a worthwhile investigation. Carlos' history included seeking large amounts of vestibular input, whirling himself, obsessing on spinning objects, banging on his ear or head to induce vibratory stimulation, crashing against the furniture, falling or throwing himself on the floor or against the wall, scratching and rubbing his arms and face until they were raw, and excessive mouthing of objects. Additionally, Carlos demonstrated a decreased tolerance of everyday noises such as the hairdryer or vacuum.

The state's OTA had already implemented structural changes within Carlos' day in an effort to help him manage his environment. These strategies included organizing his vocational work environment in zones for different activities, implementing structure and routine to his day, organizing picture card symbols to help him transition from one activity to the next, providing timers to help with preparation with transitions, and minimizing the extraneous stimuli within his environment by setting up his work station in a less distracting part of the work area.

The consulting OT confirmed the OTA's thoughts that sensory integrative strategies were appropriate. The Wilbarger Protocol, the most effective for sensory defensiveness, was shared with the assistant. As part of this program, it was emphasized that the possible fear reactions that Carlos might demonstrate be respected. If someone has functioned in a defensive manner for what could have been the past 25 years, therapy needs to be supportive and not invasive. Therapeutic listening (Frick, 1998) was also outlined for implementation based on Carlos' auditory issues. It was suggested that this program begin prior to the Wilbarger Protocol in order to begin modulating Carlos' level of arousal. In addition to the Wilbarger Protocol and therapeutic listening, the concepts of the sensory diet were discussed based on the assistant's understanding from the seminar. The plan was for the assistant to implement these strategies and call the OT to discuss observations and possible revisions.

Questions for Discussion

- If Carlos spends each day in a workshop setting, identify sensory diet activities that might be appropriate. Remember to include opportunities within self-care, vocational, and maintenance activities.

- Are there any suggestions that could be shared with the transportation staff with regard to noise on the van, seat placement, or the amount of touch provided when assisting Carlos on and off the van?

REFERENCES

American Psychiatric Association. (1994). *Diagnostic and statistical manual for mental disorders* (4th ed.). Washington, DC: Author.

AOTA. (1997). *OT services for children and youth under the Individuals with Disabilities Education Act.* Bethesda, MD: Author.

Ayres, A. J. (1972). *Sensory integration and the child.* Los Angeles, CA: Western Psychological Services.

Bauman, M. L., & Kemper, T. L. (1985). Histoanatomic observations of the brain in early infantile autism. *Neurology, 35,* 866-874.

Bauman, M. L., & Kemper, T. L. (1994). *The neurobiology of autism.* Baltimore, MD: Johns Hopkins University Press.

Beery, K. E. (1997). *The Beery developmental test of visual-motor integration—revised.* Parsippany, NJ: Modern Curriculum Press..

Blossom, B., Ford, F., & Cruse, C. (1996). *Physical therapy and OT in the public schools.* Rome, GA: Rehabilitation Publications and Therapies Inc.

Brigance, A. H. (1991). *Brigance diagnostic inventory of early development—revised.* North Billerica, MA: Curriculum Associates Inc.

Bruininks, R. H. (1978). *Bruininks-Oseretsky test of motor proficiency.* Circle Pines, MN: American Guidance Service.

Cohen, F., & Volkmar, F. R. (1997). *Autism and pervasive developmental disorders: A handbook.* New York, NY: Doubleday.

Courchesne, E., Yeung-Courchesne, R., Press, G. A., Hesselink, J. R., & Jennigan, T. L. (1988). Hypoplasia of vermal lobules VI and VII in autism. *New England Journal of Medicine, 318,* 1349-1354.

DeGangi, G. A., & Berk, R. A. (1983). *DeGangi-Berk test of sensory integration.* Los Angeles, CA: Western Psychological Services.

DeGangi, G. A., & Greenspan, S. (1989). *Test of sensory functioning in infants.* Los Angeles, CA: Western Psychological Services.

Folio, M. R., & Fewell, R. R. (1983). *Peabody developmental motor scales.* Austin, TX: Pro-ed.

Frick, S. (1998). *Listening with the whole body workshop.* Hamden, CT: Author.

Gardner, M. F. (1995). *Test of visual-motor skills—revised.* Hydesville, CA: Psychological and Educational Publications Inc.

Gardner, M. F. (1996). *Test of visual-perceptual skills—revised.* Hydesville, CA: Psychological and Educational Publications Inc.

Hanschu, B. (1997). *Evaluation and treatment of sensory processing disorders.* Bridgewater, NJ: Author.

Kanner, L. (1943). Autistic disturbances of affective contact. *Nervous Child, 2,* 217-250.

Miller, L. J., & Roid, G. H. (1994). *The toddler and infant motor evaluation.* Tucson, AZ: Therapy Skill Builders.

Ornitz, E. M., & Ritvo, E. R. (1968). Neurophsyiologic mechanisms underlying perceptual inconsistency in autistic and schizophrenic children. *Archives of General Psychiatry, 19,* 22-27.

Parham, L. D., & Fazio, L. S. (1997). *Play in OT for children.* St. Louis, MO: Mosby-Year Book Inc.

Petty, L., Ornitz, E. M., Michelman, J. D., & Zimmerman, E. G. (1984). Autistic children who become schizophrenic. *Archives of General Psychiatry, 41,* 129.

Reisman, J., & Hanschu, B. (1992). *Sensory integration inventory—revised for individuals with developmental disabilities.* Hugo, MN: PDP Press.

Rimland, B. (1985). The etiology of infantile autism: The problem of biological versys psychological causation. In A. Donnellan (ed.), *Classic readings in autism.* New York, NY: Teachers College Press.

Ritvo, E. R., Freeman, B. J., Pingree, C., Mason-Brothers, A., Jorde, L., Jenson, W., McMahon, W. M., Petersen, W., Mo, A., & Ritvo, A. (1990). The UCLA - University of Utah epidemiologic survey of autism prevalence. *American Journal of Psychiatry, 146*, 194-199.

Sponheim, E. (1996). Changing criteria of autistic disorders: A comparison of the ICD-10 research criteria and DSM-IV with DSM-III-R, CARS, and ABC. *Journal of Autism and Developmental Disorders, 26*(5), 513.

Vort Corporation. (1995). *HELP checklist*. Palo Alto, CA: Author.

Western Psychological Services. (1983). *The DeGangi-Berk test of sensory integration*. Los Angeles, CA: Author.

Western Psychological Services. (1988). *The childhood autism rating scale*. Los Angeles, CA: Author.

Western Psychological Services. (1989). *The test of sensory functioning in infants*. Los Angeles, CA: Author.

Wilbarger, P., & Wilbarger, J. (1991). *Sensory defensiveness in children ages 2-12: An intervention guide for parents and other caregivers*. Santa Barbara, CA: Avanti Educational Programs.

SUGGESTED READING

AOTA. (1989). *Guidelines for OT services in school systems.* Bethesda, MD: Author.

Blanche, E. I., Botticelli, T. M., & Hallway, M. K. (1995). *Combining neurodevelopmental and sensory integration principles: An approach to pediatric therapy.* Tucson, AZ: Therapy Skill Builders.

Case-Smith, J., Allen, A. S., & Pratt, P. N. (1996). *OT for children.* St. Louis, MO: Mosby-Year Book Inc.

Dunn, W. (1991). *Pediatric OT.* Thorofare, NJ: SLACK Incorporated.

Fisher, A. G., Murray, E. A., & Bundy, A. C. (1991). *Sensory integration: Theory and practice.* Philadelphia, PA: F. A. Davis Co.

Two Preschoolers with Sensory Integration Dysfunction

Chapter 13

Wendy Mueller, MA, OTR/L

WHAT IS SENSORY INTEGRATION?

"The organization of sensation for use"—A. Jean Ayres (1979)

Sensory integration is our unconscious ability to receive incoming information from the various sense organs. Our nervous system sorts the "data," then integrates the new information with our stored memories to generate ideas and to formulate a verbal or motor plan of action. Sensory integration is a function of our central nervous system, which organizes sensory input, channeling useful sensory data into the proper "files" in the brain and filtering out extraneous information, discarding it in the neurological "trash" (Figure 13-1).

Sensory integration is a prerequisite for occupational performance. Sensory integration is so vital to our development that we begin processing movement as early as 8 weeks in utero, and a fetus can respond to sounds as early as 4 1/2 months after conception (Steinbach, 1998). We depend on reliable sensory information to dress ourselves, drive a car, and to learn novel skills, such as in-line skating or surfing the Internet.

It is not known how many people have "perfect" sensory integration. Our individual ability to process and organize sensory information ranges on a continuum from poor to superlative processing abilities.

WHAT IS SENSORY INTEGRATIVE DYSFUNCTION?

Sensory integrative dysfunction, or SID, occurs when an individual's nervous system does not accurately interpret incoming sensory information. This faulty information processing causes the person to have incorrect perceptions of his or her body and world. Based on these misperceptions, the brain attempts to guide the individual's behavior, causing the person with sensory integrative issues to react in unexpected ways to the environment.

An exasperated mother watches in dismay as her toddler who refuses to eat "lumpy" foods pushes the cereal out of his mouth and dumps his baby cereal on the floor. A frustrated preschool teacher gives

---

KEY CONCEPTS

- Sensory integration: Unconscious ability to receive, sort, and utilize incoming information from the various sense organs.
- Sensory integration dysfunction (SID): Occurs when an individual's nervous system does not accurately interpret incoming sensory information.
- Adaptive response: General goal of sensory integrative therapy.
- Sensory integrative therapy treatment protocol: Therapists must formulate goals and select intervention methods appropriate for each individual based on the evaluation.

ESSENTIAL VOCABULARY

Adaptive response: An appropriate, purposeful action to a demand.

Auditory defensiveness: Hypersensitivity to sound.

Dyspraxia: Poor tactile, vestibular, and proprioceptive processing; makes it difficult to plan, coordinate, or sequence motor movements.

Gravitational insecurity: Over-response to gravity/movement.

Ideation: Ability to formulate responses to incoming environmental information.

Impaired auditory processing: Difficulty utilizing auditory information efficiently and effectively.

Motor planning: Ability to perform a novel/unfamiliar task.

Olfactory defensiveness: Sensitivity to odors.

Praxis: Action based on will.

Proprioception: Information the brain receives from the muscles and joints.

Sensory defensiveness: Sensitivity to more than one type of sensory input.

Sequencing: Performing tasks in the correct order.

Tactile defensiveness: Tactile information sensitivity.

Visual defensiveness: Hypersensitivity to visual information.

Matthew his fifth time out of the morning for biting and hitting other children when they come near him. She remembers the days when she was a child and thinks a "conversation" with a paddle would fix this problem. Mrs. Algebra raises her voice as she repeats the question to Jessie for the third time. She thinks to herself, "This child is not just orbiting another planet, she's in a different galaxy." Anne breaks out into a cold sweat as she hears her husband tell her the only way she can get to the location of her corporate luncheon is to take the busy eight-lane freeway. How will she arrive in one piece? All of these individuals probably suffer from SID.

WHO "INVENTED" THE THEORY OF SENSORY INTEGRATION?

A. Jean Ayres was an OT who earned a doctorate in educational psychology and completed post-doctoral work at the Brain Research Institute at UCLA. She is the founder of sensory integrative theory. Her book *Sensory Integration and the Child* (1979) explains the basic tenets of sensory integration theory and treatment. Many researchers, included in the reference section, have built upon Dr. Ayres' work, further establishing the efficacy of the use of sensory integrative principles to treat people plagued with a wide variety of medical diagnoses, including learning disabilities, autistic spectrum disorder, and schizophrenia.

WHAT ARE THE COMPONENTS OF THE SENSORY PROCESSING SYSTEM?

In an attempt to be concise and clear, this explanation vastly oversimplifies the complexity of the nervous system. It is important to understand that each system has multiple branches that connect it to other parts of the peripheral and central nervous systems. For example, the auditory system has connections to the vestibular system, the reticular formation, the cerebellum, the temporal lobe, and the parietal lobe of the brain (Frick & Lawton-Shirley, 1994).

The tactile, auditory, vestibular, proprioceptive, visual, olfactory, and gustatory systems are the primary receptor centers for various types of sensory information. These systems transport messages via nerves to other peripheral sensory receptors, the brainstem, cerebellum, and the cerebral cortex. The cortex then forwards a verbal or motor plan of action to the muscles and joints guiding our behavior in the environment (Frick & Lawton-Shirley, 1994). A description of the basic functions of each system is outlined below.

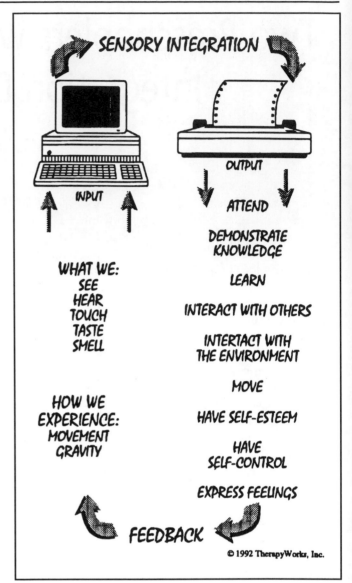

Figure 13-1. Sensory integration flowchart. (Reprinted with permission from Williams, M. S., & Shellenberger, S. (1996). *"How does your engine run?" A leader's guide to the alert program for self-regulation.* Albuquerque, NM: TherapyWorks Inc.)

The tactile system is responsible for gathering "touch" information. We have two different types of touch perception. The first type is protective touch, which allows us to determine if a stimulus is painful and to identify the temperature of a stimulus. We rely on our protective touch to warn us if a stove is hot or to register pain if a bee stings us on the arm.

The second type of touch is discriminative touch. This type of touch enables us to reach into our purse and know by feel if we have grasped our keys or our sunglasses. Discriminative touch gives us the ability to write while listening to a lecture without having to look at the movements of our pen in order to ensure we are recording the words we hear. We know what words are on the page due to our intact discriminative touch pathways.

The auditory system not only registers incoming sounds, it also relays these combinations of sound to the brain where sequences of sounds are translated into words and assigned meaning. The auditory system is closely connected to the vestibular system.

The vestibular system is located in the inner ear behind the cochlea and oval window, two key structures of the auditory center. The vestibular system is responsible for detecting our body position in space and where we are in relation to gravity. The vestibular system influences muscle tone and helps us maintain balance, coordinate the movements of the right and left sides of the body (bilateral coordination), and identifies the source of movement. For example, our vestibular system notifies us if we are hanging upside down from the monkey bars, spinning on a merry-go-round, or beginning to fall out of a chair. It also lets us know our body's location in relationship to the wall, table, or our textbooks scattered across the floor.

The vestibular system works in conjunction with the proprioceptive system. The word *proprioception* comes from the Latin word "proprius," meaning "one's own" (Ayres, 1979). Proprioception is the information our brain receives from the muscles and joints. Proprioception allows us to determine where each body part is in space, how fast it is moving, the direction in which it is moving, and the force of the motion. For example, proprioception gives us the ability to drink from a cup without looking in a mirror. We are able to guide the cup to our mouth, and miraculously, if all goes well, we do not miss our mouth or spill liquid on ourselves.

Although the vestibular and proprioceptive systems play an integral role in both motor coordination and in maintaining static or dynamic balance, we would have difficulty catching a frisbee without the assistance of our visual system. Many people think of vision in terms of acuity, which is "the eyes' ability to resolve detail, an exceedingly important skill for correctly identifying information..." (Gentile, 1997, p. 136). In actuality our eyes perform many complex movements and play a role in visual perception.

Ocular movements, including visual tracking, accommodation, and convergence, allow us to perform such tasks as reading text without moving our head, looking from the blackboard to our paper, or catching a ball.

Visual perception includes many skills, including directionality, figure ground perception, and visual form constancy. Directionality allows us to determine where our body or an object is in space and gives us the ability to utilize spatial concepts in language such as front, back, right, left. Figure ground perception helps us find our shoes in a cluttered room or to locate a needed textbook on our bookshelf. Visual form constancy assists us in recognizing that the "B" in the word "ball" is the same letter as the "B" in the word "boring."

Our sense of smell, the olfactory sense, detects odors that the brain interprets as noxious, pleasant, or neutral. Smell assists us in identifying people and in orienting ourselves in our environment. For example, you can predict your dad is coming down the stairs because you smell his aftershave, or you can tell when you are nearing your favorite pizza parlor before it comes into view as the scent of baking pepperoni wafts to your eager nose from around the corner. We are warned of fire by the smell of smoke filling the air. Smell is linked to taste. Anyone who has had a cold knows your appetite is diminished, because with nasal congestion, food just does not "taste" the same due to our inhibited olfactory function.

The sense of taste performs the valuable function of alerting us to the difference between a chocolate sundae and liver. Additionally, it plays a role in advancing our physical growth, as taste contributes to our willingness to expand our diet to include a wide repertoire of foods essential to physical growth and brain development.

How Do These Sensory Systems Interact with the Other Performance Components?

Hopefully, it is now evident to the reader that the sensory systems exchange information and collaborate with the central nervous system to enable us to perform the various activities required to fulfill our roles as occupational beings.

This section of the chapter will give a brief description of each performance component and examples of how individuals rely on these skills to perform the "job" of living.

Postural control involves muscle tone, balance, and the coordination of various reflexes. Our bodies constantly shift position in response to the forces of gravity, imposed movement, and changes in our muscle strength (e.g., muscle fatigue). If someone comes up behind us and tips our chair backward, our postural control mechanisms pull us upright and prevent us from hitting our head on the floor.

Body scheme is our internal "map" of the characteristics of each body part, the location of each body part in relation to the rest of the body, and a "file" of all of the movements made by each body part. When you play the game Twister, you are able to distinguish your left arm from your right foot because of your intact body scheme even though they may not be in their usual place.

Bilateral coordination is the ability to coordinate the movements of both sides of the body as well as the motions of the upper and lower extremities. Skills necessitating bilateral coordination include skipping, swimming, and riding a bicycle.

Eye-hand coordination requires the visual, vestibular, and proprioceptive systems to coordinate information to enable us to type, hit a tennis ball, or flip pancakes.

Oral-motor skills serve us from infancy. We coordinate sucking, swallowing, and breathing to drink from a bottle and to speak our first word. As we mature, oral-motor skills become increasingly complex to allow us to drink from a straw, blow bubbles with gum, and whistle our favorite tune.

How Is Sensory Integration Related to Occupational Performance?

Armed with our sensory processing system, we are equipped to act in the environment. Our brain filters and prioritizes incoming sensory stimuli, directing our attention to the most salient information and giving us the ability to concentrate on the task at hand.

The brain works with all of the sensory systems to achieve praxis. Praxis means "action based on will" and comes from the Greek words for "doing, acting, deed, practice" (Fisher, Murray, & Bundy, 1991). Praxis has three components: ideation, motor planning, and sequencing. Ideation is the ability to formulate responses to incoming environmental information; this may include answering a question, deciding our next move in a game of chess, or strategizing a hiding place in a game of hide-and-seek. Motor planning is our ability to perform a novel or unfamiliar task, such as completing a puzzle you have never seen before, learning to ski, or learning to write in cursive in second grade. Sequencing is the process of performing tasks in the correct order (e.g., tying shoes or pronouncing an unfamiliar word).

Without praxis, we would not be able to verbally express our thoughts or to cook a meal. We rely on praxis to help us in social situations and learn the West Coast Swing dance. Sensory processing is critical to our ability to regulate emotion and attention in various environmental contexts. Without sensory integration, we would be unable to perform the ADLs required to fulfill our life roles of child, student, parent, or OTA.

What Are the "Symptoms" of SID?

Sensory integration has received criticism from some individuals because there is no biological testing available to provide concrete diagnostic "proof" that a neurological issue exists. OTs determine the presence of SID through the use of clinical observations, standardized testing, parent report, and from information supplied by others involved with the individual's care (e.g., teacher, day care worker, etc.).

There are many suspected causes of SID, including premature birth; an anoxic episode before, during, or after birth; chronic otitis media (recurrent ear infections); or institutionalization in an underdeveloped nation's orphanage. In many cases, the cause of SID is unknown. Many parents report they experienced similar difficulties during their own childhood, but in many instances, their issues did not interfere with their performance to the degree that SID is now affecting their child at school and/or at home.

Because SID may affect any of the sensory systems we have discussed in this chapter, its manifestations vary from one individual to the next. As we look at the signs of sensory processing issues for each sensory area, keep in mind that an individual may present with processing difficulties in one or more of the sensory areas.

Tactile

There are two primary types of tactile processing problems. In one instance, the nervous system perceives touch as an uncomfortable or noxious stimulus. Tactile input includes imposed or unexpected touch and certain textures of food, clothing, or objects. The nervous system may trigger an autonomic response in the person, causing him or her to demonstrate a "fight, fright, or flight" response to tactile input. A fight, fright, or flight reaction may include physically aggressive behavior toward one's self or others, yelling, crying, or hiding. Older children may use critical or avoident language to hide feelings of anxiety or fear toward a given situation or activity. Sensitivity to tactile information is known as tactile defensiveness.

Individuals with tactile defensiveness may demonstrate any of the following behaviors: a preference to remove shoes and socks as soon as possible; complaints of discomfort due to clothing labels, seams, or the texture of a fabric; avoidance of "messy" media including sand, finger paint, or glue; unusually high or low tolerance to pain; avoidance of certain foods; physically aggressive behavior toward others (e.g., pinching, hitting, biting); and/or avoidance of group activities which place people in close proximity to one another. Tactile defensiveness may fluctuate in its severity, and, therefore, the individual may not demonstrate the same reaction to identical stimuli from one moment to the next.

A second type of tactile processing problem occurs when an individual's nervous system does not accurately register tactile information. In this instance, people typically exhibit a decreased, delayed, or absent reaction to tactile sensations. Poor tactile discrimination contributes to motor dyspraxia and visual-perceptual deficits because the individual is unable to identify the temporal-spatial qualities of tactile stimuli (Fisher et al., 1991). Signs of impaired tactile perception include a tendency to mouth toys or objects beyond expected age ranges, a decreased

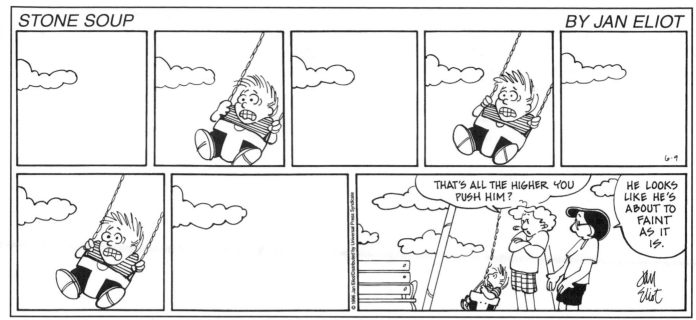

Figure 13-2. Comic strip depicting gravitational insecurity. (Stone Soup © 1996 Jan Elliot. Reprinted with permission from Universal Press Syndicate. All rights reserved.)

response to pain, messy eating, illegible handwriting, and difficulty manipulating buttons, snaps, or zippers.

Auditory

Impaired auditory processing results in the individual having difficulty utilizing auditory information efficiently and effectively. A person with auditory processing deficits may exhibit the following: deficits in sound discrimination (e.g., distinguishing "buh" from "duh"), poor auditory attention, limitations in auditory memory, difficulty with spelling/phonics, poor auditory sequencing, difficulties with selective listening, poor sound articulation, and an oversensitivity to certain sounds. Examples include a child who does not respond to the teacher's verbal directions or the child who pronounces the word gloves as "glubs" and when corrected states, "I did say that."

A child with hypersensitivity to sound may begin to cry when attending the circus and beg to go home. Another child with auditory defensiveness may cover his or her ears and complain that the humming of the fluorescent lights sounds like "bumblebees." Some individuals with auditory defensiveness report they are able to hear the blood rushing through their ears or that they can hear their heartbeat, causing them to become distracted at times during the day or to have difficulty falling asleep at night. Some children are so sensitive to sound that they resort to "shutting down" and filtering out the majority of incoming auditory information. These individuals may appear to have a hearing loss because their response to auditory information is very inconsistent. The therapist will refer a person for an audiological assessment when the status of the individual's hearing is in question.

Vestibular

As with tactile perception, one's nervous system can over or under respond to gravity and movement. People who experience gravitational insecurity "have an excessive emotional reaction to vestibular sensations even when there is no danger of falling..." (Ayres, 1979, p. 83). Individuals with gravitational insecurity are fearful of movement they cannot control (e.g., sliding, swinging, or spinning). These individuals are frequently anxious when descending the stairs or riding an escalator. They often experience motion sickness during movement-based activities. Gravitational insecurity is not imagined. It is the result of a "malfunction" of the internal structures of the vestibular system. An example of a child with gravitational insecurity is depicted in (Figure 13-2).

Another form of faulty vestibular system processing is known as an under-reactive vestibular system. People who crave vestibular input require a strong or prolonged stimulus to register movement information. Movement seekers may jump on furniture, "crash" into other people or objects, deliberately fall, fidget in their chair, and spin or swing for a long time without becoming dizzy.

Proprioception

People with impaired proprioceptive processing have difficulty performing coordinated movements and typically have decreased awareness of their body position in space. As a result, they may slump or slide in a chair, toe walk, bump into walls or door frames, step on toys on the

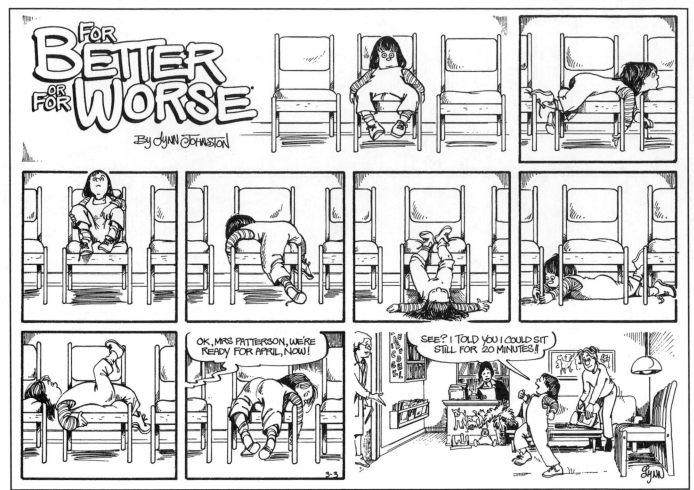

Figure 13-3. Comic strip depicting impaired proprioceptive processing. (Reprinted with permission from © Lynn Johnston Productions Inc./Dist. by United Feature Syndicate, Inc.)

floor, break the tips of pencils or crayons, or hold a pencil or crayon in a "vise" grip. To gain more proprioceptive information, people with decreased proprioceptive processing invent "excuses" to move including repeatedly asking to use the restroom or to get a drink of water. Adults with proprioceptive issues may frequent the water cooler or the vending machines.

An example of a child with impaired proprioceptive processing is depicted in Figure 13-3.

Vision

Visual defensiveness is a hypersensitivity to visual information that, usually in conjunction with other sensory processing deficits, causes the child to appear hyperactive and distractible. Because the child cannot ignore the noises, lights, and confusion of many people doing different things in the environment, he or she may not be able to perform to potential.

Individuals with visual defensiveness may avoid making eye contact with others. One child reported, "I see the colors of your eyes moving, and it makes me dizzy."

As discussed previously in this chapter, visual spatial skills help us determine directionality, complete puzzles, read, write, dress ourselves, drive, and use directional concepts in language. Many children who cannot identify left, right, up, down, front, back on themselves cannot verbally describe the relationship of one object to another.

For example, Katie attended a 4-year-old preschool class. At the first parent/teacher conference, Katie's teacher told her mother that Katie was very bright but seemed "dazed" at times. Katie's mother was startled and asked the teacher for an example. The teacher commented that when she directed Katie to the bookshelf on the right side of the room she would notice Katie wandering the left side of the room searching for the bookcase.

Olfactory

People with olfactory defensiveness are sensitive to odors. They may avoid people and appear "stand-offish" due to their inability to tolerate the scent of perfume, soap, or deodorant. Some people are so sensitive to smell they will gag or vomit in response to a specific scent. For example, my 4-year-old friend Josh gagged when he smelled parmesan cheese, preventing his family from eating in pizza places or Italian restaurants.

Some people who are hypo-responsive to olfactory stimulation report they like the smell of gasoline or smoke. They may not react to noxious odors such as sulfur and frequently report they cannot "taste" foods unless they are spicy or indicate all foods taste the same.

Gustatory

Oral defensiveness is hypersensitivity in the mouth that causes people to experience great discomfort or excessive gagging/vomiting when they encounter certain food textures or oral hygiene implements.

If a person is hypo-responsive to taste, he or she may crave hot or spicy food. Many individuals with a dulled sense of taste will put ketchup or salsa on everything or ask to suck on slices of lemon. They may drink pickle juice or lemon juice straight from the jar or bottle in attempts to "wake up" their sense of taste.

Sensory Defensiveness

If an individual has a tendency to experience a fight, flight or fright response to more than one type of sensory input, he or she has what is known as sensory defensiveness. For example, a person who is irritated by background noise and is fearful of escalators, elevators, or moving sidewalks has both auditory defensiveness and an overly responsive vestibular system.

Sensory defensiveness may cause individuals to misperceive the world as dangerous, alarming, or at the very least, irritating (Wilbarger & Wilbarger, 1991). People with sensory defensiveness may carefully construct their daily routine to avoid anxiety-provoking sensory events. An incident most people would consider trivial might cause extreme stress or anxiety for a person with sensory defensiveness. Their behavior may appear odd to others as they attempt to gain a sense of security in what they perceive as a threatening and unpredictable world.

Dyspraxia

If a child has poor tactile, vestibular, and proprioceptive processing, it is difficult for him or her to plan, coordinate, or sequence motor movements. This condition is known as dyspraxia. Children with dyspraxia have difficulty learning new skills. They gain skills by practicing a task over and over until they have memorized the necessary steps. Many children with dyspraxia have average to above average intelligence. They are very resourceful and develop elaborate coping strategies to "survive." These compensatory techniques may include avoiding tasks perceived as challenging or learning "splinter" skills in order to fit in

socially. Others may cope by down-playing the effect dyspraxia has on their lives (e.g., "Hopscotch is for babies").

EVALUATION OF SID

As discussed previously in this chapter, OTs evaluate a person's sensory processing abilities by reviewing sensory checklists, performing standardized testing, clinical observations, and by interviewing the individual or the individual's caregivers. An OT may perform a home or school visit to gather additional information about a child or if there is a reported difference in the person's sensory processing abilities and/or performance from one setting to the other.

OTs can elect to become certified in administering the Sensory Integration and Praxis Tests (SIPT). Developed by Dr. Ayres (1984), the SIPT has 17 subtests that evaluate various sensory processing abilities, including visual perception, static/dynamic balance, auditory processing, praxis, and tactile perception. The certification process includes courses dedicated to the theory and treatment principles of sensory integration. Three segments of the five-course series cover the administration, interpretation, and scoring of the SIPT.

Assessment instruments other than the SIPT that an OT may utilize to evaluate a person's sensory integrative abilities include the Sensory Profile (1999) by Winnie Dunn, PhD, the Balzer-Martin preschool screening (1992), the Test of Sensory Function in Infants (DeGangi & Greenspan, 1998), the Test of Developmental Visual-Motor Integration (VMI) (Beery, 1997), and the Draw-a-Person test (Goodenough & Harris, 1963). There are also a large number of sensory processing checklists therapists use to collect information from parents or teachers.

TREATMENT PLAN FOR INDIVIDUALS WITH SID

The general goal of sensory integrative therapy is to facilitate an adaptive response, which is "a purposeful, goal-directed response to a sensory experience... or environmental demand" (Ayres, 1979, p. 6).

No two people with SID are alike. Therapists must formulate goals and select intervention methods appropriate for each individual. Therefore, there is no "standard" sensory integration treatment protocol. It is critical that the OT closely monitor the person's response to each activity to modify the intervention plan as needed. To illustrate the variations in sensory integrative treatment, two case studies are detailed below.

The case studies include medical and developmental histories for each child. Early childhood literature emphasizes that people develop at various rates and that "milestones" are achieved within an age range vs. at a specific chronological age. For the purposes of these case studies, an expected age is given for some of the major developmental milestones. These ages are guidelines, but certainly are not absolutes in terms of expected times a child should perform a specific skill.

The average age for a child to sit independently is 6 months. A child is able to crawl at approximately 8 months of age. The average age for both walking independently and use of single words is 12 months of age.

Both case studies feature medical histories and sensory profiles common to children with SID. The cases are fictional and do not resemble an actual individual case.

Case Study 1: Johnny Doe

Johnny Doe is a 4-year, 6-month-old child referred for an OT assessment due to concerns regarding his sensory processing abilities and motor skill development.

Mrs. Doe reported Johnny was born 4 days early and was delivered vaginally. Johnny's family history includes an aunt and uncle with speech language difficulties.

Johnny's early childhood medical history is significant for chronic otitis media his first 2 years of life and frequent upper respiratory infections. His hearing is within normal limits. Per parent report, developmental milestones were achieved within expected age ranges with Johnny crawling at 4 months of age, sitting independently at 6 months of age, and walking independently at 13 months of age. Johnny has received speech language therapy since he was 2 years of age due to a severe expressive/receptive language disorder.

Mrs. Doe reported Johnny is a selective eater who prefers bland, soft foods such as cheese pizza, chicken fingers, and spaghetti with no sauce.

Mrs. Doe expressed concerns regarding Johnny's difficulty following directions and his tendency to be "forgetful." She gave the example of Johnny placing his sippy cup on the table in the den and being unable to find it "2 minutes later." She reported Johnny cannot find shoes or toys even if he just finished playing with them a short time ago. He has difficulty answering questions and does not join in with the other children in school. He becomes "terrified and nervous if we suggest arranging a play date."

Johnny's teachers note he has difficulty with cutting and handwriting. He is unable to remember the letters of the alphabet but is very good with formboard puzzles.

Johnny's sensory processing abilities were assessed utilizing a sensory history questionnaire. His motor skills were evaluated using two standardized tests: the Peabody Developmental Motor Scales (PDMS) (Folio & Fewell, 1983) and the VMI.

The PDMS is an assessment of gross and fine motor skills standardized on children from birth to 83 months of age. The PDMS divides the gross and fine motor scales into subtests.

The gross motor scale has five subtests: reflexes, balance, nonlocomotor, locomotor, and receipt/propulsion. The nonlocomotor subtest evaluates the child's ability to lift his or her head, arms, and legs against gravity. The locomotor subtest assesses skills such as crawling, walking, running, and jumping. The receipt/propulsion subtest evaluates eye-hand-foot coordination, including kicking and throwing a ball.

The fine motor scale has four subtests: grasp, hand use, eye-hand coordination, and manual dexterity. The grasp subtest assesses the child's prehension patterns, such as use of a tip-to-tip pincer grasp to pick up a Cheerio or use of a tripod grasp to hold a pencil. The hand use subtest evaluates the child's object manipulation skills. The eye-hand coordination subtest looks at the child's performance of pre-writing tasks such as cutting with scissors and copying shapes. The manual dexterity task assesses the child's ability to perform tasks utilizing both hands simultaneously.

The PDMS gives both a gross and fine motor age equivalent score. It also gives a percentile rank and a standard deviation determined by comparing the child's score to the normative data. As a point of reference, a score equal to or greater than minus two standard deviations below the mean indicates that 98% of children the same age scored higher on the PDMS than the child participating in the assessment.

Based on the results of the OT assessment, Johnny presented with:

- Tactile and oral defensiveness
- Poor tactile discrimination
- Impaired proprioceptive processing
- Decreased visual tracking
- Visual perceptual deficits
- Impaired auditory processing
- A hypo-reactive vestibular system
- Dyspraxia
- Decreased upper and lower extremity muscle strength
- Decreased balance
- Impaired bilateral coordination
- Decreased oral-motor strength and coordination

At a chronological age of 54 months, Johnny achieved an age equivalent score of 32 months on the PDMS gross motor subtest. This score was in the second percentile for his age and was greater than two standard deviations below the mean. He achieved an age equivalent score of 44 months on the PDMS fine motor subtest. This score was in the first percentile for his age and was greater than two standard deviations below the mean.

The VMI is a 27-item test designed to evaluate visual-motor integration. It is 'normed' for children 3 through

18 years of age. The test results yield a standard score, a percentile rank, and an age equivalent

On the VMI, Johnny's perceptual age equivalent was less than 3 years. His standard score was 83. The mean standard score on the VMI is 100 plus or minus 15. His score was in the 13th percentile for his age.

Based on the assessment results, recommendations included OT three times per week, implementation of an intensive daily home program, continued speech language intervention, and a vision examination due to his visual tracking/visual perceptual difficulties.

Goals for treatment included:

- Normalizing Johnny's response to tactile input including unexpected touch and tolerating glue, sand, or finger paint on hands and tags/labels in clothing.
- Expanding Johnny's diet to include mixed texture foods (e.g., yogurt with fruit), chewy foods (e.g., meat other than chicken nuggets), and vegetables.
- Improved gradation of movement and improved tactile discrimination as evidenced by applying an appropriate degree of pressure on the page when writing, completing seat work or homework without complaints of hand "cramping" due to holding the pencil too tightly, and improved letter formation.
- Improved oculomotor control and visual perception as evidenced by his ability to copy from a blackboard in a timely manner, find a desired object in a cluttered room, and perform age-appropriate dressing skills.
- Accurately sequence multi-step tasks.
- Hold a pencil with an age-appropriate grasp pattern.
- Alternate feet when descending stairs.
- Walk six consecutive steps on a balance beam.
- Skip.
- Ride a bike with training wheels.

A typical treatment session includes a "warm-up" period of vestibular/proprioceptive activities and oral-motor activities. The purpose of these activities is to increase Johnny's organization of behavior and postural control. Favorite activities are jumping into a large ball pool to find hidden small toys or swinging prone in a hammock using a reacher to grab small Koosh balls. The reacher/Koosh ball activity also involves upper extremity strength and eye-hand coordination.

After approximately 10 to 15 minutes of this preparatory work, Johnny typically engages in upper extremity strengthening activities such as finding coins in putty, cutting putty with scissors to make "pizza" or "cookies," wheelbarrow races, making mazes with a hole punch, or popping bubbles with a trigger sprayer. The last portion of the session typically focuses on visual perceptual activities including dot-to-dot or seek-and-find puzzles, balloon volleyball, "I Spy" games, or non-formboard puzzles.

Johnny participates in individual OT three times per week for 1 hour per session. One of his treatment sessions is a therapeutic horseback riding group. Johnny's aunt, who is his primary caretaker, implements an OT home program for 30 minutes to an hour each day. Per his therapist's recommendation, Johnny also participates in individual swimming lessons, vision therapy to address difficulties with visual tracking, and gymnastics.

After 3 months of intervention, Johnny's mother and aunt report he is now dressing himself independently. He is "keeping better track of his things" and is "becoming much more social." His aunt commented, "He left my side at a birthday party and didn't check in with me for over an hour—that's huge." He is now asking for cut-color-paste workbooks and is "doing more" on the playground. He is beginning to ask to have people over to play. His articulation has improved "more with 3 months of OT than in the past year of speech therapy." His family also notes his ability to follow directions "the first time we ask" has "greatly improved."

Case Study 2: Maya Mueller

Maya is a 3-year, 1-month-old child referred for a speech language and OT assessment by her pediatrician due to concerns regarding Maya's communication and motor skill development.

The Muellers moved to the United States 10 years ago from a foreign country. They reported it was difficult for them to seek "outside" help for Maya, due to the differences in the cultures. They stated they chose the evaluating OTs based on recommendations from family friends.

Mrs. Mueller reported Maya was born at 38 1/2 weeks gestational age after a 17-hour labor via Cesarean section delivery due to fetal distress.

Maya began to babble between 9 and 12 months of age and began using jargon at 2 years of age. Mrs. Mueller reported Maya currently does not have any true words in her expressive vocabulary. She makes her needs and preferences known by gesturing, crying, or vocalizing.

Maya sat independently at 6 months of age, crawled independently between 6 and 7 months of age, and began to walk independently at 12 months of age.

In response to questions regarding Maya's oral-motor skill development, Mrs. Mueller reported Maya is a selective eater whose diet has become progressively limited. At the time of the assessment, Maya was eating white rice and crackers. She would also drink juice and water. She avoids "any foods that require a lot of chewing, such as pizza." Mrs. Mueller reported Maya used to eat anything and that she was desperate to "get Maya to eat again." The family is vegetarian per custom.

In response to questions regarding Maya's social-emotional development, Mrs. Mueller indicated Maya enjoys swinging and listening to books. She is easily distracted and does not "stick with" an activity longer than a few seconds. She likes letters, Barney, and spinning objects in her hands. Maya prefers to play with her parents and cries when in the company of family friends or in a crowded environment. The Muellers stated they no longer go to friend's homes because "as soon as we pull into the driveway, Maya begins to scream and does not stop until we return home." She typically ignores other children.

Mr. and Mrs. Mueller indicated they had been concerned about Maya for the past 6 months. They brought their concerns regarding Maya's lack of speech to Maya's pediatrician at her 1-year-old checkup. Her pediatrician recommended the Muellers "wait a few more months for Maya's language to develop."

The Muellers began to talk with friends sharing their concerns about Maya's development. At the advice of family friends, whose child was similar to Maya, the Muellers took Maya to their home country for several months. The friends had told the Muellers that their child had begun to talk after spending 2 months "at home."

The Muellers kept extending their stay in their home country hoping Maya would begin to speak. They returned to the United States and made another appointment with the pediatrician. She then referred the Muellers for speech language therapy. The speech language pathologist, after speaking with the Muellers by phone, persuaded them to bring Maya for a joint occupational and speech language therapy assessment.

The Muellers had enrolled Maya in a church preschool program, hoping the "social exposure" would alleviate her "anxiety toward other children." Mrs. Mueller said the teachers called her the first morning wondering if "it was okay for Maya to sit in the corner and spin puzzle pieces." They told Mrs. Mueller if anyone "got near her she screamed." After Maya's fourth day, the school told Mrs. Mueller that Maya was not ready for school and suggested they bring her back next year.

When asked to complete a sensory history questionnaire, Mrs. Mueller stated, "I tried, but it was just too overwhelming." The therapists gathered information about Maya through clinical observations and parent interview. Although reluctant to utilize standardized testing with Maya, the therapists were forced to, as the insurance company required a report including "age equivalent and percentile scores."

When asked specific questions from the sensory questionnaire, Mrs. Mueller indicated Maya was reluctant to walk barefoot on the grass her first 18 months of life, that she never plays in her food, dislikes smooth or creamy foods, and never "gets into anything in the house." Mrs. Mueller remarked, "I've never had to baby proof my house. Maya has never tried to open a cabinet or drawer." Mrs. Mueller expressed concerns regarding Maya's refusal to use a spoon or fork. When presented with a utensil at meals, Maya would throw it on the floor and eat with her hands.

The OT presented Maya with toys from the PDMS in order to gain the needed information for the insurance company. Maya's scores on the PDMS were affected by her limited interest in the OT and in many of the test items.

The examiners had a great deal of difficulty engaging Maya in any type of reciprocal verbal or play exchange. She would briefly look at one of the examiners and would tolerate hand-over-hand assistance to perform a motor activity such as stacking rings but would quickly walk away from the task or go to her mother for a hug.

Maya was noted to utilize "avoidance techniques" such as hugging her mother, crying, or walking away from the examiners. She participated in a maximum of one back-and-forth exchange.

Maya preferred to spin objects in her hands and to swing. She began to jump in place with her head angled downward and flapping her hands at the sight of the swing. Mrs. Mueller reported Maya "does that when she is excited or stressed." When asked how frequently Maya spins objects at home, Mrs. Mueller indicated Maya will "spin toys for hours."

At a chronological age of 37 months, Maya achieved an age equivalent score of 22 to 23 months on the PDMS fine motor scale. This score was in the first percentile for children Maya's age. The score was greater than two standard deviations below the mean.

Clinical observations made during the assessment were helpful in determining the underlying factors affecting Maya's performance. She switched hand use at midline, an indicator of decreased bilateral integration, a function of the vestibular system.

Maya held the crayon in an immature pronated grasp. A pronated grasp is when the child holds the crayon in the fist with the thumb angled downward. We would expect a child to demonstrate an emerging tripod grasp pattern between 36 and 41 months of age. Maya's continued use of a pronated grasp was most likely due to decreased hand muscle strength.

Maya had limited interest in coloring. She scribbled briefly on the paper. Although she did observe the therapist make vertical lines on the page, she made no attempts to copy the therapist. After observing the therapist, she walked away and began to wander around the room. She then picked up a small block she had brought with her from the lobby and began to spin it rapidly in her hands.

Maya's gross motor skills were screened utilizing portions of the PDMS gross motor subtest. Maya was unable to catch a tossed ball thrown directly to her by her mother. She watched her mother instead of the ball and appeared startled when the ball entered her visual field.

This reaction suggested decreased visual tracking. Maya threw the ball by dropping it with two hands, indicating decreased motor planning.

Maya was unable to imitate a skip and could not pedal a tricycle. She straddled the balance beam with her feet, but her mother reported Maya was able to walk a wide high beam in her gymnastics class. Her performance of these tasks suggested decreased vestibular/proprioceptive processing with subsequent difficulty in the areas of bilateral coordination and motor planning. Her inability to generalize a skill she had mastered in a different setting is typical of a child with dyspraxia.

The therapists performed an oral examination due to concerns regarding Maya's limited diet. During the examination, she vigorously resisted intra-oral stimulation. Mrs. Mueller reported Maya "projectile vomits" when she eats mashed potatoes. Maya gagged when her hard palate was touched with an infant toothbrush, and she demonstrated a gag on the middle third of her tongue, suggesting a mild to moderate degree of oral hypersensitivity.

After 1 hour of testing, Maya began to cry and hid her face in her mother's lap. Therefore, testing was discontinued at that time.

Based on the results of the assessment, it appeared Maya's performance was affected by a number of factors including:

- Decreased upper and lower body strength
- Decreased balance
- Impaired bilateral coordination
- Dyspraxia
- Impaired eye-hand coordination, including decreased visual tracking
- Tactile and auditory defensiveness
- Impaired vestibular and proprioceptive processing
- Impaired auditory processing
- Mild to moderate oral hypersensitivity, which may affect nutrition/physical growth
- Oral apraxia
- Decreased oral-motor strength

Goals of therapy included improving Maya's sensory processing, increasing her upper and lower extremity muscle strength, increasing the strength of her oral-facial musculature, improving her joint attention, and increasing her verbal and nonverbal turn-taking skills.

Recommendations included speech language and OT three times per week with implementation of a daily home program. The therapists also told the Muellers about several preschool programs in the area that would understand Maya's needs and would provide her with therapy at school. The Muellers elected to start with individual speech language and OT.

After contacting Maya's pediatrician, the therapists also referred the Muellers to a developmental pediatrician to rule out a diagnosis of autistic spectrum disorder. The pediatrician stated she did not agree that Maya had autism, but that she would not oppose the referral. She also commented she did not feel Maya had "motor coordination problems."

Maya began treatment immediately. The OT and OTA conducted a home visit and provided the Muellers with suggestions to implement with Maya at home. Maya participated in a co-treatment with the speech language pathologist and the OT because of her limited physical endurance and due to family request. The Muellers traveled more than 25 miles to bring Maya to therapy.

Treatment activities by the OT/OTA team included vestibular input in the form of swinging to increase Maya's ability to efficiently process movement and to stimulate expressive language. Cause-and-effect toys were introduced and the therapists practiced turn-taking with Maya. Oral-motor toys were utilized along with specific oral-motor exercises to strengthen Maya's oral-facial muscles and to decrease her oral hypersensitivity. The therapists addressed Maya's motor planning difficulties by providing her with hand-over-hand assistance when exposing her to new activities. Although Maya initially "fussed" when motored through a task, she began to tolerate the intervention and watched her hands as the therapist guided her through a task.

The first week of treatment, the Muellers came to every appointment. The second and third weeks of intervention, the Muellers began to cancel appointments for unknown reasons.

The therapists talked with Mrs. Mueller at the next session. Mrs. Mueller admitted, "I need to tell you some things about our culture. I did not tell you at first, because I was afraid you would not work with Maya." Mrs. Mueller confided that if Maya was sleeping when it was time to leave for therapy, Mrs. Mueller would let her sleep and cancel the session. She explained it was against their culturally related parenting beliefs to wake Maya if she wanted to sleep. Furthermore, the home program "was not going well." Maya would resist her parents and begin to cry. Mrs. Mueller explained her husband could not stand for Maya to cry and that "forcing children to do things against their will" was another "violation" of their culture.

The therapists empathized with Mrs. Mueller and thanked her for sharing her concerns with them. The therapists then discussed possible options with Mrs. Mueller regarding the direction of Maya's intervention program.

Mrs. Mueller stated she and her husband agreed they wanted the therapists to "push Maya" but felt it was difficult for them to implement the same techniques at home. She requested increasing Maya's therapy to five times per week because it was "just so hard to work with her at home."

Maya had an appointment with a developmental pediatrician who diagnosed Maya with autism. The OT accompanied the Muellers to the assessment at their request.

After the assessment, the Muellers asked the OT if autism was "a serious illness." They asked if medication was available to treat "this problem" and if it was "curable." The therapist provided the Muellers with information about autistic spectrum disorder.

Maya began daily speech language and OT intervention. The therapists encouraged Mr. and Mrs. Mueller to attend the sessions to help them practice activities to try with Maya at home.

After 2 months of intervention, Maya began to speak utilizing jargon. Single words began to emerge, immersed in jargon. For example, Maya would say, "EE, EE No." She began to eat dry cereal and cheese.

Her motor skills began to improve as well. The Muellers reported Maya "emptied three of the drawers of clothing in her bedroom. Yesterday, she went upstairs and turned on the faucet." The Muellers had taken Maya to a birthday party expecting to "leave at any moment." They were pleasantly surprised when Maya "did not cry at all. She sat by the other children and watched them." Friends were "amazed" at the change in Maya.

The Muellers began to investigate the preschool programs in the area and elected to enroll Maya in a private preschool program based at the clinic where she was currently receiving individual speech language and OT.

The program included daily speech language and OT. It also incorporated therapeutic horseback riding, swimming, and gymnastics into the children's day. Maya's class had five other children with various medical diagnoses, including SID, mild cerebral palsy, and developmental dyspraxia. The adult-to-child ratio in the program was one to one. After 1 month in this program, Maya's working vocabulary increased to 10 words. She began to engage in one- to two-step structured play at home. Her parents indicated they "had not seen Maya spin a toy in weeks."

THE ROLE OF THE OTA IN SENSORY INTEGRATIVE TREATMENT

Sensory integration is one of the many specialty areas of practice in OT. A therapist may choose to advance his or her knowledge base by attending continuing education courses or by pursuing an advanced degree where courses in sensory integrative theory and treatment are part of the curriculum.

Sensory integrative assessment and treatment is based on skilled clinical observation and drawing conclusions based on the principles of sensory integrative theory. The treatment process is dynamic, requiring constant revision and adaptation based on the child's response to each carefully selected activity.

Because the purpose of each activity is not always clear to the casual observer, a person implementing a sensory integrative treatment approach must be well-versed in the tenets of sensory integration theory and must be able to give an explanation of the purpose and goal of each activity.

Each treatment session involves an assessment of the child's response to each presented activity. For example, if a child becomes green and complains of a stomach ache after swinging for 5 minutes, the treating therapist must know this is due to overstimulation of the vestibular system. The therapist must quickly engage the child in activities with a heavy proprioceptive component in attempts to alleviate the effects of excessive vestibular stimulation.

Sensory integrative assessment requires advanced clinical reasoning; therefore, evaluation should be conducted by an OT with advanced training in sensory integration theory and treatment.

An OT or an OTA should implement sensory integrative treatment (with advanced training in sensory integrative theory and treatment with a child). An OTA who has mastered competency criteria may utilize sensory integrative treatment activities outlined in a treatment plan by an OT.

REFERENCES

Ayres, A. J. (1979). *Sensory integration and the child.* Los Angeles, CA: Western Psychological Services.

Ayres, A. J. (1984). *Sensory integration and praxis test.* Los Angeles, CA: Western Psychological Services.

Balzer-Martin, L. A., & Kranowitz, C. S. (1992). *Balzer-Martin preschool screening program.* Washington, DC: Kranowitz/Balzer-Martin.

Beery, K. E. (1997). *Developmental test of visual-motor integration.* Parsippany, NJ: Modern Curriculum Press.

DeGangi, G., & Greenspan, S. I. (1998). *Test of sensory function in infants.* Los Angeles, CA: Western Psychological Services.

Dunn, W. (1999). *Sensory profile.* San Antonio, TX: Psychological Corp.

Fisher, A. G., Murray, E. A., & Bundy, A. C. (1991). *Sensory integration: Theory and practice.* Philadelphia, PA: F. A. Davis Co.

Folio, M. R., & Fewell, R. R. (1983). *Peabody developmental motor scales and activity cards.* Chicago, IL: Riverside Publishing Co.

Frick, S. M., & Lawton-Shirley, N. (1994). Auditory integrative training from a sensory perspective integrative perspective. *Sensory Integration Special Interest Section Newsletter, 17*(4).

Gentile, M. (1997). *Functional visual behavior.* Bethesda, MD: AOTA.

Goodenough, F. L., & Harris, D. B. (1963). *Goodenough-Harris drawing test*. San Antonio, TX: Psychological Corp.

Steinbach, I. (1998). *Samonas sound therapy*. Kellingham, Germany: Techau Verlag.

Wilbarger, P., & Wilbarger, J. L. (1991). *Sensory defensiveness in children aged 2-12*. Denver, CO: Avanti Educational Programs.

SUGGESTED READING

Hannaford, C. (1995). *Smart moves*. Arlington, VA: Great Ocean Publishers.

Kranowitz, C. S. (1998). *The out-of-sync child*. New York, NY: Skylight Press.

Two Children with Cerebral Palsy

Chapter 14

Tara J. Glennon, MS, OTR/L, BCP

INTRODUCTION

Cerebral palsy (CP) is a category name for brain injury that occurs prior to, during, or just after birth. The causes of the damage are often associated with intracranial hemorrhage, loss of oxygen, infections, trauma, delivery complications, or metabolic disorders. In some situations, however, the cause of the CP is unidentifiable, and thus termed *etiology unknown*. The reader should appreciate that medical and technological advances have both increased and decreased specific instances of CP. It is logical for one to understand that medical testing and pre-emergency interventions have decreased the incidences of brain injuries. However, medical interventions have also resulted in a higher frequency of babies surviving a fragile pregnancy. These babies, surviving despite low birth weight and prematurity, often show a higher incidence of abnormal tone and motor issues. Despite the cause(s), the neurological effect results in motor deficits that can be observed by early childhood. The specific location of the brain damage results in distinct types of motor and tonal problems. Thus, there are differing types of CP reported. Each of these types of CP is presented in Table 14-1.

FRAMES OF REFERENCE

Despite the frame of reference utilized on behalf of the child with CP, any interventionist must always consider the child's role within the environment. Occupational behavior is the basis of our profession. It is imperative that environmental adaptations be completed and opportunities presented so that the child can acquire the skills necessary to meet the demands of environment. This concept is universal to many frames of reference, based on developmental principles, acquisitional considerations, and coping concepts so that the child is able to take care of his or her own needs.

The most common intervention strategy for this diagnosis, despite the specific type of CP observed, is the neurodevelopmental treatment (NDT) approach. This approach, developed by Dr. and Mrs. Bobath in the 1940s, was originally designed for children with CP and is pri-

ESSENTIAL VOCABULARY

Ataxic: Characterized as a disturbance of balance secondary to abnormal muscle tone.

Athetoid: Characterized as fluctuating tone with decreased proximal stability.

Cerebral palsy: Collective term for brain injury prior to, during, or just after birth.

Family centered: The child functions within the family as a unit.

Hypotonic: Low tone that often masks under-lying spasticity or athetosis.

Neurodevelopmental: Developmental theory that emphasizes symmetry and righting reactions.

Occupational behavior: Acquiring skills to meet the demands of the environment.

Spasticity: High tone often resulting in synergistic patterns of the upper and lower extremities.

KEY CONCEPTS

- Medically based services: Paid for by insurance carrier upon medical necessity.
- School system practice: Guided by federal law for a free and appropriate education.
- Medical vs. educational services: Differences in service delivery models and team approaches.
- OT/OTA collaboration: Intricate interactions between two practitioners who each have necessary information and understanding of performance.

Table 14-1

Types of Tone

Spastic; Hypertonic

Tonal Patterns

- Presents as low tone in the trunk and high tone more distally
- Increased flexor patterning of the upper extremities (UEs)
- Extensor patterning of the lower extremities (LEs)
- Tone increases with effort or quick movements, emotion, excitement, and attempts at speech
- Severe tone, constant co-contraction

Movement Patterns

- Mild/moderate cases: child is able to walk but may demonstrate stereotypical movements as total movement synergies, associated reactions noted with movement attempts, range limitations occur more distally
- Decreased midrange control
- Primitive reflexes persist, such as ATNR, STNR, TLR, positive support, Moro, and startle
- Moderate/severe: decreased postural reactions, protective responses, and righting and equilibrium reactions; joint tightness and contractures can lead to orthopedic deformities

Related Issues

- Postural issues may affect respiration, suck-swallow-breath, and oral motor control
- Seizure disorders occur in approximately half the individuals with CP, most likely with spasticity
- MR, visual perceptual difficulties, hypersensitivity to environmental stimuli
- Play skills slow to develop
- Psychosocial issues: self-esteem, behavioral, and social skills

Hypotonic; Low Tone; Flaccid

Tonal Patterns

- Markedly low at birth or in infancy
- Low tone typically masks underlying spasticity, athetosis, or ataxia
- Flat or "pancake" chest, which makes the child prone to upper respiratory tract infections

Movement Patterns

- Affects trunk and all limbs with resulting hypermobile joints
- Decreased gradation of movement may be noted to utilize anatomic structures rather than active muscular control
- Decreased righting, equilibrium, and protective extension responses
- Primitive reflexes persist

Related Issues

- Decreased tactile, proprioceptive, and vestibular processing
- Decreased postural control affects respiration and the suck-swallow-breath mechanism
- Decreased oral motor status secondary to decreased stability
- Can also be diagnosed learning disabled or MR
- May demonstrate decreased motivation, frustration, have difficulty with change, and poor self-image
- May be fearful of movement

Ataxic

Tonal Patterns

- Described as a disturbance of balance
- Underlying muscle tone usually hypotonic or slightly increased in the lower extremities and more distally
- Tone changes with emotion and excitement

Movement Patterns

- Dysmetria: clumsy, unstable, and uncoordinated; presents as low tone in the trunk and high tone distally
- ROM is not an issue
- Decreased coordination, control of muscles, and balance
- Lack of a point of stability negatively influences the execution of equilibrium and righting reactions
- May need to utilize a wide base of support
- Uses more gross patterns
- Decreased performance of fine and gross motor skills

Related Issues

- Oral control is compromised, may use his or her teeth to stabilize cup
- Decreased articulation and food manipulation in mouth
- Nystagmus
- Sensory problems
- May have diagnosis of MR
- Difficulty developing social relations
- Difficulty with pre-vocational tasks and life skills

Table 14-1, continued

Types of Tone

Athetoid

Tonal Patterns

- Characterized by writhing, worm-like movements
- Fluctuating tone
- Demonstrate decreased proximal stability
- Abnormal tone noted in all extremities

Movement Patterns

- Movement in extreme ranges
- Movements appear bizarre and purposeless
- Movements may be uncontrollable
- Lack midrange control

- Demonstrates increased movements with emotion and excitement
- Secondary joint fixing when attempting to increase stability
- Hypermobile distal joints that can sublux

Related Issues

- Possible hearing loss
- Possible LD
- Less likelihood of MR than with other types of CP
- Emotionally labile
- Easily frustrated
- Possibly having poor self-image and low self-esteem

---

mary within the medical model. Although NDT is considered a developmental theory, it does not encourage the development of typical motor milestones. The theory emphasizes foundational skills such as symmetry, righting and equilibrium reactions, and weight shifting as precursors to acquiring motor skills. The NDT frame of reference outlines specific, intricate treatment strategies that focus on precise handling techniques to promote normal movement patterns. Extensive clinical experience and a strong foundational knowledge of normal and abnormal movement patterns provide the framework of treatment implementation. In preparation for work with children diagnosed with CP, these complex intervention strategies are outlined in an 8-week, advanced certification course offered to OTs, PTs, and speech language pathologists. Despite the complexities of direct therapeutic intervention, the NDT frame of reference consistently emphasizes carryover within the natural context of the child's day and participation in functional tasks. The role of the OTA can be quite extensive within home- or school-based therapy, as well as within institutional environments. The intricacy of this frame of reference requires intense cooperation between the OT and OTA.

The use of sensory integration techniques is also critical when understanding the child's responses to movement inputs and other sensory experiences. Sensory integration theory emphasizes the importance of sensory processing as a foundation for learning within all developmental sequences. Motor skill acquisition is among the most identifiable of these sequences. NDT and sensory integration techniques are often utilized together.

Dr. Mary Reilly developed a theory of play which has expanded how we value the play experience. She believed that play gave meaning to the daily life of a child and provided opportunities to learn rules, develop interactions, and form the basis for adult competencies. As clinicians working with a child diagnosed with CP, the play experiences chosen must provide opportunities for the child to grow and develop socially and emotionally. The child with CP, therefore, presents a unique challenge that may require the use of environmental modifications, technology, adaptive equipment, and toy modification so that the child's curiosity is stimulated. The focus is providing the child with the possibility of pressure-free mastery of the environment. As we attempt to provide this accessibility to play experiences, the therapist may also wish to remember the biomechanical approach. ROM, strength, and endurance must be factors in the designing of play experiences. The more accessible the activity, the more the child will be invested, and the more meaningful and organizing the activity is for the child.

ASSESSMENT

Within the arena of pediatric practice, the evaluation process is complex. When presented with a child with CP, the collaboration between the OT and OTA is quite involved. For this reason, this section is offered to the OTA not only to understand his or her role within this process, but to appreciate the evaluation tools completed by the OT.

The first step in the assessment process is determined by who is asking for and paying for the evaluation and for what reason. There is a distinct difference between medically and educationally based services, and, therefore, the evaluation tools must reflect those differences. Within the medical realm, standardized evaluation tools, analysis of adaptive living skills within the home environment, and the identification of underlying quality of skills would be emphasized. The educational system focuses on functional outcomes within the academic environment to determine eligibility for services (AOTA, 1989a, 1989b). Through either evaluation process, the collaboration between both therapists allows for the identification of strengths and weaknesses, possible causes of problems, intervention needs, and appropriate plans for intervention. The role of the OTA can be essential if managed effectively with the OT.

Quite often, when concerns are raised about a child's performance, a screening might occur. The screening is often considered to be the initial step in the evaluative process, in order to rule in or out the need for specific evaluations. However, within the medical realm, a screening is not generally utilized when a child has a diagnosed condition, for it is assumed that the child will demonstrate rehabilitative or occupational concerns. A child with CP, therefore, moves directly to the assessment process. Within the educational environment, a screening may occur in order to determine if the child's deficits are interfering with classroom performance. If the child's classroom functioning is compromised, the child would be moved on to the assessment phase. As this screening is not formalized, it can typically be completed by the OT or OTA. Observations of functional performance within the classroom environment, conversations with the teacher to determine his or her concerns regarding the child's performance, and chart review of other team member evaluations to document areas of deficits can be completed by the OTA as the initial phase in the evaluation process (Blossom, Ford, & Cruse, 1996).

For the child with CP, the degree of involvement would determine the appropriate assessment tools (Case-Smith, 1993; Case-Smith, Allen, & Pratt, 1996). For example, if the child is severely involved, there are two distinctly different types of evaluation tools that would need to be reviewed for possible use. First, newly available standardized assessment tools regarding the quality of movement are uniquely appropriate for the child with motor impairments. These include Miller and Roid's (1994) Toddler and Infant Motor Evaluation (TIME) and the Alberta Infant Motor Scale (AIMS) authored by Piper and Darrah (1994). Given the complexity and intricacy of these tools, an occupational or physical therapist's implementation, judgment, and rating are necessary. However, while these tools provide valuable information regarding the movement patterns of these children, they do not necessarily address occupational performance or movement within the context of functional life tasks (Dunn, 1991).

The second cluster of evaluation tools, standardized instruments commonly utilized with other children, is available to the OTR in order to assess fine motor, visual motor, or perceptual skills. However, these tools do not typically provide for the needed modifications with regard to a child with significant motor impairments. Therefore, in addition to the standardized qualitative observations of motor performance mentioned above, criterion-referenced tools, non-standardized assessments, and adaptive skill checklists are often appropriately utilized for this population of children. Several of these tools can be completed by the OTA and shared with the supervising therapist for review and analysis. Again, the role of the OTA within the evaluation process is substantiated due to the need for extensive information regarding functional skills within a variety of environments. For it is this information, related to occupational performance, which will substantiate the need for intervention and focus the plan of action.

As part of the overall assessment process, the OTA might utilize non-standardized tools for a child with CP. These include gathering historical information from the chart regarding other medical assessments and/or teacher reports and completing interviews with parents and/or teachers. In addition, questionnaires should be implemented which might identify areas of difficulty not readily observed within a clinic or school environment, investigate child/family history, document developmental milestones, obtain pre- and post-natal birth history, and outline pertinent hospitalizations. A specific inventory/observation tool that may be used is the Sensory Integration Inventory of Individuals with Developmental Disabilities (SII-DD) (Reisman & Hanschu, 1992). This tool is not age specific and is designed as a formalized questionnaire that can be completed by the family or educational staff. The SII-DD is used to identify sensory processing issues which present as behaviors that might interfere with functional participation within the environment. The results of the questionnaire need to be interpreted by the OT secondary to the complicated and evolving theory of sensory integration.

Based on the fact that children with CP are frequently unable to functionally complete a task or demonstrate poor quality of skills, the certified assistant should develop competencies in and implement a criterion-referenced assessment. These tools are designed to gain descriptive information of functional domains of performance, outline components of skills that are present or absent, and describe the child's current functioning, while providing guidelines for future skill emergence. The following is a list of criterion referenced assessments that would be appropriate for a child with CP.

1. The *Brigance Diagnostic Inventory of Early Childhood Development* (1991), a tool for children birth through 7 years, can be used for the child with CP. This assessment is particularly appropriate for school settings as it allows for other disciplines to complete additional sections related to

other domains of functioning. Domains appropriate for OT include fine motor, dressing, and feeding. The OTA is able to complete these portions of the evaluation and share the findings with the OT for analysis and coordination with other assessment findings.

2. The *Hawaii Early Learning Profile (HELP)*, published by the Vort Corporation (1995), outlines skills for two age groups: birth to 3 years and 3 to 6 years. This tool is specifically designed for children with multiple handicaps or developmental delays and can be used for severely delayed children up to 12 years of age. As this evaluation tool provides an in-depth task analysis of all daily living skills (e.g., dressing, feeding, fine motor, and visual motor skills), it is an appropriate tool for the OTA to complete.

3. Therapy Skill Builders publish comprehensive books authored by Rhoda Erhardt in 1994. The *Erhardt Developmental Prehension Assessment (EDPA)* and the *Erhardt Developmental Vision Assessment (EDVA),* highly descriptive approaches to observing children birth to 6 years, are particularly appropriate for children with CP. The intricacy of these tools, due to the quantified observations, is appropriate for the OT to complete. Both age levels and outlines of the sequences of development are provided.

Case Study 1—Lauren, a 1 1/2-Year-Old Child with Spastic Type CP

Background Information Concerning Early Intervention

Federal legislation from the 1980s significantly impacted services to young children. Based on a collection of principles that recognizes that the family is the constant in the child's life, a family-centered system was created, placing the emphasis of services on the child within the context of his or her environment. The focus of early intervention services is to promote interaction, collaboration, and sharing of information between the family and the professionals (AOTA, 1989a). Through these interactions, the professionals can recognize and appreciate family strengths and individuality, with respect for diversity and various cultural backgrounds, while attempting to meet the family's concerns. For these reasons, the evaluation is typically completed by two professionals. This team utilizes permitted standardized evaluation tools to look at many variables, such as the degree and type of disability, personality, temperament, and

behavior of the child, as well as family interactions, needs, and strengths. This allows the parents to express their concerns and the priorities of their child's intervention program. The OTA, regardless of the level of experience, would not be appropriate to evaluate the child's needs as extensively as the early intervention process mandates. As attempts are generally made to minimize the number of professionals entering the family's home, it would not be appropriate to perform a joint evaluation with the OT. Additionally, the system intends to foster relationships with critical individuals, thus decreasing the number of people with which the family needs to interact.

This process of outlining the child's needs, as seen by the parents, results in the formal document of services called the Individual Family Service Plan (IFSP). This plan ensures that partnerships with the family are established and family goals are outlined and prioritized. The IFSP is reviewed at 6-month intervals until such time as the child no longer requires intervention or until the child turns 3 years and exits the program. Throughout this process, the team must decide what is the most natural environment for the services to be delivered. Typically, the child's home or day care environment is the most appropriate. However, there are situations where clinic-based services, which emphasize specialized play group experiences or intensive therapeutic services, can also be outlined. Regardless of the location, it is of primary importance that the interventionist function as an educator for all people who are naturally a part of the child's life.

For these reasons, the early intervention specialist must be flexible and responsive to family-identified needs in an ongoing situation. Additionally, because communication is key, typically there are primary interventionists identified so that the family is not bombarded with the input of many people. The transdisciplinary model of one primary interventionist or the interdisciplinary approach of a small team of people who collaborate and prioritize goals together is most often utilized. The role of the OTA within this model is dependent on several factors. First, the level of experience is critical. If one is delivering services within the home environment, with no others immediately available for discussion and collaboration, the practitioner must be sufficiently adept at answering all of the parent's potential questions (Finnie, 1974). Therefore, the therapist must have suitable experience in order to manage the situation effectively. If the child receives services within a clinic setting, with many professionals or the supervising OT readily available, the OTA has the necessary supports, and is therefore an appropriate service provider. The next series of considerations include the priorities identified by the parents, the extent of the child's limitations, and the other service delivery personnel identified to participate in the child's plan. In order for the OTA to be identified as the OT service provider, all of these factors would need to be discussed and resolved to the satisfaction of the entire team of professionals working on behalf of the child.

Case Presentation

Lauren, the only child of William and Sarah, has been determined eligible by the state's birth to 3 system for therapy services following a referral from her pediatrician. The parents, who own their own business and work from home, have identified several priorities for their child. Positioning and handling at home to make caring for her easier during functional tasks such as mealtime, bathing, dressing, and play was a major concern. Additionally, they felt that intensive physical, occupational, and speech language therapies should be provided away from the home environment. Their concern, secondary to the fact that they work within the home, was that they would be unable to work effectively if Lauren was having difficulty with the therapies. They appeared fragile in terms of the difficulties that lie ahead of Lauren and did not believe that they would be able to endure her possible crying or struggling with the therapeutic processes. Instead, they would prefer the nanny bring Lauren to her therapies and focus their attentions on follow through within the home environment.

The OTA employed by the early intervention facility had 3 years' experience working with children and had worked intricately with the OT throughout. Because of this and along with the fact that the primary intervention would take place within the clinic setting, she was assigned this case following the eligibility process. The team of therapists working directly with the child, completed the HELP so that a baseline of each domain of functioning was established and progress could be measured by this tool in the future.

The priorities identified by the parents shaped the goals recorded on the IFSP. These goals, outlined for a 6-month period, focused on functional tasks. Each professional, in combination with the parents and team, outlined the behavioral objectives that would be utilized to measure Lauren's progress toward the goal areas. For Lauren, as with all children, a behavioral outcome is required to identify an observable, behavioral statement and to identify under what conditions or circumstances the child would be expected to master the behavioral statement. For all outcomes, criteria were documented to determine how the team would measure Lauren's success. Lauren's behavioral outcomes were as follows.

1. When provided with upright support within her mother's ring sitting position on the floor, Lauren will:
   - Push her arm three quarters of the way through a sleeve (shirt, coat) as it is held open for her, in three out of four attempts.
   - Pull the shirt down over her head as it rests on top of her head, using two hands, in three out of four attempts.
   - Push her leg into the pant opening as her leg is held at the beginning of the opening by the caregiver in an effort to achieve correct placement, in three out of four attempts.
2. When in a 90-90-90 sitting position in her Rifton chair with foot rests, hip strap, shoulder harness, and tray, Lauren will reach for and obtain a preferred toy using palmar grasp in four out of five consecutive attempts.
3. While in a supported side-lying position, Lauren will activate a single switch positioned 6 to 12 inches in front of her, with the hand or the upper arm, to activate a preferred toy for at least 30 seconds.

NDT therapeutic intervention within the one-to-one situation focused on postural control and weight shifting as it allowed for more functional reach patterns. Weight bearing and trunk rotation activities were consistently incorporated so as to decrease the tonal influence on upper extremity movements (Blanche, Botticelli, & Hallway, 1995). Throughout these sessions, the practitioner focused on expanding play opportunities for Lauren, as well as increasing participation in daily living tasks following therapeutic handling techniques. Although Lauren's nanny was present during all sessions to allow for training and carryover, several visits were made to the home. During these sessions, positioning for function and handling techniques were outlined. The practitioner utilized home programming sheets from the OT files in order to outline what the parents could do at home. These sheets included information concerning relaxation of muscles, encouraging movements in as normal a pattern as possible, positioning in proper alignment to prevent deformities, lifting and carrying alternatives which minimized abnormal tonal responses, and positioning options for play (Figure 14-1) and daily task involvement. When in the home, the practitioner needs to be as supportive as possible. This includes respecting and encouraging beneficial ways in which the family was already facilitating the child's development, making suggestions that were practical and relevant to their family life, and making sure not to give the family more to do than their time permitted.

CASE STUDY 2—MARY, A 5 1/2-YEAR-OLD DIAGNOSED WITH MILD, HYPOTONIC CP

Background Information Concerning School System Practice

In the early 1970s, OT services were mandated within the educational system. Although these laws have been

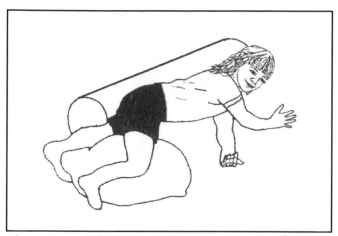

Figure 14-1. Side-lying position.

revised, expanded, and redefined since that time, OT has always remained part of the law as a related service for the child to benefit from special education (AOTA, 1989b). A related service is defined as that which is necessary to support the special education instruction. OT, as an educationally based related service, is not intended to be a medical service. Despite the rehabilitative concerns, the therapist must determine if the therapeutic intervention is necessary for educational performance.

The intent of special education is to educate the child in the typical classroom with peers who do not have special needs. This part of the law is referred to as the least restrictive environment (LRE). For the child with CP, this creates a unique challenge. The role of OT is critical in outlining modifications and adaptations within the classroom environment, so that the child is able to be educated with his or her peers.

As with any federally funded program, a legal document must be designed in order to outline the necessary services. From birth to 3, this was called the IFSP; the child within the family as the focus; whereas in the school system, the Individualized Education Plan (IEP) is the legal document that addresses the child as part of his or her educational environment. The IEP is designed through the process of a group identified as the Pupil Planning and Placement Team (PPT). Members of this team include parents, special and regular educators, an administrator, special service providers such as OT personnel, the student if appropriate, and other invited members which could include an attorney, parent or child advocate, or other parent support. The IEP serves as a tool for measuring progress, ensuring communication, and providing ongoing evaluation of the child.

The IEP, which is updated at least every year, must include the child's current level of educational performance, annual goals, short-term/behavioral objectives, the services required to meet objectives, and criteria to assess whether objectives have been met. It is imperative that the goals and objectives be specifically related to education. Each year, at the annual IEP meeting, the previous goals are measured to determine progress, continued services are decided, and new goals are developed as appropriate. At that time, the roles of the OT and OTA are to collect data to answer these questions. Throughout each of these phases, the OT staff must remember to translate technical information into educational terms so that interdisciplinary team members can utilize this information effectively.

For the child with CP, educationally based OT services are uniquely appropriate for the certified assistant. Striving to provide the child with functional skills for use within the educational environment focuses on environmental modifications and adaptive skill development. When considering the child's level of physical involvement, environmental issues include seating and positioning, utensil adaptation, modification of learning and play/leisure materials, use of technology to access learning materials, and/or accessibility in and around the school building. Self-care activities within this environment are also critical in allowing the child every opportunity to meet his or her own needs and master occupational performance.

Although the services discussed within this section are prescribed through educational laws, OT must also address what might be considered more medically based or rehabilitative in nature, if these issues impact activities within the educational environment. These concerns might include safety secondary to possible seizures, oral motor skill development in order to ensure safety during lunch and snack time routines, strength and ROM as related to participation endurance, wheelchair training for building accessibility, and/or postural control in order to maintain an upright, "ready for learning" position.

Case Presentation

Mary, the second of Barbara and Joseph's three children, began special education services at age 3, as outlined by the educational laws. Upon entrance, Mary, diagnosed with mild, hypotonic CP, was identified as having fine motor, visual motor, and oral motor concerns that were determined to have potential negative effects on her educational program. Since that time, Mary has received OT services by the OT staff to address the above mention issues.

At present, Mary is entering kindergarten and is to be included within the regular classroom. Based on the issues identified within Mary's current IEP, several types of service delivery methods were discussed by the team. For OT, direct and monitoring were determined to be appropriate, while consultation to the team was inherent in the monthly team meeting process.

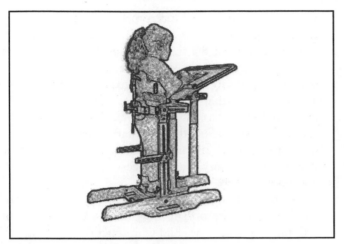

Figure 14-2. Stander with tray.

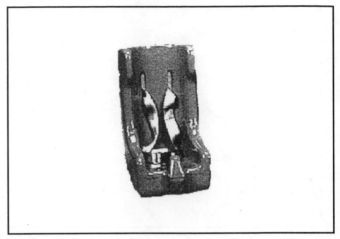

Figure 14-3. Tumbleform seat.

Prior to arrival in kindergarten, the OT department, with the assistance from physical therapy, was responsible for ordering appropriate positioning devices which would allow Mary access to educational materials and situations. Both therapists determined that Mary would require a Rifton chair, stander with a tray (Figure 14-2), and tumbleform supportive seating device (Figure 14-3) for use during floor time, daily circle time, and music class. The therapists ordering and providing these devices for Mary's use were accountable for the functional and safe implementation of this equipment. Therefore, both therapists designed a program for use, in-serviced the classroom staff, and outlined a system to monitor how the equipment was being used within the classroom. For OT, the focus was on how this equipment supported Mary's ability to participate in educational activities.

Mary's direct services, the most basic form of service provision that implies hands-on contact, was discussed by the team. While Mary's parents were not opposed to pull-out services, if necessary, they would prefer for her interventions to occur within the classroom environment.

This thought was consistent with the inclusion model outlined on her IEP. For the OTA assigned to Mary's case, the scheduling of intervention was critical. Since fine and visual motor goals were outlined on Mary's IEP, it was determined that the therapist would provide services within the classroom during morning "drawing" time and during free play. This would allow the therapist to address the fine and visual motor skills as they naturally occur for all of the children. During the first weeks of the school year, the OTA set up the tabletop situation where Mary does her work. Lowering the table to the proper height, ensuring that her feet were able to be firmly placed and supported on the floor when sitting all the way back in her chair, and providing a tabletop surface which was angled approximately 30 degrees, was com-

pleted. The 90-90-90 position was encouraged for all functional tasks presented to Mary.

The part of Mary's IEP that outlined oral motor goals was also discussed by the team. Although Mary was physically able to get food to her mouth, either with her fingers or with the spoon, safety was a concern during feeding. Therefore, two methods needed to be outlined for meal and snack time at school. For snack in the classroom, Mary was provided with foods that were safe for her to eat independently. This allowed Mary to sit at the table with her friends and develop socialization skills that might typically occur during mealtime. During lunch time, when the other children went to the cafeteria, Mary would receive therapeutic feeding. The discussions that led to this decision involved several factors:

1. The cafeteria was particularly loud and distracting for Mary.

2. Oral-motor skills were identified as a primary concern.

3. Therapy would be intrusive.

When therapeutic feeding strategies were discussed, Mary's parents felt that direct therapy for feeding was inappropriate for lunchroom implementation. The decision was based on the fact that the intense intervention might be disturbing for Mary to receive in view of the other children. For Mary, delayed oral movements, low tone, and postural issues affecting the suck-swallow-breath mechanism made choking a possibility. Additional difficulties Mary presented included drooling, food loss, decreased tongue movements, decreased involvement of cheeks to manage food, and limited ability to chew. These issues required both NDT and sensory integrative approaches (Blanche, Botticelli, & Hallway, 1995).

The oral motor interventions were designed and implemented through the collaboration of OT, OTA,

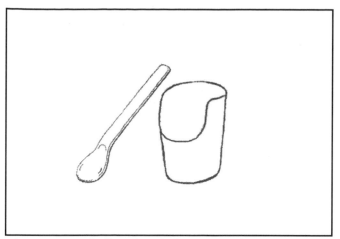

Figure 14-4. Shallow-bowled spoon and cut-out cup.

speech language pathologist, teacher, and parents. In addition to direct intervention by the therapy staff, a plan for training all staff included a written plan and videotape of a session. Daily implementation of strategies could be ensured when all staff involved with program implementation were adequately trained.

The first issue, proper positioning, was one of the most critical issues for Mary due to decreased tone and limited postural control. Providing stabilization allowed Mary to concentrate on eating rather than maintaining her posture. It also allowed for alignment of internal organs necessary for digestion and for ease of swallowing to prevent aspiration. The program also identified that the person feeding Mary should ideally be directly in front of Mary, at or below eye level, to allow for observation of jaw, mouth, and tongue movements. This also enhanced midline orientation and facilitated interaction between Mary and the caregiver.

The actual feeding part of Mary's program was quite specific to prevent variation and reduce safety concerns. A shallow-bowled spoon was provided as it was the appropriate size to fit between her teeth, was rubberized, and had a shallow bowl (Figure 14-4). This shallow bowl, along with the feeder placing small to moderate amounts of food on the spoon, allowed for greater ease when Mary attempted to remove the food from the spoon. The program emphasized presenting the spoon at midline and pressing the bowl of the spoon on the front third of tongue. This technique facilitated the proper tongue movements to manage and propel the food backward for Mary to swallow safely. The feeder was not to remove the spoon until Mary's mouth was ready to close, waiting for the lips to close around the spoon. Then the spoon was to be removed straight out.

For cup drinking, Mary's juice was thickened with gel thickener, yogurt, or applesauce, as she demonstrated difficulty managing and swallowing thin consistencies. The recommended technique was to bring the cup to the lips, rest the cup on Mary's lower lip, and wait for Mary to come to the cup to obtain the juice. Instructions were provided to watch fluid flow, easily observed with the use of a cut-out cup (see Figure 14-4), and provide jaw control during this process. Jaw control variations, outlined on the home program sheets, were outlined to teach normal jaw movements, provide proprioceptive feedback during drinking and swallowing, and promote lip/jaw closure and gradation.

SUMMARY

The diagnosis of CP, the category name for brain injury resulting in abnormal muscle tone, is a unique challenge for the OTA. The multiple issues involved, including postural control, upper extremity functioning, oral motor skills, daily living skills, and ability to access the environment, emphasize the need for intense cooperation between the OT and OTA. Each professional collects specific information with respect to the individual's level of functioning, with synthesis necessary in order to develop a comprehensive plan of action. Several frames of reference are appropriate, some requiring more intensive training than others. For example, NDT outlines specific handling techniques to promote normal movement patterns. For this approach, extensive clinical experience is considered optimal. Occupational behavior, on the other hand, is inherent in the role of the certified assistant and is the basis of our profession.

Also important for the delivery of OT services, the interventionist must remember to view the child within the context of his or her environment. Varying laws regulate how services are delivered, based on the environment in which the child must function. These laws need to be clearly understood and adhered to. Working with this population of children is not only intricate, but fascinating in all its complexities.

CLINICAL PROBLEM-SOLVING

Barry, a 35-year-old man who is severely medically involved, has spastic type CP and significant oral motor difficulties. He resides in a group home for the mentally retarded and has a history of frequent pneumonia. Based on his medical status, oral motor programming is critical to prevent aspiration. The procedures mentioned above continue to be appropriate, but the carryover portion of feeding intervention would need to be more structured. Based on the fact that there are three shifts of caregivers, and the therapists are not always available, training and monitoring are critical. Frequent in-service sessions need to be implemented, and documentation of training must be part of the record for liability reasons and to keep track of the schedule of training sessions. Photos and diagrams, easily accessible to the caregiver, would assist with correct implementation of the plan. The formal program, outlined in the chart with specific detail, must be consistently followed by every caregiver working with Barry. Therefore, a formal chart of documentation would need to be outlined so that the therapist can track implementation. What suggestions could be used to develop this?

Carlos, a 6-year-old Hispanic boy, presented with athetoid type CP, average intelligence, and primitive oral motor patterns. He was the youngest of five children, ages 6 through 12. Although the therapist made many attempts to facilitate independence during self-care activities, Carlos' mother, Alicia, continued to complete these tasks for him. At school, he was fed using the strategies designed by OT. These techniques were shared with the staff and Carlos' family. However, Alicia continued to feed Carlos with a bottle at home. As the therapist assigned to this case began to understand the cultural background and values of Carlos' family and his role as the youngest child, she began to modify her original plans. The revised plan, intended to elicit a match with Alicia which respected her cultural beliefs, first focused on Carlos' health and safety. Then, by designing activities which would not significantly disrupt the family's routine at home, play and leisure were expanded. Alicia enjoyed watching Carlos learn to play with toys and interact with his siblings. As Carlos demonstrated increased curiosity, motivation, and independence, other activities were added. What activities could be suggested to enhance the mother-son relationship?

Brian, a 13-year-old boy with athetoid type CP, presented with perceptual and motor deficits, as well as a seizure disorder which resulted in unanticipated drop seizures. He received medically based occupational and physical therapy services within a clinic environment. During physical therapy, Brian worked toward independent ambulation with the use of a walker weighted at the base for stability. At school, Brian received only OT services. Since he was able to independently negotiate the school environment with his wheelchair, he was not eligible for educationally based physical therapy. Toward the end of the school year, as Brian had mastered the use of the walker, his mother requested that he be able to use the walker in school. The school administrator asked OT to develop safety mechanisms for using the walker. First, data was collected regarding the seizures to determine if any precipitating events could be identified. It was determined that seizures were most associated with the onset of illness, lack of sleep, and when over-aroused. The protocol for walker use that was outlined, identified that communication between home and school would be imperative so that illness or decreased sleep were identi-

fied, and the walker would not be used. Additionally, Brian was restricted from using the walker in the hallway when changing classes and in the cafeteria. These situations were identified as too over-arousing, with many people moving erratically and too much noise. When using the walker in specified situations, Brian would have to wear a hard helmet for protection, as well as be closely supervised by educational staff. What other options might be available?

John, a 13-year-old with ataxic type CP, has received OT since the age of 2. Early on, his direct OT program focused on NDT techniques to gain more control of his extremities for functional use. As John advanced in the grades and continued difficulty with controlled upper extremity was observed, the use of technology gained importance. At the most recent IEP meeting, the parents and team decided to focus on vocational skills needed for the upcoming years. John's regular and special education teachers presented the district's curriculum for review by the team. Secondary to motor, perceptual, and cognitive limitations, the role of the OT outlined by the team included environmental modifications, task analysis, assistive technology, and assistance with program development. This consultative role was considered to be more beneficial to the team rather than direct services. What might the consultant suggest for modifications?

REFERENCES

AOTA. (1989a). *Guidelines for OT services in early intervention and preschool services.* Bethesda, MD: Author.

AOTA. (1989b). *Guidelines for OT services in school systems.* Bethesda, MD: Author.

Blanche, E. I., Botticelli, T. M., & Hallway, M. K. (1995). *Combining neurodevelopmental and sensory integration principles: An approach to pediatric therapy.* Tucson, AZ: Therapy Skill Builders.

Blossom, B., Ford, F., & Cruse, C. (1996). *Physical therapy and OT in the public schools.* Rome, GA: Rehabilitation Publications and Therapies, Inc.

Brigance, A. H. (1991). *Brigance diagnostic inventory of early development—revised.* North Billerica, MA: Curriculum Associates Inc.

Case-Smith, J. (1993). *Pediatric OT and early intervention.* Newton, MA: Andover Medical Publishers.

Case-Smith, J., Allen, A. S., & Pratt, P. N. (1996). *OT for children.* St. Louis, MO: Mosby-Year Book, Inc.

Dunn, W. (1991). *Pediatric OT.* Thorofare, NJ: SLACK Incorporated.

Erhardt, R. P. (1994). *Developmental hand dysfunction: Theory, assessment, and treatment* (2nd ed.). Tucson, AZ: Therapy Skill Builders.

Finnie, N. R. (1974). *Handling the young cerebral palsied child at home.* New York, NY: Penguin Books USA, Inc.

Miller, L. J., & Roid, G. H. (1994). *The toddler and infant motor evaluation*. Tucson, AZ: Therapy Skill Builders.

Piper, M., & Darrah, J. (1994). *Alberta infant motor scale*. Oakland, NJ: W. B. Saunders.

Reisman, J., & Hanschu, B. (1992). *Sensory integration inventory—revised for individuals with developmental disabilities*. Hugo, MN: PDP Press.

Vort Corporation. (1995). *HELP checklist*. Palo Alto, CA: Author.

SUGGESTED READING

AOTA. (1997). *OT services for children and youth under the Individuals with Disabilities Education Act*. Bethesda, MD: Author.

Dunn-Klein, M., & Delaney, T. A. (1994). *Feeding and nutrition for the child with special needs*. Tucson, AZ: Therapy Skill Builders.

Henderson, A., & Pehoski, C. (1995). *Hand function in the child: Foundations for remediation*. St. Louis, MO: Mosby-Year Book, Inc.

Parham, L. D., & Fazio, L. S. (1997). *Play in OT for children*. St. Louis, MO: Mosby-Year Book, Inc.

Sheda, C., & Small, C. (1990). *Developmental motor activities for therapy: Instruction sheets for children*. Tucson, AZ: Therapy Skill Builders.

World Health Organization. (1993). *Promoting the development of young children with CP*. Geneva, Switzerland: Author.

A Second-Grader with Conduct Disorder

Chapter 15

Linda Florey, PhD, OTR, FAOTA

INTRODUCTION

Conduct disorder is the diagnostic name given to repetitive and persistent patterns of behavior in which the basic rights of others, societal norms, or rules are violated. These patterns of behavior cause significant impairment in social, academic, or occupational functioning (American Psychiatric Association [APA], 1994). Physical and verbal aggression is common (Earls, 1994). Children may display bullying, physical cruelty to people and to animals, and may deliberately destroy the property of others. There are two subtypes based upon age. Childhood onset occurs before the age of 10 and typically involves physical aggression and disturbed peer relationships. Adolescent onset occurs after 10, and these youth tend to have more norma-

tive peer relationships but may engage in illegal and criminal behavior (Kazdin, 1995). Childhood onset is considered to be the more severe form of the disorder.

Conduct disorder is more common in boys than girls (APA, 1994). Children and adolescents with conduct disorder typically have low self-esteem and, to hide this, may portray themselves as tough and uncaring. Learning disabilities are common. They are likely to show academic deficiencies and diminished social skills with both peers and adults. There is no single cause of conduct disorder. Children with behavior problems have symptoms that place them on the border of several neurological, psychiatric, and psychoeducational categories (Lewis, 1996). The course of conduct disorder is variable, but children with early onset are at increased risk for antisocial personality

KEY CONCEPTS

- Conduct disorder: A psychiatric disorder characterized by repetitive/persistent patterns of behavior that violate the basic rights of others, societal norms, or rules.
- Occupational behavior: Targets the broad parameters of play, student role, and socialization as the primary concern of OT practitioners working with children.
- Task performance: Assessment of attention span, ability to make decisions, follow directions, sequence steps, use tools/materials, and solve problems using a craft/activity.
- Individual Educational Plan (IEP): Aimed at improving the child's educational performance. It contains specific instructional objectives, services, and modifications needed to achieve the objectives.
- Behavioral frame of reference: Learning based on environmental consequences and leads to either positive or adaptive behavior or negative or maladaptive behavior.

ESSENTIAL VOCABULARY

Cognitive, motor, social complexity: Used in grading activities according to problem-solving processes, visual/motor skill, and social exchange required.

Interdisciplinary Treatment Plan: A plan of care, includes goals and interventions of all disciplines working with a patient.

Learning disability: A chronic condition of unknown cause, interferes with learning/working.

Legal hold: A court-ordered restraint often associated with a belief that an individual is a danger to self or others.

Middle childhood: The years from 6 to 12.

Post-traumatic stress disorder: Symptom pattern following exposure to an extreme situation often involving threatened death or serious injury that produces intense fear, helplessness, or agitation.

Open seclusion: Temporary placement in an isolated room with no windows or furniture, door open.

Residential treatment facility: Where individuals live temporarily for therapeutic benefit.

Social skills: Social competence, refers to the ability to produce mutually reciprocal interactions with others.

disorders and substance-related disorders (APA, 1994). These children are at great risk for premature death from violent causes (Earls, 1994).

FRAMES OF REFERENCE

The frame of reference used in this chapter is occupational behavior. This frame of reference targets the broad parameters of play, student role, and socialization as the primary concern of OTs in working with children and adolescents. Play, work, and role are major theoretical principles that contribute to an understanding of an individual's occupational behavior. There is a developmental progression in the manner in which work and play are incorporated into an occupational role. Occupational role focuses on a combination of societal expectations and individual achievements in productive daily activities or occupations of individuals. In middle childhood, the ages of 6 to 12 years, work, play, and major daily activities focus on the role of student. The role of student is much broader than solely mastering the expectations of the curriculum. This role includes the learning and mastery of both academic and social expectations, which include those formally taught in school and those informally learned on the playground, gym, and other social settings. A major clinical focus for OTs is to determine the extent to which mental illness has disrupted or impoverished occupational behavior and to identify steps to ameliorate dysfunction and to foster new learning (Florey, 1998).

Assessments and treatment techniques drawn from additional frames of reference may be used to ameliorate dysfunction in occupational role and socialization. The behavioral frame of reference is very useful in working with children with conduct disorder.

CASE STUDY 1

Tony is an 8-year, 7-month-old boy admitted to the child inpatient service of a teaching hospital for combative behavior at school and increasingly aggressive behavior at home. He had thrown furniture in the classroom, punched a teacher in the stomach, hit other children at school, and had made increasing verbal threats to harm his younger brother and mother. Tony lived with his mother, stepfather, and his 4-year-old biological brother. His mother was 6 months pregnant with another child.

Tony was born in Florida of mixed ethnicity. His mother was Latino-American and his biological father was Caucasian. Tony had been abused both physically and mentally by his biological father, who was an alcoholic. He had also witnessed beatings of his mother by his father. His parents divorced when he was 5, and his mother moved him and his brother to California to seek asylum from the father. His mother met and married his stepfather, a Latino-American who had no children of his own.

Tony had problems in the first and second grades and had been dismissed from school on three occasions for physically fighting with others. The teachers said that he routinely picked on the younger children on the playground, and they regarded him as a bully. On another occasion, they had to stop him from beating a puppy with a stick. Aside from his poor behavior on the playground and during class, he was not a good student. He achieved poor marks, but the teachers did not know if he was really trying or too busy misbehaving to concentrate on schoolwork. At home, Tony swore, broke toys, and often threatened his younger brother. His stepfather tried to be buddies with him and felt that he was just acting "normal" as anyone would if they had been abused so young. His mother became increasingly afraid that Tony might harm her and her unborn baby and her younger son. He had threatened her with a kitchen knife on two occasions.

On the day of admission, Tony had thrown a chair across the room in class and started to physically attack two other boys. The police were called, and Tony was brought into the emergency room of the medical hospital in four-point restraints and placed on a 72-hour legal hold, which meant that he had to remain at the hospital for 72 hours because he was a danger to self and others. His parents were notified. He was transferred to the psychiatric section of the hospital and admitted as an inpatient. His parents agreed to a voluntary admission, which meant that the legal hold could be cancelled.

Assessment and Evaluation Process

Tony was scheduled for an OT assessment as part of the interdisciplinary treatment plan. The length of stay on the child service is 10 to 14 days. The focus of the evaluations are to quickly determine direction for intervention as an inpatient and at discharge. The initial evaluation is documented in the chart within 48 hours of admission. Additional evaluations may be performed to probe deficit areas first identified.

The overall focus of inpatient hospitalization for the interdisciplinary team is to stabilize behavior, identify major problems, clarify diagnosis, and initiate medication trials if indicated. The treatment of long-term psychiatric problems or family issues is not done at the inpatient level but at a less expensive level of care, such as in a partial hospital program or as an outpatient.

The OTA reviewed the chart and reported the history to the OT as described in the case study section. They both introduced themselves to Tony and told him they would each meet with him separately to find out the kinds of activities he enjoyed and new ones he might like to learn. The therapists worked together and shared assessment functions to gain a view of his play and socialization.

Evaluation and Findings

The routine evaluations used include an interview regarding patterns of daily activity, play activity check list, observation of task performance, observation of social interaction, and an assessment of visual motor integration. This last assessment is routinely done as many of the children have deficits in this area and their attempts to "cover" for deficits may spark behavior problems in the school situation. The specific format, purpose, the responsible OT personnel, and the results or findings follow.

Evaluation by the OT

Typical day interview and McDonald Play Activity Inventory—Revised (MPAI-R). This assessment included a semi-structured interview and structured checklist.

The purpose was to determine patterns of daily living, school, play activities, and chores; to determine whether play activities are dominantly gross motor, fine motor, social group, or solitary passive.

Findings

Tony refused to answer questions about chores, school, and play stating, "It's none of your business." Information was gained through a brief interview with the mother during visiting hours and through probing play activities listed on the MPAI (McDonald, 1987) with Tony. His mother reported that he was able to handle his self-care and that he had responsibilities at home of setting the table, making his bed, and cleaning the garage with his stepfather. He received an allowance of $2 per week, which he spent on candy. She said that he had behavior problems in school and had trouble controlling his temper with other children. He did not do well sharing TV time at home with her younger son and always wanted things his way. There were not any boys his age in the neighborhood, so she knew he did not have any friends there and assumed he did not have any at school because of his behavior.

The MPAI can be used for purposes of sorting children's interest into the four categories of gross motor, fine motor, social group, or solitary passive, or it can be used as a probe to elicit information from children who do not or are unable to spontaneously identify activities in which they like to engage. In this case, it was used as a probe and seemed less threatening to Tony. The activities circled were distributed nearly equally in all areas and included a mix of sports, crafts, card and team games. He also used the items to indicate activities he wished to do in the future. For example, he circled "play baseball," saying that he wanted to be on a team. He circled several items con-

cerning friends. When asked what he and his friends did, he named two of the children on the unit and referred to a game they had played earlier in the hospital day. When asked about friends away from the hospital and at home, he said "I just told you."

The OT noted that he was unwilling to give information, his interests included a mix of activities he had done and those he wished to do, and that he did not have any friends.

Evaluation by the OTA

The Beery-Buktenica Developmental Test of Visual-Motor Integration (VMI) is a structured test using form copying. The purpose is to determine developmental or age equivalent status of visual-motor skills. The evaluation was completed by the OTA.

Findings

Tony printed his name on the VMI booklet, and then threw it on the floor saying, "I'm not doing this shit." The OTA gave him a count of five to pick it up or he would have a time out of the area. This is part of the general behavioral program for non-compliance and will be covered under the treatment activities/techniques section. After the 2 minute time-out, the OTA picked up the book and again explained the purpose as seeing how his eyes and hands worked together and that it was not a test of his drawing ability. He achieved an age equivalent score of 5 years, 9 months, indicating impairment in visual-motor integration.

Evaluation by Both the OT and the OTA

Task performance was evaluated by both practitioners using both checklists and observations.

The purpose of the checklist was to determine decision-making, ability to follow directions, attention span, and to solve problems.

Findings

Tony was observed working on craft projects on two separate occasions. The OT initially gave him a choice of two "failproof" activities of stain-a-frame or copper tooling with a template. Easy one-step activities are initially given to assess task performance to give children a feeling of success and promote positive feelings about OT. Tony selected copper tooling and a pirate picture from template choices. He eagerly started out and then said that he had "messed up" and wanted to start over. When assured that he had not made any mistake, he seemed unsure and needed to be coached and encouraged to finish. The OTA worked with Tony and one other boy on making a treasure box by gluing puzzle pieces on a cigar box. He said he thought this was dumb, asked to change to another shape box in the middle of the project, but again completed it with encouragement and firm guidance. The COTA explained that all children learned activities as part of their program.

Both therapists noted that he was able to select from alternatives and he was able to attend to the activity. He frequently thought he had made a mistake on projects that contained little margin for failure, and he needed encouragement and coaxing to complete projects. He did not display any pleasure with his end product.

Evaluation by Both the OT and OTA

Further observation of socialization in OT area, recreation area, and on the inpatient unit was completed using a semi-structured guide.

The purpose of the guide is to determine frequency and content of interactions with peers and adults.

Findings

Tony was observed during structured activities such as dodge ball and community meeting as well as informal activities on the unit. Tony displayed two styles of interaction with peers. He was either isolative and distanced himself from others unless specifically included in activities, or he was intrusive, bossy, and dominating with others. With adults, he was mainly negative and oppositional, testing and challenging the limits. At other times, he was pleasant and laughed, but he seemed to convey a general demeanor of distrust and responded best one to one with an adult working with him in a playful manner. He also seemed to gravitate toward the male staff on the unit.

GENERAL GOALS

The OT summarized the evaluation findings and presented them to the treatment team. The primary concerns identified by the OT and OTA were his social distancing and/or bossiness with peers, lack of peer friendships in the home setting, fear of failure in task situations, and poor visual motor integration. Nursing and recreation therapy had observed similar social interaction problems with peers, and, additionally, Tony had two open seclusions for physical aggression against peers and attempting to kick staff. School testing revealed that he was functioning below grade level in all areas. Psychology had completed cognitive testing, and, although Tony was in the dull normal range, there was a 15-point differential between verbal and performance IQ, with verbal higher, suggesting a potential learning disorder.

The team was concerned that placement in a regular class might not be the best option for Tony, given his behavioral difficulties and the potential of a learning disorder. They felt that the mother and stepfather should request an IEP at school. The OT decided to pursue additional visual motor testing in this short hospitalization to tease out more information that might be useful for securing services as part of his IEP. The psychiatrist on the team had administered a depression inventory in which Tony had scored as clinically depressed. This was not surprising, as he was not doing well in school and had interactional difficulties. Depression was also not unusual with children with conduct disorder and was often manifest as irritability and rage. The physician was also concerned with the potential for post-traumatic stress disorder given his early history of physical abuse. Tony was placed on a small dose of antidepressant medication to help with the depression. Social work was concerned with the stepfather's minimizing Tony's aggression and treating it as "normal" and "macho."

General OT goals included that Tony initiate positive contacts with peers, that he resolve problem situations by using words instead of fighting, and that he successfully complete simple projects to gain a feeling of accomplishment and mastery in tasks. Additional visual motor testing to determine if his difficulties were more in the visual or motor realm was also a goal. Nursing was teaching principles of behavior management to the parents to deal with Tony's noncompliance and aggression, and social work was also working with the parents to help them initiate an IEP and to help the stepfather gain a more realistic picture of Tony's problems.

TREATMENT ACTIVITIES/TECHNIQUES

There is a behavioral program on the child inpatient service to ensure consistent expectations for behavior and consequences for loss of control for all children by all staff. Children are given a prompt or reminder for unacceptable behavior, and, if they fail to comply, are then given a 2-minute time out of the area or activity to cool off. If they are unable to voluntarily take the time out and if their behavior continues to escalate, they may be placed in the seclusion room, which is barren—containing no windows or furniture. The door of the room is open or closed depending on the severity of the tantrum or behavioral dyscontrol. Children are released into the milieu after they have calmed to the point that they can talk about the events that led to their escalation.

OT program planning for individual patients is completed within the context of the existing program, which is broadly designed to promote goals for most child patients while addressing individual needs. Program planning is guided by the four following principles (Florey, 1998).

1. Play and task environments should be populated with peers. It is critical for children to be able to work within a peer group, and it is the peer group in which many children with psychosocial dys-

function have difficulty. In the peer group, children learn and practice the sharing of materials, equipment, space, and the attention of others.

2. Social skills learning should be part of the task and play environments. Social skills are part of social competence in which social skill is one component. Social competence refers to mutually reinforcing social relationships and these are developmental in nature (Cartledge & Milburn, 1995; Cox & Schopler, 1996). In middle childhood, fostering positive social relationships may include sharing and compromising, giving affection and praise to others, helping others, learning to enter ongoing peer activities, and changing behavior in response to the needs of others.

3. Programs should be conducted within natural childhood activities dominated by toys, crafts, and games and embedded within natural childhood models. The overall process of the activity should be emphasized and not the final product. The end goal of toys, crafts, and games focuses on ways in which children can benefit, such as sharing materials, engaging in social banter, and achieving a sense of pride in workmanship rather than simply making a coin purse. Florey and Greene (1997) suggest that activities be graded according to cognitive complexity (problem-solving process required), motor complexity (motor and visual motor skill required), and social complexity (social exchange such as opportunities for peer interaction and cooperatively using space and materials). Often, social goals with children cannot be attained, as the activity may be too complex along other dimensions, which triggers poor social strategies.

Natural models for this age range include club, scout, and small group formats that have a distinctive identity. Children of this age seek to belong and be part of a larger social environment. At the UCLA Neuropsychiatric Hospital, a Cub Scout den chartered under the Boy Scouts of America has been in operation since 1971 and there has been an informal liaison with the Girl Scouts as well. With dramatically shorter lengths of stay, both boys and girls are combined into a general scout program. The children wear t-shirts and shirts representative of scouts and work on scouting principles, such as citizenship, rather than specific badges and pins.

Groups are conducted on the inpatient unit, in other parts of the hospital, and in the immediate community to gain an idea of how the children are able to maintain safety and social cues in less restrictive spaces.

4. Expectations for behavior should be explicit and known. Expectations for behaviors are best phrased as rules. Children of this age are beginning to understand rules and enjoy constructing rules. Rules for general safety and conduct as well as consequences for rule violations should be known. Principles of the behavior management system may be incorporated in the rules.

Tony was involved in a number of OT programs during his 10-day hospitalization. These included community meetings, friendship club, the scout troop, and lunch cooking group, which the OTs co-lead with recreation therapy. He was also involved in task/craft, newspaper, free play, baking groups, and in a special group that focuses on spiritual needs of children in which the OT and OTA work with the chaplain. The OT and OTA work together in most of the groups but also divide functions. Tony's mother attended two OT sessions, and the OT worked with her to learn how to present activities at his level and to set limits on his noncompliant and aggressive behavior while the OTA served as a model. Parental participation was arranged in conjunction with nursing, and it gave parents an opportunity to practice the behavioral strategies in an activity context.

His participation and specific goals in the baking, task, and free play groups are reviewed, as these give a snapshot of his typical patterns of behaving in different situations.

Baking Group

Tony worked with three other children in preparing after dinner snacks for all of the children on the inpatient unit. The purpose was to simulate being part of a family work group. Specific goals for Tony included working with others in taking turns, sharing, and using words to express his anger instead of physically fighting. The group was baking and frosting cupcakes. The OT and OTA had organized the tasks so that as one pair mixed the cake batter, the other pair placed cupcake papers in tins, and both pairs then filled the cups. At first, Tony did not want to participate and then rapidly changed to wanting to do everything. He needed specific direction as to what his job was and required prompts to stay within those limits. The group played a simple table game while the cupcakes were baking and cooling. Tony wanted to dominate the game, choosing the color of his marker and announcing that he would go first, but was responsive to suggestions to settle color and turns in a fair manner. Throughout the game, he tried to cheat by moving ahead spaces, became angry, and denied that he was cheating when his errors were pointed out to him. He needed continual prompting to keep from dominating his peers. He worked better on frosting the cupcakes, a solo task, in which each member was responsible for frosting and decorating a set number of cupcakes.

Task Group

The OT led the task groups. The goal for him was to follow directions, complete a simple craft, and say one good thing about how he had done. Tony's response was typical throughout his stay. During task groups, he would typically refuse to engage, saying that the craft was "stupid" or babyish. With encouragement and cajoling, he would engage. He made real or imagined mistakes and had little tolerance for any error or frustration. When he made an error, he wanted to begin again instead of attempting to fix his mistake and when told that the mistake could be corrected, threw the project across the table. He would allow the OT to fix the mistake, and then he could continue after a great deal of encouragement. He could not find anything good to say about his performance and when the OT suggested that he was learning to try hard things, he replied, "Whatever, I guess." Tony was very sensitive to failure of any kind and anticipated failure in most activities that he attempted.

Free Play

The OTA set up the free play situation, which was a mix of board games, creative media, dress-up clothes, and selected crafts. The purpose of the session was to observe how children were able to select play activities without an adult directing them, and how they approached settling any disputes that occurred. Three to four children were in the group. There were few stated rules for this group except for the obvious ones of no hitting or fighting. The OT began the sessions by saying that the number one rule of the playroom was to have fun, but in order to have fun, they would have to share materials and take turns. She also told them that they had responsibilities in that they had to return play items to their storage spaces and they had to clean up for themselves. She also stated that although she was in the playroom, she would not be able to teach a craft or play a game with anyone, as she was making a list of needed supplies. The goal for Tony was to observe his overall pattern and see to what extent he could negotiate positively with peers on his own.

Tony either isolated himself and wandered around the playroom touching materials, or he gravitated toward the play of others. He seemed to have little capacity to generate ideas on his own. He abruptly entered situations in which others were playing and announced that he would play too. He was bossy, domineering, and had very little tolerance for doing anything other than his way. The OTA needed to prompt him several times to stop annoying others before the situation escalated to Tony losing control. It was as if he had two modes: loner or boss, and he needed the modeling of others to select play activities.

There was a meeting of all the disciplines with the mother and stepfather at discharge in which different team members presented their findings and recommendations. The team told the family that Tony's persistent pattern of aggressive behavior was called *conduct disorder* and that there were many factors that contributed to this clinical picture. Conduct disorder was a name given to a cluster of symptoms known collectively by this name and there was no one cause. He may have sustained some "soft" neurological damage during periods of physical abuse and this may contribute to a learning disorder. A learning disorder is suspected when there is a difference in verbal and performance IQ, which often suggests a processing problem. The poor performance picture also fit with the OT-extended testing on motor and visual tests of in which he was below age equivalent in both components but lower in fine motor areas. Although he did not display any pronounced fine motor deficits in simple tasks, his fear of making a mistake and exposing a deficit may have made him hesitant to attempt new activities.

The team explained that a learning disorder may help explain some of his behaviors in the school setting, as he had a very low tolerance for frustration and his behavior focused attention on his interactional rather than academic difficulties. He also showed some evidence of depression, a disorder of mood, which may have been due to a poor self image. The physician recommended that he be continued on the antidepressant initiated early in the hospital stay.

Tony also had an ingrained distrust of adults, which made it difficult for adults to like engaging with him. His peer interactional difficulties and his noncompliance leading to aggression were paramount and evident in the reports of all clinical disciplines. His stepfather was still of the conviction that he was only sticking up for and asserting himself, but he did agree that without strict limits on his aggressive outbursts, there could be danger to the younger son in the family, his pregnant wife, and the newborn baby.

The team focused on discharge recommendations centering on the school and home. They recommended that Tony have an IEP. The team felt he may qualify for a learning disabled class and would probably need additional testing in the school system to pinpoint the learning problem. He would also qualify for an emotionally disturbed (formerly called "seriously emotionally disturbed" in the school system) class based on his behavioral difficulties, but it was the hope of the team that dealing with his underlying learning disorder may help with his behavioral difficulties. The therapist recommended that he have OT in the school to address his fine motor difficulties, and that structured social skills be included in the IEP so that he could learn positive ways of working with other children.

At home, the team advised the parents to continue the behavioral training program they had learned in the hospital, which was a system of earning privileges for good behavior and the withdrawal of privileges for poor behavior. He also needed to be included in family chores and needed some special time with both his mother and his stepfather so that he could begin to trust adults. The occupational and recreation therapists suggested games and activities that Tony and his parents could easily do together in their special time with him (e.g., cards, baking cookies, planting flowers, playing catch). This was important for him, as Tony made working with him difficult, and pushing people away was part of his strategy of not getting hurt first. It was also important to find activities in which he could succeed so that he could begin to generate some positive feelings about himself. The OT also recommended that Tony attend a camp for children with behavior problems in the summer. This camp worked exclusively with children with social problems and had daily structured activities in which competition with others was eliminated. The focus instead was on process, and this would be a good direction for Tony.

CLINICAL PROBLEM-SOLVING

Case Study 2

Ben is a 9-year-old boy admitted to the child inpatient service for increasingly violent and aggressive behavior and a suicidal threat. Ben was admitted from a residential treatment center where he had been for the past 3 months. He was born out of wedlock to an 18-year-old girl who had abused alcohol and cocaine during her pregnancy. He had been removed from the mother and placed in a foster home at that time, as the mother was unable to care for him. He had had no contact with his biological mother. He had been adopted by his first foster mother.

Ben's behavior problems began in preschool. He was aggressive and hyperactive and at age 5, was diagnosed as having attention deficit hyperactive disorder. He was placed on a stimulant to control his hyperactivity. Ben had been suspended from schools on several occasions because of fighting and destroying school property. His adopted mother had other children in the home, and she was increasingly unable to handle his behavior problems. He had been moved from one foster home to another as foster parents were unable to handle his impulsive and aggressive behavior. He had also been placed on an antipsychotic medication in addition to the stimulant because of his increasing rage attacks. He was placed in a group home for children for behavior problems but had run away. He was placed in a locked residential treatment facility, as this was felt to be the most therapeutic option for him. He was admitted to the inpatient service because he had thrown furniture, hit staff, and was threatening to kill himself by jumping out of a two-story window.

How would the OT and OTA evaluate Ben? What effect does in-utero exposure to drugs and alcohol have on an individual? What types of recommendations does one make to a residential treatment facility? Is there a way to influence this negative and self-defeating cycle that Ben is exhibiting?

REFERENCES

American Psychiatric Association. (1994). *Diagnostic and statistical manual of mental disorders* (4th ed.). Washington, DC: Author.

Cartledge, G., & Milburn, J. (1995). *Teaching social skills to children and youth* (3rd ed.). Boston, MA: Allyn and Bacon.

Cox, R., & Schopler, E. (1996). Social skills training for children. In M. Lewis (Ed.), *Child and adolescent psychiatry: A comprehensive textbook* (2nd ed.). Baltimore, MD: Williams & Wilkins.

Earls, F. (1994). Oppositional-defiant and conduct disorders. In M. Rutter, E. Taylor, & L. Hersov (Eds.), *Child and adolescent psychiatry: Modern approaches* (3rd ed.). Oxford, England: Blackwell Scientific.

Florey, L. (1998). Psychosocial dysfunction in childhood and adolescence. In M. Neistadt & E. Crepeau (Eds.), *Willard & Spackman's OT* (9th ed.). Philadelphia, PA: Lippincott.

Florey, L., & Greene, S. (1997). Play in middle childhood: A focus on children with behavior and emotional disorders. In L. D. Parham & L. Fazio (Eds.), *Play in OT for children*. St. Louis, MO: C. V. Mosby.

Kazdin, A. (1995). Conduct disorder. In F. Verhulst & H. Koot (Eds.), *The Epidemiology of Child and Adolescent Psychopathology*. Oxford, England: Oxford University Press.

Lewis, D. (1996). Conduct disorder. In M. Lewis (Ed.), *Child and Adolescent Psychiatry: A Comprehensive Textbook* (2nd ed.). Baltimore, MD: Williams & Wilkins.

McDonald, A. (1987). *The construction of a self-report instrument to measure play activities and play styles in 7 to 11 year old children*. Unpublished master's thesis. University of Southern California.

A Third-Grader with Attention Deficit Hyperactivity Disorder

Sue Triplett Hunt, MA, OTR

INTRODUCTION

Attention deficit hyperactivity disorder (ADHD) is now the official term used to describe both attention deficit disorder (ADD) and ADHD. *The Diagnostic and Statistical Manual of Mental Disorders* (4th ed.) (American Psychiatric Association, 1994) has identified three subtypes of ADHD:

1. Predominantly inattentive type
2. Predominantly hyperactive and impulsive type
3. The combined type

ADHD is one of the most common mental health disorders among children today, occurring more often in boys than girls. Children with ADD/ADHD are persistently more impulsive and less attentive than their same-aged peers.

There is no exact cause of ADD/ADHD, however, research suggests that it may be

KEY CONCEPTS

- Diagnosis: Must be made by a physician according to three patterns of behavior.
- ADD/ADHD: No exact cause, may be biological or neurological. Common behaviors: inattention, impulsivity, emotional instability, and excessively high level of activity.
- Assessment: May involve various parent and/or teacher checklists, sensory histories, observations, and evaluation of related performance areas such as fine motor, self-help, and play skills.
- Frames of reference: Coping, occupational, and sensory integration are commonly used.
- Eligibility for related services: Children who are not eligible for services under the Individuals with Disabilities Education Act may be eligible under Section 504 of the Rehabilitation Act.
- Section 504 of the Rehabilitation Act of 1973: This federal law guarantees reasonable accommodations to individuals attending federally funded programs. Anyone regarded as having a disability is eligible for these accommodations.
- Environmental adaptations: Might include such things as preferential seating, use of a desktop easel, or special paper.
- Home visit: Visit to the home to determine any needed modifications for play, self-help, social interactions, routines, etc.
- Consultation: Sharing of expertise by one team member to another.
- Recommendations and strategies: Specific suggestions to assist the child, teacher, and caregiver with identified concerns.
- Follow-up: Therapist returns to the setting to offer suggestions for any new or continuing concerns.

ESSENTIAL VOCABULARY

Distractibility: Difficulty paying attention to the task at hand while "tuning out" other, less relevant information.

Hyperactivity: Excessive level of activity.

Impulsivity: The inability to regulate emotions or behavior, giving little consideration to the consequences of a behavior before doing it.

Inattention: Lack of attention span or concentration.

Level of arousal: Varying states of alertness.

Organizational skills: The ability to organize materials, space, and time in order to complete a task.

Reasonable accommodations: Modifications and adaptations to accommodate or provide access to activities.

Social skills: Behaviors including greeting, taking turns, listening, and maintaining a topic during social interactions.

biologically and neurologically based. A child with ADHD will frequently have a parent, sibling, or other family member with similar behavior and educational history, indicating that there is a genetic predisposition for this disorder. Other factors that have been suggested as contributing to ADHD include prematurity, prenatal toxic exposures, and prenatal damage to the fetal nervous system, although no scientific evidence indicates that these factors cause ADHD (Kaplan & Sadock, 1998).

The symptoms of ADHD range from mild to severe and may be inconsistently displayed. Inattention, impulsivity, and emotional instability are among the most common issues for people with ADHD. Although children with ADHD may be able to pay attention to activities that are highly motivating to them, they often have difficulty completing tasks that are unfamiliar or that require organization and sustained focus. Impulsivity interferes with the development of age-appropriate social skills, as these children often interrupt or act before thinking about the possible consequences of their words or actions. Poor safety awareness is also a common concern for families of children and adults with ADHD, as they are not only impulsive, but seek out novel experiences. Limited interpersonal awareness is another common trait of individuals with ADHD, as characterized by angry outbursts, blaming others for problems, and over-sensitivity to criticism.

Many positive traits can be associated with people with ADHD. These characteristics may include high energy, creativity, perseverance, resourcefulness, high intelligence, risk taking, spontaneity, and high verbal skills.

A psychiatrist, pediatrician, neurologist, or a family physician can make the diagnosis of ADHD. According to DSM-IV, three patterns of behavior must be identified in order for an accurate diagnosis to be made. These patterns are:

1. The pattern must appear before the age of 7.
2. The pattern must continue for at least 6 months.
3. The behaviors must negatively affect at least two areas of the child's life, such as school, home, or social settings.

The typical age of onset of ADHD is between 2 and 7 years (Barkley, 1990), however, many children with ADHD will not show symptoms that interfere with daily functioning until later childhood. The physician may recommend medication for some children with ADHD. Commonly prescribed medications include Ritalin (Novartis, Basel, Switzerland), Dexedrine (Smith-Kline Beecham, Philadelphia, PA), and Cylert (Abbott Laboratories, Inc., North Chicagop, IL). These medications are intended to modulate attention and impulsivity. Educational and psychosocial interventions are generally used in conjunction with medication.

Research indicates that although the primary symptoms of ADHD tend to diminish during the adolescent years, some behaviors may remain, including low self-esteem, restlessness, impulsivity, low self-confidence, and impaired social interactions. Often, as adults, these individuals show less hyperactivity, but are accident prone and impulsive (Kaplan & Sadock, 1998).

FRAMES OF REFERENCE

Depending on the nature of the symptoms, various frames of reference can be implemented for the child with ADHD. The coping frame of reference may help the therapist identify the child's learning style, as well as to identify the kinds of environmental adaptations that may be necessary for improved occupational performance. Using this frame of reference, the therapist may assist the child in acquiring new skills for self-regulation, social interactions, and organization.

Another frame of reference appropriate for this group would be the occupational frame of reference. This frame addresses adaptive functioning and social competence. Interventions within this frame might include a social skills group, helping the student to organize school materials, and offering strategies for completing daily routines, so that eventually new habits are established.

A sensory integrative approach may be used for the client with tactile, vestibular, and proprioceptive processing issues. Often children with ADHD have difficulty calming down, alerting, or organizing themselves. Interventions that may help these children learn to maintain an optimum level of arousal include deep pressure touch and heavy work. Interventions designed to provide opportunities for organizing and sequencing motor tasks, enhancing postural control, or promoting awareness of body position in space may be useful for the child demonstrating difficulty with handwriting or physical education activities. It should be noted that not all children with ADHD have problems with sensory processing.

ASSESSMENT

One useful tool when assessing a child with ADHD is a behavioral checklist. Several behavioral checklists are available. These checklists provide a good starting point to gain insight into the behaviors that are interfering with the child's daily life. The parent or teacher can complete the *Achenbach Child Behavior Checklist* (Achenbach & Edelbrock, 1983). This tool is designed for children ages 4 to 16 years. The *Connors' Parent Rating Scale* or the *Connors' Teacher Rating Scale* (Connors, 1990) is also completed by either the teacher or the parent and is for children from 3 to 17 years of age. Both the OTA and the OT should review the checklist and keep in mind that the behavior of children with ADHD fluctuates from place to place and time to time.

Another helpful tool is the sensory history. Poor sensory processing can lead to social problems, disturbances in sensory modulation, and sensory avoidance behaviors. Several sensory histories have been published for collecting data on sensory functioning, including the *Touch Inventory for Elementary School-Aged Children* (Royeen & Fortune, 1990), *Teacher Questionnaire on Sensorimotor Behavior* (Carrasco & Lee, 1993), and *Sensory Profile* (Dunn, 1999). These histories can be filled out by parents and teachers and should be reviewed and interpreted with an OT.

Frequently, children with ADHD will have immature fine or gross motor skills. In these instances, a motor assessment may be utilized. The *Peabody Developmental Motor Scale* (PDMS) (Folio & Fewell, 1983) assesses both fine and gross motor skills in children from 1 month to 7 years. The *Bruininks-Oseretsky Test of Motor Proficiency* (BOTMP) (Bruininks, 1978) assesses gross motor skills including speed, agility, balance, bilateral coordination, strength, and upper limb coordination. The fine motor portion of the BOTMP tests response speed, visual-motor control, upper limb speed, and dexterity. Both the PDMS and BOTMP can be administered under the supervision of an OTR after practicing the administration of the test on several typically developing children. An OTR should review and interpret the results of either motor assessment. In addition, clinical observations of muscle tone, posture, reflex development, and strength should be completed in collaboration with the OT.

Another common concern for the child with ADHD is visual-motor integration skills. Visual-motor integration skills can be evaluated using the *Test of Visual Motor Skills—Revised* (TVMS-R) (Gardner, 1995), the *Developmental Test of Visual Perception* (DTVP) (2nd ed.) (Hammill, Pearson, Voress, 1993), or the *Developmental Test of Visual-Motor Integration—Revised* (VMI-R) (Beery & Buktenica, 1997). Tests of visual perception may also be indicated, and these include the *Motor Free Visual Perceptual Test* (1996) and the *Test of Visual-Perceptual Skills (Non-Motor)—Revised* or the *Test of Visual-Perceptual Skills (Non-Motor) (Upper Level)* (Gardner, 1992, 1996). These can be administered and scored by the OTA, with assistance from the OT. Although these scores may be used to plan intervention, best practice in school-based therapy indicates that goals and objectives be functional and not directed at improving test scores.

When concerns are specifically directed at handwriting, it is necessary to evaluate several performance areas. Assessment of visual perception and visual-motor integration using the previously mentioned tools should be completed along with observations of handwriting and functional hand use. The therapy assistant, in collaboration with the OT, can administer handwriting assessments. Two commonly used handwriting evaluations are the *Evaluation Tool of Children's Handwriting (ETCH)* (Manuscript: *ETCH-M* and Cursive: *ETCH-C*) (Amundson, 1995), *Children's Handwriting Evaluation Scale* (CHES), and *Children's Handwriting Evaluation Scale for Manuscript Writing* (CHES-M) (Phelps, Stempel, & Speck, 1984, 1987). Both of these handwriting tools evaluate speed and legibility of writing. Analysis of results should be a cooperative effort of the OTA and the OT. *Assessment of Hand Skills in the Primary Child* by Benbow (1995) may be useful in determining the specific performance components that interfere with handwriting. This tool is appropriate for COTAs to utilize after watching the video and observing several typically developing children performing these tasks.

An observation of the child in various settings is critical. Structured settings, such as the classroom and non-structured settings, such as the playground or cafeteria, should be observed. In addition, specific adaptive tasks, such as dressing, playing, safety awareness, and organizing personal belongings, should be addressed.

SECTION 504 OF THE REHABILITATION ACT OF 1973

When a student with a disability is not eligible for special education services, yet has difficulty participating in and benefiting from educational programs, he or she may be eligible for OT services under Section 504 of the Rehabilitation Act of 1973. Under Section 504, anyone who is identified as having a physical or mental impairment that substantially limits a major life activity, has a record of the impairment, or is regarded as having such an impairment, is eligible for reasonable accommodations. Any program receiving federal funding is required by law to make reasonable accommodations. These accommodations might include menu modifications, therapy services, or environmental adaptations for these individuals.

CASE STUDY

Nathan is a third-grader in Mr. Roth's class at Webster Elementary School. He lives at home with his mother and a 13-year-old sister, Elizabeth. Nathan's mother, Mrs. L., has become increasingly concerned with Nathan's recent behavior at home. Although he had never been an "easy" child, Mrs. L. had always excused his rambunctious behavior on the fact that he was "just being a boy" and was subjected to various family stressors. When Nathan was 5, his father moved out of the house after dropping out of a rehab program for cocaine addiction. It was a very stressful time for the family and Mrs. L. was forced to return to work a few months earlier when her husband's drug abuse had become so out of control that he was fired from his job. During this time, Nathan became even more distractible and irritable. Mrs. L. noticed that he could not seem to stay focused long enough to play a simple game with his sister or sometimes even finish a sandwich at lunch. He was always "flitting" around the house, never seeming to get engaged with a toy or activity. His arguments with his sister quickly escalated to name calling and angry outbursts. He would often throw a tantrum if he didn't get his way.

As a baby, Nathan had always been fussy and had not begun sleeping through the night until he was almost 6. Now at 7 ½, he seemed very immature in contrast to how Elizabeth had behaved at that age. Recently, during a visit to the pediatrician for his asthma, Nathan created a scene in the waiting area when another child would not immediately give up the remote-controlled car that Nathan wanted to play with. When Mrs. L. mentioned her concern over Nathan's high level of activity and difficulty staying with certain tasks to the pediatrician, he asked for her input as he completed a behavioral checklist. The pediatrician also asked Mrs. L. to give another checklist to Nathan's teacher the next day. Using the information from both Mrs. L. and Mr. Roth, the pediatrician diagnosed Nathan as having ADHD.

Mr. Roth had also been concerned about Nathan's behavior in school. Nathan had begun to fall behind in classroom work, despite the fact that Mr. Roth felt that Nathan understood the material and was a bright student. Nathan's assignments were often crumpled and torn, sometimes barely legible. Nathan's personal space was often disorganized. Sometimes he did not get started on an assignment until long after the others, as he was unable to locate his pencil, workbook, scissors, etc. Math was especially difficult for Nathan; he was unable to copy equations from the board and could not align numbers or letters on the lines of primary paper. Mr. Roth indicated that soon the class would be beginning cursive writing instruction, and that he was concerned this would be difficult for Nathan. He also noted that Nathan was out of his seat so often that he was disrupting the whole class. Problems on the playground were reported, too. He seemed to lack all judgment on the equipment, standing on the top rung of the jungle gym, jumping off the teeter-totter in mid-air, and running wildly into groups of children. Fortunately, he seemed to have excellent gross motor skill and coordination and always regained his balance and landed on his feet.

Soon after the diagnosis was made, Mr. Roth requested permission from Mrs. L. for a meeting with the Child Study Team to identify possible services to help Nathan at school. At the meeting, Mrs. L. and the team determined that Nathan was still managing to function within the normal range for his grade, and that he did not require special education services, thus making him ineligible for services under the Individuals with Disabilities Education Act. However, the team felt that he might benefit from some services and modifications in order to continue to meet the academic requirements of the third grade curriculum. A referral to OT was made.

Assessment

After meeting briefly with Mr. Roth before school, the OTA reviewed the behavior checklists that Mr. Roth and Mrs. L. had filled out. She noted Nathan's high activity level, his lack of organizational skills, and problems with handwriting. Using this information, she and the OT determined that the following assessments would be useful:

- Sensory profile completed by Mrs. L. and Mr. Roth.
- Classroom observation including:
  - Postural control, upright posture, feet on floor, using hands to support head, etc.
  - Unusual behaviors during writing, such as chewing on the pencil or task-avoidant behaviors, etc.
  - Environmental factors, such as improper chair or desk height, cluttered walls or work areas, etc.
  - Organization of materials and workspace.
  - Visual concerns, squinting, rubbing eyes, using his finger to visually track while reading, etc.
- Collection of handwriting samples and class assignments to:
  - Determine which tasks are more problematic—copying from the board or composing.
  - Note letter formation, alignment, orientation, spacing, and slant.
- Playground, physical education, and cafeteria observation of:
  - Social skills
  - Organizational skills
  - Distractibility/off-task behavior
  - Safety awareness
  - Use of gross motor equipment
- Observation in art room.
- Home visit or phone interview with Mrs. L. related to play and self-care skills.
- Explanation and discuss sensory profile.
- Administration of Test of Visual-Motor Integration Skills.
- Assessment of Hand Skills in the Primary Child.

The OT and OTA designed a plan for assessing and observing Nathan based on the therapy assistant's previous experience with the various tools being utilized. The

COTA administered and scored the TVMS-R and completed the Benbow observations. The OTR did classroom, gym, art, and playground observations. The sensory profile was explained to Mrs. L and sent home for her to complete. The OTR also scheduled a consultation visit with Mr. Roth during his planning period.

Results of Assessment and Observations

The sensory profile did not indicate any significant sensory processing problems, however, it was reported that Nathan would occasionally become overly excited and had difficulty calming down. Neither his mother nor the teacher felt that this behavior was interfering with his performance at school.

The classroom observation provided information regarding Nathan's disorganization, distractibility, and level of activity/arousal. Nathan's postural control was adequate for the task of writing; however, his desk and chair height needed to be adjusted. Pencil grasp was immature. Nathan's desk and workspace were disorganized, and he had difficulty finding papers, pencils, etc. During writing tasks, Nathan found many other things to do, sometimes completely avoiding the assignment until the class was moving on to another activity. Work samples indicated that copying was more difficult than creating. Letter formation, alignment, orientation to line, and spacing was problematic.

On the playground, social skills were a concern. Nathan was unable to successfully participate in child-directed games. This appeared due to his limited ability to take turns and stay on task. He quickly became angry and would either antagonize other kids or abandon that game and attempt entering another. Social skills were also an issue in the cafeteria. Nathan typically moved through the lunch line without waiting his turn. He had difficulty listening during conversations at the lunch table and often blurted out information not related to the conversation.

Nathan scored within 6 months of his age on the TVMS-R, and no further testing was done in this area.

When observed using the Benbow assessment, Nathan was unable to maintain a palmar arch or adequately separate the two sides of his hand. Precision rotation was also difficult and impaired his ability to use math manipulatives.

Intervention

Under Section 504, an accommodation plan is recommended. Formal, written goals and objectives are not required (Figure 16-1). The therapist and assistant collaborated with Mrs. L. and Mr. Roth to design Nathan's plan. Direct OT was recommended on a short-term basis to address Nathan's handwriting and organizational skills. Handwriting was an area the OTA had spent considerable time learning about. She had attended conferences and reviewed various handwriting programs. *Loops and Other Groups: A Kinesthetic Writing System* (Benbow, 1990) was determined to be an appropriate program to use with Nathan. The OTA and OT volunteered to provide in-service training to third-grade teachers who were interested in using this curriculum in their classrooms. Other interventions designed to help Nathan with handwriting included trial use of adaptive equipment such as pencil grips, clipboards, raised line paper, highlighters, and graph paper. Nathan's seat and desk height were adjusted. The OTA implemented these interventions in the classroom.

The therapy assistant designed various strategies to help Nathan with organizing his materials and workspace. She provided organizational strategies that could then be maintained and monitored by Mr. Roth. These strategies included:

- Use of a three-ring notebook with Velcro closures.
- Use of self-adhesive hole reinforcers for torn papers.
- Pocket folders for homework marked with "Done" on one side and "To Do" on the other.
- Pocket folders that are color-coded for specific subjects.
- Use of a compartmental tray for art supplies, with clearly marked areas for various materials.
- Name labels on all materials.
- Use of a small pocket notebook to keep track of homework assignments.
- Checklists for Nathan to refer to regarding materials he needs to bring home, steps to completing assignments, etc.

A "Lunch Bunch" group was recommended for improving socialization skills. This group consisted of three or four of Nathan's peers who were chosen by the teacher. The children ate lunch together for a 1-week period. Different students joined Nathan every week. Strategies for improving listening skills, turn-taking, reading facial expression, staying on topic, and manners were introduced, modeled, and reinforced by more socially mature students and the intermittent attendance of the OTA.

The OTA and OT created activities for developing palmar arches, improving precision rotation, and separating the two sides of the hands. These activities included various manipulatives, age-appropriate games, and crafts that could be used during math, cooperative learning activities, and "down time" in the classroom. Activities and materials were changed often, as novelty is a key factor in maintaining interest and attention. In addition, the OTA offered suggestions for crafts and games that corresponded to the general curriculum during monthly consultations with Mr. Roth.

Student: _____ DOB: _____ [Insert School District Name] Meeting Date: _____
INDIVIDUALIZED EDUCATION PROGRAM

MODIFICATIONS/ADAPTATIONS IN REGULAR EDUCATION - INCLUDING NONACADEMIC AND EXTRACURRICULAR ACTIVITIES - AND COLLABORATION/SUPPORTS FOR SCHOOL PERSONNEL

Modifications/Adaptations in Regular Education - Including Nonacademic and Extracurricular Activities	Sites/Activities Where Required and Duration	Required Supports for Personnel and Frequency and Duration of Supports
Materials/Books/Equipment: ☐ Alternative Text ☐ Consumable Workbook ☐ Modified Worksheets ☐ Manipulatives ☐ Access to Computer ☐ Tape Recorder ☐ Supplementary Visuals ☐ Large Print Text ☐ Spell Check ☐ Calculator ☐ Assistive Technology: (specify) _____ ☐ Other: (specify) _____		_____
Tests/Quizzes/Time: ☐ Prior Notice of Tests ☐ Preview Test Procedures ☐ Test Study Guide ☐ Simplify Test Wording ☐ Oral Testing ☐ Limited Multiple Choice ☐ Student Write on Test ☐ Shortened Tasks ☐ Hands-on Projects ☐ Reduced Reading ☐ Alternative Tests ☐ Objective Tests ☐ Extra Credit Options ☐ Extra Time–Written Work ☐ Extra Time–Tests ☐ Extra Time–Projects ☐ Extra Response Time ☐ Modified Tests ☐ Pace Long Term Projects ☐ Rephrase Test Questions/Directions ☐ Other: (specify) _____		_____
Grading: ☐ No Spelling Penalty ☐ No Handwriting Penalty ☐ Grade Effort + Work ☐ Grade Improvement ☐ Course Credit ☐ Base Grade on IEP ☐ Base Grade on Ability ☐ Modified Grades ☐ Pass/Fail ☐ Audit Course ☐ Other: (specify) _____		_____
Organization: ☐ Provide Study Outlines ☐ Desktop List of Tasks ☐ List Sequential Steps ☐ Post Routines ☐ Post Assignments ☐ Give One Paper at a Time ☐ Folders to Hold Work ☐ Pencil Box for Tools ☐ Pocket Folder for Work ☐ Assignment Pad ☐ Daily Assignment List ☐ Daily Homework List ☐ Worksheet Formats ☐ Extra Space for Work ☐ Assign Partner ☐ Other: (specify) _____		_____
Environment: ☐ Preferential Seating ☐ Clear Work Area ☐ Study Carrel ☐ Other: (specify) _____		_____
Behavior Management/Support: ☐ Daily Feedback to Student ☐ Chart Progress ☐ Behavior Contracts ☐ Parent/Guardian Sign Homework ☐ Positive Reinforcement ☐ Collect Baseline Data ☐ Set/Post Class Rules ☐ Parent/Guardian Sign Behavioral Chart ☐ Cue Expected Behavior ☐ Structure Transitions ☐ Break Between Tasks ☐ Time Out from Positive Reinforcement ☐ Proximity/Touch Control ☐ Contingency Plan ☐ Other: (specify) _____		_____
Instructional Strategies: ☐ Check Work in Progress ☐ Immediate Feedback ☐ Pre-teach Content ☐ Have Student Restate Information ☐ Extra Drill/Practice ☐ Review Sessions ☐ Review Directions ☐ Provide Lecture Notes/Outline to Student ☐ Use Manipulatives ☐ Modified Content ☐ Assign Study Partner ☐ Computer Assisted Instruction ☐ Monitor Assignments ☐ Provide Models ☐ Repeat Instructions ☐ Support Auditory Presentations with Visuals ☐ Multi-Sensory Approach ☐ Highlight Key Words ☐ Oral Reminders ☐ Display Key Vocabulary ☐ Visual Reinforcement ☐ Pictures/Charts ☐ Visual Reminders ☐ Provide Student With Vocabulary Word Bank ☐ Mimed Clues/Gestures ☐ Concrete Examples ☐ Use Mnemonics ☐ Personalized Examples ☐ Number Line ☐ Other (specify) _____		_____

Note: When specifying required supports for personnel to implement this IEP, include the specific supports required, how often they are to be provided (frequency) and for how long (duration).
(e.g. "the speech/language pathologist will meet with the student's classroom teacher for 20 minutes each week for the school year, to plan language activities which can be used in the classroom.")

Figure 16-1. Page 8 of the Connecticut State Individualized Education Program, August 1998, *Modifications/Adaptations in Regular Education: Including Nonacademic and Extracurricular Activities and Collaboration/Supports for School Personnel.* (Reprinted with permission from the Connecticut State Individualized Education Program.)

Once adaptations and materials are in place within the classroom, OT would meet on a regular basis with various school personnel and Mrs. L. to brainstorm and plan further modifications, as needed.

Home Visit

A home visit was requested by Mrs. L. to address several issues. Mrs. L.'s priority was for Nathan to become more independent in his morning routine. It was very difficult to constantly monitor him, as she also had to get herself and Elizabeth ready for work and school each morning. Nathan required constant redirection to continue getting dressed, eat breakfast, and pack his backpack. He often got to school without his homework or with inadequate clothes for the season. The OTA recommended that brief, colorful lists be designed and placed in strategic places to serve as a reminder of the things he needed to do while he was in that particular place. She also recommended that Nathan be required to pack his backpack and lay out appropriate clothes for the weather the night before, again utilizing the brief checklists. A timer was suggested to help Nathan stay on task for each segment of his morning routine. Mrs. L. would set the timer for the appropriate amount of time needed for a particular task, and this would allow her to quickly check in on his progress.

Another team idea was to involve Nathan in an extracurricular activity. This would provide opportunities outside of school to practice his newly acquired social skills and to enhance his self-confidence and self-esteem. Knowing Nathan's love of the water, Mrs. L. enrolled him in the town's recreational swimming program for one night each week. Not only did Nathan have the opportunity to learn new strokes and gain skills, he also seemed to come home very relaxed and proud of his new accomplishments.

Follow-Up

The OTA made several visits to the classroom over the next 6 months. She and Mr. Roth utilized a form they

INPUT SHEET

To: _____

From: _____

Date: _____

Student: _____

Activity	Comments
Activity	Comments
Activity	Comments
Activity	Comments

Special Notes:

Next Week/Session:

Figure 16-2. Input sheet. (Reprinted with permission from Sanderson, C. (1999). *Input sheet for classroom consultation*. Therapist developed unpublished worksheet.)

referred to as an "input sheet" (Figure 16-2), which proved to be very helpful. Mr. Roth and various other teachers involved with Nathan were encouraged to leave Input Sheets in the OTA's school mailbox regarding tasks that were causing problems for Nathan at school. The OTA could then discuss the concerns with the OT before offering suggestions in writing on the bottom half of the input sheet. The sheet would then be returned to the teacher. These sheets were also helpful for communicating with Mrs. L., so that she might utilize some of the strategies at home. Input sheets were kept in a notebook so that problems, progress, and plans could be documented on a regular basis.

Program Discontinuation

Consultation continued throughout the school year. Nathan's fine motor skills improved through the use of toys, games, and manipulatives that were highly motivating. Nathan's handwriting also improved; however, he continued to require cueing to slow down and more carefully orient his letters. Nathan was also more able to effectively organize his time and space. Initially, he relied heavily on environmental adaptations, such as lists and pocket folders, but within a few months had memorized many of the simple checklists and could organize his materials for

most projects. Mrs. L. also noticed changes at home. She had become aware of how important structure was for Nathan. She felt that many of the strategies offered had been instrumental in his increasing independence with self-help skills.

Socially, Nathan continued to have some difficulty, although he remained very popular among the more outgoing kids in his class. His impulsivity caused him to say hurtful things, but he had become more aware of other's feelings and would be quick to apologize upon recognizing his insults. The Lunch Bunch club continued, and various resource room, classroom, and special education staff participated on a rotating basis.

A meeting was held prior to school starting the following year to discuss strategies that were helpful with Nathan's new teacher. The input sheets provided a review of both successful and unsuccessful interventions. The OTA assisted the teacher in designing new "cue cards" and other organizational strategies appropriate to the fourth-grade curriculum. The OTA made two visits to the classroom in the first month of school to help problem-solve any issues related to handwriting and organization of materials, etc. A phone call was also made to Mrs. L., who felt that things were going well thus far. At this point, OT was discontinued with the understanding that if further issues arose, additional consultative visits might be requested.

ADULTS WITH ADHD

For many adults with ADHD, the hyperactivity they experienced in their childhood will have diminished, however, other symptoms of ADHD may persist. There are many adults with ADHD who have developed strategies for staying on task, attending to things not intrinsically interesting, and organizing their time. Strategies such as the use of tape recorders to record important meetings and colored files for organizing written materials are effective. The use of bill-paying software, oversized calendars placed in prominent locations, and daily planners may also be effective for the adult with ADHD.

CLINICAL PROBLEM-SOLVING

Clarissa is an 8-year-old girl recently diagnosed with ADHD. Clarissa has great difficulty tuning out noise or activity in the classroom. She is constantly moving about the room, unable to sit still for more than 1 or 2 minutes. Her high level of activity has significantly impacted her performance at school. She has been identified as in need of special education services secondary to her ADHD. Clarissa has been referred for OT. Completion of a sensory profile indicates that she has problems in the area of sensory processing, in particular, with regulating her overall state of arousal. The OTR observed Clarissa in the classroom. Clarissa was so busy that it was impossible for her to engage in classroom assignments and discussions, despite the fact that she had a lot to contribute. OT was recommended by the team to address her sensory processing skills and her ability to modulate her level of arousal. What treatment approaches might be used in this case?

The OT and OTA designed an intervention plan that included use of a "sensory diet" for use in the school environment. The OTA and OT offered strategies that could be easily incorporated into her daily routine such as listening to calming music through headphones during silent reading or while completing written work. Other strategies included the use of heavy work activities interspersed throughout the day. The Alert Program (Williams & Shellenberger, 1996) was also implemented for use in individual and group sessions with the OTA. This program offers strategies for teaching children or adults how to regulate their own level of alertness. The OTA taught visual imagery and relaxation techniques to Clarissa. The therapist and the therapy assistant met periodically to discuss how Clarissa was progressing. They also met with the classroom teacher to brainstorm ways to address self-regulation issues in the classroom.

Eric, a second grader, was referred to OT due to his clumsiness at school. His teachers noted problems with the organization and sequencing of tasks. Upon evaluation by the OT, it was determined that Eric had poor balance, immature bilateral hand skills, motor planning problems, and poor visual-motor integration. Physical education was especially difficult for Eric. His self-esteem was suffering due to poor performance during team sports. What treatment approaches might be used in this case?

The team recommended therapy, and the therapists worked together to design an intervention plan. Handwriting, ball handling, and balance skills were targeted. The OTA provided direct weekly therapy for 6 months to concentrate on these skills. The OTA also provided consultation to school staff to address classroom performance in the area of handwriting. Can you think of activities that would address his self-esteem issues? Handwriting? Balance? Ball handling skills?

Ray is a 22-year-old man who has been referred to OT by his psychologist. He has recently taken a job as a traveling sales representative and is having difficulty preparing for trips and sales calls. Recently, he has forgotten important information presented at sales meetings and frequently misses meetings and appointments. What suggestions can you make to help Ray become more prepared and organized for his new job?

REFERENCES

Achenbach, T. M., & Edelbrock, C. (1983). *Manual for the child behavior checklist and revised child behavior profile*. Burlington, VT: University of Vermont, Department of Psychology.

American Psychiatric Association. (1994). *Diagnostic and statistical manual of mental disorders* (4th ed.). Washington, DC: Author.

Amundson, S. J. (1995). *Evaluation tool of children's handwriting: Manuscript and cursive examiner's manual*. Homer, AK: OT KIDS.

Barkley, R. A. (1990). *Attention deficit disorder: a handbook for diagnosis and treatment*. New York, NY: Guilford Press.

Beery, K. E., & Buktenica, N. A. (1997). *Developmental test of visual-motor integration* (4th ed. rev.). Parsippany, NJ: Modern Curriculum Press.

Benbow, M. (1990). *Loops and other groups: A kinesthetic writing system*. San Antonio, TX: The Psychological Corp.

Benbow, M. (1995). *Assessment of hand skills in the primary child. Video*. Albuquerque, NM: Clinician's View.

Bruininks, R. (1978). *Bruininks-Oseretsky test of motor proficiency examiner's manual*. Circle Pines, MN: American Guidance Service.

Carrasco, R. C., & Lee, C. E. (1993). Development of a teacher questionnaire on sensorimotor behavior. *Sensory Integration Special Interest Newsletter, 16*(3), 5-6.

Connecticut State Department of Education (1998, August). *Connecticut State Individualized Education Program: Modifications/Adaptations in Regular Education-Including Nonacademic and Extracurricular Activities and Collaboration/Supports for School Personnel*. Hartford, CT Connecticut State Department. of Education; 8.

Connors, C. K. (1990). *Connors' rating scales manual. Conners' teacher rating scales. Connors' parent rating scales*. North Tonawanda, NY: Multi-Health Systems, Inc.

Dunn, W. (1999). *The sensory profile user's manual*. San Antonio, TX: The Psychological Corp.

Folio, R., & Fewell, R. (1983). *Peabody developmental motor scales and activity cards manual*. Austin, TX: Pro-Ed.

Gardner, M. F. (1992, 1996). *Test of visual-perceptual skills (non-motor) and test of visual-perceptual skills (non-motor): Upper level*. Burlingame, CA: Psychological and Educational Publications, Inc.

Gardner, M. F. (1995). *Test of visual-motor skills-revised and test of visual-motor skills: Upper level adolescents and adults*. Burlingame, CA: Psychological and Educational Publications, Inc.

Hammill, D. D., Pearson, N. A., & Voress, J. K. (1993). *Developmental test of visual perception (2nd ed.) examiner's manual*. Los Angeles, CA: WPS.

Jones, C. B. (1998). *Sourcebook for children with attention deficit disorder: A management guide for early childhood professionals and parents*. San Antonio, TX: Communication Skill Builders.

Kaplan, H. I., & Sadock, B. J. (1998). *Synopsis of psychiatry: behavioral sciences/clinical psychiatry* (8th ed., p.1197). Baltimore, MD: Williams & Wilkins.

Phelps, J., Stempel, L., & Speck, G. (1984, 1987). *Children's handwriting evaluation scale and children's handwriting scale for manuscript writing*. Dallas, TX: CHES.

Royeen, C. B., & Fortune, J. C. (1990). TIE: Touch inventory for school aged children. *Am J Occup Ther, 44,* 165-170.

Sanderson, C. (1999). *Input sheet for classroom consultation*. Therapist-developed unpublished worksheet.

Williams, M. S., & Shellenberger, S. (1996). *How does your engine run? A leader's guide to the Alert program for self-regulation*. Albuquerque, NM: Therapy Works.

SUGGESTED READING

Asher, I. E. (1996). *OT assessment tools: An annotated index* (2nd ed.). Bethesda, MD: AOTA.

Colarusso, R. P., Hammill, D. D., & Mercier, L. (1996). *Motor-free visual perception test-revised*. Novato, CA: Academic Therapy Publications.

Dornbush, M. P., & Pruitt, S. K. (1995). *Teaching the tiger: A handbook for individuals involved in the education of students with attention deficit disorders, Tourette syndrome or obsessive-compulsive disorder*. Duarte, CA: Hope Press.

Ermer, J., & Dunn, W. (1998). The sensory profile: A discriminant analysis of children with and without disabilities. *Am J Occup Ther, 52*(4), 283-290.

Jones, C. B. (1994). *Attention deficit disorder: Strategies for school-age children*. San Antonio, TX: Communication Skill Builders.

Porr, S. M., & Rainville, E. B. (1999). *Pediatric therapy: A systems approach*. Philadelphia, PA: F. A. Davis.

Reif, S. (1998). *The ADD/ADHD checklist: An easy reference for parents and teachers*. Paramus, NJ: Prentice Hall.

Smith, J. C., Allen, A. S., & Pratt, P. N. (1996). *OT for children* (3rd ed.). St. Louis, MO: Mosby.

Stancliff, B. (1998). Understanding the "whoops" children. *OT Practice,* 18-25.

A Teenager with Depression

Chapter 17

Linda Florey, PhD, OTR, FAOTA

INTRODUCTION

Depression is a disorder of mood in which there is diminished interest and loss of pleasure in most activities. Somatic complaints and social withdrawal are common. Associated symptoms include disturbances in sleep, appetite, psychomotor agitation (irregular action or unrest) or retardation, and decreased concentration. Adolescents experience hopelessness and feelings that things will never change for the better. The most serious complication of depression is suicidal thoughts, including recurrent thoughts of death or actual attempts at suicide (Weller, Weller, & Svadjian, 1996). Children and adolescents with depression usually have multiple problems, such as educational failure and impaired psychosocial functioning. Prominent risk factors include family disharmony, learning difficulties, and parental psychiatric disorder. Numerous causes may lead to the expression of depressive symptoms. The overlap of depression and other psychiatric diagnoses has been one of the most consistent findings of research studies. Depression has been associated with conditions as diverse as conduct disorder, anxiety states, learning problems, hyperactivity, drug use, and anorexia nervosa (Harrington, 1994).

KEY CONCEPTS

- Mood disorder: A psychiatric disorder characterized by disturbance of mood involving either elation or depression.
- Asperger's disorder: A psychiatric disorder characterized by severe and pervasive impairment in social interaction and restricted and stereotypic patterns of behavior and activities.
- Occupational behavior: A frame of reference that targets the broad parameters of play, student role, and socialization as the primary concern of occupational therapy practitioners working with individuals of this age.
- Task performance: An assessment of attention span, ability to make decisions, follow directions, sequence steps, use tools and materials, and solve problems using a craft or activity.
- Pervasive developmental disorders (PDDs): Psychiatric disorders characterized by severe and pervasive impairment in social interaction, communication, and other areas of development in addition to stereotypic behavior, interests, and activities.
- IEP: A plan aimed at improving the child's educational performance. It contains specific instructional objectives including specific services and modifications needed to achieve the objectives.

ESSENTIAL VOCABULARY

Allen Cognitive Levels: Six levels of cognitive ability with corresponding expectations for functional capabilities for daily living.

Depression: A psychiatric disorder characterized by disturbance in mood—diminished interest and loss of pleasure in most activities.

Psychomotor agitation: Irregular action, unrest, or disquiet.

Role dysfunction: Inability to perform and adjust adaptively to social expectations associated with roles of player, student, worker, homemaker, volunteer, or retiree.

Social skills: One of the skills of social competence that refers to the ability to produce mutually reciprocal interactions with others.

Somatic complaints: Complaints focused on bodily functions such as loss of energy and reduced sleep.

Visual-motor integration: Ability of the eyes and hands to work together effectively and efficiently.

FRAMES OF REFERENCE

The frame of reference used in this chapter is occupational behavior. It is the same one used in the chapter on the child with conduct disorder and theoretical considerations are addressed in that section (Chapter 15). This frame of reference targets the broad parameters of play, student role, and socialization as the primary concern of occupational therapists in working with children and adolescents. In adolescence, work, play, and major daily activities focus on the role of student, which includes concerns with mastery of social learnings and expectations as well as academic learnings. A major clinical focus for occupational therapists is to determine the extent to which mental illness has disrupted or impoverished occupational behavior and to identify steps to ameliorate dysfunction and to foster new learning (Florey, 1998).

Assessments and treatment techniques drawn from additional frames of reference may be used to better understand and ameliorate dysfunction in occupational role and socialization. The cognitive disability frame of reference is very useful in uncovering cognitive deficits and their impact on daily activities. This frame of reference targets deficits in functional capabilities as a result of biological and chemical changes in the brain. There are six levels of cognitive ability and corresponding expectations for functional capabilities for daily living. Identifying the cognitive level is helpful in guiding the team in developing behavioral expectations and goals that are realistic for the patient (Allen, 1998).

CASE STUDY 1

Michael is a thin, poorly groomed, 17-year-old boy admitted to the inpatient unit of the adolescent service because of self-mutilation of his arms and legs with a razor blade. He said that he was not trying to commit suicide, but that he had made the deep cuts to his body to see how his "body worked." He was not on any drugs when he made the cuts, although he admitted to using pot in the past as it helped him relax. He wore green nail polish and dressed in black. Michael said that he dressed this way and was unshaven because he was "Gothic."

Michael is an only child and grew up with his mother in a rural community near the coast in central California. His mother and father divorced when he was young and he had not had any contact with his father since the divorce, which occurred when he was 3. Michael's mother reported that his father had been diagnosed with bipolar disorder. His mother worked during the days, and she felt that he was somewhat of a "latchkey" kid. His mother reported that he never had many friends that he played with as a child, but she assumed that he had made some

friends in school. He had always received good grades until 2 years ago when his grades slipped from As and Bs to Cs and Ds. He was also spending a lot of time on the weekends on the Internet. His mother was concerned with his change in grades and the increase in isolative behavior and took him to a physician who placed him on an antidepressant.

Michael's grades improved in the next few years but she was concerned with his general physical appearance of dressing Gothic and his increasing time spent on the Internet. His mother learned that Gothic was a term used to represent a particular style of dress and detached demeanor in which dressing in black was prevalent and a cynical view of life dominated. She described him as a loner and was concerned that he was becoming too dependent on the Internet and computer games. When he was not on the Internet, he read scary novels. His hygiene was poor and she had to remind him to bathe and to shave. He picked at his food and often roamed the house at night. One night, his mother found him bleeding in the bathroom from cuts he had made on his arms and legs with a razor blade.

Assessment and Evaluation Process

As part of the interdisciplinary treatment plan, Michael was scheduled for an occupational therapy assessment. A screening process to determine the need for occupational therapy was not performed as it is the expectation of the facility that all patients receive an assessment to determine the focus and frequency of occupational therapy intervention. The evaluation is documented in the chart within 48 hours of admission, and the focus is on determining direction for intervention both as an inpatient and at discharge. Additional evaluations may be performed following 48 hours to probe deficit areas first identified.

The length of stay on the adolescent service is 10 to 14 days. The overall focus of inpatient hospitalization for the interdisciplinary team is to stabilize behavior, identify major problems, clarify diagnosis, and initiate medication trials if indicated. The treatment of long-term psychiatric problems is not done at the inpatient level, but rather at a less expensive level of care such as in a partial hospital program or as an outpatient.

The OTA reviewed the medical chart and reported the history to the occupational therapist as described in the case study section. The first step in the assessment process was for both the OTA and OT to meet briefly with Michael to explain occupational therapy services and the evaluation process and to gain an impression of his social interaction within the peer group. The OTA and OT first observed him briefly in the day room of the inpatient unit. He sat apart from the other adolescents who were engaged in various activities such as card and board games and did not look around or show interest in his surroundings. The OT and OTA both introduced themselves and their roles in the inpatient setting. At that meeting, Michael's eye contact was sporadic and he responded to questions about the inpatient unit activities with one line responses. His face was "mask-like" in that he maintained a blank look and did not show any animation in expression. His grooming was poor and he had body odor. The therapists shared assessment functions, which was often typical for them.

EVALUATION AND FINDINGS

The routine evaluations used include an interview regarding daily living activities, an assessment of task performance, the Allen Cognitive Level, observation of social interaction, and an assessment of visual motor integration. The specific format, purpose, the responsible occupational therapy personnel, and the results or findings follow.

A Daily Living Interview is a semi-structured interview designed to determine patterns of function in daily living, school, and leisure activities.

The OT found that Michael was difficult to interview. His response to open-ended questions regarding time use was that he did not know exactly what he did or when he did it. He did not volunteer any information, and the OT had to probe each area. The OT obtained a skeleton of his typical day as one of arising in the morning, taking the bus to and from school, and then getting on the Internet once he reached home. He said that he did not have many friends at school, but that he had one friend on the Internet. He was unable to identify any parts of school that he liked or disliked but said that he liked to read and write on his own. He particularly liked reading Stephen King novels. Aside from the Internet, he played games on the computer. He said he did not like sports, did not have any hobbies, and hated crafts. When asked about his self-care routine, he said he did not have a regular time when he did anything. Michael was asked if he helped out around the house, and he replied that he used to and that sometimes he did if his mother made him. He replied that he could fix himself a meal, and that he had made spaghetti and quesadillas (flour tortillas filled with cheese) on his own. When asked what kind of work he might like to do, he said that he wanted to go to college and be a writer. On the weekends, he said that he liked to go to the beach by himself, watch the waves, and smoke.

The OT noted that Michael had a restricted and rigid pattern of interests, no regular or meaningful social contacts, and that he did not assume responsibility for his self-care or helping around the house. He also did not do well with open-ended questions but needed categories identified for him such as, "What hobbies do you have?" and then he could answer.

A task performance checklist to determine decision-making, ability to follow directions, attention span, ability to sequence steps, and ability to solve problems was used by the OTA.

Michael was given the choice of two board games to play with the therapist or making a craft project. He said that he didn't want to do anything, but the OTA selected a board game and he agreed to play with her. They played Parcheesi (Milton Bradley, Pawtucket, RI), and the OTA observed that he demonstrated more animation than she had seen. He quickly learned the game and seemed to like the strategy involved. The OTA noted that he attended well to the game and was able to concentrate and plot game moves. He was not able to initiate or make a decision on his own but did respond and participate once a decision was made for him.

The OTA used a semi-structured guide in observation of socialization in occupational therapy area, recreation area, and on the inpatient unit.

The purpose was to determine frequency and content of interactions with peers and adults.

Michael was observed during structured activities such as a community meeting, recreation activities, and informal activities on the unit, including mealtime. The OTA observed that his pattern of interaction with others was consistent in all settings. He isolated himself from his peers and if forced to sit next to a peer at meals or in a meeting, he did not initiate any contact. The other adolescents on the unit "gave him space" and did not talk with him, as he did not respond to their questions or comments. His eye contact was generally poor and sporadic but was better when he was with an adult rather than peers. He would respond to questions of adults, and he would engage in board games with them. He refused to play shuffleboard, volleyball, ping pong, or any physical games.

The OT used the Allen Cognitive Level test of leather lacing stitches to determine an initial estimate of Michael's ability to function and to master new learning.

Michael said that he did not want to do this lacing and reminded the therapist that he hated crafts. She told him that this was perfect for him, as it was not a craft at all but rather a way to check out his ability to solve problems on something he had not done a million times. He participated in the process and achieved a score of 5.6, indicating that he was at the level of exploratory actions and could problem-solve by trial and error but had difficulty anticipating the results of his actions. He was able to learn new activities, but needed assistance with activities requiring him to plan ahead. The therapist concluded that this cognitive level was typical of many adolescents and that many needed assistance in planning and structuring their time.

Lastly, the OTA administered the Beery-Buktenica Developmental Test of Visual-Motor Integration (VMI), a structured test using form copying.

The purpose of the VMI is to determine developmental or age equivalent status of visual motor skills

Michael achieved an age equivalent score of 12 years, 3 months, indicating some impairment in this area. This did not seem to interfere with his daily functioning as in handwriting and ability to handle small objects on board games, but it may have contributed to his dislike of crafts, which typically require visual-motor skill.

The OT and OTA decided that additional assessments, such as vocational surveys, were not warranted until deficits in social and daily functioning were addressed. They speculated that remediation of his functional pattern would require a significant period of time.

General Goals

The OT and OTA summarized their findings and presented them to the treatment team. The team was headed by a psychiatrist and other members included a nurse, psychologist, recreation therapist, social worker, speech and language specialist, and a school consultant. The primary concerns of the occupational therapists were his poor eye contact, poor grooming, lack of identified friendships or social contacts, lack of observed ability to initiate social contact or to initiate activities on his own, and his restricted and rigid pattern of interests. His strengths included his ability to learn new activities and to participate in social and activity situations if they were expected of and set up for him.

The treatment team as a whole was concerned not only with his knife cuts, disorganized routine, sleep and appetite disturbances, and social isolation, which were all part of the syndrome of depression, but they were also concerned with his prolonged history of poor social interactions and his restricted and rigid pattern of interests. The team considered that they may be dealing with an adolescent with two disorders: depression and Asperger's disorder, which is one of the PDDs characterized by severe and pervasive impairment in social interaction and restricted and stereotypic patterns of behavior and activities. Michael was placed on a trial of new antidepressant medication and the team was asked to observe for increasing signs of social interaction and increase in interests as the depression lifted.

General occupational therapy goals for Michael included enhancing social interaction with others by including him in groups and having him initiate contact with others, improving his self-care and sense of responsibility in keeping his room and area clean, and improving his time management by having him engage in purposeful activities.

Treatment Activities/Techniques

The OT program is broadly designed to meet the needs of most adolescents. One goal of the program in short-term hospitalization is to simulate selected social and task expectations that adolescents encounter in the community to gain a sense of how they function in these situations for continuing assessment purposes and for discharge recommendations. The goals for individual patients are implemented individually and within small group programs. Placing the program within small groups of adolescents is critical in working with adolescents with psychiatric disorders, as it is in the peer and social group that difficulties are most evident. Strategies for dealing with others are an integral part of the group focus. Program planning is also accomplished within the context of the interdisciplinary team in order that there are individualized yet consistent expectations for all adolescents.

Throughout his hospitalization of 14 days, Michael was included in a boy's grooming group co-led with nursing, a room check program, a cooking group, and craft/recreation groups co-led with recreation therapy. The OTA and OT worked separately or together depending on the needs of the group. Michael's participation in these groups and his specific goals in each one are briefly reviewed.

Boy's Grooming Group

This group of six adolescents met daily with a nursing staff and the OTA. Expectations for self-care were given but there were choices the adolescents had within those expectations, and they were also able to set a special goal for themselves. General expectations included bathing or showering daily, shaving if necessary, combing hair, and brushing teeth. Michael selected showering in the evening each day, combing hair daily, and shaving every other day. He could not think of any special goals so the occupational therapists suggested removing his green nail polish and cleaning his nails. Michael instead selected flossing his teeth but toward the end of the second week, he finally removed the green nail polish. His overall self-care improved: he bathed and combed his hair daily and his body odor was no longer offensive.

Room Check Program

This group was led by the OT. The occupational therapist gave points for clean and organized rooms, and the adolescents then used the earned points for extra privileges, which included such areas as selecting the music on the radio during some OT groups or going on special outings. Michael was to have his bed made, shirts and jeans hung in the closet, other clothing folded and placed in drawers, countertops clean, and books and games orderly. He had only one book that he brought with him and was responsive to keeping his clothing organized. He earned points and privileges, but could not decide what privilege to select and said that he really did not care about that.

Cooking Group

Both the OT and OTA worked together in the weekly lunch and snack groups of four to six adolescents, as two individuals were needed to assess functional and social behavior and to direct the tasks. Both groups were held in the occupational therapy kitchen, which is a small space with no opportunity to isolate oneself. In the first lunch group, Michael and another male peer were asked to make the salad together. His peer was friendly and outgoing and asked Michael a number of questions regarding the task at hand, to which he had to respond. In the second lunch group and in the snack groups, he continued to respond to peer questions and even initiated some communication with his peers regarding the task. He would also respond to questions during these mealtimes, but he seemed awkward and unable to initiate casual mealtime talk with others. When he did, he directed his comments to the OTs.

Craft/Recreation Groups

The OTA was responsible for the task selection within these groups. Michael did not wish to participate, but the OTA told him that he had to attend this group with the other adolescents and that he had to select something to do with his time. Initially, he was unable to spontaneously select anything, and this pattern persisted throughout his hospital stay. He demonstrated no ability to initiate activities on his own. His mood seemed better, as his face was less mask-like; but despite the decreasing depressive mood, he seemed unable to initiate activities for himself other than reading. A computer was not made available to him, as he would further isolate himself from others. He was responsive to selecting among choices of board games or outdoor activities that did not involve sports (e.g., shuffleboard), however, by discharge, he was participating in volleyball.

Discharge Planning

At discharge, there was a meeting with the mother and all the disciplines, in which each discipline presented its findings and recommendations. The team explained to the mother that Michael had two psychiatric disorders: mood disorder, and depression and Asperger's disorder. Asperger's disorder is one of the disorders in the PDD spectrum characterized by severe and sustained impairment in social interaction and the development of restricted and repetitive patterns of behavior, interests, and activities. Unlike autistic disorder, which is also in the PDD spectrum, there are no significant delays in areas other than social interaction, such as language and adaptive skills (American Psychiatric Association, 1994). The Asperger's disorder explained the long history of social isolation, lack of friendships, and his restricted pattern of interest and behavior centered around the Internet and computer in general. Michael was uneasy in the company of others, especially peers. He was more responsive to adults and even initiated contacts with adults toward the end of hospitalization. His cutting himself to "see how his body worked" was not a typical suicide threat.

Michael was also depressed, which accounted for his decreasing concentration in his studies and his changing grades, his mask-like face and generally depressed mood, his cutting on himself for any reason, and his deterioration in self-care, including sleeping and eating patterns. His inability to initiate and plan activities on his own, other than the computer, was probably attributable to both disorders.

The OTs were concerned that Michael maintain his self-care and responsibilities and that he receive some social skill training to learn some of the rudiments of working with others that he had never learned. The OT explained to the mother that Michael had difficulty initiating tasks but that he had been responsive to specific expectations and directions and that he would probably need her or someone to organize his time and expectations. The OTA gave the mother a list of standards for self-care he had accomplished in the hospital and discussed with the mother specific expectations for caring for his room and for assisting her with preparation of the evening meal and other chores. The mother was very responsive to this and said that she had done this when he was younger and he had done well. She had stopped, as she assumed he knew how to organize his time and tasks. The OT also recommended that Michael have an IEP to address his social awkwardness and to learn social skills. There was such a program in his school system.

The OT told the mother that Michael had seemed to enjoy low key recreation activities, such as shuffleboard and board games, and that a few of these activities could be expectations for him to engage in on the weekends. He would also be in the company of others on these occasions. This would represent an expansion of his interests and behavior beyond the computer. She suggested that the mother determine if any such programs were offered through YMCA or youth groups in their community with the eventual goal of having Michael participate on his own on a regular basis. The OT and OTA both advised an approach of gradualism in that expecting too much of him at once would be too uncomfortable for him. They suggested that the mother initially play board games with him and at the same time introduce him to one other setting to which he was expected to go one time on the weekend. His mood was improving, and although his social awkwardness persisted, this was the time to introduce gradual changes in his daily pattern.

CLINICAL PROBLEM-SOLVING

Case Study 2

Imagine Michael at age 27. Do you think he went to college and that he is now a writer? What type of work might he be doing? Would living in a rural or urban setting make any difference? Will he still need someone to organize his time and his tasks for him? Has his social communication improved? What kinds of issues might be arising and might need to be addressed?

Case Study 3

Ann is a short, attractive 15-year-old African-American girl admitted to the adolescent inpatient service for threatening to kill herself with her stepfather's gun. She had recently given birth to a baby, whose father was her stepbrother. The stepbrother had sexually abused her for years, and Ann had become pregnant. The Department of Family and Social Services had become involved, and the stepbrother had been arrested and removed from the home. The stepfather was furious with Ann, as he blamed her for ruining the family and said she had probably done something provocative to lead his son on. The admitting diagnosis was depression secondary to post-traumatic stress disorder due to sexual abuse.

What are the major concerns of the OTR and COTA with Ann? How would the evaluations differ from those used with Michael, or would they? Are there some cultural stereotypes concerning women operating here? What might discharge concerns and recommendations center on?

REFERENCES

Allen, C. K. (1998). Cognitive disability frame of reference. In M. Neistadt & E. Crepeau (Eds.), *Willard & Spackman's OT* (9th ed.). Philadelphia, PA: Lippincott.

American Psychiatric Association. (1994). *Diagnostic and statistical manual of mental disorders* (4th ed.). Washington, DC: Author.

Florey, L. (1998). Psychosocial dysfunction in childhood and adolescence. In M. Neistadt & E. Crepeau (Eds.), *Willard & Spackman's OT* (9th ed.). Philadelphia, PA: Lippincott.

Harrington, R. (1994). Affective disorders. In M. Rutter, E. Taylor, & L. Hersov (Eds.), *Child and adolescent psychiatry: Modern approaches* (3rd ed.). Oxford, England: Blackwell Scientific.

Weller, E., Weller, R., & Svadjian, H. (1996). Mood disorders. In M. Lewis (Ed.), *Child and adolescent psychiatry: A comprehensive textbook* (2nd ed.). Baltimore, MD: Williams & Wilkins.

A Young Adult Car Mechanic with Traumatic Brain Injury

Chapter 18

Deanna Proulx-Sepelak, OTR/L

INTRODUCTION

Traumatic brain injury, or TBI, is a term commonly used throughout the medical profession to describe an event that physically alters the composition of the skull cavity and, more importantly, its contents. This term is often interchanged with others such as "head injury," which is formally defined by Mosby's *Medical, Nursing, and Allied Health Dictionary* (1994) as "any traumatic damage resulting from blunt or penetrating trauma of the skull that can include vessels, nerves, and/or meninges that are torn, bleeding and edematous." This definition has been analyzed more specifically to include several separate subcategories:

- Diffuse axonal injury—Injury occurs as a result of the stretching in the axons of the nerves within the brain resulting in coma; often not evident on CT scans.

- Closed head injury—Skull is not fractured; injury occurs as a result of contusions or internal hemorrhage; evident on CT scans.

- Depressed skull fracture—Outer skull remains intact, however, fragments from the inner surface have dislodged and compress or lacerate the brain itself.

- Compound skull fractures—Outer tissues are torn, skull is open, and there is likely to be direct trauma with brain tissues (Morris, Pedley, & Rowland, 1995).

The effects of these types of injuries are life-altering not only to the client but to his or her family members, loved ones, friends, and the caregivers who nurture the often times slow recovery process.

As reported in a study by Sniezek, Sosin, and Waxweiler (1995), TBI is one of the leading causes of death among United States residents between the ages of 15 and 24 years, mostly male (average

ESSENTIAL VOCABULARY

Acceleration/deceleration: Forces acted upon the brain that result in injury.

Community re-entry: Simulated or actual activities used to prepare a client for discharge into the public community.

Coup/contrecoup: Refers to points of actual contact made between the brain and the skull encasement in the event of a trauma.

Executive function: Higher level, multistep, cognitive functions or abilities requiring skill/precision.

Homunculus: Commonly used illustration representing anatomical structures and functions of the primary motor and/or sensory areas of the brain.

Memory notebook: Used with clients who have sustained a brain injury resulting in memory loss.

Neural plasticity: Innate healing ability of the brain via "re-routing" neural pathways in an effort to compensate for areas of tissue damage.

KEY CONCEPTS

- Patterns of recovery: The Rancho Los Amigos (RLA) Scale of Recovery and the Glasgow Coma Scale measure progress.
- The interdisciplinary approach: Professionals from multiple disciplines address common concerns.
- Continuum of care in brain injury management: OT services begin with coma level functioning to community re-entry.
- TBI: Deformation of the brain's soft tissue as a result of an external, traumatic force.

annual rate: 33 per 100,000) and those residents age 65 years and older (average annual rate: 31 per 100,000). Approximately 2 million residents of the United States sustain a brain injury annually, ranging in severity from concussion to coma to even death. Of this population, an average of 56,000 are fatally injured, approximately 373,000 are hospitalized, and of those who do survive, almost one-third result in lifelong disabilities (Silverman Saunders, 1996). Sniezek et al. (1995) also report that as of 1992, 44% of the deaths associated with TBI were attributable to firearms, as compared with 34% due to motor vehicle accidents (previously the leader) and 9% to falls. The Centers for Disease Control and Prevention have predicted that firearms will become the leading over-all single cause of death within the United States by the year 2001 and is already the leading cause of death related to TBI as of 1995 (Mitka, 1998). It is through these statistics that we see the "nature of the beast" and the demand for skilled personnel to provide assistance to all who have been touched by the event of TBI.

NEUROANATOMY OF HEAD INJURY

The brain itself can be likened to several different analogies in order to describe the mechanisms of injury in which it is susceptible. The preferred analogy lies in that of a gelatinous mold suspended in a fluid-like substance that is entirely encased within a roughly lined cavity. With this analogy, the gelatin mold represents the brain, the fluid is cerebrospinal in nature, and the roughly lined cavity represents the inner surface of the skull. In normal stasis, the brain remains relatively protected. Its primary role is to direct all conscious and unconscious functions of the body via the central nervous system. These functions are classically "mapped" within the brain itself and vary in degree of complexity from heart rate, respiration, and arousal to concept formation, generalization, and overall executive function. One specific type of map is common-ly referred to in the realm of neurology as a homunculus of the brain (Figures 18-1 and 18-2).

This homunculus illustrates the mapping of higher cortical functions specific to the primary motor and sensory cortices (Hole, 1984). By understanding the normal neuroanatomical structures and functions of an intact brain, one can better understand and analyze the effects of injury specific to its location within the skull.

In the event of an injury, the brain is jarred from its normal stasis and makes direct contact with the roughly lined skull encasement. This phenomena is also described as an acceleration and deceleration of the brain itself, which causes coup and contrecoup. These terms are used to describe the actual points of the brain that make direct contact with the skull. Often, these two points are at directly opposite poles. Coup describes the exact point

where the injury occurred and acceleration was generated by the external force, and the contrecoup describes the point opposite of coup where the brain decelerates or rebounds off the skull encasement (Trombly, 1995). Therefore, with one external force or injury to the skull, two areas of the brain are injured. In comparing this type of injury to that of a single area or focal injury, such as seen with a cerebrovascular accident, we can more clearly understand why the latter manifests itself on only one-half of the body, while with head injury, it is much more com-mon to see bilateral disabilities.

As indicated earlier, understanding the neuroanatomy and mechanisms of injury to that anatomy, the COTA and OTR are at an advantage in their ability to accu-rately treat a client's strengths and weaknesses. For example, a client has sustained a head injury to the frontal lobe in a motor vehicle accident and has a tra-cheostomy, which is inhibiting his or her ability to com-municate. Based on the understanding of neuroanato-my, even without a means of communication, the thera-pist can be suspicious of a degree of memory deficit from the frontal lobe and possible visual deficit from the occipital lobe as result of coup and contrecoup. This small bit of information regarding the possible areas of weakness can have a very large impact on the degree of success you will have during your initial interaction with a client who has sustained a TBI.

THE RECOVERY PROCESS

It is true that everyone is individual in his or her response to an injury. It is uncommon to see any two injuries to the brain that present exactly alike, though sim-ilarities do exist. These similarities are frequently referred to as stages of recovery after a brain injury. So similar, in fact, that two separate objective methods have been adopted to assess and measure an injury to the brain: the Rancho Los Amigos Scale (RLA) (Booth, Kodimer, & Malkmus, 1980) and the Glasgow Coma Scale (Jennett & Teasdale, 1981).

The RLA was first introduced at the Rancho Los Amigos Hospital in Downey, CA, and formally devel-oped into an objective evaluation tool via the outlining of similarities in behaviors observed at each stage. This evaluation, specific to cognitive awareness, is outlined at eight different levels and graded along a continuum from most primitive and basic reflexes up to higher level executive functioning. These levels are indicative of the more commonly observed behaviors expected from a client at any particular time in the recovery process (Figure 18-3).

The Glasgow Coma Scale is the evaluative measure of choice for physicians presented with a client who has sus-tained an acute TBI. This method is more indicative of

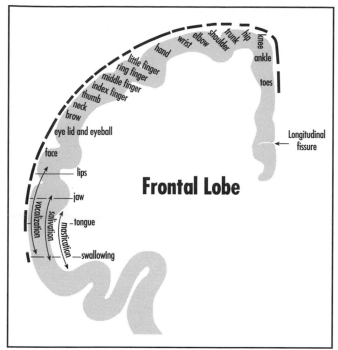

Figure 18-1. The homunculi of the primary motor cortex: frontal lobe. (Adapted from Hole, J. W., Jr. (1984). *Human anatomy and physiology.* Dubuque, IA: Wm. C. Brown Publishers.)

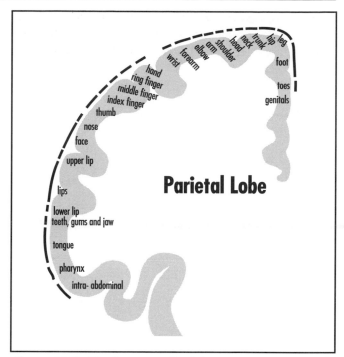

Figure 18-2. The homunculi of the sensory areas: parietal lobe. (Adapted from Hole, J. W., Jr. (1984). *Human anatomy and physiology.* Dubuque, IA: Wm. C. Brown Publishers.)

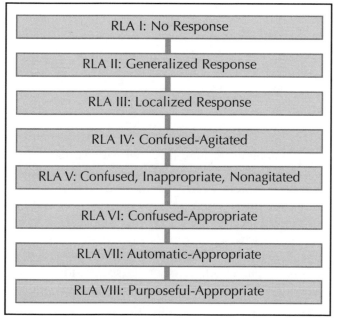

Figure 18-3. Rancho Los Amigos Scale of levels of cognitive functioning. (Adapted from Booth, B. J., Kodimer, C., & Malkmus, D. (1980). *Rehabilitation of head injured adult: Comprehensive cognitive management.* Downey, CA: Professional Staff Association of Rancho Los Amigos Hospital.)

the severity of brain injury and therefore, the predicted outcome (Pedretti & Zoltan, 1990). With this measure, points are awarded based on three different types or levels of response: motor, verbal, and eye opening. The points are accrued based on the quality of responses, and a rating is then applied overall.

The patterns of recovery within the brain and the appropriate utilization of OT intervention collaboratively are designed to facilitate healing and promote function.

Although the RLA and the Glasgow Coma Scale outline generalizations of behaviors or expectations, each presents clinicians with a much clearer outline of the treatment for a client with a brain injury. In theory, the brain remains a relatively mysterious organ affixed at the very center of our being. We are aware of its capacity to heal and compensate for weakness through neural plasticity; we also have become rather skilled at saving the lives of those with brain injuries who may not have previously been saved. Yet we as the clinicians, continue to struggle with its management over the entire duration of recovery. Some clients progress much quicker than others. Some will skip a stage or two; some will remain stationary in any one particular stage for an extended period of time. Some become fixed at any one point and no longer progress.

It is crucial for OTAs and OTs to develop a familiarity with both the RLA and the Glasgow Coma Scale in order to best maximize the choice of treatment techniques available. Too often clients are asked to perform tasks that are not congruent with the current level of function, and this results in a sense of failure to both the caregiver and the client. Although each client has been objectively judged to be at a particular RLA or Glasgow level, we are constantly reminded of the individual and the dynamics behind his or her specific injury through his or her level of success with a particular task or activity of daily living. These subtle differences often create the complexity associated with the success, or lack thereof, in treating a client with a brain injury.

Frames of Reference

It would be a fallacy to say that any one particular frame of reference is applied to OT intervention with the treatment of a client who has sustained a head injury. Rather, a diverse spectrum of frames available are used at various levels of recovery appropriate to the behaviors and symptoms manifested by each individual. In translation, this simply indicates the ongoing need for re-evaluation and restructuring of the environment necessary to progress to the next recovery level while also attending to all of the deficits presented at any given time. For example, you may be treating a client following a brain injury at the RLA IV level who requires a memory notebook applying the cognitive-perceptual frame, a token system for using the notebook appropriately in the behavior modification frame, and an overall endurance training program within the biomechanical frame in order to address the client's needs specific to that particular point of recovery. Some of the more commonly used ones are as follows: biomechanical, sensory integration, behavior modification, Model of Human Occupation, cognitive-perceptual, cognitive disabilities, and neurodevelopmental frames of reference.

Interdisciplinary Approach

The model in which treatment is generally delivered to clients who have sustained a brain injury is the interdisciplinary model. This model is commonly used due to the complexity and diversity of needs with which a client may present. In the interdisciplinary model, a team is formed of several different professional domains who meet on a routine basis in order to best plan the delivery of services while maintaining a focus on the client and family needs (Hoeman, 1996). For example, an interdisciplinary team working within a brain injury division may include, but is not limited to, the following: the medical doctor; the neuropsychologist; the primary nurse; the occupational, physical, and/or speech therapist; the social worker; the dietitian; and the case manager. This routine collaboration of specialists allows for the continuous planning of the most optimal treatment in accordance with all strengths or weaknesses while allowing for a forum of support and structure so often necessary to the treating team members working with this population.

Evaluation, Goals, and Treatment: Case Applications

The complexity of the injury itself is very important to remember at this particular point of the text. Each individual presents differently, having his or her own set of specific strengths and weaknesses that can change frequently throughout the duration of treatment. This treatment is also provided along a continuum of care based on the client's changing needs, including a combination of the following: acute hospitals, rehabilitative hospitals, subacute care facilities, transitional living facilities, day treatment programs, outpatient care centers, and home care agencies. It is due to this fact that the presentation of evaluative procedures, goal setting, and actual treatment intervention strategies are best outlined according to the RLA measure.

CASE STUDY 1

Client

Michael, a single, 24-year-old man.

Diagnostic History

Unbelted passenger in a head-on motor vehicle accident. Thrown from the vehicle resulting in a compound skull fracture and TBI.

Service Delivery

It is important to note here that with Michael's case, both the OT and OTA worked collaboratively to address his needs. The OTA cared for much of Michael's direct therapeutic intervention with supervision from the OT and handled much of the family education. This working relationship acted as a means of support and clarification for the OTA based on having already succeeded in demonstration of competency skills specific to the treatment facility.

RLA Level I

Setting

Acute hospital.

Referral

The acute care hospital routinely refers all clients with TBI to occupational and physical therapy as soon as the individual is medically stable.

Evaluations

Client is currently in the coma state and unresponsive; therefore, formalized evaluations are inappropriate and not implemented.

Goals

The general goal at this stage of recovery is to elicit any response to external stimulation while preventing long-term deformities, such as contractures.

Treatment

Treatment at this stage of recovery is focused on prevention. The OTA or OT will provide the following:

- Passive range of motion (PROM) to all joints to prevent contractures and normalize tone.

- Promote proper positioning and educate other caregivers of its importance in promoting normalized tone, preventing contractures, and preventing decubitus formation. Bilateral resting hand splints were implemented.

- Creation of an immediate surrounding environment that is familiar. Michael's family members were asked to bring many items from his apartment that had been part of his regular routine including familiar music, pillows, blankets, and photographs.

- A sensory kit was utilized routinely to attempt to promote a response from Michael to external stimulation.

- Education is very important to both the family and the other caregivers. Michael's family required training regarding the role of occupational therapy, proper positioning, use and application of splints, including the wear schedule, importance of eliciting a response thereby using a familiar surrounding. It is also important here to consider the need for support systems available to the family, make necessary referrals, and act as a resource when necessary.

RLA Level II

Setting

Acute hospital and subacute care facility.

Evaluations

Michael has progressed to the next level of recovery based on his ability to elicit a reflexive response to noxious stimuli. Type of evaluations are nonformalized and are concentrated in the objective documentation by the OTA or OT reflecting motor-sensory responses to noxious stimuli via touch, smell, sound, and light.

Goals

The general goal of this stage of recovery is to increase arousal based on responses to sensory stimulation as measured by the frequency, duration, and quality.

Treatment

Treatment at this stage is very similar to that of RLA Level I. The OTA or OT will provide the following:

- PROM to all joints as previously described.

- Continuation of the positioning techniques that have been implemented, including splints, etc.

- Emphasis on familiar surroundings remains very important and is a vital piece of treatment of which the family is an integral piece. Continue to explore and generate ideas directly with the family members.

- Utilization of the sensory kit to promote a response to external stimulus continued on a routine basis and was also carried over by the family.

- Education and reinforcement of the carryover in techniques with Michael's family and caregivers continues to be a focus of treatment. Structure is important in the management of all stages of recovery, and here is emphasized through consistency in the sensory techniques used to elicit the responses for all who are in contact with Michael.

RLA Level III

Setting

Subacute care facility or rehabilitative hospital.

Referral

Occupational therapy at this level is a standard referral from the medical doctor overseeing Michael's care.

Evaluations

At this level, the therapist(s) can expect to be able to establish a means of simple communication with the client in order to progress toward more formal evaluation procedures. In Michael's case, he is now able to respond with simple head nodding of "yes" or "no." With this skill established, the OTA and/or OT will need to determine the accuracy of those responses prior to implementing a more formal evaluation, such as sensation. This determination was achieved through asking simple yes/no questions of Michael in which the answers are already known such as: "Are you married?" or "Are you a man?" Nonformal, functional skills can also begin to be assessed by the OT, including basic activities of daily living (ADLs), such as washing or dressing.

Goals

1. Promote the recognition of significant others.
2. Promote orientation to person, place, and time including what has happened to bring the client to the hospital.
3. Promote sensory stimulation to increase arousal and attending skills.
4. Promote highest level of independence with ADLs.

Treatment

- A highly structured environment is key for success in treatment. For Michael, a memory notebook was compiled including information such as his name, age, the date, where he was, why he was there, photos, names of common caregivers and significant others, and most importantly, the schedule he would need to follow on a daily basis. This notebook was referred routinely as a means of directing Michael's thinking, to provide him with a source of information, and to introduce his deficit areas as a means of developing insight. At this stage of recovery, Michael's level of arousal and insight continue to be considerably deficient. With this in mind, the memory notebook was initiated with a heavy emphasis on family and caregivers to carryover throughout Michael's day and make its use more routine. This responsibility will shift to Michael at a later stage of recovery and is implemented here to promote a smooth transition at that time.

- Focus was also placed on Michael's ability to perform ADL skills. On a routine basis, the therapist would work closely with Michael in an early morning session to provide the visual and auditory cues necessary to facilitate independence in his ability to perform his morning routine. Michael's family remained an integral part of therapeutic intervention by providing the therapist with a list of meaningful vocational and avocational tasks familiar to him. These tasks were used to engage Michael, increasing his ability to attend for longer periods of time. One such successful task used with Michael at this level was disassembling and reassembling a small motor, part of his vocational responsibilities prior to the accident. Although Michael was able to attend to a simple computer-generated task for only 5 minutes at a time, he could sit for up to 20 minutes at a time reassembling a motor with 100% accuracy.

- Education is important at any stage of recovery. At this particular stage, it is common for significant others to have a lot of questions based on how their loved one is functioning. Once awake from coma state, families are often frightened by what is observed and confused about what to expect. The role of the therapist here is to provide resources and information regarding support groups, make the necessary referrals as appropriate, and educate about the recovery process following a brain injury. It is crucial for family members to receive accurate information regarding realistic expectations for recovery. The most successful forum for this type of discussion is in a family conference. This is an opportunity for all immediate caregivers, including the COTA and OTR, to discuss with family members all matters at hand so as not to have inconsistencies in information provided.

RLA Level IV

Setting

Rehabilitative hospital.

Referral

As level IV can present with significant agitation, rehabilitation hospitals are often equipped with special units or programs specific to those needs. The team may recommend a referral for these types of special services at this level of recovery.

Evaluations

At this level, the therapist can expect agitated, inappropriate behaviors with confusion; therefore, it is once again difficult to formally evaluate. The OTA and OT will instead utilize objective documentation of behaviors observed and possible precursors to that behavior. Evaluation of functional skills is possible, however, safety must always be considered for both the client and the caregivers. The Comprehensive Occupational Therapy Evaluation Scale (COTE) or a Routine Task Inventory (RTI) can be implemented and scored by the OTA under the supervision of the OT for a more formal evaluation of functional skill at this level. Practitioners should also take note of the surrounding environment during evaluations at this level. Both treatment and evaluations should be provided in a quiet, calming environment rather than a busy, noisy environment to minimize distraction and possible agitation.

Goals

1. Increase the duration of time that the client is able to attend to a task without an agitated outburst.
2. Monitor client's interactions with others or in small groups and ensure appropriateness of participation.

3. Increase client's overall orientation to person, place, and time, fostering insight into current strengths and weaknesses.
4. Ensure safety of the client, the therapist, and all others in immediate area in the event of an agitated outburst.
5. Promote independence in all basic self-care areas.

Treatment

- Safety is of the utmost importance during this stage of recovery. Michael would often have agitated outbursts throughout the day as a result of his current level of confusion. These outbursts were characterized by aggressive posturing, verbal harassment, and the throwing of objects at the therapist, family members, and other caregivers. These outbursts often occurred following any attempt to orient Michael to the accident and his injuries. His comments reflected his level of insight and were commonly associated with his perception of being locked up for no apparent reason. When these outbursts occurred, Michael would often flee from the area and the therapist would passively follow a short distance behind to ensure his safety.

- All of the highly structured treatment sessions were planned for Michael based on his interests and conducted in the least distracting environment. Numerous alternatives were prepared to account for his low frustration tolerance and impatience. In the event that Michael would disengage from any one particular task, the therapist would attempt to re-engage with a different task. Michael's interests were key in engaging him during treatment sessions and often included automotive or cooking skills in the absence of any sharp items.

- All members of the treating team and the family were informed of the importance in the uniform use of the memory notebook. The responsibility of this item was now shifted from caregivers and family to Michael himself. The contents were expanded to include a token economy system as a means of modifying Michael's behavioral outburst. With a given number of tokens achieved through actively participating in therapeutic sessions, Michael's family agreed to provide him with certain positive reinforces such as video games and short, supervised outings approved by the doctor.

- The utilization of bilateral upper extremity splints for positioning at night was discontinued at this stage due to the safety risks and poor carryover due to limited insight.

- Education is again a critical piece at this level of recovery. Emotional outbursts and inappropriate acts or comments occur not only in the presence of family but directed to the family members themselves. Family must be educated regarding the fact that these behaviors are a result of the injury. It is important to continue to emphasize the need for support and the benefits of that support. With Michael, education was provided to the family regarding how to manage emotional outbursts, what seems to be catalysts to these outbursts, the use of the memory notebook for re-orientation, need for constant and direct supervision due to the lack of insight as well as the degree of confusion, and the importance of carryover with the token economy system devised.

RLA Level V

Setting

Rehabilitative hospital.

Evaluations

At this level of recovery, the agitation and inappropriate impulses experienced by the client have subsided, yet the confusion and decreased attention persist. Standardized evaluative procedures can be attempted by the OTA who has either demonstrated service competency for the specific evaluation or is under the supervision of the OT. These include, but are not limited to, the following: manual muscle testing, goniometry, Motor-Free Perceptual Test, Kohlman Evaluation of Living Skills (KELS), COTE, Cognitive Assessment of Minnesota (CAM), and the Rivermead Behavioral Memory Test.

Goals

1. Facilitate independent use of memory notebook for orientation and daily routine.
2. Increase insight into strengths and weaknesses via repetition.
3. Increase attention span and ability to problem solve in functional situations.
4. Maximize level of independence with ADLs using compensatory strategies for initiation.
5. Promote the use of appropriate social skills within interactive group environments.
6. Facilitate the use of visual-motor skills based on repetition of simple commands.

Treatment

- At this point of recovery, Michael was able to sit with the therapist in the clinic for a 30-minute treatment session involving simple tabletop tasks when given a short break each 10-minute interval. During this break, Michael would walk one lap around the department and return to the table as a means of managing his irritability and decreased attention span.

- A focus of Michael's treatment at this stage was placed on perceptual-motor skills. Worksheets that included simple one- or two-step directions were used promoting both perceptual and cognitive skills, such as form constancy, right-left discrimination, scanning, dexterity, generalization of learning, initiation, attention, recognition, sequencing, and appropriate interpersonal skills.

- Michael began to work in a small group based on the development of orientation skills on a daily basis. Here, the therapist expected Michael to remain for the 20-minute duration of the group and conduct himself appropriately to both the other group members and the group leader. At first, these group meetings were supervised by the primary therapist in the event that Michael would leave the group and the group leader was not able to follow. Within 2 weeks, Michael was performing this function appropriately without supervision.

- The development of insight regarding Michael's strengths and weaknesses was a crucial component at this stage of recovery. This was achieved through the use of functional activities, such as dressing and cooking. For example, Michael would commonly arrive to therapy in the clothes he had worn the previous day. If approached, Michael would defend himself and state that the therapist must be mistaken. To address this area, repetition was used. The therapist created a section of the memory notebook that was added to at the beginning of each session and included what Michael was wearing. In a short time, Michael was able to independently refer to the memory notebook and identify this as a problem.

RLA Level VI

Setting

Rehabilitative hospital or transitional living facility.

Referral

As Michael became prepared for discharge from inpatient services, the OTA and OT spoke with the case manager to arrange for the continuation of appropriate occupational therapy intervention on an outpatient basis.

Evaluations

At this stage of recovery, the client will present with an increased attention span and will be better able to participate in standardized evaluation procedures. As some were indicated previously in RLA Level V, these evaluations include, but are not limited to, the following: KELS, COTE, CAM, Bay Area Functional Performance Evaluation (BaFPE), Lowenstein Occupational Therapy Cognitive Assessment (LOTCA), Test of Visual Perceptual Skills, and possibly a home evaluation prior to discharge as deemed appropriate. Each formal evaluation represented can be provided by the OTA who has demonstrated service competency or alongside the OT as with, for example, the home evaluation.

Goals

1. Increase ability to independently manage a daily schedule.
2. Increase independence with IADL tasks.
3. Increase higher level cognitive skill ability, including associations, categorization, generalizations, and problem-solving in novel situations.
4. Increase overall safety awareness through independent carryover of compensation techniques for any lingering confusion and disorientation.

Treatment

- The underlying basis of all treatment at this level is based on principles of repetition and the creation of a highly structured environment to promote success. Emphasis has been removed on the use of a token economy as a form of behavior modification and reinforcement of expected outcomes.

- The focus of Michael's current treatment became based in the awareness of the external environment and his daily routine. The therapist took on a more passive role, allowing for the "control" to be decided upon by Michael. These steps were made to facilitate the soon coming adjustment to a transitional living facility where Michael would be solely responsible for his self-care and getting to all scheduled appointments independently with appropriate requests for assistance if necessary. It was important to introduce Michael to these expectations. He became responsible for getting himself to and from all of his scheduled therapy appointments without the assistance of a transportation staff member. It was also very important that he manage his time accordingly in order to be able to perform this task independently.

- The complexity of all tasks that were addressed in the clinic were graded in order to provide the optimal amount of challenge, including such tasks as supervised cooking, actual hospital navigation using maps or signs, and money management skills.

- Education at this point was provided to the family regarding compensation techniques that are successful in promoting Michael's independence with emphasis placed on the importance of carryover. A family conference was again conducted where all members of the team, including the OT and OTA, discussed with the family Michael's discharge plan to the transitional living facility. Here, he would be expected to care for his own needs between Monday and Friday with only occasional supervision, then transition to home with weekend, overnight visits.

RLA Level VII

Setting

Transitional living facility or day treatment program.

Referral

The outpatient OTA/OT team began services after speaking with the case manager and family members. The transition is made even smoother if the previous OTA/OT team is able to meet with the new OTA/OT team to discuss current status in detail and any particular treatment strategies that were successful specific to Michael.

Evaluations

Michael's residual weaknesses include his executive functioning skills and overall endurance at this level of recovery. More rigorous, multistep evaluation procedures are then implemented focused on addressing Michael's need to return to work.

These evaluations include, but are not limited to, the following: Minnesota Rate of Manipulation Test, Purdue Pegboard Test, Jebson Hand Function Test, Crawford Small Parts Dexterity Test, Hooper Visual Organization Test, and a referral for a driving evaluation as deemed appropriate. Once again, these evaluation procedures can be provided by either the OTR or the OTR and COTA collaboratively.

Goals

1. Independence with daily routine.
2. Integration of cognitive ability into community re-entry skills.

3. Identify return to work status and address components identified as weaknesses.
4. Incorporate physical and emotional skills into meaningful activity.

Treatment

- At this point in Michael's treatment, the focus became community re-entry and return to work. On a routine basis, Michael joined a small group of other clients who had sustained head injuries. In this group, members were responsible for planning and implementing a community outing on a weekly basis. Clients were given a goal sheet that had been contributed to by each member of the treating team and required Michael to complete certain tasks while in the community. These tasks included asking for assistance, following directions, or identifying means of transportation. Michael was given the freedom of navigation within the community on these trips with supervision only, however, was solely responsible for completing the task at hand within the time frame allotted.

- The therapist contacted Michael's employer to request a copy of his previous job description. The long-term plan is for Michael to return to this capacity of work and, therefore, it is necessary to practice these functions. The job description was broken down into components and performed individually until mastered. Upon mastery, steps were added to heighten complexity of the task, working toward independence in performing all components of the job description.

- Education at this stage of recovery included both Michael and his family. It is often at this stage that clients begin to experience grief over their loss based on the development of insight. This grief is often very difficult for families to manage as a result of their own grieving process over their loss of who Michael previously was and who he is now evolving into. Education regarding coping skills, role adjustment, and support services is very important, making sure to refer to other professionals as necessary.

RLA Level VIII

Setting

Day treatment program or outpatient rehabilitation.

Evaluations

Many clients will not regain this level of functioning as a result of their injury. Mild brain injuries have a higher capacity to reach this level, however, Michael has not.

Evaluations at this point target specifically the return to productive living and include intensive vocational testing as a means of exploring alternative job functions. It is common for a vocational counselor to be added to the treatment team as a specialist at this point of recovery.

Goals

1. Increase tolerance to stressful situations.
2. Implement the independent use of compensatory strategies to address residual memory, social, and IADL skills.
3. Participation in a support group therapy environment.
4. Maximize automatic reactions to environmental stimuli.
5. Successful return to a productive living situation, including work or school.

Treatment

- The focus of treatment here would address residual deficit areas and implementation of compensatory strategies. Tasks that include work roles or IADL tasks are often addressed.
- Community re-integration is continued at this stage with higher expectations and a greater level of independence.
- Ideally, the client will return to work in a smaller capacity while continuing therapy intervention in order to overlap in skills necessary to master.
- Education continues for both clients and families in the form of support groups as a means of addressing loss and grief.

CLINICAL PROBLEM-SOLVING

Although Michael's recovery process has not reached the RLA VIII level, he is a success story for others who have sustained a brain injury. After 18 months of intensive therapeutic intervention, Michael was able to return to a supervised living situation, independently manipulate his immediate environment for use of public transportation, and maintain the job he had been performing prior to the injury. He was now 28 years old, the better portion of 2 long years had passed. Not all clients who sustain brain injuries are able to attain these goals. A key function of Michael's recovery was the supportive investment of his family and his employer, who together enabled his success alongside the treating team. Michael will continue to learn following his injury and may eventually reach the RLA level VIII over time; the capacity of the brain to heal does not have a time limit. He may continue with outpatient therapy, group therapy, and even one day

return to living independently. However, until then, he is proud of what he has achieved and those around him know he worked harder than many of us are ever asked to in order to achieve what he has at this point in his life.

Important to reinforce here are the compounding effects of the individual when treating a brain injury. For example, what if Michael's recovery had reached its highest stage at level V? What if Michael was married and the provider for his 2-year-old son? Would these factors have influence on the previously outlined occupational therapy intervention? Yes, the treatment plan would be considerably different to accommodate for these factors had they occurred.

Had Michael reached recovery level V and had ceased to make the gains characteristic of level VI, treatment and discharge plans as outlined previously would be changed dramatically. At this level, Michael would require direct supervision 24 hours per day. More than likely he would need cueing to complete his ADLs efficiently. He would be unable to conduct necessary IADLs without assistance and may pose a significant safety risk if responsible for any cooking. His insight would continue to be compromised and, therefore, he may be highly resistive to any limits placed on him. Michael's family would require extensive education prior to discharge to consider factors such as hiding car keys and unplugging the stove in order to limit safety risks associated with limited insight. The family would also require more of a support system than described earlier to address psychosocial issues around Michael's injury, his need for constant supervision, and the possibility of external services to assist with his care.

Had Michael been married and the father of a 2-year-old, other factors would need to be integrated into the treatment plan. Considerations would be made vocationally and financially regarding the impact of his inability to work during his recovery. Attention would need to be paid to his wife's capacity to handle all tasks required of a household and associated with providing sole care of a 2-year-old. Encouragement would be provided to the wife by the entire treatment team regarding possible support systems and need for assistance from various other family members if possible. Often times it is very difficult to include the spouse in treatment and provide necessary education due to the time constraints associated with being a sole child caregiver while also working to accommodate for any loss of income. These types of scenarios present with very difficult and individualized issues that arise continuously throughout the recovery process and require specific integration into the treatment plan.

SUMMARY

TBI remains in a league of its own. It is an extremely complex diagnosis requiring a multitude of professional intervention and skill. Brain injury robs a person of him- or herself; the person prior to the injury often disappears and in his or her place evolves a different person who may only resemble the first. The mechanism of brain injury has changed over time, yet its prevalence remains stable and the need for intensive, precise, and individualized treatment continues. It is thought that these are the very same reasons that COTAs, OTRs, and many other disciplines find this subspecialty area extremely rewarding. It is not often that a therapist is granted the privilege to work this closely with his or her client for weeks or months at a time, actually influencing each stage of recovery. It is becoming an even more rare occasion in the event of managed care service delivery models. As therapists within this practice domain, we are given a true opportunity to help those who are in need. We are able to guide their recovery and become part of an experience which they, their families, and ourselves are not likely to soon forget.

DIRECTORY OF RESOURCES CURRENTLY AVAILABLE

American Brain Tumor Association
2720 River Rd.
Des Plaines, IL 60018
800-886-2282

Brain Injury Society
1901 Ave. N., Suite 5E
Brooklyn, NY 11230
718-645-4401
www.virtualtrials.com/bis/

National Head Injury Foundation
Connecticut Ave. N.W., #812
Washington, DC 20036
800-444-6443

National Resource Center for TBI
Phoenix Project
P.O. Box 84151
Seattle, WA 98124
206-329-1371
www.neuro.pmr.vcu.edu

REFERENCES

Anderson, K. N., Anderson, L. E., & Glanze, W. D. (1994). *Mosby's medical, nursing, and allied health dictionary.* St. Louis, MO: Mosby-Year Book Inc.

Booth, B. J., Kodimer, C., & Malkmus, D. (1980). *Rehabilitation of head injured adult: Comprehensive cognitive management.* Downey, CA: Professional Staff Association of Rancho Los Amigos Hospital.

Hoeman, S. (1996). *Rehabilitation nursing process and application.* St. Louis, MO: Mosby.

Hole, J. W., Jr. (1984). *Human anatomy and physiology.* Dubuque, IA: Wm. C. Brown Publishers.

Jennett, B., & Teasdale, G. (1981). *Management of head injuries.* Philadelphia, PA: F. A. Davis.

Mitka, M. (1998). Good news on guns—But not for everyone. *JAMA, 280*(5), 403.

Morris, J. R., Pedley, T. A., & Rowland, L. P. (1995). Head and spinal cord trauma. In *The Columbia University College of Physicians & Surgeons Complete home medical guide.* New York, NY: Crown Publishers, Inc.

Pedretti, L. W., & Zoltan, B. (1990). *Occupational therapy: Practice skills for physical dysfunction.* St. Louis, MO: C. V. Mosby Co.

Silverman Saunders, C. (1996). Heading off head injury. *Current Health, 23*(1), 20-22.

Sniezek, J. E., Sosin, D., & Waxweiler, R. J. (1995). Trends in death associated with TBI, 1979 through 1992: Success and failure. *JAMA, 273*(22), 1778-1781.

Trombly, C. (1995). *Occupational therapy for physical dysfunction.* Baltimore, MD: Williams & Wilkins.

A Telephone Repairman with Spinal Cord Injury

Chapter 19

M. Laurita (Lita) Fike, MA, OTR

INTRODUCTION

There are between 230,000 and 450,000 people living with SCI, or spinal cord injury, in the United States, and each year one-third to one-half of these people are hospitalized (Woodruff & Baron, 1994). Nearly 10,000 new SCIs occur every year, and while 10% to 15% of these patients are admitted to specialty SCI hospitals, the rest are treated at community rehabilitation facilities or general hospitals. Because of the complexity of this health condition, OT practitioners are highly likely to be involved in the care of people with SCI on both initial admission and subsequent re-admissions (National Spinal Cord Injury Association [NSCIA], 1998).

DEFINITION

Part of the central nervous system, the spinal cord is a band of motor and sensory nerves that travels through the vertebral canal, extending from the base of the brain

KEY CONCEPTS

- Levels of spinal cord injury (SCI): The level at which the spinal cord is injured determines which peripheral sensory and motor nerves are affected (quick method of estimating the remaining functional abilities of the patient).
- Complications: In addition to loss of feeling and movement, SCI results in a variety of secondary complications, including blood pressure problems, breathing difficulties, incontinence/other bladder problems, and loss of skin integrity. These complications increase the complexity of treatment planning and intervention.
- Precautions: Because of the various complex problems with SCI, therapists must observe precautions in bringing the patient to an upright position, ROM activities of the neck and shoulders, length of sitting time, and environmental temperature.
- Intervention strategies: Treatment for patients with SCIs involves increasing endurance and strength in remaining performance components (biomechanical approach) and the provision of and training in the use of techniques and equipment that substitute for lost functions (rehabilitative approach).
- Adaptive equipment: A manual and/or power wheelchair for mobility is the most common type of equipment prescribed for use by patients with SCI. Other types of equipment include wrist-hand orthoses, mouthsticks, hand controls in cars, and environmental control systems.
- Community reintegration: Comprehensive treatment programs for patients with SCI include helping them develop methods or plans for public or private transportation, home assessment and adaptation, and return to school or work.

ESSENTIAL VOCABULARY

Autonomic dysreflexia: Nervous system disorder triggered by a variety of stimuli. May result in dangerous, high blood pressure.

Decubitus ulcers: Skin breakdown from unrelieved pressure on the skin, frequently over bony prominences.

Heterotopic ossification: Abnormal calcifications at shoulder, elbow, hip, or knee joints, resulting in redness, swelling, limitations in ROM, and pain.

Orthostatic hypotension: Sudden drop in blood pressure upon changing from supine to sitting or sitting to standing, resulting in dizziness and fainting.

Paraplegia: Loss of movement in lower body and legs.

Self-catheterization: Insertion of a flexible plastic tube into the urethra by the patient, permitting the bladder to be emptied and controlled.

Tenodesis: Fingers naturally flex when the wrist is extended and extend when the wrist is flexed. When combined with a splint holding the thumb and fingers rigid, this permits patients with SCI to have finger grasp and release functions.

Tetraplegia: Loss of movement in both arms and legs.

to just below the waist. The nerves that exit from and return to the spinal cord through the spinal vertebrae carry neuronal information to and from the brain and various parts of the body. SCI refers to damage to the spinal cord that stops the information flow and results in a functional deficit, that is, a loss of ability to move, to control bodily processes (such as respiration and control of bladder or bowel), or to feel sensation (NSCIA, 1998).

ETIOLOGY

The National Spinal Cord Injury Statistical Center (NSCISC) (1998) reported that since 1991, the majority (35%) of SCIs result from motor vehicle accidents (MVAs). Acts of violence (gunshot, knife, or stabbing wounds) account for another 30.4%. The percentage due to violence has been steadily increasing, while the percentage due to MVAs is decreasing. Falls rank third in cause at 19.5%, although after age 45, falls account for nearly half of all SCIs. Sports injuries cause 8.9% of SCIs, and two-thirds of these are from diving injuries. Various other causes, including vascular accidents, tumors, and infectious diseases, account for 6.9% (Go, DeVivo, & Richards, 1995).

The specific SCIs derived from the causes include compression and hyperextension (stretch) cord injuries, fractures and dislocations of the vertebrae that crush or transect the cord, and penetration of the cord.

PREVALENCE

Data from the NSCISC suggest that, in addition to the numbers noted above, another 5,000 people suffer SCIs but die before they can be treated. SCI primarily affects young adults, with the mean age increasing since 1973, when it was 28.6 years. Since 1990, the mean age has been 34.5 years. Males outnumber females four to one, and this has remained the same during the time such statistics have been collected (DeVivo et al., 1991; Go, DeVivo, & Richards, 1995).

Over the past 25 years there has been a significant change in the ethnic distribution. In 1973, Caucasians accounted for 77.5% of SCI, African-Americans 13.5%, Hispanics 6%, and other ethnic minorities were 3%. But since 1990, the incidence of injuries among African-Americans has increased to 28.7%, and among Hispanics to 10.5%, while that among Caucasians has fallen to 56.2% (NSCISC, 1998).

LEVELS OF INJURY

SCIs are initially classified as complete or incomplete. In a complete injury, the damage prevents the passing of any neuronal information between the brain and various parts of the body. This indicates a total loss of movement and sensation. In an incomplete injury, some nerve pathways, either sensory or motor, may be preserved. However, incomplete injuries can also result in devastating functional losses. Three types of incomplete injuries are:

1. Central cord lesion—This occurs when the central portions of the cervical spinal cord are damaged; the patient usually has less functional return in the arms and upper body than in the legs.

2. Brown-Sequard lesion—In this type of injury, one-half of the cord is transected (hemisection); the patient loses postural stability, motor function on the same side as the lesion, and the ability to feel pain and temperature changes on the opposite side.

3. Anterior cord lesion—The anterior structures of the cord are injured, and the patient loses the ability to move below the level of the lesion. The patient also loses the ability to feel pain or temperature changes, but the senses of touch, proprioception, and vibration are preserved.

When the injury occurs to the spinal cord as it passes through spinal vertebrae in the neck, known as the cervical (C1-C8) vertebrae, loss of function generally involves the respiratory system, the trunk, bowel, bladder, sexual function, and both the arms and the legs. This type of SCI has traditionally been called quadriplegia, but in the newer, international classification, it is termed tetraplegia, referring to involvement of all four limbs.

SCIs that occur through the thoracic (T1-T12) vertebrae usually affect the chest and the legs. Damage to the spinal cord at the level of lumbar vertebrae causes loss of control of the legs, bowel, bladder, and sexual function. At the sacral level, there is some functional loss involving the legs, bowel, bladder, and sexual function. Injuries at the thoracic, lumbar, and sacral level are generally termed paraplegia, meaning involvement of the lower half of the body.

The SCI is normally described by referring to the first letter of the skeletal level (cervical, thoracic, lumbar, sacral) and the number of the most distal uninvolved segment of the spinal nerve segment with full function, for example, C4 or T3 (American Spinal Injury Association [ASIA], 1992).

Historically, the incidence of tetraplegia has been slightly higher than that of paraplegia, but current trends indicate that incomplete paraplegia is increasing, while complete tetraplegia is decreasing. Since 1991, the incidence of SCI by neurological category is as follows:

- Complete paraplegia—28.9%
- Incomplete tetraplegia—28.6%
- Incomplete paraplegia—21.8%
- Complete tetraplegia—18.4%%

Approximately half of all SCI result in tetraplegia, but the proportion of tetraplegics increases dramatically after age 45, accounting for 66% of all injuries after age 60 and nearly 90% of all injuries after age 75. Further, 92% of all sports injuries result in tetraplegia. Most people who suffer SCI at or above C3 still die at the time of the accident, and those who survive are usually ventilator dependent for life (DeVivo et al., 1991).

INITIAL MEDICAL AND REHABILITATIVE TREATMENT

Patients are generally admitted to the emergency room, where physical examination is followed by neurological examinations to determine the level of injury. Medications such as methylprednisolone, a steroid, are frequently given to reduce swelling at the site of the injury; this is believed to reduce the severity of the damage to the spinal cord, particularly in cases of incomplete injury. The injured spine must be immediately stabilized, either surgically, with internal fixation, or with traction on bed frames designed to immobilize the patient. Patients with cervical injuries may require halo traction, which involves a metal band attached to the skull, held in place with metal rods affixed to a plastic body jacket. Patients with paraplegia may require only a plastic jacket or brace (Yarkony, 1994).

Patients with tetraplegia must also receive respiratory assistance; those with C1-C3 lesions will require a ventilator. Patients are also catheterized. At least one-half of patients admitted to emergency rooms with SCIs also have other injuries, including brain injuries, and these injuries will be treated as well, with the patient usually moving to the intensive care unit. If the patient's spine is stabilized, rehabilitation generally starts within 48 hours of admission. After the patient's medical condition has normalized, the patient with SCI transfers to a rehabilitation unit or hospital, where inpatient treatment will last 1 to 3 months (Yarkony, 1994). In 1992, patients with tetraplegia averaged 95 hospital days, while those with paraplegia stayed an average 67 days. This is a significant reduction in hospital stay from 1973, when on average, tetraplegia treatment lasted 6 months, and paraplegia treatment lasted 3 months (NSCISC, 1998).

PROGNOSIS

According to the National Spinal Cord Injury Database (NSCISC, 1998), overall, 85% of SCI patients who survive the first 24 hours are still alive 10 years later. This is compared with the 10-year survival of 98% of the non-SCI population, given similar age and sex. Historically, the most frequent cause of death among people with SCI was renal failure. However, medical advances in urologic management have reduced the number of deaths due to this cause. The current most common causes of death include pneumonia, pulmonary emboli, and septicemia. An increasing number of people with SCI are now dying of unrelated causes, such as cancer or cardiovascular disease, which is similar to the general population.

Life expectancies for persons with SCI are increasing, but are still somewhat below those for people with no SCI. Mortality rates are significantly higher in the first year following injury than in subsequent years.

Almost all people with SCI return to private residences after rehabilitation; less than 6% go into nursing homes or to other hospitals. Those who go into nursing homes tend to be elderly or have very high cervical injuries with no resources for home care.

At the time of injury, more than half of patients age 16 to 59 are employed, while the rest are students, homemakers, or unemployed. Eight years after injury, about one-third of persons with paraplegia and one-fourth of persons with tetraplegia are employed. People who return to work within the first year of injury tend to return to work at the same job, for the same employer. Those who return to work after the first year either work for different employers or were students who found work. The National Spinal Cord Injury Database has not yet evaluated the impact of the Americans with Disabilities Act on the re-employment of persons with SCI.

PRECAUTIONS AND COMPLICATIONS

SCI is a complex health problem because of the multiple systems affected. The OT practitioner must be aware of a large number of potential medical problems and must observe many precautions, during both the evaluation and the treatment stages of the patient's care.

Autonomic Dysreflexia

Autonomic dysreflexia is an autonomic nervous system disorder that can be triggered by a variety of stimuli and may result in dangerously high blood pressure. The patient may complain of a sudden headache; he or she may exhibit sudden sweating and reddening of the face, restless behavior, increased spasticity, or a sudden drop in pulse rate. This is a medical emergency and immediate intervention is required. The OT practitioner should bring the patient to a sitting position if he or she has been prone or supine in order to lower the cranial blood pressure. The urinary catheter and drainage bag should be checked to make sure that urine is flowing. If the catheter is clamped, it should be released. If the drainage bag is full, it should be emptied. Tight clothing should be loosened, and the OT practitioner should check for other sources of skin irritation, such as a clothing gather or cushion roughness. In the hospital, nursing personnel should be notified as quickly as possible; in community or home care, the home care nurse or the patient's physician should be contacted by phone for further directions in patient care (Jones, 1986; Trombly, 1989).

Range of Motion Restrictions

Patients with SCIs should not receive evaluations or treatments involving passive ROM past 90 degrees at the shoulder, nor should manual muscle testing or strengthening exercises be provided to the shoulder muscles until advised by the physician. The shoulder muscles affect movement of the cervical and thoracic spine, and this must be avoided until the spine is fully stabilized (Schneider, 1990).

Patients with lower tetraplegia are potentially able to use their arms and wrists for tasks requiring manual dexterity, by taking advantage of natural tenodesis. When the wrist is extended, the fingers and thumbs assume a flexed position. When the wrist is flexed, the fingers extend. This motion can be used, with or without the assistance of a splint, to substitute for hand grasp and finger pinch tasks. It is important that wrist extensors and finger flexors be allowed to tighten in order to provide as much power as possible to the tenodesis grasp. Therefore, the OT practitioner must never extend the wrist and fingers at the same time, nor flex the wrist and fingers at the same time. ROM exercises for full flexion of the fingers should only be done with the wrist in extension, and for full extension of the fingers, with the wrist in flexion (Hill & Presperin, 1986).

Othostatic Hypotension

A SCI not only affects the motor and sensory spinal nerves, but also the autonomic nervous system, which is responsible for regulating blood pressure in response to position changes. Patients with SCI will usually have been immobilized in a supine or prone position to stabilize the spine, and when they first attempt to sit up, will experience sudden drops in blood pressure that may result in dizziness, nausea, and fainting. If the patient experiences these symptoms during treatment, the OT practitioner should recline the patient in bed or tip the wheelchair back to allow for increased cerebral blood flow. The OT practitioner should work with the patient and other health care providers to provide a consistent and slow introduction of moving the patient from bed-lying to sitting, until the patient develops adequate sitting tolerance (Kovich, 1986).

Respiratory Impairment

Patients with tetraplegia will experience respiratory difficulties due to paralysis of the phrenic nerve and diaphragm, and often require tracheostomy with assisted ventilation. Patients with C1-C3 require permanent assisted respiration. Patients with tracheostomies often have difficulty in coughing to clear their respiratory passageways and will need suctioning at various times, including during OT treatment. The OT practitioner must be alert to signs of need for suctioning, such as an unproductive cough or rasping, congested sounds during respiration, and must either learn to perform suctioning as required or must contact the appropriate personnel in a timely manner (Daniel & Strickland, 1988).

Hypothermia and Hyperthermia

As in the case of orthostatic hypotension, patients with SCI may have impaired thermal control due to damage to the autonomic nervous system. They may have difficulty maintaining an even body temperature and must avoid prolonged exposure to heat and humidity and to moderate to severe cold. The OT environment should be mild, and exercise must be discontinued if air-conditioning is unavailable during hot and humid months. The OT practitioner must be alert for signs that the patient is suffering subnormal body temperature or is overheating, and contact nursing as appropriate for intervention (Trombly, 1989).

Sensory Losses

Patients with SCI will have sensory loss below the level of the lesion and are in danger of suffering pressure ulcers (decubiti) as well as other injuries to the skin. OT practitioners should observe standard precautions for sensory loss and should encourage patients to use vision to compensate for sensory loss.

During transfers and bed mobility, patients as well as their caregivers must avoid shearing stress or friction injuries to the skin by lifting the body away from surfaces, rather than sliding.

Patients should use a wheelchair cushion whenever seated for long periods of time, including when out of the wheelchair. They should also perform weight shifts every 15 to 20 minutes throughout the day in order to relieve pressure.

While in bed, patients should reposition every 2 hours, unless on an alternating pressure mattress or other pressure reduction device.

Patients should also inspect their skin daily for evidence of pressure injuries, using a curved handle mirror to inspect the buttocks. The stages of pressure injury development are as follows:

- Stage I—The skin is intact but stays reddened for over 20 minutes after the pressure is relieved. The reddened area is often warm to touch. At this level of injury, the treatment is primarily prevention of further injury by increasing the amount of cushioning, by removing the irritant causing the pressure, or by increasing the number of weight shifts and repositioning periods.

- Stage II—The skin is broken, but the injury is confined to superficial areas. Treatment consists of removing the pressure until the skin heals completely. This means if the buttocks area is involved, the patient must not sit, and must be positioned in prone or side-lying at all times.
- Stage III—The pressure wound has extended into deeper levels of the skin.
- Stage IV—The wound area has extended into the level of muscles.

Treatment at stages III and IV typically requires surgical debridement and may require grafting. Again, until the area has healed, the patient must not put any pressure on the wound site. Decubitus ulcers can be life threatening if infection develops, and the cost of surgical care and hospitalization is staggering (Garber, 1985; Garber & Krouskop, 1982).

Heterotopic Ossification

This condition involves abnormal calcification around joints, usually the elbows or knees, but may also involve hips and shoulders. Symptoms include swelling and redness, as well as limitations in joint ROM. Above the level of the lesion, the patient may also experience pain or tenderness. OT practitioners should report the symptoms to the patient's physician (Kovich, 1986).

Spinal Shock and Spasticity

Immediately after the SCI, the patient experiences flaccid paralysis, which may last for days, weeks, or months. However, once the spinal shock is reduced, the patient at T-12 or above may experience mild to moderate spasticity caused by the reflexive motor synapse through the spinal cord. Muscle relaxing medications are often very effective in relieving spasticity. However, the OT practitioner must assist the patient in managing spasticity to increase the patient's functional independence. Spasticity in the hips and legs, for example, can be triggered deliberately by patients to assist in lower extremity dressing. However, it can also cause problems during transfers. The OT practitioner must teach the patient to use positioning and other techniques to inhibit spasticity. In addition, the patient must do regular ROM exercises to prevent contractures (Hollar, 1995).

EVALUATION TOOLS

After initial stabilization, all members of the treatment team will evaluate the patient. Initial OT evaluations are generally based on occupational performance components, which may include:

- Functional ROM
- Upper extremity strength testing
- Dexterity and coordination testing
- Sensory testing
- Muscle tone testing
- Assessment of sitting tolerance and trunk balance

These tests are most often completed by the OT; however, qualified OTAs may contribute to the evaluations by gathering data, particularly in such areas as dynamometer and pinch strength tests and dexterity tests such as the nine-hole-peg test (Daniel & Strickland, 1988).

The OT practitioner also evaluates occupational performance to the extent that is possible with patients who have suffered such catastrophic functional losses. Patients with paraplegia will be evaluated regarding their ability to perform basic activities of daily living (BADLs). Some tasks, such as washing the face, brushing teeth, combing hair, shaving, and self-feeding will be accomplished by these patients with little difficulty once they are able to assume a full sitting position. While prone or supine for spinal stabilization, however, patients with paraplegia may need equipment positioned for them in order to be independent in these tasks. Other BADLs, such as toileting, bathing, and lower extremity dressing, will require both adaptive techniques and special equipment in order for the patient to become independent. Training in these areas will begin once the patient is able to tolerate sitting for 2 to 4 hours.

Patients with tetraplegia will be unable to do most BADLs without training in the use of special equipment or adaptive techniques. For lower level tetraplegia, the use of a universal cuff around the palm of the hand may permit self-feeding and facial hygiene after equipment set-up. High-level tetraplegics will be dependent in most BADLs, even with adaptive equipment. Therefore, evaluation of BADLs is generally deferred until sitting tolerance is achieved and initial treatment for strengthening has begun. Either OTs or OTAs may conduct BADL evaluations.

After the patient with SCI has achieved sitting tolerance and initial treatment has begun, OT practitioners will also gather information regarding the patient's education and vocational history, avocational interests, psychological adaptation to the injury, and personal goals. OTAs will often conduct these assessments in consultation with their supervising therapist.

During ongoing treatment and prior to discharge, patients will participate in assessment of their instrumental activities of daily living (IADLs). These usually involve evaluations regarding mobility needs, including manual and/or powered wheelchairs, home care and safety, environmental accessibility, and driving assessments.

OTAs may contribute to these assessments by gathering measurement data and by specific communication with the patient and the patient's family, such as filling out questionnaires and drawing floor plans with them. Patients are often referred to community resources for driving assessments and training.

OTs and OTAs should work together with the patient to develop an individualized treatment plan based on the patient's goals and the results of the various evaluations (Daniel & Strickland, 1988; Farmer, 1986; Hollar, 1995).

CASE STUDY

Assessments and Evaluations

John R. is a 24-year-old, right-dominant, Mexican-American who was working for the local telephone company when he fell and sustained a C-6 fracture. He was admitted to a the county general hospital, where his medical condition was stabilized and he was placed in head tongs with traction in a suspension bed for 2 weeks. In the suspension bed, John's position was changed from supine to prone every 2 hours to relieve skin pressure. During this time, he was referred to the general rehabilitation services in the acute care wing of the hospital. His OT team consisted of an OT and an OTA. Because John was in traction and confined to bed, the initial activities of assessment of sitting tolerance and skin integrity and prescription of wheelchair were deferred. Instead, while John was in the supine position, the OT evaluated John's hand, wrist, and elbow ROM and sensation. She then fitted John with a universal cuff for his right hand, which had good wrist extension and pronation. She also adapted and applied a wrist-driven orthosis to his left hand, which was weaker than his right.

At the next session, John was in the prone position, and he was able to move his arms freely below the bed. The OTA was then able to evaluate his ability to wash his face, brush his teeth with a toothbrush in the universal cuff, and feed himself a snack of finger foods using both hands. The OTA also took an occupational history, helped John fill out a leisure interest list, and discussed his goals for therapy. Based on these initial assessments, and a review of the assessments by the physician and the rest of the team, the two OT practitioners felt they had enough information to design an early intervention program for John.

Frames of Reference

The central nervous system, of which the spinal cord is a part, does not regenerate, and although many scientists are engaged in research to develop methods to encourage regeneration, at this time there is no cure for SCI. This means that health care providers have no methods to directly restore the motor and sensory functions that are lost when the spinal cord is transected. Treatment therefore consists of methods to enhance and increase remaining functions, which is considered a biomechanical treatment approach, and methods to provide substitutions for abilities that have been permanently lost, known as the rehabilitative treatment approach (Trombly, 1989).

In the OT intervention for SCI, the OT practitioner focuses on occupational performance and generally utilizes the biomechanical and rehabilitative approaches simultaneously. However, to simplify discussion, these methods will be presented separately.

The biomechanical approach includes activities and exercises which target occupational performance subcomponents. For example, intervention may involve training or instructions designed to increase muscle strength, improve or prevent loss of joint ROM, increase endurance for daily activities, enhance dexterity and manipulative skills, and prevent loss of skin integrity. In most instances, the therapeutic goal will only be achieved through repetition and practice. The skill of the OT practitioner is required to provide intervention that will motivate and satisfy the patient despite the occasional monotony of repetition (Trombly, 1989).

The rehabilitative approach consists of teaching alternative methods for achieving satisfactory occupational performance (e.g., teaching a patient to transfer to the toilet from a wheelchair) and providing equipment that will assist the patient in accomplishing tasks that he or she can no longer do without assistance (e.g., a wheelchair may provide the patient with mobility). Although most of the compensatory techniques and equipment provided to people with SCI are readily identified, the OT practitioner may need to be creative in obtaining equipment and modifying techniques to benefit the specific needs of the patient (Trombly, 1989). Table 19-1 presents intervention strategies based on occupational performance and performance components at the various levels of SCI and has been compiled using information from Daniel and Strickland (1988), Hill (1986c), Adler (1996), Trombly (1989), and Wilson et al. (1984).

Treatment Programming

Treatment for patients with SCI can be effectively carried out in both individual and group settings. During individual treatment, the OT practitioner usually works on goal-setting and goal-revision, personal hygiene and dressing skills, equipment measurement and fabrication, and patient and family teaching. An early morning care program is particularly useful for practicing BADL skills, such as bathing, dressing, and bowel and bladder care, at realistic times. Some hospitals have also developed late evening care programs, often involving family members,

Table 19-1

Treatment Approaches for Patients with Spinal Cord Injury, Based on Level of Injury

SCI Level with Muscles and Movements Available	Occupational Performance Areas	Biomechanical Intervention	Rehabilitative Intervention and Equipment Needed
C-1 to 3 Head and neck muscles innervated by cranial nerves Patient can: Talk, chew, swallow, blow	Dependent for respiration BADLs: Directs others for all self-care IADLs: Can use environmental control unit to move bed, turn on TV, answer phone, open doors Directs others for all other IADLs Mobility: Can use power w/c controlled by sip and puff or head motion Communication: Word processing by electronic typewriter or computer Can use speakerphone with automatic dial Leisure: Can play computer and electronic games, use mouthstick for art activities, read using page-turner Work: Operate computer, phone services by voice only	Joint ROM to all joints once spine is stabilized Increase sitting tolerance and increase general endurance by increasing length of time patient sits and engages in activities. Monitor for fatigue; observe precautions for hypotension and skin pressure Identify available muscles; provide manual resistance to help strengthen head, neck, and facial muscles Work to improve strength in blowing, in rhythm with respirator Provide activities involving use of mouthstick and or head pointer to increase strength and endurance	Requires ventilator at all times Head support needed during prolonged sitting Education must be provided to patient regarding directing own care, including the selection and training of own attendants in future The involvement of family and friends in the educational process is also important Patient must receive training in use of all equipment, including instructing others in set-up Environmental control unit (ECU) operated by computer, mouthstick, head pointer, head switch or tongue switch Power w/c with tilt and recline for pressure control, for inside use. Requires supervision for outside use Computer or word processor with switches operated by mouthstick (requires maximal assistance) or head pointer, head or tongue switch (requires set-up and minimal assist)
C-4 Diaphragm and trapezius Patient often has independent respiration; has scapular elevation	BADLs: Can drink independently after set-up with long straw Directs others for all self-care	All interventions as for C1 to 3 Provide manual resistance to trapezius, to increase strength/mobility of neck	May increase level of independence similar to C-5 if using externally powered flexor hinge splint and electric mobile arm support,

Table 19-1, continued

Treatment Approaches for Patients with Spinal Cord Injury, Based on Level of Injury

SCI Level with Muscles and Movements Available	Occupational Performance Areas	Biomechanical Intervention	Rehabilitative Intervention and Equipment Needed
	IADLs: Can use environmental control unit to move bed, turn on TV, answer phone, open doors Directs others for all other IADLs **Mobility:** Can use power w/c controlled by sip and puff, chin control, or head switch **Communication:** Word processing by electronic typewriter or computer Can use speakerphone with automatic dial **Leisure:** Can play computer and electronic games, use mouthstick for art activities, read using page-turner **Work:** Operate computer, phone services; can use mouthstick to operate other equipment, such as tape recorder, adding machine	Provide respiratory exercises in conjunction with respiratory and physical therapy to increase strength and endurance of diaphragm	but this is expensive and uncommon Equipment needs similar to C-1 to 3, but can operate chin controls, has better neck control and endurance, and can use mouthstick for long periods Needs mouthstick holder As for C–1 to 3, education must be provided to patient regarding directing own care, including the selection and training of own attendants in future Patient must receive training in use of all equipment, including instructing others in set-up Office or school equipment may need minor modifications to operate by mouthstick
C-5 Infraspinatus and deltoid, biceps brachialis, brachioradialis, supinator Patient has shoulder abduction to 80 to 90 degrees, external rotation; elbow flexion and supination; use of gravity can substitute for shoulder adduction, internal rotation, and pronation	**BADLs:** Patient can feed self, do facial hygiene and make-up, and can assist with dressing and bathing after set-up, with use of adaptive equipment **IADLs:** Can use hand controls to move bed, turn on TV, answer phone, open doors, and operate other equipment	Joint ROM to all joints once spine is stabilized Increase sitting tolerance and increase general endurance, increasing length of time patient sits up and engages in activities. Monitor for fatigue; observe precautions for hypotension and skin pressure	Equipment needs for BADLs include mobile arm support, wrist orthosis and universal cuff for utensils, toothbrush, comb; plate guard, long drinking straw, dycem to stabilize plate and glass; long-handled bath sponge Requires joystick-controlled power w/c with tilt and recline for pressure relief Needs manual w/c, can op-

Table 19-1, continued

Treatment Approaches for Patients with Spinal Cord Injury, Based on Level of Injury

SCI Level with Muscles and Movements Available	Occupational Performance Areas	Biomechanical Intervention	Rehabilitative Intervention and Equipment Needed
	such as electric lifts. Directs others for all other IADLs Mobility: Need power w/c for long distances. Can use manual chair with quad pegs for short distances Communication: Word processing by electronic typewriter or computer and phone using typing stick or orthosis Leisure: Can play computer and electronic games, use orthosis for art activities, read using page-turner Work: Operate computer, phone services; can use orthosis to operate other equipment, such as tape recorder, adding machine	Provide activities and exercises that will increase strength of shoulder and elbow muscles in all available ranges. Practice activities in which patient uses gravity to accomplish full range Provide activities that will increase patient's dexterity in use of orthosis and typing sticks, particularly to increase typing speed	erate for short distances using quad pegs on wheels Requires gel or air cushion Needs adaptation for orthosis or cuff to utilize typing stick May need adaptations to operate equipment if it requires holding down several keys at one time As for the above SCI patients, education must be provided to patient regarding directing own care, including the selection and training of own attendants in future Patient must receive training in use of all equipment, including instructing others in set-up
C-6 Pectoralis major, serratus anterior, lattisimus dorsi, pronator teres, radial wrist extensors Patient can flex shoulder and reach forward; additional movements include shoulder internal rotation, extension, and adduction, and pronation and extension of the wrist—this provides the patient with tenodesis grasp, a major increase in function	BADLs: Can feed self, do facial and hair grooming using tenodesis grasp, although may also use universal cuff for some activities. Wrist-driven hinge orthosis (WHO) is also used at this level, giving more power and control to the tenodesis grasp. Can bathe self using tub bench and long shower hose. Dressing can be done independently with modified techniques Bowel and Bladder Care: Can insert suppositories for	Joint ROM to all joints once spine is stabilized. Major precaution: preserve tenodesis grasp as noted before Increase sitting tolerance and increase general endurance by increasing length of time patient sits up and engages in activities. Monitor for fatigue; observe precautions for hypotension and skin pressure Provide activities and exercises that will increase the strength of shoulder, elbow,	May use universal cuff, or WHO for BADLs and IADLs. Some equipment may need enlarged handles. Rocker knife may be useful. Will need tub bench and long shower hose, and equipment for bowel and bladder programs Will need training in adapted techniques for dressing Can use manual w/c, but may need power w/c for long distances. Will need training in independent

Table 19-1, continued

Treatment Approaches for Patients with Spinal Cord Injury, Based on Level of Injury

SCI Level with Muscles and Movements Available	Occupational Performance Areas	Biomechanical Intervention	Rehabilitative Intervention and Equipment Needed
	bowel program using adaptive device. Can transfer independently to toilet. Can empty own catheter bag and clamp. Requires assistance for intermittent catherization	and wrist muscles in all available ranges, noting particularly the position of fingers during tenodesis. Will need to increase endurance for operating manual w/c	side-to-side weight shifts for pressure relief, and use of sliding board for transfers
			Will need special driver's education for operating an adapted motor vehicle
	IADLs: Can operate TV, radio, phone, typewriter, computer using tenodesis grasp, or orthosis, and typing stick. Can do light housekeeping and cooking. Needs w/c accessible kitchen	Provide activities to increase patient's dexterity in donning and doffing clothing, any orthosis, and use of typing sticks, particularly to increase typing speed and ease of equipment operation	May need assistance in acquiring car adaptations
	Mobility: Can use manual chair for short distances. May need power w/c for long distances. Can drive car using hand controls and adapted steering wheel		
	Leisure: Can play table games, such as cards, table tennis with some adaptations. Can participate in some w/c sports		
	Work: Can operate very light-weight hand tools, computers, office equipment; can perform desk and phone jobs		
C-7 Triceps, extrinsic finger extensors, flexor carpi radialis Patient can now do elbow extension and can actively extend fingers, as well as flex wrist	In general, the patient with C-7 SCI functions much as the C-6, except most occupational performances are easier. At the C-7 level the patient can do a push-up transfer and weight shift because of the triceps. Primary mobility is with manual w/c	Biomechanical intervention is much the same as for C-6, with emphasis on strengthening the additional muscles and increasing endurance of operation of manual w/c	May need wrist splint for self-feeding or no adaptations. Will need training as above for dressing. Needs equipment for management of bowel and bladder Requires manual w/c and training in push-up weight shifts for pressure relief and push-up transfers

Table 19-1, continued

Treatment Approaches for Patients with Spinal Cord Injury, Based on Level of Injury

SCI Level with Muscles and Movements Available	Occupational Performance Areas	Biomechanical Intervention	Rehabilitative Intervention and Equipment Needed
			Will need special driver's education for operating an adapted motor vehicle. May need assistance in acquiring car adaptations
C-8, T-1 (T-2,3,4) Intrinsics, including thumb, extrinsic finger flexors and thumb flexors, extrinsic thumb extensor, ulnar wrist flexors and extensors Patients at this level have UE control with fine motor and prehension	BADLs and IADLs are similar to C-7, but are easier. Patient is able to dress from a sitting position	Similar to C-7	Independent in UE tasks without orthosis, including management of bowel and bladder. Requires manual w/c and needs special driver's education for operating an adapted motor vehicle. May need assistance in acquiring car adaptations
T-5 to T-11 Intercostals begin to come in, as well as long muscles of back Patients at these levels are beginning to establish functional trunk control in sitting; they are able to lean forward without using UE. Limited ambulation with long leg braces may be possible	Independent in most BADLs and IADLs. Can stand with assistance and do moderately heavy work while seated. Endurance is increased due to better respiratory reserve	Aggressive strengthening to upper extremities and trunk. Work at standing table with leg braces to increase overall endurance	Independent in self-care and home-care from w/c. Requires manual w/c since ambulation is still difficult. Will need hand controls for motor vehicle
T-12, and Lower Full function of intercostals and abdominal muscles At L-4, low back muscles, hip flexors, and quadriceps come in Patients at these levels have full trunk control, more endurance, and increasingly easier ambulation with long leg braces and crutches	Similar to T-5, 6. Has better endurance, can use outdoor lawn and recreation equipment, such as rider mower or snow mobile with hand controls	Aggressive strengthening for all available muscle groups. At L-4, standing and ambulating during IADLs will be useful in increasing both leg strength and endurance	At the higher levels, patients will still need manual w/c for long distances and for convenience. May or may not need hand controls in motor vehicle at L-4. Still lacks voluntary control of bowel and bladder

which focus on undressing, personal hygiene, and preparation for bed, including positioning and padding to prevent pressure sores. These programs are often organized and staffed by OTAs (Hollar, 1995).

Early Treatment Programming

John is a young, single male diagnosed with a C-6 lesion resulting from an injury at work. John had told the OTA he wanted to be as independent as possible in taking care of himself. The OT and OTA decided to use both the biomechanical and rehabilitative approaches, working to increase John's endurance and upper extremity strength while providing him with the adaptive equipment he needed to substitute for weak hand function. The OTA worked with John on early morning self-care and self-feeding, using the universal cuff, wrist orthosis, and utensils with built-up handles. Because John had also expressed an interest in woodworking, the OTA also started John on a small bird house kit, which required sanding and painting; she increased the length of time John worked on his project as his endurance improved. At the end of the 2 weeks, when the traction was removed and he was placed in a body jacket with a head brace, John was able to feed himself independently in the prone position after set-up. He was also able to wash his face, brush his teeth, comb his hair, and work at his project for 2 hours daily without fatigue. At this time his OT team measured him for a hospital wheelchair and cushion and started his sitting program. Within 2 days, John was able to sit up in the wheelchair for 2 hours without symptoms. He was then transferred to the rehabilitation unit, where he was reassessed by his new OT treatment team.

In spinal injury rehabilitation settings, group treatment can be very effective because patients are able to see each other at various stages of rehabilitation. Patients can help one another problem-solve and provide emotional support for each other (Fike, 1984). Typical groups might include a leisure interest group, in which crafts and games are used not only to develop avocational interests, but also to develop strength and endurance. For example, mouthstick drawing, painting, ceramic glazing, and computer games help develop strength of head and neck muscles and sitting endurance, as well as manipulative skills of the mouth and tongue. For patients with paraplegia, leatherwork and light woodworking can help develop upper extremity strength, as well as provide opportunities for the patient to work on weight shifting and trunk balance (Hollar, 1995).

Lunch groups offer patients the opportunity to practice self-feeding skills, including the use of adapted equipment. Home skills groups involve cooking and other light house-keeping skills; for patients with tetraplegia, these groups offer the opportunity for decision-making and supervision of others in carrying out tasks for them. Some institutions offer "mat classes," in which patients with C-6 and lower level injuries can practice putting on outer clothing, such as slacks, shirts, and shoes. Community integration groups assist patients in making the transition from hospital to home, including the use of public transportation and management of architectural barriers (Hill, 1986a).

Transitional Treatment Programming

Upon transfer to the rehabilitation unit, John found himself surrounded by other patients with SCIs, amputations, strokes, and head injuries. This was initially surprising to John, but he continued to state he wanted to be as independent as possible. The physical therapy department, with consultation from the OT team, had ordered a wheelchair for John, but he would use the hospital chair until his own arrived. The OT team fitted his chair with a tray and worked with him until he could remove and attach it himself. He was expected to join other patients in the lounge for meals, where he became increasingly independent, working with the OTA to apply his own adaptive equipment, select his food from the cafeteria line, and bring it to the table using a wheelchair tray. He also joined two groups run by OTAs, one in the morning, a mat class which worked on self-dressing skills with three other patients who had SCIs, and an afternoon home-care group, which worked on meal preparation, laundry, and house-keeping tasks as they would need to be done from a wheelchair. Since John lived by himself in an apartment, he needed to learn to use standard equipment as much as possible, so he had his treatment program in an unmodified kitchen area. Fortunately for John, his incomplete injury was proving to have spared some peripheral neurons; his right hand functioned at the C-7 to C-8 level, while his left remained at the original diagnostic level of C-6. John was therefore able to develop more independence than might be expected for a complete C-6 injury. For example, he proved to have good trunk balance and was able to completely dress himself, transfer to his wheelchair, and manually push his wheelchair using regular rims rather than quad-pegs. Two nights a week John also participated in community reintegration groups supervised by OTAs, in which the patients arranged for their own public transportation with modified vans and attended local community events such as baseball games.

Even in community hospitals, it is effective to work with patients who have spinal injuries in mixed diagnosis groups and not just from the necessity imposed by pressures from health maintenance organizations. The motivation, psychological support, and assistance in problem-solving that group members offer each other should not be underestimated (Fike, 1984).

From the beginning of the patient's admission to rehabilitation services, treatment must be coordinated with the treatment team members. This includes not only the doctor, nurses, physical therapists, and others involved in the patient's care, but also the patient and the patient's designated family members. Care must be taken to schedule services so that the patient is challenged, but not overwhelmed or overfatigued. The patient and family must be involved in setting goals and should be kept informed at all times of changes in program or treatment.

When the team anticipates discharge, a plan should be established to help the patient make the transition, including short-term visits to the anticipated home-setting. This provides the patient with opportunities to try his or her new skills in a realistic setting and to build self-confidence. When the patient returns to the hospital, any encountered difficulties can be the focus of the final sessions of treatment. It may also be important to assist the patient in contacting the state department of vocational services for possible assistance in returning to school, occupational training, or previous work settings (Hill, 1986b).

Planning for Discharge

Since John had been injured on the job, his medical and rehabilitation expenses were being covered by workers' compensation. The representative from the workers' compensation board met with the treatment team and John early in his treatment program to begin planning for discharge. John's apartment was on the third floor, but his building had an elevator and was wheelchair accessible. John was given a weekend pass, in which he returned to his apartment, accompanied by a friend. There John tried out the skills he had been working on in the hospital and returned on Monday with a list of accomplishments and challenges. The OT team worked with John to overcome the problems he had found at home by suggesting ways he could modify his environment and by helping him select adaptive equipment for his home. The workers' compensation representative also met with John's employer, the public telephone company. John would not be able to return as a linesman, but other jobs were available within the company that involved deskwork, including customer representative and operator. The OT met with the personnel director of the telephone company to obtain various job descriptions. Then she, the OTA, and John established pre-vocational goals, including increasing fine motor skills and more efficient operation of computers and calculators. John was able to use departmental equipment to work on his goals while hospitalized.

Psychological and Cognitive Implications

Throughout the treatment program, the cognitive and emotional needs of the patient must be considered and addressed. SCI is a massive trauma to the neurological system, and a certain percentage have simultaneous brain injuries. These dual injuries may cause changes in the cognitive status of the patient, necessitating modifications in training and rehabilitation, similar to programs developed for patients with TBIs (Brown, 1992; Hollar, 1995).

Paralysis, dependence on ventilators, the loss of mobility, the loss of bowel and bladder control, the changes in sexual function, all result in massive disturbances to the patient's self-image, to self-esteem, and to occupational role effectiveness. The treatment program must be designed to incorporate methods that will address these needs, as well as the physical and functional problems (Jordan, Wellborn, Kovnick & Salzstein, 1991). The use of group treatment to provide group support and the OT practitioner's skillful use of active listening and interpersonal skills may be effective in designing a holistic treatment program for patients with SCI (Fike, 1984).

Providing Group Support

Early in John's rehabilitation program, he had difficulty discussing personal or private issues with either of his two female OT practitioners. He avoided eye contact when discussing bowel and bladder concerns and became extremely embarrassed when the topic of sexuality was discussed. John had broken up with his long-time girlfriend just 2 weeks before his injury. He had one brother who visited him regularly, but the rest of his family was in Mexico. Several friends also visited and attended his therapy and some of the recreational events with him. The OTA in charge of the evening recreational program decided to ask a male social worker to be a guest speaker one evening to discuss sexuality following SCI or other traumatic injuries. John's brother and a friend attended, as did several other patients and their family members. As the group began to ask questions and discuss their concerns, John gradually joined the discussion. At the following OT sessions, John was then able to ask for specific information regarding sexual activity, which the OTA was able to provide in a matter-of-fact manner using materials from the departmental resource library. While nursing had taken care of his bowel program and catheterization, John also wanted to be more independent in this area. Since these topics had come up during the group discussion, John now felt comfortable asking the OTA about equipment for these personal needs. He was able to use the equipment in the privacy of his room and report back on his progress. John was discharged at the end of 4 weeks on the rehabilitation unit, approximately 6 weeks after his injury. His plans included on-the-job training as a service representative at the phone company. He was independent in his BADLs and IADLs and in using public transportation. His one, unmet goal was driver education, and this was to be arranged on an outpatient basis.

Follow-Up and Chronic Care Needs

Patients with SCI may be followed as outpatients for several months to 2 years, and some may continue to show improvements in strength, endurance, and self-care skills during this time (Yarkony, Roth, Heinemann, Lovell, & Wu, 1988). Other patients may be involved in prevocational or vocational training or may return for additional training in orthotics use or use of other equipment. Some research has suggested that OTs tend to supply patients with more equipment than is actually used by patients after discharge. Therefore, equipment needs should periodically reassessed (Garber & Gregorio, 1985).

Some patients will return for tendon transfers to improve grasp, although this surgery is not as common as it has been in the past. Those patients who do choose to have tendon transfers will need training to learn to use the transferred muscles in new ways (Hollar, 1995).

Despite maintaining appropriate routines in self-care, patients with SCI are susceptible to respiratory infections, urinary tract and kidney infections, and the development of skin breakdown. Patients with SCI may also develop contractures and may lose function due to increases in spasticity. Re-hospitalization is common (NSCISC, 1998). On these occasions, the OT practitioner may take advantage of the opportunity to make modifications in equipment or self-care techniques or to provide other treatment as indicated by evaluation.

As improvements in medical care have increased the survival rate of patients with SCI, there has also been an increase in the numbers of elderly people with SCI. As this population ages, they will experience the normal decrease in strength, endurance, and physical fitness, as well as such age-associated problems as joint degeneration and skin fragility (Yarkony, Roth, Heinemann, & Lovell, 1988). During re-hospitalization, changes in status due to aging should be considered at these times, with appropriate modifications in equipment and adaptive techniques.

CASE STUDY: FOLLOW-UP CARE

John returned for driver education and driver training using a modified sedan, which he accomplished in 1 month. John owned a relatively new car, a four-door Ford. Since he already had a job lined up, the Department of Vocational Services was willing to modify the vehicle by purchasing and fitting the car with hand controls. The department also modified the car to accommodate a roof-based lift system that electrically lifted John's wheelchair to the roof of his car and stored it under a plastic cover. John returned to the rehabilitation unit every 6 months for 2 years. During that time he had no incidences of skin breakdown, no respiratory problems, and he remained independent in his self-care. After 2 years, John returned to Mexico to be closer to his family and was lost to further follow-up.

CLINICAL PROBLEM-SOLVING

1. Consider a mother of two young children who has an injury similar to John's, or an elderly man with a T1 injury.
2. How might group treatment enhance the therapy program for patients with SCI?
3. What problems may these patients with SCI experience after discharge?

REFERENCES

Adler, C. (1996). Spinal cord injury. In L. W. Pedretti, (Ed.), *OT: Practice skills for physical dysfunction* (4th ed.). St. Louis, MO: Mosby-Year Book.

American Spinal Injury Association (1992). *Standards for neurologic classification of spinal injury patients.* Atlanta, GA: Author.

Brown, D. J. (1992). Spinal cord injury: The last decade and the next. *Paraplegia, 30,* 77-82.

Daniel, M. S., & Strickland, R. L. (1988). *OT protocol: Management in adult physical dysfunction.* Rockville, MD: Aspen Publishers.

DeVivo, M. J., Richards, J. S., & Stover, S. L. (1991). Spinal cord injury: Rehabilitation adds life to years. *West J Med, 154,* 602-606.

Farmer, A. R. (1986). Evaluation. In J. P. Hill (Ed.), *Spinal cord injury: A guide to functional outcomes in OT* (pp. 7-18). Rockville, MD: Aspen Publishers.

Fike, M. L. (1984). The role of OT in psychological rehabilitation of the physically disabled. In D. W. Kruger (Ed.), *Rehabilitation psychology* (p. 221). Rockville, MD: Aspen Publishers.

Garber, S. (1985). Wheelchair cushions for spinal cord individuals. *Am J Occup Ther, 39,* 722-725.

Garber, S., & Gregorio, T. (1985). Upper extremity assistive devices: Assessment of use by spinal-cord injured patients with quadriplegia. *Am J Occup Ther, 44*(2), 126-131.

Garber, S., & Krouskop, T. (1982). Body build and its relationship to pressure distribution in the seated wheelchair patient. *Archives of Physical Medicine & Rehabilitation, 63,* 17-20.

Go, B. K., DeVivo, M. J., & Richards, J. S. (1995). The epidemiology of spinal card injury. In S. L. Stover, J. A. DeLisa, & G. G. Whiteneck (Eds.), *Spinal cord injury: Clinical outcomes from the model systems* (pp. 21-55). Gaithersburg, MD: Aspen Publishers.

Hill, J. P. (1986a). Group programs. In J. P. Hill (Ed.), *Spinal cord injury: A guide to functional outcomes in OT* (pp. 225-228). Rockville, MD: Aspen Publishers.

Hill, J. P. (1986b). Putting it all together: Discharge planning. In J. P. Hill (Ed.), *Spinal cord injury: A guide to functional outcomes in OT* (pp. 225-228). Rockville, MD: Aspen Publishers.

Hill, J. P. (1986c). *Spinal cord injury: A guide to functional outcomes in OT* (pp. 225-228). Rockville, MD: Aspen Publishers.

Hill, J. P., & Presperin, J. (1986). Deformity control. In J. P. Hill (Ed.), *Spinal cord injury: A guide to functional outcomes in OT* (pp. 49-86). Rockville, MD: Aspen Publishers.

Hollar, L. D. (1995.) Spinal cord injury. In C. A. Trombly (Ed.), *OT for physical dysfunction* (4th ed.). Baltimore, MD: Williams & Wilkins.

Jones, R. (1986). Bladder and bowel management. In J. P. Hill (Ed.), *Spinal cord injury: A guide to functional outcomes in OT* (pp. 145-168). Rockville, MD: Aspen Publishers.

Jordan, S. A., Wellborn, W. R. III, Kovnick, J., & Salzstein, R. (1991). Understanding and treating motivation difficulties in ventilator-dependent SCI patients. *Paraplegia, 29*(7), 431-442.

Kovich, K. (1986). Related disorders. In J. P. Hill (Ed.), *Spinal cord injury: A guide to functional outcomes in OT.* Rockville, MD: Aspen Publishers.

National Spinal Cord Injury Association. (1998). *Fact Sheet #1.* Available: http://www.erols.com/nscia/resource/factshts/fact02.html (1999, Jan.8).

National Spinal Cord Injury Statistical Center (1998). *Spinal Cord Injury FAQ.* Available: http://www.sci.rehabm.uab.edu/shared/faq.data.html (1999, Jan. 8).

Schneider, F. S. (1990). Traumatic spinal cord injury. In: Umphred, D. S. Neurological Rehabilitation (2nd ed.) (pp. 423-484). St. Louis: C.V. Mosby.

Trombly, C. A. (Ed.). (1989). Spinal cord injuries. In: Occupational therapy for Physical dysfunction. (3rd ed.) (pp. 555-570). Baltimore: Williams & Wilkins.

Wilson, D. J., McKenzie, M. W., Barber, L. M., and Watson, K. L. (1984.) Spinal cord injury: A treatment guide for occupational therapists (rev. ed.). Thorofare, NJ: SLACK Incorporated.

Woodruff, B. A., & Baron, R. C. (1994). A description of non-fatal spinal cord injury using a hospital-based registry. *Am J Prev Med, 10*(1), 10-14.

Yarkony, G. M. (1994). *Spinal cord injury: Medical management and rehabilitation.* Gaithersburg, MD: Aspen.

Yarkony, G. M., Roth, E. J., Heinemann, A. W., & Lovell, L, (1988). Spinal cord injury rehabilitation outcome: The impact of age. *Journal of Clinical Epidemiology, 41*(2), 173-177.

Yarkony, G. M., Roth, E. J., Heinemann, A. W., Lovell, L., & Wu, Y. (1988). Functional skills after spinal cord injury rehabilitation: Three-year longitudinal follow-up. *Archives of Physical Medicine & Rehabilitation, 69,* 111-114

A Teacher's Aide with Schizophrenia

Chapter 20

Margaret Drake, PhD, OTR/L, ATR-BC, CPAT, FAOTA

INTRODUCTION

Schizophrenia is a brain disease. This disorder has been found in all cultures (Ninan, Mance, & Lewine, 1998; Torrey, 1988). While symptoms of the disease have been recognized for centuries, schizophrenia was not given this name until the beginning of the 20th century (Kaplan & Sadock, 1996; Stoudemire, 1998). In the classification used in the United States, a person must have experienced the general symptoms of schizophrenia for 6 months and strong symptoms for at least 1 month before the diagnosis becomes official (American Psychiatric Association, 1994). Approximately 1% of the population develops schizophrenia, though only half of this group gets treatment. Equally as many women as men develop schizophrenia (Kaplan & Sadock, 1998), although the onset of schizophrenia for males usually happens earlier than for females (Kaplan & Sadock, 1998; Lewine et al., 1998).

Males often have their first episode in their teens, while females are more likely to experience the disease after age 25. This debilitating mental disorder affects 1% of the population worldwide and takes up a large percentage of US hospital beds (Kaplan & Sadock, 1998)

There are four types of schizophrenia. When the person is unresponsive to the environment either from being over-excited or in a stupor, this is called *catatonia*. *Undifferentiated* refers to a type of schizophrenia in which the person may have symptoms of schizophrenia but not paranoia, catatonia, or disorganization. In *disorganized* schizophrenia, the person appears to have no system of thought or communication pattern for appropriately interacting with others. *Residual* schizophrenia is typically comprised of remaining chronic symptoms, which are usually the negative ones, after the major dysfunctional aspects of the disease have disappeared.

KEY CONCEPTS

- Brain disease: Schizophrenia has structural differences, blood-flow differences, and chemical differences.
- Schizophrenia affects the individual, the family, and society.
- Stigma: The name "schizophrenia" has had a stigma associated with it for many decades.
- Positive symptoms: These include hallucinations, disorganized speech, loosened associations, and bizarre behavior. *Positive* implies that these features are an excess added unto the patient's existing personality.
- Negative symptoms: These features represent a loss of normal function, such as decreased emotional response, loss of enjoyment in life, decreased cognition interfering with meaningful communication, and little interest in activities or socializing.

ESSENTIAL VOCABULARY

Delusion: A firmly held, false belief with no basis in fact. Common delusions are paranoid, grandiose, religious, or feeling everything, including TV stories, refer to him- or herself.

Disorganized speech: Phrases and ideas expressed follow no theme or line of thought and may include perseveration (involuntary repetition of words or phrases), neologisms (newly coined words), or clanging (words are made to rhyme despite their meaning in the sentence).

Flattened affect: Incongruous absence of appropriate emotional response.

Hallucination: A false sensory perception. Can occur in all sensory systems; the most common are auditory hallucinations.

Illusion: A misinterpretation of a real experience, such as a mirage in which it appears water is on a road that is known to be dry.

Loose associations: Ideas switch from one subject to another unrelated topic.

Psychosis: Out of touch with reality, disorganized thinking resulting in loss of functional capacity.

FRAMES OF REFERENCE

Theories or frames of reference commonly used with persons diagnosed as schizophrenic are the lifestyle/adaptive performance model, the neuromotor behavior model, and the cognitive disabilities model.

The lifestyle/adaptive performance model includes ideas from anthropology, history, economics, psychology, politics, and physiology to explain mental illness. It describes four domains: self-care, intrinsic gratification, interpersonal relationships, and making contributions to others' welfare as being important aspects of humanity (Fidler, 1996).

The neuromotor behavior model includes ideas such as sensory integration, the biochemistry of medication, and neurodevelopmental treatment. These theories focus on the necessity of biological balance for proper neurological function. The neurological system is considered the basis of mental dysfunction (Neistadt & Crepeau, 1997).

The cognitive disabilities model focuses on discovering what cognitive capabilities a client has and providing the person with appropriate activities for his or her level of function. How information is processed in the neurological system indicates whether or not the person has cognitive dysfunction. This can be determined by his or her performance. The cognitive performance level achieved is often used as a predictor of future function (Allen, Earhart, & Blue, 1992).

CASE STUDY

Lindy came from a loving, well-educated family. She is a white female born and raised in a large metropolitan area. From birth she was a loving child but was considered somewhat slow in reaching developmental milestones.

When Lindy had a high fever at age 6, her mother was unable to prevent convulsions on the way to the hospital, despite the fact that her mother was a health care professional. Following this episode, Lindy was noticed by her teacher, as well as her two sisters and parents, to have more behavioral problems. Within a few months after this episode, her father, who was a community college teacher, died of a heart attack. This unexpected event put a great deal of stress on all family members. By the time Lindy was 12, her emotional outbursts and frequent shoplifting episodes persuaded her family to place her in a residential treatment facility run by a religious order. Lindy functioned well in this structured setting, which provided special education, recreation, and religious instruction. When she came of age, she was no longer eligible for this placement. She hovered on the borderline diagnostically between moderately mentally retarded and merely somewhat slow. She continued to have intermittent seizures that could be controlled with a medication adjustment.

During the next 5 years, she moved back and forth from living with her mother to living in a group home for the mentally handicapped. She attended a day treatment program in a center that prepared clients for employment. At the center, she met a male who was a little more disabled than herself and with the reluctant permission of their two families, they married. This union lasted a little over a year. Both families had been supportive, but the new husband and wife needed even more daily assistance and supervision as a couple than they had as individuals. After the divorce, Lindy returned to the treatment center and reestablished her residence in a group home. Eventually, at age 28, Lindy was employed as a teacher's aide in a public school special education class for the severely and profoundly retarded. Lindy was physically tall and strong and well-suited to the work of lifting the immobile, severely, and profoundly retarded students with whom she worked. Near the beginning of the second year in this class, Lindy began to experience episodes of crying and frequent arguments with her supervising teacher. Her coworkers found her sitting on a bench during a noon recess talking to herself as she sat on a bench near the playground. Her mother learned of this incident and took Lindy to see the family doctor. The family doctor thought she needed to see a psychiatrist. The psychiatrist to whom she was referred thought Lindy needed to reduce her stress. With the support of her sisters and mother, Lindy requested and was given a leave of absence from her job as teacher's aide. During this leave, she was hospitalized at a private psychiatric hospital and diagnosed with schizophrenia.

Referral

This hospital was a 60-bed facility. There were three 20-bed units: one for substance abusers, one for newly admitted acute care psychiatric patients, and one for those being treated in more specialized programs such as eating disorders, obsessive compulsive disorders, dissociative disorders, depression, and schizophrenia.

In this particular hospital, the psychiatrist wanted all her newly admitted patients to receive OT, if possible. Lindy received a referral to OT. Notices of new referrals were placed in the OT message box. The OTA picked up all the referrals each morning. She and the OT decided together how to go about screening and evaluating the new clients. They used a variety of evaluation tools depending upon which they thought fit the client. Eclecticism, using whichever theory seemed to fit the individual patient, was the basis for evaluation and treatment choices in this setting. This meant that sometimes they used the lifestyle performance model and sometimes they used the cognitive disabilities or neuromotor behavior model. Sometimes patients had the benefit of being evaluated by assessments from more than one model.

Lindy had been put on a regimen of a new antipsychotic medication.

Assessment and Evaluation Process

The OTA did many of the screening interviews as she had developed competence through workplace learning. She used the Life Style Performance Profile Occupational History (Hemphill, 1982) as a guideline for interview questions. From this assessment she learned about Lindy's recent job and that she thought her best asset was her physical strength and capability to do heavy lifting. She felt badly about her recent problems communicating with her supervising teacher. She had enjoyed the socialization she shared in the teachers' lounge and with the other aides while loading and unloading students from vans and buses. Lindy had also enjoyed the approval from her family while she had been employed. The aide position was the only gainful employment she had ever had. The most difficult part of this job was the boredom with the simple curricula used in the classroom for the severe and profound students. Lindy tired of the feeding routines that took up so much of the school day. She was able to discuss the classes she had enjoyed in the residential school from which she had graduated. Because the school had been so structured with little time for leisure, Lindy had not developed any particular leisure preferences, other than swimming. She had won swimming medals in the Special Olympics. Aside from references to her work, Lindy was unable to summarize any of her activities for a typical week.

The OTA discussed this information with the OT. It was decided to assess Lindy using the Allen Cognitive Levels test. The OTA administered the test. Lindy scored 4.2, as she was able to do the three whip stitches but could not figure out how to fix the mistake made by the OTA. The OT verified these findings by doing the Routine Task Inventory (Allen et al., 1992). Lindy was able to dress herself appropriately, but left the label hanging out of her t-shirt. When combing her hair she missed part of the back of her head. Nursing reported that she did not need supervision when bathing but she needed to be reminded to do it at the scheduled time. She needed three reminders to clean up after herself in the bathroom she shared with a roommate. Lindy was excited about joining the daily exercise group and promised to be there on time. She had no trouble at mealtime apart from eating too quickly and interacting only when others spoke to her. The medication nurse reported that Lindy required explanations each time she took her medication. Housekeeping was not a routine she could manage without assistance and supervision. She could heat a can of soup for herself but left the dishes on the table and the dirty pot in the sink until reminded to clean up. Lindy reported running out of money before each payday. She had been able to ride her bicycle on the familiar route from the group home to the school until she began to have seizures and the doctor told her to discontinue riding to avoid injury from falling.

General Goals

From the screening and assessment, the following goals were designed when Lindy sat down with the OT and OTA:

1. To practice initiating conversation with others during mealtime.
2. To make a daily budget to spread her 2 weeks' salary to last until the next payday.
3. To increase her tolerance for aerobic exercise from 5 to 10 minutes.
4. To complete at least one dish for the weekly meal prepared by the cooking group.
5. To decrease the reminders about cleaning up after herself to one reminder per day.

Treatment Activities/Techniques

To accomplish goal 1, a game was devised in which patients were to ask another patient a question during mealtime. This became a round robin exercise in which the person to whom the question was asked would respond to each of the questions asked by previous participants at the table as well as responding to his or her own question. After each had responded to all the questions, a new round would start. The psychiatric technicians were instructed in how the game was played and took over supervision during mealtime.

To accomplish goal 2, Lindy was given play money in the amount of her regular paycheck. She was then asked to divide the money into 14 equal piles and put them into separate envelopes. She then took one envelope and divided it into the cost of breakfast at a fast-food restaurant, lunch in the school cafeteria, $20 for the group home operator where she usually had her evening meal, and $2 for other needs such as toothpaste, sanitary pads, etc.

To accomplish goal 3, Lindy was included in the aerobic exercise group that met daily in the dayroom for a half hour before lunch. Initially, she did the low impact aerobics with several older patients, however, by the end of the first week, she was spontaneously joining in the regular aerobic exercises.

To accomplish goal 4, on Friday, the regular cooking group session planned a spaghetti luncheon. Lindy chopped enough carrots, radishes, green peppers, and green onions to mix nicely with the two heads of lettuce that she tore into bite-sized pieces. Then she mixed two envelopes of ranch dressing mix with a pint of no-fat yogurt to complete the salad. The other patients declared it a tasty, crisp salad.

To accomplish goal 5, Lindy was enlisted in a pact with her roommate, in which they would remind each other and record how many reminders it took. The one who achieved the fewest reminders as verified by nursing would be taken by the OTA to the gift shop to look around or out unto the grounds for a walk on the marked exercise trail.

These rewards were chosen by Lindy and her roommate.

Discharge Planning

After the second week, the treatment team met to discuss Lindy's future. The medication appeared to be decreasing Lindy's auditory hallucinations. She was less argumentative. The OT reported that her cognitive level had improved to 4.4 on the Allen Cognitive Levels test. This meant that she was able to follow a routine as long as nothing unusual happened. It was decided by the psychiatrist in consultation with the OT, nurse, and social worker that Lindy could return to the group home and to the treatment center, but not to her aide job until her cognitive level had improved to level 4.8. This would require that she return every 2 weeks for an evaluation by the OT and other treatment team members.

CLINICAL PROBLEM-SOLVING

Often other factors, especially performances contexts, change the focus of the OT treatment. The following stories were designed to stimulate clinical problem-solving.

Lindy was able to maintain her independence while living in a group home for up to 6 months at a time. She appeared to have the type of schizophrenia in which stability on one medication could not be maintained for more than 6 months. Episodes of psychotic behavior recurred regularly. These recurrences were sometimes linked with Lindy's involvement with a series of boyfriends whom she met in the group home or at the activity center where she eventually went for daytime supervision. She was never able to return to her teacher's aide job. What activity could the OTA in the activity center provide to engage Lindy's interest and distract her from inappropriate come-ons to male clients?

A 35-year-old white male patient named Tom, whom Lindy met at the activity center, was diagnosed as a paranoid schizophrenic when he was 18 years old. He had been in many treatment facilities since that time. At the time he met Lindy, he was living at home with his parents because the last group home where he had lived had evicted him when he attacked another male patient. He and Lindy had a short intimate relationship. He functioned at a higher cognitive level than Lindy and was able to persuade her to join him in evading the rules. The two of them would meet at the bus stop and ride the metropolitan transit bus together to the activity center. They would touch and arouse each other while sitting in the rear seat. Sometimes, they would get off the bus at a stop short of their final destination and go into the public park restroom to have sexual relations. When Tom began to demonstrate jealousy by threatening to hurt other male clients in the activity center when they spoke to Lindy, he was told by the staff that they must discontinue their relationship. The case managers for both Tom and Lindy were informed. What activities could the OTA use to engage him and distract him from his involvement with Lindy? How could she arrange the scheduling or the environment to keep the two of them apart?

In the activity center, there was a 46-year-old African-American female schizophrenic named Millie, with a dual diagnosis. She was an alcoholic and a schizophrenic. During an exercise class at the center, she began to become friends with Lindy. The two women lived in group homes only two blocks apart. The OTA and other staff members thought that by encouraging this relationship, they would be protecting Lindy from Tom. One morning, the group home operator called the activity center to notify them that the previous evening Lindy had returned late and was drunk. Neither Lindy nor Millie were supposed to drink alcohol while taking the antipsychotic medication prescribed. What other information should the OTA find out before talking to Lindy and Millie? How could Lindy be protected from repeating the drinking episode with Millie?

Lindy's roommate in the group home was a 40-year-old Hispanic female with schizophrenia named Helena who sometimes had catatonic episodes. These episodes usually occurred after she had been on a holiday visit to her family home in a rural area more than 100 miles from the group home. Her large family would fail to supervise her medication regime because there were so many people visiting. In the confusion, Helena's medication would be forgotten. When the family realized that Helena had not had her previous doses of medication, they would have her just double the dose. This erratic medication regimen would throw Helena into a catatonic stupor. By the time she returned to the group home, she often could not be aroused. At this time, the group home operator would ask Lindy to awaken her roommate for meals. Lindy would be unable to do this and would become upset and fearful that she would have to adapt to a new roommate. Helena did not attend the activity center. How could the OTA assist Lindy in solving this problem?

REFERENCES

Adams, W. (Ed.). (1993). Volunteers needed to attack stigma. *NAMI Advocate, 14*, 9.

Allen, C. K, Earhart, C. A., & Blue, T. (1992). *OT treatment goals for the physically and cognitively disabled*. Rockville, MD: AOTA.

American Psychiatric Association. (1994). *Diagnostic and statistical manual of mental disorders* (4th ed.). Washington, DC: Author.

Costanzo, G. (1993). Letter to the editor. "Neurobiological disorder" lessens stigma. *NAMI Advocate, 14*, 1.

Fidler, G. (1996). Lifestyle performance: From profile to conceptual model. *Am J Occup Ther, 50*, 139-147.

Goodman, L. A. (1997). Physical and sexual assault history in women with serious mental illness: Prevalence, correlates, treatments, and future research directions. *Schizophrenia Bulletin, 23*, 685-696.

Hemphill, B. (1982). *The evaluative process in psychiatric OT*. Thorofare, NJ: SLACK Incorporated.

Kaplan, H. I., & Sadock, B J. (1996). *Concise textbook of clinical psychiatry*. Baltimore, MD: William & Wilkins.

Kaplan, H. I., & Sadock, B. J. (1998). *Kaplan and Sadock's synopsis of psychiatry* (8th ed.). Baltimore, MD: Williams & Wilkins.

Lewine, R., Haden, C., Caudle, J., & Shurett, R. (1998). Sex-onset effects on neuropsychological function in schizophrenia. *Schizophrenia Bulletin, 23*, 51-61.

Miller, L. J. (1997). Sexuality, reproduction, and family planning in women with schizophrenia. *Schizophrenia Bulletin, 23*, 623-635.

Neistadt, M. E., & Crepeau, M. B. (1997). *Willard & Spackman's OT* (9th ed.). Philadelphia, PA: Lippincott.

Ninan, P. T., Mance, R. M., & Lewine, R. R. J. (1998). Schizophrenia and other psychotic disorders. In A. Stoudemire (Ed.), *Clinical psychiatry for medical students* (3rd ed.) (pp. 153-185). Philadelphia, PA: Lippincott-Raven Publishers.

Stoudemire, A. (1998). *Clinical psychiatry for medical students* (3rd ed.). Philadelphia, PA: Lippincott-Raven Publishers.

Torrey, E. F. (1988). *Surviving schizophrenia* (2nd ed.). New York, NY: Harper & Row.

A Mother and Caterer with Multiple Sclerosis

Chapter 21

Barbara L. Kornblau, JD, OT/L, FAOTA, DAAPM, ABDA, CDSM, CCM
Lori T. Andersen, EdD, OTR/L

Introduction

Multiple sclerosis (MS), a chronic and often disabling disease of the central nervous system (National Multiple Sclerosis Society, 1998), involves the myelin sheaths that surround the brain and spinal nerves. When the myelin sheath functions properly, it serves to insulate the nerve cells, facilitating the speed of transmissions along the nerves. In an individual with MS, the myelin sheath, normally a soft or fatty material, becomes sclerotic or hardened, thus slowing the transmissions. No one knows exactly why this happens.

Etiology

Although many scientists studying the cause of MS looked to allergies, viruses, infections, genetics, environment, and other agents as possible causes, its etiology remains a mystery. Most evidence, however, points to the generally accepted theory of MS as an autoimmune or body-attacking-itself response (National Multiple Sclerosis Society, 1997b).

Another popular theory looks at environment as a cause of MS. Studies show individuals residing in northern areas of the United States report a higher incidence of MS than among those residing in southern states. Those who change regions prior to the age of 15 take on the same risk as those residing in their new home region. Those who move after age 15 show the same incidence as their previous home. This suggests exposure to an environmental factor in childhood may trigger MS later in life (National Multiple Sclerosis Society, 1997b).

A third theory, as yet unproven, looks at a variety of viruses as a cause of MS, since viruses often cause demylination and inflammation. Though not contagious to others, the virus theory examines the idea that a virus could cause this immune system to attack the body. Finally, genetic factors, another yet unproven theory, show one's chances of contracting MS increases several fold if a family member contracts the disease. While scientists cannot pinpoint a specific genetic cause of MS, some studies suggest genetic material of individuals with MS contains some common

Key Concepts

- Multiple sclerosis (MS): Chronic, disabling disease of the central nervous system.
- Occupation: Daily activities that provide meaning and/or purpose.
- Canadian Model of Occupational Performance (CMOP): A conceptual framework that looks at the interaction between person, environment, and occupation.
- Canadian Occupational Performance Measure (COPM): An assessment that emphasizes a client-centered approach by determining client's valued occupations and goals.

Essential Vocabulary

Autoimmune: Condition in which the body attacks itself.

Diplopia: Double vision.

Exacerbation: Increase in symptoms.

Myelin sheath: Covering of nerve fibers.

Remission: Lessening of symptoms.

genetic markers which, with future advances in genetic techniques, may show an increased susceptibility to MS (Adams, Victor, & Ropper, 1997; National Multiple Sclerosis Society, 1997b).

EPIDEMIOLOGY

The Multiple Sclerosis Society, the organization dedicated to ending the devastating effects of MS, estimates in the United States MS affects between 250,000 and 350,000 or more individuals. MS occurs more in woman than men (approximately 2:1) and with increased frequency in whites of northern European ancestry, minimally in African-Americans and Asians-Americans, and virtually never in some populations, such as Eskimos. MS often strikes individuals in the prime of life, during young adulthood, with two-thirds of the cases of MS showing an onset between ages 20 to 40 (Adams, Victor, & Ropper, 1997; National Multiple Sclerosis Society, 1997a).

CLINICAL SIGNS AND SYMPTOMS

When one speaks of MS, one speaks of a disease of unknown origin, whose unpredictable symptoms, both visible and hidden, vary in severity from individual to individual. The variability of symptoms and the similarity of its symptoms with other neurological disorders often trick physicians into confusing MS with other conditions, such as systemic lupus erythematosus or vertigo. Physicians often make the diagnosis of MS as a last resort, after the other possible diagnostic labels prove incorrect. This sometimes takes up to anywhere from 5 to 10 years. Though magnetic resonance imaging (MRI) can confirm the diagnosis in most cases, pressure to curb high priced diagnostic tests often influences physicians to look for alternative methods of diagnosis.

In order to make a formal diagnosis of MS, physicians must find two basic signs in their patients. One must show a history of at least two attacks separated in time where the symptoms come and go, commonly referred to as "exacerbations" and "remissions." One must also show signs of damage to two or more parts of the myelin sheaths of the central nervous system (Hall, Rohaly, & Shneider, 1995).

IMPACT ON OCCUPATION

Individuals with MS may experience sensory, motor, and cognitive symptoms (Table 21-1) (Reingold, 1996). Sensory symptoms usually include visual difficulties such as blurred vision, diplopia or double vision, and blank spots (Schapiro & Langer, 1994). Other sensory symptoms may include parasthesia and/or numbness, vertigo, and on rare occasions, auditory disturbances (Schapiro & Langer, 1994). Motor symptoms may include spasticity, gait and balance difficulties, paralysis of some degree, weakness, intention tremor, ataxia, bladder dysfunction, bowel problems, and sexual dysfunction (Schapiro & Langer, 1994). Cognitive symptoms may include problems with short-term memory and attention span.

When MS strikes, its symptoms can cause a variety of interruptions in one's occupational performance. The fatigue and other motor and sensory symptoms may interfere with independent performance of activities of daily living. For example, an individual may find dressing overwhelmingly fatiguing.

The cognitive symptoms acting alone or in concert with motor and sensory symptoms can contribute to difficulties in the workplace. An individual may lack the ability to remember details required for work or may find it difficult or impossible to concentrate on job responsibilities. Some symptoms may interfere with safe task performance or the patient's safety in general. For example, short-term memory problems may cause an individual working in a restaurant to leave the stove on.

Symptoms may also impair the ability to perform occupations—the meaningful and purposeful activities in one's life (Finlayson et al., 1998). Hobbies and other meaningful and purposeful activities may need to take a back burner when symptoms make performance impossible.

Motor, sensory, and cognitive symptoms can also interfere with or change one's role as worker, parent, spouse, homemaker, and others. For example, a mother may find she can no longer care for her baby or a husband may find his wife now needs to bathe him, thus altering their previous roles. OT intervention can minimize the effects of MS on one's occupation—those activities and tasks of everyday life given value and meaning by the individual performing them—and one's roles (Finlayson et al., 1998).

Not all individuals diagnosed with MS will find themselves with the same symptoms or experience the same impact on occupational performance or role changes. Following diagnosis, MS generally follows one of four patterns. Affecting about 20% of individuals with MS, the mild or benign sensory pattern causes few episodes over the course of one's life from which most people completely recover (Hall, Rohaly, & Schneider, 1995; National Multiple Sclerosis Society, 1997c). The relapsing/remitting or exacerbation/remitting pattern causes those affected to experience a sudden onset of symptoms or attacks followed by partial or total recovery over time. This pattern affects approximately 20% to 30% of individuals with MS (Hall et al., 1995; National Multiple Sclerosis Society, 1997c).

Table 21-1

Signs and Symptoms that Individuals with Multiple Sclerosis May Experience

Sensory	Motor	Cognitive
Blurred vision	Spasticity	Short-term memory difficulties
Diplopia (double vision)	Gait and balance difficulties	Shortened attention span
Blank spots in the visual field	Paralysis of some degree	Difficulty concentrating
Parasthesia or numbness	Intention tremor	Emotional ability
Vertigo	Ataxia	
Auditory disturbances (rare)	Bladder dysfunction, bowel problems	
	Sexual dysfunction	
	Incoordination	
	Fatigue	

The remitting/progressive or relapsing/progressive pattern starts out following the relapsing/remitting pattern but after time becomes chronic or slowly progressive, hence its name, secondary progressive MS (Hall et al., 1995; National Multiple Sclerosis Society, 1997c; Reingold, 1996). Approximately 40% of individuals with MS experience this pattern. Finally, approximately 10% to 20% of all individuals with MS follow the chronic progressive or primary progressive pattern, which comes on slowly and progresses without remission (Hall et al., 1995; National Multiple Sclerosis Society, 1997c; Reingold, 1996).

MEDICAL TREATMENT AND PRECAUTIONS

Physicians use a variety of medications to treat the symptoms of MS (Schapiro & Langer, 1994). These medications may cause side effects for the individuals taking them, such as increased fatigue. Some environmental conditions, such as extreme heat or cold, may affect the impact of the symptoms on one's life. Others claim stress serves to exacerbate their symptoms (Hall et al., 1995).

REFERRAL SOURCES

Individuals with MS may receive referrals for OT services from case managers, the state vocational rehabilitation services, certified rehabilitation counselors, the National Multiple Sclerosis Society, primary care physicians, physiatrists, neurologists, rehabilitation nurses, and others.

FRAMES OF REFERENCES

The CMOP provides a framework for OT practice. This model, which emphasizes client-centered practice, looks at the interaction among people, their occupations and roles, and the environment in which they live (Townsend et al., 1997). In the client-centered approach, the client plays a central role setting goals and prioritizing treatment to enable occupation.

As MS is a chronic progressive disease, the rehabilitative frame of reference is often used. When motor, sensory, and/or cognitive impairments cannot be remediated, clients are educated in compensatory methods, given adaptive devices/equipment, and/or the environment is adapted to enable occupation (Dutton, 1995).

CASE STUDY

Mrs. Ryeman Simon is 31 years old and was recently diagnosed with MS (Table 21-2). Mrs. Simon stated she experienced incoordination and numbness in her dominant right hand. She also complained of constant fatigue. Mrs. Simon is married and has two children, one boy age 9 and one girl age 7. She works as a catering manager at a large resort hotel on the grounds of Rocky Raccoon's Fantasy World. She and her family live in a two-story house. This house has a basement where the laundry room is located. Two weeks ago, Mrs. Simon had an exacerbation of symptoms and was admitted to the hospital where the diagnosis of MS was finally made. She continues to be out on sick leave following her discharge from the hospital.

Mrs. Simon states she needs her husband to assist her to bathe and dress, as she quickly fatigues while doing these tasks. Mrs. Simon has always assumed responsibility for all the cooking, laundry, and housecleaning activities. Her family has now taken over these duties. She enjoys working in her flower beds and garden in the backyard. However, she stopped gardening because she lacks

Table 21-2

Mrs. Simon's Signs and Symptoms

Balance difficulties
Difficulty walking
Incoordination
Numbness in right upper extremity
Fatigue

energy and cannot get up and down from the ground without help. Mrs. Simon has worked for Rocky Raccoon's Fantasy World for 7 years and is a well-liked employee, winning Employee of the Month awards 12 times. As catering manager, she is responsible for all arrangements for catered events at the Bandit Hotel. This includes coordinating events with resorts' sales managers and their clients, ordering all food, and coordinating outside vendors who provide decorations or entertainment. Her job requires her to schedule and supervise 12 employees. These employees need direction in arranging the room set up for specific events, setting tables, and serving food. Mrs. Simon's doctor has a note for her to give to her boss. It reads as follows: "Mrs. Simon is able to return to her job with the following work restrictions: no work around steam and heat, no prolonged standing, no work over 40 hours of work per week, no lifting over 20 pounds. Mrs. Simon fatigues easily." She knows she will have to return to work shortly and is scared to death of returning to her job since she is having so much difficulty just caring for herself and her family. She knows some things must change in order for her to continue to care for herself and her children, manage her home, and do her job again, but she does not know what changes need to be made.

Referral

Mrs. Simon's was referred to an outpatient clinic by her health maintenance organization (HMO) physician for an OT evaluation. This HMO authorized the evaluation but requires the OT to phone in with the recommended plan of treatment to obtain authorization for additional visits.

Assessment and Evaluation Process

Prior to Mrs. Simon's first visit, the OT reviewed the medical evaluation that the referring physician sent with the prescription ordering OT. With knowledge of the MS disease process and specific deficits documented by the referring physician, as well as limited background information on Mrs. Simon's occupational roles, the OT then gathered several assessment tools in preparation for Mrs. Simon's first visit to the outpatient clinic. The "apartment" in the outpatient clinic was the setting for the OT evaluation. Mrs. Simon arrived at that outpatient facility using a straight cane to assist with her ambulation. The OT introduced herself and the OTA. She explained the purpose of OT to Mrs. Simon. Mrs. Simon displayed a positive attitude and appeared receptive to making necessary modifications to her lifestyle in order to resume her roles.

In starting the evaluation process, the OT asked about Mrs. Simon's past medical history and recent medical problems that resulted in her hospitalization. She also inquired about Mrs. Simon's occupational roles and related tasks. Mrs. Simon was a good historian and gave accurate information. Using a client-centered approach, the OT administered the COPM. The COPM determines which occupations are most important to the client and the client's perception of performance in these occupations. The COPM documented that Mrs. Simon's priorities include: managing her own self-care, caring for her family (cook, clean, and launder), returning to her job as a catering manager, and tending to her flower gardens. The OTA helped Mrs. Simon fill out an activity configuration to illustrate a routine day prior to her hospitalization. Figure 21-1 shows the activity configuration.

Mrs. Simon's typical weekday included helping the children off to school before going to work, picking the children up at an after school program before going home to prepare dinner, clean up, and fix lunches for the next day. Her weekend consisted of housecleaning, laundry, driving the children to and from various activities, and preparing meals. Mrs. Simon also explained her work requires a great deal of walking, especially in and out of the kitchen area as she coordinates schedules of employees and catered events. She would often assist with the set up of decorations and food, carrying items that sometimes weigh up to 30 pounds.

The OTA then assessed Mrs. Simon's ability to dress and undress herself. Mrs. Simon needed assistance to unbutton and button her shirt, as well as assistance to manage the zipper and snap for her jeans. She needed contact guard assist to maintain her standing balance while standing to pull up her pants. She also needed assistance to tie her running shoes.

Mrs. Simon stated she needs Mr. Simon's assistance to step in and out of the bathtub. The OT determined Mrs. Simon needed moderate assistance to maintain standing balance while stepping in and out of the bathtub. Mrs. Simon stated that as she is unable to get up and go down to the bottom of the tub. She stands while Mr. Simon helps her to bathe so she does not lose her balance. She also mentioned she has difficulty holding onto the wet bar of soap.

Time	Monday	Tuesday	Wednesday	Thursday	Friday	Saturday	Sunday
6-7 a.m.	Shower; dress	Shower; dress	Shower; dress	Shower; dress	Shower; dress		
7-8 a.m.	Make breakfast; wash dishes; get children off to school	Make breakfast; wash dishes; get children off to school	Make breakfast; wash dishes; get children off to school	Make breakfast; wash dishes; get children off to school	Make breakfast; wash dishes; get children off to school	Shower; dress; make breakfast; wash dishes	Shower; dress; make breakfast; wash dishes
8-9 a.m.	Make beds; drive to work	Make beds; drive to work	Make beds; drive to work	Make beds; drive to work	Make beds; drive to work	Make beds	Make beds
9-10 a.m.	Work	Work	Work	Work	Work	Drive children to activities	Church
10-11 a.m.	Work	Work	Work	Work	Work	Laundry	Church
11-Noon	Work	Work	Work	Work	Work	Cleaning	Change clothes
12-1 p.m.	Work	Work	Work	Work	Work	Make lunch; wash dishes	Make lunch; wash dishes
1-2 p.m.	Work	Work	Work	Work	Work	Drive children to activities	Drive children to activities
2-3 p.m.	Work	Work	Work	Work	Work	Laundry	Gardening
3-4 p.m.	Work	Work	Work	Work	Work	Cleaning	Gardening
4-5 p.m.	Work	Work	Work	Work	Work	Gardening	Gardening
5-6 p.m.	Pick up children; make dinner	Pick up children; make dinner	Pick up children; make dinner	Pick up children; make dinner	Pick up children; make dinner	Pick up children; make dinner	Pick up children; make dinner
6-7 p.m.	Eat dinner	Eat dinner	Eat dinner	Eat dinner	Eat dinner	Eat dinner	Eat dinner
7-8 p.m.	Wash dishes	Wash dishes	Wash dishes	Wash dishes	Wash dishes	Wash dishes	Wash dishes
8-9 p.m.	Other chores, such as laundry, grocery shopping, clothes shopping, etc.					Family activity	Family activity
9-10 p.m.	Make lunches	Make lunches	Make lunches	Make lunches	Family activity	Family activity	Make lunches
10-11 p.m.	TV	TV	TV	TV	TV	TV	TV

Figure 21-1. Activity configuration.

When the OT assessed her ability to manage in the kitchen, Mrs. Simon required minimal assistance with standing balance when bending to the lower cabinet to get out pots and pans and when reaching into the lower part of the refrigerator to get items. She is unable to complete meal preparation tasks, as she fatigues quickly. When making the queen-sized bed, Mrs. Simon was only able to perform half of the task before fatiguing. Mrs. Simon was able to place laundry into the washer and dryer, but needed contact guard assist with balance when attempting to take laundry out of the washer and dryer. She stated that she is not doing the laundry at home because she gets tired going up and down the stairs to the basement laundry room and cannot carry the clothes up or down the stairs.

The OTA used a dynamometer and a pinch meter to assess Mrs. Simon's grip and pinch strengths. Mrs. Simon's right grip strength measured 26 pounds compared to the left side of 42 pounds. Her three-point pinch strength in her right hand measured 7 pounds compared to 10 pounds in her left hand. The OTA used the nine-hole peg test to assess fine motor coordination. Results of this assessment showed a mild deficit in finger dexterity. Sensory tests completed by the OT revealed diminished sensation for light touch and stereognosis in Mrs. Simon's right hand. This deficit was demonstrated in functional tasks as Mrs. Simon had difficulty with manipulating buttons and tying her shoes. Mrs. Simon also demonstrated difficulty with writing. Her writing was shaky, letters were poorly formed, and she fatigued quickly.

Treatment Planning

Problem List

1. Mrs. Simon requires minimal assistance in self-care activities, grooming, bathing, and dressing.
2. Mrs. Simon requires minimal assistance to safely transfer in and out of bathtub.
3. Mrs. Simon requires maximal assistance with meal preparation tasks.
4. Mrs. Simon requires maximal assistance in light household cleaning activities and laundering activities.
5. Mrs. Simon is unable to participate in gardening activities.
6. Mrs. Simon is unable to perform work tasks of catering manager.

Treatment Goals

1. Mrs. Simon will be independent in self-care activities (grooming, bathing, and dressing) using adaptive aids and energy conservation techniques as needed.
2. Mrs. Simon will independently and safely transfer in and out of bathtub using safety grab bars.
3. Mrs. Simon will be independent in meal preparation tasks using energy conservation techniques, work simplification, and adaptive aids as needed.
4. Mrs. Simon will be independent in light household cleaning activities and laundering activities using energy conservation techniques, work simplification techniques, and adaptive equipment as needed.
5. Mrs. Simon will be independent maintaining her tabletop flower garden and flower window boxes using energy conservation techniques and adaptive equipment as needed.
6. Mrs. Simon will be independent in performing her job of catering manager using energy conservation techniques, work simplification techniques, and adaptive equipment as needed.

Treatment Methods

1. Education in principles of energy conservation and work simplification techniques and incorporation of principles into daily living tasks.
2. Assistance to obtain a safety bath bench and education in care and use of safety bath bench.
3. Safety education and transfer training.
4. Education and assistance in reorganizing various environments such as the bathroom, bedroom, kitchen, and work area to promote safety and independent performance.
5. Education in the disease process of MS and precautions.

The OT calls the HMO to obtain authorization for two visits per week for the next 4 weeks. The HMO authorizes two visits per week for the next 3 weeks.

Treatment Implementation

As endurance is a major limiting factor in Mrs. Simon's daily life, the OT discusses Mrs. Simon's daily routine and makes several recommendations to modify her routine to enable Mrs. Simon to complete all priority tasks with less fatigue. This involves educating Mrs. Simon in energy conservation and work simplification techniques. These techniques include:

1. Participate in activities while seated.
2. Organizing the work area, obtaining all supplies, tools, and equipment prior to starting the task
3. Minimize energy expenditure by combining tasks and eliminating unnecessary tasks.
4. Use electrical appliances to do work.
5. Use lightweight tools that do not require as much energy to lift.
6. Arrange materials so that gravity assists with task completion.
7. Take rest breaks before fatigue stops participation in an activity.
8. Have others do the task for you (Trombly, 1995).

The OTA provides Mrs. Simon's with a button hook with a zipper pull on one end. This facilitates her independence with clothes closures. The OTA shows Mrs. Simon how to use this adaptive aid and has Mrs. Simon practice using them. They discuss the arrangement of Mrs. Simon's bedroom. The OT suggests the easy chair in the bedroom become the center of her dressing area. She also suggests Mrs. Simon enlist the help of her husband and children to prepare their own lunches for work and school, respectively. She suggests Mrs. Simon choose her clothing for the next day and lay the items out next to her "dressing" chair each night before work. She also suggests that Mrs. Simon consider showering in the evening to spread out tasks. This would give Mrs. Simon all night to rest.

To ensure safety and independence in bathtub transfers, the OT explains to Mrs. Simon the necessity to obtain safety grab bars for the bathtub. She provides Mrs. Simon with the name of several hardware stores where she can purchase the safety grab bars. Mr. Simon knows a reliable handyman who can install them. The OT indicates the placement and angle of the safety grab bars in Mrs. Simon's bathtub. The OT also recommends Mrs. Simon obtain a safety tub seat to sit on while she bathes and a hand-held shower head to help her save energy while bathing. The Multiple Sclerosis Society provides durable medical equipment to people with MS who have the need for such equipment. Mrs. Simon was also cautioned not to shower with very hot water, as this would contribute to fatigue. The benefits of a full terry cloth robe to dry off after bathing were described. One need only to wrap oneself in the robe to dry off, rather then expending energy using a towel and reaching and rubbing the body to dry off. The OT also recommended soap on a rope or soap in a pump bottle so that she would not have difficulty with dropping the soap while bathing.

For grooming activities, the OTA suggests Mrs. Simon place a stool in her bathroom vanity area so that she may sit and conserve energy while brushing her teeth, fixing her hair, and putting on make-up. Sitting while doing these activities also protects her from falling.

The OT asks Mrs. Simon to outline her kitchen set up. The OT makes several recommendations to Mrs. Simon on how to put needed tools and items in easily accessible areas. The OT explains that those items Mrs. Simon uses least frequently for meal preparation should be placed on the higher cabinet shelves, and further back in the cabinets. Those items most often used should be placed in areas where Mrs. Simon can reach them without excessive bending or having to move other items to access them. Those items in the refrigerator that are most often used should be placed on the higher shelves in the front. If the family buys items in larger containers, these items may be split up into smaller containers. For example, a gallon of milk can be poured into two one-half gallon containers so that Mrs. Simon can lift them more easily. Electrical appliances such as food processors and electric mixers can help with food preparation while saving energy. With a little planning ahead, Mrs. Simon can gather all needed supplies and use a wheeling cart to help transport those supplies to the designated work area.

A kitchen stool placed near a kitchen counter can enable Mrs. Simon to sit while preparing foods. The OT also suggests Mrs. Simon consider enlisting family assistance on the weekend to make larger amounts of food that can be frozen or refrigerated for use throughout the week. In this way, Mrs. Simon will not have to prepare a meal each weekday evening; she can merely heat a meal. The children can assume such chores as setting and clearing the table and loading and unloading the dishwasher to help Mrs. Simon save her personal energy.

The OTA discusses ways to enable Mrs. Simon to do some light housekeeping activities. She recommends Mrs. Simon use a lightweight vacuum throughout the house, including the kitchen area. She further recommends that Mrs. Simon sit while vacuuming and dusting, moving to another seat only when unable to reach another area of the room. She has Mrs. Simon practice this in the ADL apartment, demonstrating how Mrs. Simon can move her body while seated in order to reach much of the surrounding area with the vacuum. For making the bed, the OTA shows Mrs. Simon how to sit at various places on the edge of the bed while making one trip around the bed to straighten the sheets, blankets, and bedspread.

Discussion reveals Mr. Simon is handy and he previously considered installing a laundry chute. He will do this to eliminate the need to carry dirty laundry to the basement. Mrs. Simon can make one trip to the basement to sort the clothing and start the laundry. Other family members can take responsibility to place laundry in the dryer, and when dry, carry it upstairs to a work area where Mrs. Simon will iron and fold clothing. Family members are then required to take their own clothes to their rooms.

Mr. Simon has also begun construction of a gardening table and several flower boxes. Mrs. Simon can sit at the table and tend to her boxes. The wheeled cart can transport flower boxes to and from desired locations, as well as to transport a water can to water flowers.

To facilitate Mrs. Simon's return to work, the OT and OTA will review with Mrs. Simon the specific functions involved in her job. Reviewing the specific tasks and comparing them to the work restrictions outlined by Mrs. Simon's physician will help determine which tasks Mrs. Simon can perform and which ones she cannot perform. Mrs. Simon may require reasonable accommodations in order to perform her job. These may include dictation, or voice activation for the computer at work or other assistive technology. Other accommodations Mrs. Simon may require may include a shortened workday, flexible work schedule, or a rearrangement of her work station. The OTA can work with Mrs. Simon to develop the skills she needs to advocate for herself to acquire needed accommodations from her employer. The OT, with the assistance with the OTA, can provide consultation to the employer, if needed, to facilitate the reasonable accommodation process and Mrs. Simon's smooth transition back into the workplace. This may include an on-site workplace evaluation to further explore essential job tasks and how they can be modified or accommodated to enable Mrs. Simon to perform her job.

Discharge Planning

The OT and the OTA made plans to make a visit to Mrs. Simon's home to ensure that Mrs. Simon is able to implement and carryover ideas and concepts learned in the clinic. The whole family was also invited to the clinic for an educational session on how Mrs. Simon has redesigned her lifestyle, how she uses adaptive equipment and compensatory techniques to manage her daily living tasks, and how they can help. Mrs. Simon was also given information on how to contact the National Multiple Sclerosis Society and the local chapter for support and information.

CLINICAL PROBLEM-SOLVING

In OT, treatment plans are individualized for each patient or client. Patient/client goals, stage in life, roles, and the context in which he or she lives are some of the factors that guide the treatment planning process. How will you change your treatment plan for each change listed below?

1. Mrs. Simon tells you that while she was out on sick leave she received notice that she was "let go" from her job.

2. Mrs. Simon explains to you that in her culture it is expected that she perform all housekeeping tasks. Housekeeping work is considered a woman's work; men do not help with these activities.

3. During the initial interview, you find out that Mrs. Simon is employed as a short order cook at one of the resort restaurants. Her job requires her to cook over a hot stove and be on her feet all day long.

4. Mrs. Simon is a 70-year-old retired nurse. Her grown children live more than 500 miles away in another state. She is the primary caretaker of her elderly husband. Her husband requires maximal assist with all his self-care, bed mobility, and transfers.

REFERENCES

Adams, R. D., Victor, M., & Ropper, A. H. (1997). *Principles of neurology* (6th ed.). New York, NY: McGraw Hill.

Dutton, R. (1995). *Clinical reasoning in physical disabilities.* Baltimore, MD: Williams & Wilkins.

Finlayson, M., Impey, M. W., Nicolle, C., & Edwards, J. (1998). Self-care, productivity and leisure limitations of people with multiple sclerosis in Manitoba. *Canadian Journal of Occupational Therapy, 65*(5), 299-308.

Hall, H. L., Rohaly, S. M., & Shneider, M. A. (1995). Multiple sclerosis. In M. G. Brodwin, F. Tellez, & S. K. Brodwin, (Eds.), *Medical, psychological, and vocational aspects of disability* (pp. 455-471). Athens, GA: Elliot & Fitzpatrick, Inc.

National Multiple Sclerosis Society. (1997a). MS information epidemiology. Retrieved February 13, 1999 from: http://www.nmss.org.msinfo.cmsi/epidemiology.html.

National Multiple Sclerosis Society. (1997b). MS information etiology. Retrieved February 13, 1999 from: http://www.nmiss.org/msinfo/cmsi/etiology.html.

National Multiple Sclerosis Society. (1997c). MS information prognosis. Retrieved February 13, 1999 from: http://www.nmss.org/msinfo/coursetakes.html.

National Multiple Sclerosis Society (1998). MS information diagnosis. Retrieved February 13, 1999 from: http://www.nmss.org/msinfo.howdiagnosed.html.

Reingold, S. C. (1996). *Multiple sclerosis clinical research overview.* National Multiple Sclerosis Society. Unpublished handout.

Schapiro, R. T., & Langer, S. L. (1994). Symptomatic therapy of multiple sclerosis. *Current Opinion in Neurology, 7,* 229-233.

Townsend, E., Stanton, S., Law, M., Polatajko, H., Baptiste, S., Thompson-Franson, T., Kramer, C., Swedlove, F., Brintnell, S., & Campanile, L. (1997). *Enabling occupation: An OT perspective.* Ottawa, Ontario: Canadian Association of OTs.

Trombly, C. A. (1995). Retraining basic and instrumental activities of daily living. In C. A. Trombly (Ed.), *OT for physical dysfunction* (4th ed., pp. 289-318). Baltimore, MD: Williams & Wilkins.

A Self-Help Group Leader with Anxiety

Chapter 22

Margaret Drake, PhD, OTR/L, ATR-BC, CPAT, FAOTA

INTRODUCTION

Anxiety disorders are among the most common disorders experienced by people who live outside the hospital. They affect approximately 7% of the U. S. population (Granoff, 1996). These same people with anxiety often overuse the health care system because of the physical symptoms of their distress (Nagy et al., 1998). Symptoms can include afflictions of the circulatory system, such as heart palpitations, chest pain, chills, hot flashes, sweating, or faintness. Symptoms of gastrointestinal distress, such as nausea or diarrhea, are also common (American Psychiatric Association, 1994). Anxiety often blends with other emotions, such as guilt and anger, so that it is difficult to delineate it from other basic emotions of fear, love, and hate. Anxiety encompasses a future-oriented attitude in which one expects negative events and hopes to be prepared for them. Depressed people are almost always anxious, but anxious people are not necessarily always depressed. One way in which many students experience this emotion is *test anxiety* (Rapee & Barlow, 1991).

FRAMES OF REFERENCE

Theories or frames of reference commonly used in the treatment of anxiety are listed below.

- Neuromotor behavior model—This model assumes that biology is at the foundation of all human behavior, as demonstrated through the responses of the neurological system. Manipulation of the neurobiological system will change the person's experience and response to anxiety. This theory includes such ideas as those in sensory integra-

KEY CONCEPTS

- Fight or flight reaction: Although people may not need to physically flee from danger, they may feel the need to do so while being unable to identify the direct source of their fear.
- Stress reaction: A stress cycle: 1) initial surprise at an event, 2) getting used to the situation followed by 3) exhaustion. If the individual does not allow 4) the resting phase of the cycle to occur, eventually, dysfunction sets in.
- Disturbance of attention: An individual focused on internal feelings from the autonomic system is less able to focus on the external environment and therefore becomes inattentive (Rapee & Barlow, 1991).
- Information processing disturbance: Anxiety interferes with the normal transfer of the biochemical impulses carrying information in the central nervous system (Rapee & Barlow, 1991).

ESSENTIAL VOCABULARY

Agoraphobia: Fear of being out in the open or being unable to escape a situation.

Compulsion: Uncontrollable impulse to perform an act one would not normally feel the need to do. It relieves anxiety produced by an obsession.

Obsession: Tendency to have a recurrent unwanted thought.

Panic: Sudden acute fear or anxiety.

Phobia: An irrational fear of places, situations, or things.

Post-traumatic stress: The state of tension some time after a stressful event in which the individual belatedly experiences the stressful event and again feels the feelings as though it were still happening.

tion, the biochemistry of medication, and neurodevelopmental treatment.

- Cognitive behavioral model—This model assumes that behavioral responses are learned and can be unlearned. Psychiatric units adhering to this model often think of the entire unit as a teaching situation (Sanderson & Wetzler, 1995). Some of the ideas are consistent with Maxwell Andersonn's milieu therapy in which all doctors, staff, and patients are considered teachers and students learning together. The patient is expected to respond to rewards, such as privileges to leave the psychiatric unit, or punishments, such as loss of telephone privileges.

- Lifestyle/adaptive performance—The four core domains—self-care, intrinsic gratification, interpersonal relationships, and helping others—are needs that must be satisfied for an individual to be healthy. This model includes ideas that anxiety comes from imbalance in biopsychosocial responses of the individual toward the environment. Humans have an unconscious drive to action. Self-understanding is an important concept for health (Fidler, 1996). When a person feels endangered, he or she avoids the danger by developing the symptoms of anxiety. Consequently, anxiety is considered a way to avoid knowing one's self and what one really fears.

CASE STUDY

Ella Mae was born in a rural area of the South. She was the youngest of eight children born to a Scotch-Irish miner and his Cajun wife in a village owned by the mining company. The family was always in poverty due to low wages and no union benefits for miners in that region. Ella Mae was a good student compared to her brothers and sisters, however, schooling was not emphasized, as the parents did not make the connection between education and wages. Consequently, at age 16, when she could legally drop out of high school, Ella Mae did so. She took a factory job in a nearby crossroads village. At this small factory, she met a man nearly 10 years older and was soon pregnant. The Vietnam War was beginning to escalate. Her new husband realized he could have a living wage and home for his family if he joined the army. After his boot camp, Ella Mae was able to join him at his station in Texas. Her two children were born there on the army base. Compared to the poverty stricken life of a miner's daughter, the army life felt rich. After his first stint in the service, he re-enlisted. Though Ella Mae realized her husband was drinking more, she had no thought of what to do, as her own father had frequently been drunk on payday. Eventually, when her husband took dis-

charge rather than be shipped to Asia, the family moved back to the city near where they had met. At a family reunion shortly after their return, Ella Mae had a sinking sensation when she saw her father begin to fondle her 3-year-old daughter. This episode stimulated her memory of her father fondling her at that same age. This distressing memory was upsetting and denied by her mother. After a discussion with her older sister, Ella Mae was convinced that indeed her memory was correct as her sister had also caught their father fondling her 3-year-old daughter. This situation caused much family distress as the two factions disbelieved each other.

Ella Mae soon became aware that her husband was not able to function without the structure of the army base. He had not found a job after their return home. After a year of conflict, she left him despite the fact that she knew he would be unable to provide child support. She began to work at a variety of low-paying jobs and took evening classes at the local community college in order to achieve her GED (general education diploma). Her low wages caused her to be unable to pay for the upkeep on her car. When the car broke down, she was unable to get to her job, as it was not on the bus line. Consequently, she lost the job. The apartment she and her two children were living in had the heat and lights turned off during winter. Eventually, she was evicted for non-payment of rent. She then persuaded her older sister to allow her and her two children to live in one of the sister's bedrooms for the remainder of the winter months. She withdrew from night school at the community college. Her sister's home was only a block from the bus line so Ella Mae was able, through some concerned friends, to find a job in a church office also near the bus line. This job did not pay well, but Ella Mae got her first opportunity to learn some computer skills. She began to meet church members who accepted her into their midst. A few months later, she joined the church, saved enough money to repair her car and began to feel like a citizen again. She began to make friends with some other women in the church. These women were exploring ideas of feminist theology. These ideas appealed to Ella Mae, who had never felt particularly valued for her thoughts.

Ella Mae had always been somewhat plump, but now she began to gain weight at a rapid pace. She smoked and generally had some unhealthy habits. One evening, she and one of her new friends attended a special class in a home about earth-based spirituality. There she met a rather obese man, and these two found many things in common. Within a few weeks, they were living together and finding an acceptance as a fat couple that neither had experienced before as a single person. His job as an electrical engineer, which had seemed secure, suddenly came to an end when his company closed their local operation. Within a few weeks, his computer electronic expertise secured him a job in the Washington, D.C. area. Ella Mae decided to move with him.

After arriving in the area of the national capitol, Ella Mae found a job in a bookstore that suited her well as she liked to read, however, the other parts of the job—record keeping, stocking the shelves, standing for hours at the cash register—were too demanding. She failed to go to work one day after an evening of smoking marijuana with her engineer housemate. She lost the job. Her housemate had not put her on his health insurance plan, so she had no health insurance. She began to have panic attacks. She was far from family and friends. She found a women's health clinic that would give her a reduced rate for a doctor's visit. The doctor prescribed Valium for her panic attacks. The combination of addictive Valium and recreational marijuana soon made her feel unable to exist without some sort of drug-induced state. As she spiraled into depression, the relationship with her housemate began to deteriorate. When he became physically abusive, she decided to leave. She had enough money to take the bus home, where her now-married daughter lived with her newborn son and husband. After a frantic weekend, in which the daughter no longer felt able to cope with her own family and her weeping, panicky mother, she took her mother to the emergency room at a local private hospital. Ella Mae was furious with her daughter for "dumping her" at the emergency room. Nonetheless, she was able to get evaluated for medication and stopped experiencing the muscle cramping that occurred when she did not take the Valium, to which she had become addicted.

Referral

The psychiatric unit in the private hospital had 20 beds for general psychiatry and a 10-bed gero-psychiatric wing as well. By this time in her life, Ella Mae was 37 years old. On her third day in the psychiatric unit, the doctor wrote an order for an OT evaluation. Ella Mae had become calm enough to be able to participate in the group activities on the unit.

The OT arrived at 8:00 a.m. and attended the therapeutic milieu community meeting in the day room. This was the OT's first introduction to most of the patients as she could not read their charts before the early meeting. Ella Mae was sitting sullenly in the corner of the day room. She did not participate in the group's discussion about smoking privileges. The OTA was unable to attend these early morning community meetings because she arrived at 11:00 a.m. and carried on the OT activities program until 8:00 p.m.

Assessment and Evaluation Process

The OT and OTA used a treatment theory mixture of the cognitive behavioral model, which matched the milieu therapy approach used by the entire psychiatric staff and the lifestyle performance model. Every patient referred to OT was scored on the Comprehensive Occupational Therapy Evaluation Scale (COTE), an assessment of 25 different behaviors (Brayman, et al., 1976; Early, 1993). The OT would evaluate each new patient during a morning task group using the COTE scale scoring form. Initially, Ella Mae just sat in the task group and declined to participate in the available crafts. She would jiggle one leg, then the other, then drum her fingers on the table. After the 90-minute session was about half through, she began to ask another woman patient named Ruth about the small doily she was embroidering. When the OT asked Ella Mae if she would like to try embroidery, Ella Mae responded by turning her face away and continuing to talk to Ruth, ignoring the OT. After the session was over, the OT asked Ruth if she thought Ella Mae might like to embroider and if she might be willing to teach her. Ruth, a depressed patient, protested that she didn't feel she was good enough to teach Ella Mae. With the OT's encouragement, she agreed to try to teach her at the next session if Ella Mae agreed. Ella Mae's initial score on the COTE scale was 65 out of a possible 100. The higher the score, the sicker the patient. Her greatest difficulty was in the task behavior areas of *engagement, interest in activities,* and *interest in accomplishment.*

General Goals

The OT and OTA met with Ella Mae that afternoon, and the OT reported her findings on the COTE scale. Ella Mae's passive-aggressive attitude from the morning session remained during most of the 15-minute goal-setting session. The OT explained the assessment/goal-setting process as Ella Mae sat looking away from the two therapists. Finally, the OT said that it was mandatory for them to have Ella Mae's input into her goals. Ella Mae burst out, "I just want to get out of this loony bin!" The OTA calmly responded, "The quickest way for that to happen is for you to help us make your treatment goals." Then the OT explained that the three areas that were most problematic for Ella Mae were in the task behavior areas of *engagement, interest in activities,* and *interest in accomplishment.* She asked Ella Mae to share whether she saw these as a problem and how she might be helped. Ella Mae asked for an explanation of the three terms. The OT explained that *engagement* meant to become involved in activity and how Ella Mae had just sat during the morning session. Ella Mae responded, "How is that supposed to help me get out of here?" The OT explained that occupations such as embroidery and sanding wood helped calm some people, and since anxiety was the type of problem Ella Mae was dealing with, her doctor had thought she could benefit from such activities and had referred her to OT for that reason. Ella Mae then agreed that perhaps she would try this new approach to her panic attacks and chronic anxiety. After more discussion, the patient, OTA, and OT agreed on the following goals:

1. To join the *stress management group* to learn time management, relaxation techniques such as guided imagery, and the benefits of group discussions.

2. To explore a wide range of activities to discover Ella Mae's specific areas of interest.

3. To engage in daily activity in a small group of people to achieve calmness.

4. To work to complete at least one different new craft every 2 weeks.

Since caffeine is associated with greater anxiety (Nagy et al., 1998), Ella Mae additionally agreed to decrease her caffeine intake, which had often been six cola drinks per day.

Treatment Activities/Techniques

The following morning, Ruth, patiently showed Ella Mae how to separate the embroidery threads, how to use the needle threader to thread the needle, and how to slide the embroidery hoop over the cloth. Ella Mae's initial stitches were irregular and loose, but as she practiced, the quality of her stitching improved quickly.

In the afternoon *stress management group*, the whole group filled out an *activity configuration* in which each day's schedule for a week is shown in two block segments from 7:00 a.m. until 1:00 a.m. the next morning (Early, 1993). Ella Mae's activity configuration sheet showed that she stayed in bed until 11:00 a.m. most days and spent the afternoon doing errands such as buying cigarettes, calling her sister on the telephone, babysitting for her daughter, or reading novels. These were things she wanted to do. Social interaction was an area where she confessed she did almost nothing with other people. Ella Mae protested that she felt she did not socialize very well, and it always made her anxious to be with a group of people she did not know well. The other patients in the group discussed having similar feelings, though they agreed they always felt a little better after spending time with others. Ella Mae's evening schedule was mostly watching TV, smoking cigarettes, drinking colas, and trying to get to sleep. After all the patients had shared their schedules and told how much of it they felt they really wanted to do, a discussion ensued in which they agreed to support each other in trying to regularize their sleep/wake schedules. They spontaneously made a telephone list and put the hours in which they would be willing to accept calls from the other patients in the group. They hoped that they could help each other by talking on the phone when they could not sleep.

The following day after the OT session, Ella Mae asked to take her embroidery with her to the dayroom to work on outside of OT. The OT agreed to this and informed the nurses and psychiatric technicians that Ella Mae had a needle and embroidery scissors that she would have to turn into the nurse's station after she finished using them. This was to prevent any patient from attempting to inflict injury on him- or herself with the needle or scissors.

The afternoon of that second day of treatment for Ella Mae, the OTA asked the patients to fill out the Neuropsychiatric Institute (NPI) Interest Checklist (Rogers, 1988). The NPI Interest Checklist lists 80 different activities and has places for the user to mark whether he or she has a casual, strong, or no interest for each. There were only three patients in the afternoon class, a teenager with an eating disorder, Ruth (the depressed woman), and Ella Mae. Other patients who had grounds passes had gone on an outing to the walking trail and exercise stations on property in the front of the hospital building with the psychiatric technician. Ella Mae listed only a casual interest in needlework though she continued to work on her embroidered doily. She marked *strong interest* in just five areas: writing, reading, television, religion, and conversation. She had *no interest* in most activities, however, she had *casual interest* in needlework, lectures, traveling, history, and photography.

The OTA obtained a blank book for Ella Mae that afternoon so she could start a journal. The following morning, the OT showed her how to use *nature print paper* to experience the photography process. They went into the dayroom and clipped some leaves off the potted plants and took a daisy from a flower arrangement Ella Mae had received from the women in the church. She expressed real enjoyment at this printing process. The next day, Ella Mae had grounds pass privileges so she and the OTA and two patients with similar pass privileges took an instamatic camera outside to take some photographs around the hospital.

Discharge Planning

The social worker had arranged for Ella Mae to be designated as an occupant of one of the indigent beds that the hospital was obliged to provide for the community. She was allowed to stay in the hospital 5 days. On the morning of the day in which she was to be discharged, she finished the embroidered doily. In the treatment team meeting, Ella Mae told the whole staff about her plans:

- To live at her sister's rather than her daughter's.
- To meet with the psychiatrist bi-weekly for medication management.
- To go to the state employment office and get the necessary forms to start looking for a job.
- To attend the *stress management group* in OT as an outpatient, one time per week for 1 month.
- To keep her list of other patients and telephone numbers by her telephone.

CLINICAL PROBLEM-SOLVING

The first evening at home in her sister's house, Ella Mae was unable to calm herself for sleep. First, she tried a relaxation exercise she had learned in the stress management group. She felt calm only while she was lying down doing the conscious breathing and the guided imagery. The moment she stopped the conscious breathing, she felt her anxiety return. Then she remembered to go to her suitcase and find the telephone list she had agreed to keep by her telephone until she had a place of her own. She did not feel she could put it up by the telephone in the kitchen of her sister's home, which always seemed so clean and rigidly arranged. Her sister filed papers with phone numbers rather than tacking them up around her telephone. Ella Mae was now feeling anxious because she was not meeting her last discharge goal of keeping the list by the telephone. How could the treatment team have better stated the last discharge goal?

The first number on the list was Rosie, a 30-year-old Hispanic woman who had also been discharged that same day. Rosie had shared in group therapy that she was married and that her husband worked at night as a weather technician at the local TV station. Ella Mae expected to hear Rosie's voice but when the phone was answered, it was her husband and he sounded irritated. Ella Mae asked to speak to Rosie. Her husband asked who she was and why she was calling so late. Ella Mae explained that Rosie had agreed to be available to talk if someone on the phone list needed to talk. Rosie's husband said gruffly, "Well, I'll see if she's stopped this crying jag she's on." After several minutes in which Ella Mae could hear a muffled conversation, she heard Rosie's querulous voice. Rosie explained that when her husband had started to leave for his night shift, she had felt panicky. When she tried to persuade him to call in sick, he got angry with her. The telephone call turned into a counseling session in which Ella Mae listened to Rosie, who had been diagnosed with panic disorder with agoraphobia. Rosie and her husband had recently moved to the city from a smaller city after he took the job at the TV station. Rosie developed the panic and agoraphobia as she attempted to deal with the complexities of living in a new larger city far from her relatives and friends. As they talked, Ella Mae was able to persuade Rosie to meet the next day at a restaurant on the bus line, halfway between their two homes. She explained the bus system as Rosie had never had the opportunity or need to use public transportation. After several minutes, Rosie asked Ella Mae to wait while she told her husband goodbye. Then Ella Mae and Rosie spent an hour on the phone before they hung up and went to bed. What might have been an appropriate discharge goal for the staff to discuss with Rosie?

The two women met the following day and began to discuss ways to help each other. Ella Mae had the four remaining outpatient OT sessions to assist her, but Rosie had no such luxury on her husband's rather skimpy health insurance plan. They talked about starting a support group. Ella Mae said she would tell the OTA and OT about their conversation and ask for their advice.

Two days later when Ella Mae had the opportunity to discuss this plan with the OTA in the stress management group, the OTA suggested setting a regular time, arranging a place, and sending an announcement to the calendar section of the local newspaper. They brainstormed the idea with others in the OT session. The first issue was to find a public meeting place that would not cost money. As the group members offered ideas, it occurred to Ella Mae that the church in which she had formerly worked and eventually joined might be a possibility. She agreed to call a church board member and ask before the next meeting. What other places offer public meeting space? How would the OTA go about helping Ella Mae identify these?

The board member Ella Mae called was a woman who had at one time been hospitalized for obsessive compulsive disorder. Ella Mae did not know this information until the woman shared it during their telephone conversation. She was a schoolteacher who had become incapacitated because she would go over and over the grades of her high school students for fear of making a mistake. Medication and some behavioral coping skills had eventually solved this problem for her. The woman was enthusiastic and agreed to bring it up at the next board meeting. She felt that since Ella Mae was still listed as a church member, there would be no rental fee. Ella Mae went on to explain that since she no longer had access to a computer, if the board agreed to allow them to meet in the church, would it be possible for her to come to the church and type an announcement for the newspaper? The board member agreed to ask the board of trustees about this issue as well. Ella Mae felt so pleased with herself for handling all these problems associated with setting up a support group. What goals should such a support group have?

That evening, when Ella Mae called Rosie to report, Rosie replied that another person who had signed their original telephone list in the hospital had called her the night before. This caller was a young Caucasian man named Boyd, who had been depressed as well as suffering from social phobia. His medication seemed to help his depression but his social phobia had not diminished. Boyd's state government job required him to make frequent presentations of projects he developed. His social phobia incapacitated him so that the last three times, he had called in sick rather than embarrass himself by being unable to successfully present his ideas. His supervisor was becoming quite irritated. Boyd had responded with enthusiasm when Rosie told him of their support group plan. What could the OTA have done in the OT clinic to assist Boyd in conquering his fear?

By the last of the four *stress management group* sessions, with the encouragement of the OTA, Ella Mae had done all the necessary work for the first session of the support group. The church board members had agreed to allow the new group to meet in one of the smaller religious education classrooms, as Alcoholics Anonymous had the use of the social hall on that night of the week. The current church secretary had allowed Ella Mae to use the computer to prepare an announcement for the calendar section of the newspaper. Additionally, she had included the same announcement in the church newsletter and put it on the e-mail list to the congregation.

At the first session of the support group, there were six people in attendance: Ella Mae, Rosie, Boyd, a woman church member who had gotten the e-mail announcement, a male church member who had learned about it from the newsletter, and a woman who had seen the listing in the calendar section of the newspaper. Ella Mae started the meeting by asking each of the people present to introduce themselves and say why they were here. A discussion followed about the need for such a group. The next order of business was to discuss the time and place to see if it suited everyone. Lastly, they discussed a name for their new support group. After making a list of possible choices, the group voted to call it "Don't Panic." Ella Mae was praised for her leadership in arranging the meeting. The group agreed to pass the leadership around the group for future meetings. Ella Mae promised to keep sending the announcements to the newspaper as there was an obvious need for this service to others with anxiety disorders.

If a patient is not able to start his or her own support group, what other community groups might offer some support?

REFERENCES

American Psychiatric Association (1994). *Diagnostic and statistical manual of mental disorders* (4th ed.). Washington, DC: Author.

Brayman, S. J., Kirby, T. F., Misenheimer, A. M., & Short, M. J. (1976). COTE scale. *Am J Occup Ther, 30,* 94-100.

Early, M. B. (1993). *Mental health concepts and techniques for the OTA.* New York, NY: Raven Press.

Fidler, G. (1996). Lifestyle performance: From profile to conceptual model. *Am J Occup Ther, 50,* 139-147.

Granoff, A. L. (1996). *Help! I think I'm dying: Panic attacks and phobias.* Virginia Beach, VA: Eco Images.

Nagy, L. M., Riggs, M. R., Krystal, J. H., & Charney, D. S. (1998). Anxiety disorders. In A. Stoudemire (Ed.), *Clinical psychiatry for medical students.* Philadelphia, PA: Lippincott-Raven.

Rapee, R. M., & Barlow, D. H. (1991). *Chronic anxiety: Generalized anxiety disorder and mixed anxiety—depression.* New York, NY: The Guilford Press.

Rogers, J. (1988). The NPI Interest Checklist. In B. Hemphill, *Mental health assessment in OT.* Thorofare, NJ: SLACK Incorporated.

Sanderson, W. C., & Wetzler, S. (1995). Cognitive behavioral treatment of panic disorder. In G. M. Asnis & H. M. Van Praag (Eds.), *Panic disorder: Clinical, biological, and treatment aspects.* New York, NY: John Wiley & Sons Inc.

Selye, H. (1976). *The stress of life.* New York, NY: McGraw-Hill.

Three People Across the Age Span with Arthritis

Chapter 23

Lynda Bishop, MS, OTR/L

INTRODUCTION

Arthritis is an inflammatory process of a joint or joints or a noninflammatory degenerative process involving a joint or joints. Arthritis may be an acute or chronic condition and there are over 100 types of arthritis. Arthritis affects approximately 38 million people and is one of the most prevalent chronic conditions in the United States (Cook, 1999). It has been reported that women age 45 and older cite arthritis as the leading cause of activity limitation (Cook, 1999). Among the elderly population (65 years or older), the prevalence of arthritis is almost 100% (Lohman, Padilla, & Connon, 1998). The etiology of most forms of arthritis remains unclear, however, researchers believe that genetics, environment, and hormones are factors in the cause of many types of arthritis. This chapter will focus on Osteoarthritis (OA), Juvenile rheumatoid arthritis (JRA), and Rheumatoid arthritis (RA), as these types of arthritis are the diagnoses that are most likely to be seen for OT intervention.

FRAME OF REFERENCE

The Model of Human Occupation (MOHO) is a frame of reference that can guide the OTA in treating individuals with arthritis. In addition, the biomechanical and rehabilitation approaches fit well. The biomechanical approach focuses on ROM, strength, and endurance, while the rehabilitative approach concentrates on compensatory measures to achieve maximal levels of function.

OCCUPATIONAL THERAPY INTERVENTION

Many concepts of OT intervention are similar in the treatment of JRA, OA, and RA and are discussed here first before introducing the concepts specific to each disease. If an individual is limited in active range of motion (AROM) secondary to the arthritis, it is important to remember that a goal for increased AROM is not appropriate. Rather, the goal will be to maintain AROM, prevent deformity, and

KEY CONCEPTS

- Energy conservation: Principles taught to individuals incorporating efficient techniques to conserve energy while performing occupations.
- Joint protection: Principles taught to individuals to protect joints and assist in preventing deformities.

ESSENTIAL VOCABULARY

Arthritis: An inflammatory process of a joint or a noninflammatory degenerative process involving a joint.

Juvenile rheumatoid arthritis (JRA): A form of arthritis that affects children.

Osteoarthritis (OA): A degenerative disease of the joints.

Pauciarticular: A form of JRA that involves four joints or less and is generally asymmetrical.

Polyarticular: A form of JRA that involves five joints or more.

Rheumatoid arthritis (RA): A chronic systemic, autoimmune disorder.

maximize occupation. Strengthening exercises are indicated for the individual with decreased strength; however, careful consideration must be given to the amount of resistance. Building endurance is also an important goal to address. However, the person with arthritis must be reminded that regular rest periods are essential. While these performance components must be addressed, the performance areas of ADLs, work, play/leisure will be the main focus of intervention through the use of purposeful activities that are meaningful to the patient. MOHO will be incorporated in the therapy program with the individual's interests, values, roles, and habits as the deciding factors in the selection of purposeful activities.

The use of purposeful activities in OT is an excellent fit for the individual with arthritis. Apart from the fact that following a routine exercise program for upper extremity AROM and strengthening can be very tedious and boring to many individuals, exercise also gives the arthritic individual time to focus on his or her pain. However, not all individuals find exercise programs boring; to some, exercise is purposeful and enjoyable. While engaging the individual in a variety of functional activities, purposeful activity addresses AROM, strength, and endurance without the person realizing that he or she is engaged in a therapeutic program. For example, an elderly female with arthritis in both hands complained of pain in her fingers and wrists when the therapist engaged her in an exercise program using Theraputty. The patient stated that she found this activity "boring and juvenile" and "my hands hurt for ages when I'm done." This patient had been a homemaker for years. She has six children, all of whom are now married with children of their own. She has 10 grandchildren and looks forward to visits from them for Sunday dinner and large family gatherings during the holidays. She always enjoyed cooking for the family. A therapeutic program specifically designed for the occupations of this woman involved cooking, washing dishes, putting them away, and cleaning the kitchen area. This addressed areas of AROM, strength, and endurance. This program enabled this woman to perform activities that she enjoyed and took the focus off her pain.

JOINT PROTECTION

Education of joint protection is an essential part of a therapy program (Pedretti, 1996). Joint protection strategies are as follows:

1. Use large joints instead of small joints whenever possible. For example, hold a coffee cup with palms of both hands, carry a handbag on the elbow or over the shoulder instead of grasping with fingers. When rising from a chair, do not push up with fists, rather, use the palms of the hand.

2. Avoid frequent sustained grasps.

3. Do not stand or sit for long periods of time. Change positions to avoid prolonged stress of joints.

4. When performing tasks that require repetitive motions, take frequent rest periods.

5. Always respect pain. If pain is experienced, stop the activity, change position, and rest.

6. Do not lift heavy items. Use a wheeled cart.

7. Slide pots and pans on the kitchen counter rather than carry them to the stove.

In the case example above, this patient may be provided with utensils with built-up handles, shown a device for opening jars, and informed of the need to rest during prolonged activity.

An OTA may feel the urge to order adapted equipment to assist in joint protection, as there are hundreds of assistive devices sold commercially. Many of these are costly, and the assistant should not be too hasty in recommending these items. In many instances, homemade devices will work just as well at a fraction of the cost. For example, cutting a washcloth in small strips and wrapping the material around a spoon handle will enlarge the size of the spoon handle. A built up handle eliminates a tight grasp.

ENERGY CONSERVATION

Because of the need for regular rest periods, energy conservation should be incorporated into the OT program. Principles of energy conservation are as follows (Lohman, Padilla, & Connor, 1998).

1. When performing activities, sit whenever possible.

2. Take frequent rest periods.

3. Organize the home environment to avoid extra lifting, carrying, reaching, and bending. For example, place dishes, utensils, pots, and pans used for meals all in one spot on the countertop or first shelf in cupboard. Place frequently used items on the front, top shelf of the refrigerator. Arrange clothing on a chair the evening before for the next morning.

4. Plan to do chores at the time of day when stiffness and pain is least. Many people feel stiff upon arising in the morning. Therefore, chores might best be completed early in the afternoon.

5. A cart with wheels in an excellent means of transporting several items at once. For example, all cleaning supplies could be placed on the cart and wheeled to various rooms. All food items could be placed on the cart along with the proper bowls, pans, and utensils. It is also wise to prepare large quantities of food at one time and then freeze small portions.

6. Maintain correct posture and use correct body mechanics. Use leg muscles when lifting; always keep the back straight and bend at the hips and knees.

OSTEOARTHRITIS

OA affects approximately 16 million people in the United States with increasing age contributing to the susceptibility to develop OA (Cook, 1999). "Up to age 45, OA is more common in men; beyond age 55, it is more common in women" (Cook, 1999, p. 63). OA is a degenerative disease of the joints and is caused by a breakdown in cartilage and bone. It progresses slowly and is the most common form of arthritis. OA typically involves the weightbearing joints such as the hips, knees, proximal interphalangeal joints (PIPs), distal interphalangeal joints (DIPs), and carpometacarpal joint (CMC) and can range from mild to severe. While there is no known cause for OA, risk factors include obesity, sport injuries involving joints, and repetitive use of joints.

Symptoms and Management

The symptoms of OA are pain, stiffness, and limited ROM. Swelling of joints and redness may also be present (DeLisa & Gans, 1993). Medications are used to control pain; aspirin is frequently prescribed for the management of symptoms of OA. Nonsteroidal anti-inflammatory drugs (NSAIDs) are also prescribed. Weight management is indicated in the cases of obesity. In severe cases of bone degeneration, surgery might be indicated. Surgery may result in a total hip replacement or total knee replacement (DeLisa & Gans, 1993). ROM exercises and strengthening programs are also included in the management of OA.

Evaluation

The OT evaluation for the person with OA will include ROM, strength, endurance, fine motor, and observation of performance during ADLs, work, and leisure. When measuring AROM and testing strength, pain must be considered with appropriate adjustments for each made during the testing process.

Case Study 1

Mrs. Surgte is a 65-year-old married female admitted with a right total hip replacement secondary to OA. Mrs. Surgte presents as a pleasant, obese female with many complaints of pain in her right knee. She states that once she recovers from the surgery on her hip she will have her knee done. She worries that her left hip will eventually be affected by OA, as she feels "occasional twinges" at the site. Prior to the right total hip replacement, Mrs. Surgte was independent in ADLs. She reports that she does not have any hobbies. She and her husband spend much of their day watching TV. They did go to the shopping mall once or twice a week for "something to do," but Mrs. Surgte reports that she would get tired walking any distance. She had not gone to the mall for the past 2 months because "it hurt too much to walk." Mr. and Mrs. Surgte have a family dinner every Sunday for their daughter, her husband, and two young grandchildren. Mrs. Surgte enjoys cooking and looks forward to the family gathering on Sunday.

The Surgtes live in a two-story home with the bedrooms and bathroom upstairs. For the past 2 months, Mrs Surgte has been spending most of her day upstairs stating, "I did not want to go up and down the stairs much because of the pain." Her husband has been bringing breakfast and lunch upstairs, but she reports that she would come downstairs for dinner. Mr. Surgte does not like to cook and has been buying fast food. Both he and his wife have gained weight in the past 2 months.

Referral

Mrs. Surgte has been admitted to a rehabilitation unit with an estimated length of stay of 2 weeks. Orders from the physiatrist for OT are to evaluate and treat.

Assessment and Evaluation Process

The supervising OT has asked the OTA to review the medical record and introduce herself to the patient. The OTA explains OT to the patient and informs her that she is scheduled for the initial evaluation later that afternoon. Through conversation with the patient, the OTA learns that the patient would like her therapies scheduled around the soap operas she watches faithfully each day. The patient has many complaints of pain in her hip during the conversation in spite of the fact that she is lying in bed and not moving. While she is pleasant and friendly with the OTA, she states that she does not like to exercise and hopes she will not have to do too much in OT.

Mrs. Surgte arrives in OT at her scheduled time of 3:00 p.m. She immediately complains to the OT and OTA that she is missing her soap opera and hopes this will not take too long. The OT assesses the patient's AROM and strength in the bilateral upper extremities. The OT evaluates sensation. The OTA assesses the patient's transfers and functional mobility.

The OTA, through review of the medical record, conversation, and observation of the patient, felt that Mrs. Surgte was cognitively and perceptually intact. The OTA discussed this with the OT and the OT concurred. The OT had found cognition and perception to be intact through observation of the patient, conversation with the patient, and information from the OTA. Therefore, the

OT did not deem it necessary to conduct a formal cognitive/perceptual assessment.

The patient is able to dress her upper body independently. She is unable to dress the lower body secondary to hip precautions. Nursing reports that the patient is able to independently bathe her upper body except her back. She is dependent for lower body bathing. She is independent to brush her teeth and comb her hair. Toileting is with minimal assist to pull up pants over buttocks.

The evaluation results are as follows: bilateral upper extremities AROM is within functional limits. Strength is 3+/5 throughout the bilateral upper extremities. Sensation is intact as is perceptual and cognitive status. Transfers to all raised surfaces except tub are with minimal assist. Patient is dependent to transfer to tub. Functional mobility is with contact guard and verbal cues for safety. Dressing upper body is independent; lower body dependent. Bathing upper body is with minimal assist; lower body is dependent. Patient is independent to comb hair and brush teeth after set-up. Patient requires minimal assist for toileting.

The OT and OTA collaborate to develop the treatment plan for Mrs. Surgte. The OTA has contacted the physical therapist, who will be working with this patient to determine what ambulatory device that the PT thinks Mrs. Surgte will be discharged with. PT feels that the patient will need a standard walker (extra wide) for ambulation at home. At the conclusion of the evaluation process, the OTA asked Mrs. Surgte what her goals were. Mrs. Surgte stated that she would like to be able to go up and down the stairs without any pain, cook for the family, go out shopping again, and be independent so that she did not have to rely on her husband for help anymore. She also stated that she realized that she should lose weight. The OTA asked Mrs. Surgte if she had any interests other than cooking and shopping. Mrs. Surgte admitted that in the past few years she has not been as active as she had been in the past and realized that she has fallen into a daily routine that is "not very exciting." She stated that when her children were young she enjoyed doing school projects and holiday crafts with them.

The OTA and OT design a treatment plan that will address the goals important to Mrs. Surgte. Through the interview process, Mrs. Surgte's interests were learned. These interests will be incorporated through functional activities in all OT treatment sessions with Mrs. Surgte. The treatment plan includes transfer training, dressing program, functional mobility training, home and food management, and safety training. Because the bedrooms and bathroom are upstairs, and also because Mrs. Surgte will be going home with an extra wide walker, a home visit will be planned to assess the patient in her home environment.

Long-term goals set by the OT for this patient state that by discharge, the patient will:

1. Be independent in transfers to all surfaces.
2. Be independent in lower extremity dressing.
3. Be independent in functional mobility.
4. Be independent in home and food management.
5. Practice safe techniques when moving about her home environment.
6. Engage in leisure activities that will promote health and wellness both physically and psychosocially.

Treatment Activities

The OTA considers the fact that this patient does not have many interests except preparing the family dinners on Sunday. The OTA, therefore, has the patient perform functional activities in the OT kitchen, dining room, and living room such as setting the table, preparing a simple lunch, and washing the dishes. Each session will include transfers to different surfaces such as kitchen chair with arms, living room couch, and overstuffed chair with extra cushions in the dining room area.

Education on energy conservation and safe transportation of items from the kitchen to living room will be addressed. These activities address all above stated goals except dressing and bathing. The dressing and bathing program will take place in the patient's room on the unit. Note that because this patient is cognitively intact, once she is instructed in the use of assistive equipment for dressing and bathing the lower extremities, she will likely be independent in these areas after set-up. Instruction in transfers to a tub seat will be included in the OT program.

Clinical Problem-Solving

A home visit was conducted 1 week prior to discharge. Mrs. Surgte states that she is not going to attempt to go upstairs for awhile. She states she will sleep downstairs in her recliner. The house is extremely cluttered with scatter rugs throughout. There is a lot of furniture in the living room. Because Mrs. Surgte has an extra wide walker, she must walk sideways in the hallway. She also has to maneuver her walker to get through the doors to the kitchen and dining room.

What suggestions should the OTA make to Mrs. Surgte for independence in her home? What home modifications might be needed? What assistive equipment will Mrs. Surgte require upon discharge home? She will be on hip precautions for 8 weeks. Should bilateral UE strength be increased? Did the OTA incorporate enough activities in the treatment sessions? What else should the OTA focus on?

There is no bathroom downstairs. The patient's husband sat sullenly in the living room throughout the entire visit. He stated that he was not going to "pick up after her. She should do things by herself now that she got that hip fixed. I'm sick and tired of preparing her meals, I'm not going to do it anymore."

Should the OTA make any referrals for Mrs. Surgte's discharge? What, if anything, should be done about the husband's attitude toward his wife? Should the OTA incorporate the patient in leisure activities?

JUVENILE RHEUMATOID ARTHRITIS

JRA usually begins at 2 to 4 years of age. JRA affects about 71,000 children in the United States. (Cook, 1999, p. 175). There are three forms of JRA: pauciarticular, polyarticular, and systemic. Pauciarticular involves four joints or less and is generally asymmetrical (affecting a particular joint on one side of the body). Joints most commonly affected are the knee, hip, ankle, and elbow. The pauciarticular form may also cause eye inflammation called iridocyclitis. If iridocyclitis is not treated early on, it can result in blindness. Polyarticular involves five joints or more. The systemic form affects joints and internal organs and is the least common form of JRA (Cook, 1999). JRA can present as a mild condition or can be severe, leading to serious complications. Symptoms may change on a daily basis, with the child experiencing severe pain one day and mild discomfort the next. It is also significant to note that a child may experience discomfort in the morning but feel fine in the afternoon (Cook, 1999). As noted previously, there is no known cause for JRA, however, it is known that it involves abnormalities of the immune system (Cook, 1999).

Symptoms and Management

The arthritis must be present for 6 or more consecutive weeks for a diagnosis. There is no single test for the diagnosis of JRA. JRA can result in joint damage, joint contracture, and altered growth. JRA is a chronic disease that may last for many years and might have periods when the child experiences no symptoms, which is referred to as remission. Remissions may last for months, years, or forever. JRA may lead to joint deformity, altered growth, or, for children with pauciaticular JRA, there is a higher risk for chronic eye infection (Cook, 1999).

Signs and symptoms vary with each child, however, symptoms of pauciarticular and polyarticular include joint inflammation, pain, heat, altered growth, and decreased ROM. Symptoms of the systemic form include high fever that can last weeks or months, a rash on the chest and thighs, and joint inflammation that may be present with the fever or may not develop until much later. Inflammation of the heart lining, heart, or lungs may also occur. Anemia and enlarged lymph nodes, liver, or spleen are also symptoms that may be present (Cook, 1999).

ROM exercises, eye and dental care, and nutritional counseling are indicated for the child with JRA. NSAIDs are used to decrease swelling and pain. Slow-acting anti-inflammatory drugs (SAAIDs) might also be prescribed. These drugs do not immediately reduce pain or swelling. They are used to modify the natural progress of joint disease and might not be effective for weeks or months after therapy has begun (Cook, 1999).

Evaluation

OT evaluation for the child with JRA will include ROM, strength, endurance, performance of ADLs and play, and gross and fine motor skills.

Case Study 2

Johnny is a 5-year-old male with a diagnosis of JRA involving his left and right knees, left and right elbows, and both hands. Johnny was an active child with normal development. He engaged in gross and fine motor activities without difficulty. Shortly after his fifth birthday, Johnny began complaining of pain in his knees. His mother noted a little swelling in one knee and assumed Johnny had fallen or bumped his knee. She also attributed Johnny's complaints to "growing pains." Johnny's complaints diminished for a week or so and then he began complaining again. At this point, Johnny's mother did notice swelling in both knees. Johnny also reported that it hurt his hands when he had to draw in kindergarten, and he did not like to play ball because it hurt his elbows. Johnny's mother scheduled an appointment with Johnny's primary care physician. The doctor diagnosed JRA. The doctor prescribed anti-inflammatory medication, provided Johnny's mother with information on JRA, and made a referral for outpatient OT.

Assessment and Evaluation Process

The OT met with Johnny and his mother. Johnny's mother removed his coat for him and had him sit on her lap. The OT suggested that Johnny play with some of the toys in the clinic while she spoke with his mother. Johnny expressed an interest in doing this and asked his mother if it was all right. After slight hesitation, Johnny's mother gave permission but told Johnny to be very careful and play gently with the toys.

The OT observed Johnny's movements. He walked stiffly and sat down slowly and deliberately. He was guarded in all movements. He began building a tower out of blocks, occasionally letting go of the blocks and stretching his fingers.

Johnny's mother reported that her son's activity level had decreased. He tended to sit and watch TV more than in the past. In fact, she stated that she would permit Johnny 1 hour of TV a day prior to this diagnosis. "Now, because of 'my son's sickness,' I think it better that he sit quietly, so watching TV for a length of time is OK with me." Johnny's mother reported that she now dresses

Johnny and assists him with his bath. She does not allow him to play outside with the other children unless she is there to monitor him. Under no circumstances is he allowed to play ball or running games. She has asked that he be excused from playground activities at school.

The OT then turned her attention on Johnny. She got down on the floor and had him play with several toys that enabled her to observe Johnny's fine motor skills. She then had him imitate animal movements, for example, "How does an elephant move its trunk? How does a monkey scratch its back?" This gave the OT an opportunity to observe gross motor movements. Johnny enjoyed playing with the OT and a quick relationship of trust developed. This enabled the OT to conduct a formal evaluation of Johnny's ROM and strength. When it was time to leave, Johnny's mother began to prepare to put Johnny's coat on for him. The OT asked Johnny if he could put his coat on by himself. He seemed eager to show the OT that he could do this but asked his mother's permission first. Johnny was able to don his coat independently but with increased time and effort. He had difficulty buttoning the coat.

Evaluation results were as follows: The right upper extremity was within normal limits for AROM throughout except the right elbow flexion, which was limited to 80 degrees. The right fingers had edema in the PIP joints of the index, middle, and ring fingers. However, Johnny was able to manipulate various sized objects such as beads, blocks, coins, tweezers, and buttons. Strength in the right upper extremity was 3/5. The left upper extremity was within normal limits for AROM throughout with strength grossly 3/5. Slight edema was noted in the left elbow. Gross motor performance was guarded with slow, deliberate movements. The OT realized that PT will be following Johnny for gross motor issues. However, the OT includes it in the evaluation process because of its impact on ADL and play performance. Johnny was found to be intact for cognition and perception. Sensation was also intact.

OT Goals

1. Increase right elbow flexion to within functional limits.
2. Prevent contracture in right elbow flexion.
3. Increase strength in bilateral upper extremities to 4+/5.
4. Educate patient and family in joint protection.
5. Educate patient and family in energy conservation.
6. Educate patient and family in JRA related to the importance of play.

Treatment Activities

The OTA will be responsible for treatment of Johnny. In this outpatient clinic, the OTs generally do the evalua-

tions and then discuss findings with the OTA. The OT and OTA collaborate on the treatment plan. The OTA will use play as the media to treat Johnny. She will engage Johnny in fine and gross motor activities to achieve the long-term goals. The OTA will also educate Johnny and his mother on JRA. With a thorough understanding of the disease, Johnny's mother should realize that she can allow Johnny to join in many activities that she had previously believed would be harmful. The OTA will also provide Johnny's mother with information on the Arthritis Foundation and local JRA support groups for families.

Clinical Problem-Solving

Considering John's occupational performance context, suggest toys/games that would address fine and gross motor. What joint protection techniques would be especially helpful for Johnny?

Since treatment sessions alone cannot help this child reach his fullest potential, describe a home exercise program for Johnny. What concerns should the OTA have concerning Johnny's mother following through with a home exercise program?

Johnny's mother initially wanted to be involved in the entire treatment session. She hovered around Johnny and continually ask him if his joints hurt. How should the OTA deal with this?

RHEUMATOID ARTHRITIS

RA is a chronic systemic, autoimmune disorder. RA can affect the lungs, heart, and eyes in some people, and it affects 2.1 million (1 in 100) people in America. Onset is typically between ages 25 to 50; however, it can occur in all ages, and women are three times more likely to have RA than men. Presently, there is no known cause of RA, however, research has shown that genetic, environmental, and/or hormonal factors may contribute to the disease. RA is an inflammatory disease affecting joints in the body, generally in a symmetrical pattern (if one joint is affected on one side of the body such as the hand, it will be affected in the hand on the other side as well). Other parts of the body may also be affected. Accompanying joint inflammation and pain, people may experience fatigue, occasional fever, and malaise (Cook, 1999). Remissions and exacerbations may occur in the disease process (DeLisa & Gans, 1993). RA can be mild or severe, lasting variable periods of time such as a month, a few months, or years. People who have severe RA will be in the active stage of the disease for much of the time with the symptoms lasting for many years. In these cases, there may be significant joint damage and increased difficulty in performing ADLs (Cook, 1999). Today's health care system allows most people with RA to lead productive lives through medication, therapy, support groups, and patient education.

Symptoms and Management

The symptoms of RA include pain, swelling, stiffness, heat at the site, and a symmetrical pattern. Stiffness and/or pain lasts greater than 30 minutes after rest. Fatigue, occasional fever, and a general feeling of not being well are commonly experienced. Because RA is a chronic condition, depression may be experienced as well (DeLisa & Gans, 1993). Management of RA includes regular medical visits to monitor the course of the RA. Medications such as aspirin and NSAIDs are prescribed to relieve pain and decrease joint inflammation. Rest and exercise must be balanced for the person with RA. Rest helps to decrease pain and inflammation and combat fatigue. Exercise maintains ROM, increases strength, increases self-esteem, and promotes a state of well-being. Patient education brings awareness of the diagnosis and its variables and teaches individuals techniques such as joint protection and energy conservation in order that they may live a productive and fulfilling life. Support groups allow for the sharing of experiences and expression of feelings. Surgery such as joint replacement or tendon reconstruction for individuals with significant joint damage might be indicated (Cook, 1999).

Case Study 3

Mr. Caroll is an 82-year-old married male with a diagnoses of right fractured humerus and RA. He has had RA for the past 25 years. Mr. Caroll was under a doctor's care when he was first diagnosed with RA. However, when he started to feel better after a course of NSAIDs, he discontinued seeing the doctor. When his medications ran out, he felt better and thought that he was free of the RA. Over the years, if he experienced pain, he would buy over-the-counter drugs to manage his condition. If he had pain, he believed that it was part of the aging process and it was something he had to live with.

Mr. Caroll was a carpenter and had his own business. He retired at age 65, however, he continues to work with wood. He enjoys making toys for his grandchildren and simple woodwork pieces for his family. He often spends 5 hours a day in his workshop. It was here that he fell tripping over an electrical cord. The fall resulted in the fractured shoulder.

Mrs. Caroll has been a homemaker throughout her 51-year marriage. She does all the housecleaning, cooking, grocery shopping, and laundry. She is in good health and is very active in her church. Mr. and Mrs. Caroll usually go out on Saturday evenings to visit friends or attend a church function. On Sundays, they spend time with their children or grandchildren, who all live in close proximity.

Mrs. Caroll states that her husband is a very proud man. He seldom complains, however, she has observed him wince and grimace when he does his carpentry. He has difficulty eating, it seems uncomfortable for him to move his arm to bring it to his mouth, and he holds his utensil in an awkward manner. His carpentry work is not nearly the quality it used to be. Mrs. Caroll contributes this to "old age and poor vision."

Referral

Referral received from the doctor is for evaluation and treatment of the fractured humerus and RA. The orders further state A/AROM exercises for right shoulder.

Assessment and Evaluation Process

The OT and OTA collaborate in the evaluation of Mr. Caroll. The OT assesses Mr. Caroll's P/AROM and strength. The OTA assesses Mr. Caroll's ADLs through observation of him engaged in eating, dressing, grooming, brushing his teeth, functional mobility, transfers, and endurance.

A discussion between the OT and OTA determines Mr. Caroll's status as follows.

- Left upper extremity P/AROM limited to 100 degrees shoulder flexion, 110 degrees shoulder abduction, 60 degrees external rotation, and 55 degrees internal rotation. The elbow, forearm, and wrist are within functional limits for P/AROM. The digits are limited in flexion and extension but are WFL for P/AROM. Mr. Caroll is able to oppose to the middle finger. Strength at limited range is 4-/5.

- Right upper extremity AROM is limited to 50 degrees shoulder flexion, 35 degrees shoulder abduction, and 50 degrees shoulder extension. External rotation is 30 degrees and internal rotation is 25 degrees. The elbow and forearm are within functional limits for P/AROM. Strength for elbow and forearm is 3+/5. The right hand is severely deformed. The index finger has a sublux at the MP joint, the middle finger is limited in flexion to 10 degrees at the MP, 5 degrees at the PIP, 0 degrees at the DIP. The ring finger is also subluxed at the MP joint. Movement at the PIP is 5 degrees, the DIP joint is a 0 degrees. The little finger is within functional limits for AROM. The thumb is within functional limits. Opposition is to the index finger only. Mr. Caroll stated that his hand has been like this for the past several years, "getting worse each year." He stated that he holds his tools between his thumb and index finger and sometimes he "ties the bigger tools with a string in the palm of my hand."

- Dressing the upper extremities is with minimal assist to place the shirt over the right arm. Lower extremity dressing is independent. Eating is independent after set-up, however, Mr. Caroll has to use his non-dominant hand and that is awkward for him. He also had difficulty maintaining hold of the utensils. He is independent for functional mobility and transfers. Endurance is good.

OT Goals

1. Increase AROM in right shoulder to within functional limits.
2. Increase dressing to independent.
3. Educate patient in joint protection related to roles.
4. Educate patient in energy conservation related to roles.

Clinical Problem-Solving

Review the evaluation notes. Why did the OT not test Mr. Caroll's strength in the right shoulder? Is splinting indicated for Mr. Caroll?

Consider MOHO as a frame of reference for treatment specific to the occupational performance context of Mr. Caroll. What assistive equipment would Mr. Caroll benefit from? Should Mr. Caroll be told that he should no longer do woodwork because of the stress to his joints? Describe two meaningful activities the OTA could design for Mr. Caroll's treatment session.

Mr. Caroll mentions to the OTA that it has been a long time since he "cuddled up" to Mrs. Caroll because he is always so uncomfortable in bed. How can the OTA address this sexual expression performance area?

REFERENCES

Cook, A. (Ed.). (1999). *Arthritis sourcebook*. Detroit, MI: Omnigraphics, Inc.

DeLisa, J., & Gans, B. (Eds.). (1993). *Rehabilitation medicine: Principles & practice* (2nd ed.). Philadelphia, PA: J. B. Lippincott Co.

Lohman, H., Padilla, R., & Connon, S. (1998). *OT with elders: Strategies for the COTA*. St. Louis, MO: Mosby.

Pedretti, L. (1996). *OT practice skills for physical dysfunction*. St. Louis, MO: Mosby.

A Plumber and Golfer with Total Hip Arthroplasty

Chapter 24

Dairlyn Gower, BS, COTA
Marcia Bowker, OTR, CHT

INTRODUCTION

Total hip arthroplasty (THA) is the surgical replacement, formation, or reformation of the hip joint. It is performed to restore motion and preserve the necessary stability to a stiffened or painful joint. Technological advances and advancement in surgical procedures have resulted in more successful long-term outcomes. Arthroplasty of the hip is usually necessary because of degenerative joint disease, rheumatoid arthritis, or other disease process or trauma. The most significant outcome is the impact THA can make in the quality of an individual's life, not only in providing the individual with pain-free function, but also in decreasing medical costs to society by decreasing nursing home use due to the disability this type of dysfunction can cause.

Surgical procedures vary depending on many factors, including severity of joint involvement, previous hip surgery, and preferences of the physician. Complications resulting from surgery can include infection, pneumonia, nerve injury, loosening or breakage of the prostheses within the bone, pulmonary embolism, deep vein thrombosis, and blood clots (American Academy of Orthopaedic Surgeons, 1996; Wheeless, 1996). Treatment implementation can also vary depending on the type of surgery performed, as well as the individual's age, health, and motivation.

THA, the procedure described in this case study, is often necessary as a result of an individual's decreasing functional mobility and/or progressive pain. THA can improve the patient's quality of life by decreasing pain and increasing ROM and mobility, therefore, improving the patient's ability to perform ADLs. Although time frames can differ based on various factors, the prognosis is generally good after an approximate 5- to 7-day hospitalization and a 2- to 3-month recovery period. Patients can expect continued healing to occur at the greater trochanter, including decreased pain and improved strength, over 6 to 12 months. An individual who is independent before undergoing a THA should continue to be independent after surgery. In some instances, the patient may prefer to have some assistance if total independence is not a high priority, such as

KEY CONCEPTS

- Arthroplasty: Creation of an artificial joint.
- Prosthesis: Replacement part, an artificial substitute.

ESSENTIAL VOCABULARY

Acetabulum: The cup-shaped depression on the hip bone where the head of the femur attaches.

Anterolateral: In front and to one side.

Greater trochanter: The bony prominence that gives attachment to the hip abductor muscles.

Methylmethacrylate: A self-curing, acrylic resin adherent, which is applied in paste form and becomes bone-like when hardened.

NSAID: Non-steroidal anti-inflammatory drug, such as ibuprofin or aspirin.

Posterolateral: In the rear and to one side.

Thrombosis: A clotting within a blood vessel that may cause sudden blood insufficiency to the tissues supplied by that vessel.

Trendelenburg's gait: A gait pattern that can be the result of weakness of the hip abductor muscles.

assistance from a family member or a short-term nursing home stay for rehabilitation, particularly for older or weaker patients prior to returning home.

As mentioned previously, indications for THA are varied but tend to include conditions that cause pain and limit mobility, although pain is generally the primary indicator. These include:

- Osteoarthritis and rheumatoid arthritis at the hip joint
- Certain types of hip fractures
- Hip joint tumors
- Hip pain that has failed to respond to conservative treatment, such as NSAID medication, for over 6 months or that limits the ability to perform routine activities (Health Answers, 1999)

In the surgical procedure, a metal prosthesis replaces the worn head and neck of the femur; a high-density polyethylene socket component replaces the worn acetabulum (socket of the hip that receives the head of the femur). These items are shown in Figure 24-1. The components are attached to the bones of the pelvis and femoral head by means of methylmethacrylate, a self-curing, acrylic resin adherent, which is applied in paste form and becomes bone-like when hardened (Brashear & Rainey, 1978). Most procedures involve a cemented femoral stem and an noncemented acetabular component. Noncemented techniques can be also be utilized, where the prosthetic parts are intimately driven into the bone. This intimate contact allows the bone to grow into the texture of the metal component. In younger patients, generally under 50 years of age, the THA procedure is usually uncemented.

Preoperative planning for THA includes x-rays, assessment of type and size of component needed, and a thorough medical examination, which may include assessment of cardiac and pulmonary function, awareness of any pre-existing medical conditions that require anticoagulants, anesthesia consultation, preoperative exercises, and/or donation of patient's own blood for use in surgery if needed.

The surgery is performed using general or spinal anesthesia. The orthopaedic surgeon makes an incision along the affected side, exposing the hip joint. The head of the femur and the acetabulum are cut out and removed. The prosthetic ball and stem are inserted in the femur, and the prosthetic socket component is placed in the enlarged pelvis cup. The components are placed, using either the cemented or uncemented technique, and the muscles and tendons are repaired. Surgical procedures vary for hip arthroplasty and are largely due to physician preference. Two common procedures are the anterolateral and posterolateral approaches (Pedretti, 1996).

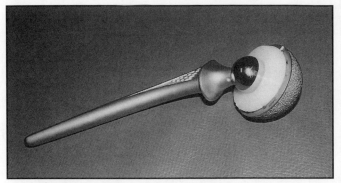

Figure 24-1. Prosthesis components.

The anterolateral approach is slightly more stable, but does split the hip abductor muscles off the greater trochanter, and the patient will experience some abductor weakness. Therefore, abduction strengthening is the most important aspect of postoperative physical therapy to lessen the incidence of Trendelenburg's gait. Specific instabilities resulting from the anterolateral approach and positions that patients need to avoid include hip external rotation, excessive hyperextension, and adduction.

The posterolateral approach does not take off the hip abductors, so there is less abductor weakness but is slightly more unstable. Specific instabilities resulting from the posterolateral approach and positions that patients need to avoid include movement over 90 degrees of hip flexion, adduction, and internal rotation (American Academy of Orthopaedic Surgeons, 1996). With both approaches, patients are strongly advised not to cross their legs until they have physician authorization; a simple concept to teach patients is to keep their knees about a shoulder width apart. If patients do not adhere closely to precautions, they are at risk for interruption of good soft tissue and muscle healing, thus increasing the risk for hip dislocation. Hip dislocation is a possibility because the new joint capsule, sometimes referred to as a pseudocapsule because it is mainly formed by scar tissue, forms over a period of 6 to 8 weeks. This is the most critical time to reinforce with patients the importance of adhering to precautions. Regardless of the approach, the success of recovery relies on the compliance of the patient for approximately the first 3 months after surgery.

Patients generally experience moderate to severe pain after surgery but by the second to third day post-surgery are placed on oral analgesic medications that sufficiently control pain. Patients also return from surgery wearing anti-embolism stockings, which reduce their risk of blood clots, and are also generally placed on chemical anticoagulation medications by their surgeon. Physical therapy treatment commonly begins the day of surgery.

FRAMES OF REFERENCE

A biomechanical frame of reference is useful for addressing medical issues. Any frames that address performance areas are helpful for returning clients to prior functioning. A multidisciplinary team facilitates quick recovery.

The team members involved in the care of the patient with hip arthroplasty usually include the following: primary physician, orthopaedic surgeon, nursing staff, OT and physical therapy practitioners, dietitian, pharmacist, and social worker (American Academy of Orthopaedic Surgeons, 1996). The role of the team is to facilitate the healing of the trochanter and soft tissues and to facilitate the development of a capsule around the joint for future stability, as well as to teach proper body mechanics, mobility, positioning, and techniques related to carrying out daily activities during the recovery period.

CASE STUDY

Carl was born June 22, 1918 in Duluth, MN. A self-employed plumber, he is married and has adult children. At the age of 57, Carl had a rapid onset of osteoarthritis. Because of his right hip pain and stiffness, he began experiencing difficulty in fulfilling his job requirements, which included getting in and out of his truck and lifting, twisting, and pulling at odd angles. At age 65, Carl became semi-retired, doing only minor plumbing jobs with the assistance of one of his sons. His wife continued to be involved in the business, managing records and the bookkeeping system.

The next year, the family physician referred Carl to an orthopaedic surgeon, who discussed the option of a THA. Carl chose not to have surgery at the time because he did not want to have it until it was "necessary." He was also concerned about the expense and lost time from work during recovery.

At the age of 72, Carl was experiencing extreme hip pain, decreased joint mobility (especially limited hip abduction), stiffness, and a painful gait. Carl, his wife, and the orthopaedic surgeon decided it was time to have THA surgery. Being able to play "a good game of golf" was Carl's primary source of motivation. Surgery was scheduled during the winter to ensure that Carl would have adequate recovery time before the golf season.

Assessment

The orthopaedic surgeon made a referral for OT services according to standard postoperative orders of the facility. The protocol (specific plan of action) used for OT evaluation, planning, and treatment was originally developed by the OT and OTA in cooperation with their facility's orthopaedic surgeons. This protocol identifies general precautions and procedures for performance of ADLs, but is flexible enough to be easily adapted to the patients individual needs, lifestyle, and home situation, as well as the specific surgical procedure.

Using a structured questionnaire and checklist, the OTA performed a preliminary chart review. The chart review allowed the OTA to screen for possible complicating factors that may impair the patient's progress, such as pre-existing conditions of rheumatoid arthritis, cancer, cardiac or pulmonary disorders, or dementia. This information was then used in consultation with the OT regarding evaluation of performance components such as AROM, strength, and cognition, which may be needed to establish realistic goals.

Program Planning

Once Carl demonstrated general competence in ambulation in physical therapy, the OT and the OTA established an individualized plan for OT treatment. The long-term goal for Carl was to return home, demonstrating independence in all ADLs with all movement precautions observed. Overall functional independence is expected to be the same and, for most individuals, improved after a THA, as the patient should now be demonstrating an increase in pain-free ROM. General short-term goals during the hospital stay should be, but are not limited to, the following:

1. Demonstrate understanding of specific precautions and bending restrictions.
2. Demonstrate independence in lower extremity dressing through utilization of adaptive equipment.
3. Demonstrate independence in basic homemaking skills, such as meal preparation, work simplification, and energy conservation.

The action plan developed jointly by the OT and the OTA for Carl's treatment appears in Figure 24-2.

Treatment Implentations

Standing orders at the hospital where Carl was a patient indicate that OT is to be initiated on the third to fourth day after surgery, unless otherwise indicated by the physician. Physical therapy was initiated the day of surgery to begin mobilization. Carl's treatment program included therapeutic exercise, mobility, and gait training. During the first 3 days, Carl used a walker and then advanced to using crutches.

On the third day after surgery, the OTA scheduled an initial visit with Carl. The purpose of OT intervention

Post-Surgery	Action Plan
Day 2	Chart review by OTA; review findings with the OT and establish plan.
Day 3-4 (depending on ambulation status)	**A.M. Treatment Session** Initial OT contact; explain OT and treatment protocol; assessment using activity inventory. Provide patient with written list of post-surgical precautions; review precautions with patient and family members. Instruct patient in lower extremity dressing. Assistive devices may include sock aid, elastic shoelaces, reacher, dressing stick, long-handled shoe horn. Instruct patient in tub/shower and toilet transfers. Assistive devices may include a raised toilet seat or commode chair, tub chair, long-handled bath sponge/brush, and grab bars. **P.M. Treatment Session** Instruct patient in basic home management, work simplification, and energy conservation techniques. Assistive devices may include a utility cart, high stool, crutch or walker bag or pail, and a firm, sturdy arm chair.
Day 4-5 (depending on which post-surgical day treatment was started)	Patient demonstrates dressing techniques; patient repeats back precautions and limitations; discuss and clarify any questions or concerns the patient or family may have. Provide patient with a list of area vendors for rental or purchase of commode, raised toilet seats, or grab bars.

Figure 24-2. Action plan.

and the plan of care were explained. During this time, the home activity inventory (Figure 24-3) was completed by Carl and the OTA to gain information about Carl's living arrangements, physical layout of the home, household activities generally performed, previously pursued leisure activities, abilities in self-care, and an inventory of specific patient concerns. Carl's wife was present and stated that she would like to attend her husband's treatment sessions to gain a better understanding of his OT program. The OTA gave Carl and his wife a copy of precautions and limitations he must follow. She highlighted the specific precautions related to his type of surgical procedure. All items were discussed and procedures were demonstrated whenever possible. Questions were answered and Carl and his wife indicated that they understood the importance of observing the precautions and limitations during the performance of all daily living activities. The list of precautions is

shown in Figure 24-4. The OTA brought a variety of assistive devices, including a reacher, elastic shoelaces, a long-handled shoe horn, a dressing stick, and a sock aid to Carl's room. Some of these items are shown in Figure 24-5. Using the dressing devices, she demonstrated how to do lower extremity dressing tasks such as putting on underwear, pants, socks, anti-embolism stockings, and shoes. Use of a sock aid is depicted in Figure 24-6.

Carl chose to use the reacher, dressing stick, and sock aid. His loafer-style shoes were easy for him to put on without any assistive devices. After practicing, Carl was able to do lower extremity dressing safely, without flexing his hip beyond 90 degrees and without rotating his hip. Although Carl had already been taught how to assume a standing position in physical therapy, the OTA reminded him to extend his knee and bring his foot forward and use his arms to push up on the chair arm rests as shown in

The Elderly with a Hip Arthroplasty

This inventory is designed to provide your occupational therapist with information about your home living environment and activities. With this information, your therapist is able to identify what area he/she can best serve you in preparation for your return home.

Personal Care
Can you dress yourself? _____ Areas of difficulty_____

Can you feed yourself? _____ Areas of difficulty_____

Can you perform bathing/grooming tasks independently?_____

Were you independent in the above areas prior to your hospitalization? _____

Areas of difficulty _____

Is there someone available to help at home: _____ If yes, who? _____

Physical Layout
Do you reside in an: Apartment, House, Other _____

Is there an elevator? _____

Number of floors _____ Steps inside house _____ Steps into house _____

Location of: Bedroom _____ Bathroom _____ Tub _____

Shower _____ Combination _____

Any areas of particular concern regarding physical layout? _____

Household Responsibilities
Which of the following activities are you currently able to perform? Cooking _____   Grocery shopping_____

Cleaning_____ Laundry_____ Dish washing_____

Pet care _____ Trash carryout _____ Snow shoveling_____

Care of lawn _____ Gardening _____ Maintenance _____

Other _____

Meal Preparation
Are you able to prepare meals?_____ Areas of difficulty_____

How many meals do you prepare daily? _____ For how many people? _____

Is there someone available to help? _____

Are the following available for your use? High kitchen stool _____ Kitchen cart _____

Microwave_____ Other_____

Transportation
Do you drive? _____ Is there someone available to drive, if necessary? _____

Who?_____

Employment
Are you employed? _____ Retired _____

Type of occupation _____

Present work status _____

Work duties (include use of stairs, lifting, bending) _____

Recreation
List hobbies/recreational activities _____

Activities discontinued because of medical condition _____

_____

_____

Figure 24-3. Home activity inventory. (Reprinted from Ryan, S. E. [1993]. *Practice issues in OT: Intraprofessional team building.* Thorofare, NJ: SLACK Incorporated.)

Precautions and Limitations Following Your Total Hip Replacement

After your surgery, there are positions and activities that can cause dislocation of your hip. Special precautions must be followed for the next 6 to 8 weeks or until your doctor lifts restrictions.

Sitting
- Sit on a firm, straight-back armchair. Avoid recliners or stools. Do not sit on soft or armless chairs. Use additional pillows or cushions or add a board under chair cushions to provide a firm surface on which to sit.
- Keep your knees apart; avoid extreme spreading of the legs. Hip width is adequate.
- Do not cross your legs at the knee, ankle, or in any other way.
- Do not lean forward when sitting.
- Do not sit for long periods of time. Try to walk around or lie down every 30 minutes.
- Do not lift knee of surgical leg higher than hip level.

Standing
- Do not stand with toes pointed inward or outward.
- Do not bend forward at the trunk more than 90 degrees.
- Do not kneel.
- When doing a task while standing, always face what you are doing and do not over-reach or twist with your upper trunk.
- When standing up from a chair, first move to the edge of the seat, keeping your surgical leg far in front of the non-surgical leg.

Dressing
- Do not bend over 90 degrees at the hip to put on socks, underwear, or trousers. You will be taught to use adaptive equipment (elastic shoe laces, long-handled shoe horn, and reacher).
- The surgical leg is dressed first and undressed last.
- Do not wear a girdle or panty hose.

Toileting
- Do not sit on low toilets. Use a raised toilet seat or an over-the-toilet commode to ease getting up and down.

Bathing
- You may take a shower. You will be shown an appropriate method to do this.
- You will need to sponge bathe if you do not have a shower or bath chair of some type. It is important to sponge bathe from a seated position to avoid falls.
- A long-handled bath sponge or brush is useful for washing the lower extremities.

Homemaking
- Avoid bending and stooping to low cabinets, ovens, and dryers. Avoid making low beds.
- Use long-handled mops, dustpans, and brooms to wash floors, sweep, and dust low areas.

Car
- The car should not have bucket seats.
- Make sure that there is adequate leg space.
- Transfer: The car should be away from the curb; back up to the passenger seat, sit down, slide straight back on the seat, and have someone assist you to move both legs as a unit into the car. Reverse the procedure to get out of the car.

Precautions Specific to You
-
-
-

Figure 24-4. Precautions list.

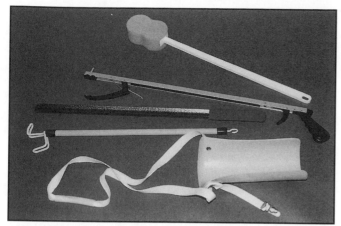

Figure 24-5. Equipment.

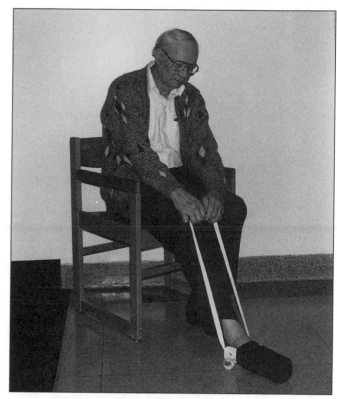

Figure 24-6. Carl using the sock aid. (Reprinted from Ryan, S. E. [1993]. *Practice issues in OT: Intraprofessional team building.* Thorofare, NJ: SLACK Incorporated.)

Figures 24-7 and 24-8, being careful to observe other precautions as well.

Next, Carl, his wife, and the OTA went to the OT bathroom area to learn shower/tub and toilet transfers. Carl indicated that the shower in their home had a 3-inch step at the entrance. Carl was shown a number of assistive devices, including a tub chair, grab bars, and a long-handled bath sponge. Carl decided that he would like to have a grab bar installed in his shower, not only because of his current situation, but also as a long-term safety device. As a plumber, he was aware of the importance that the grab bars be securely fastened to the wall studs in his bathroom so that the bars could not come free and cause a fall. He stated that he had a chair at home that he could use in the shower. Carl was instructed to walk to the step of the shower and turn so that he was facing away from the shower stall. He was then told to reach for the chair, sit, and lift his legs into the shower stall. Carl thought the long-handled bath sponge would "come in handy" at minimum cost.

The OTA talked with Carl and his wife about toilet use and learned that the toilet in their home was low. Using a toilet of this type would cause hip flexion beyond 90 degrees. Carl would need to use an over-the-toilet commode chair or a sturdy raised toilet seat. His wife indicated that a commode chair could be borrowed from a relative. The OTA also provided Carl and his wife with a list of local vendors who provide rental and sales of raised toilet seats, over-the-toilet commodes, and grab bars for the home. The OTA taught Carl to "back up" to the commode until he could feel the back of his knees touch. He was then instructed to reach for the arm rests, bring his surgical leg forward, and lower himself to the commode. This activity concluded the morning session, and the time of the afternoon session was confirmed.

That afternoon, Carl and his wife met the OTA in the OT kitchen. Instruction was provided in basic home management, work simplification (methods for making tasks easier to accomplish), and energy conservation techniques (methods for reducing exertion). Although Carl's wife normally assumed most of these tasks, she was employed by their plumbing business 4 hours a day, 4 days per week between 10:00 a.m. and 2:00 p.m. Thus, Carl would have to prepare his own lunch and clean up and perform other ADLs independently. During this treatment session, the OTA also demonstrated specific tasks, such as using a reacher, sliding items on a countertop, transporting items on a utility cart, and using a bag or pail in conjunction with a walker or crutches. Effective methods for removing and storing items in the refrigerator were also stressed, as well as using a high stool to sit on during meal preparation and dish washing. Carl was then asked to make a sandwich and a bowl of soup and to clean up, incorporating the techniques he had been taught. He completed these tasks successfully, requiring only infrequent reminders. Carl also indicated that he already had a utility cart and an ice cream pail at home for transporting items.

More general work simplification and energy conservation techniques were discussed with Carl, and important safety factors were stressed. Emphasis was placed on the following principles, which must be adhered to at home:

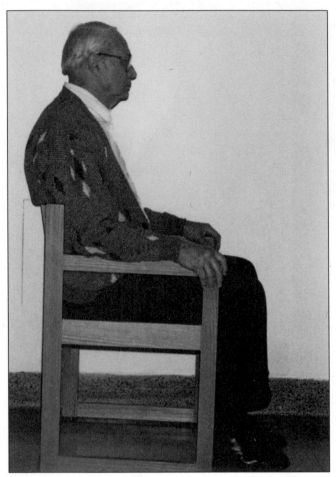

Figure 24-7. Carl standing up. (Reprinted from Ryan, S. E. [1993]. *Practice issues in OT: Intraprofessional team building.* Thorofare, NJ: SLACK Incorporated.)

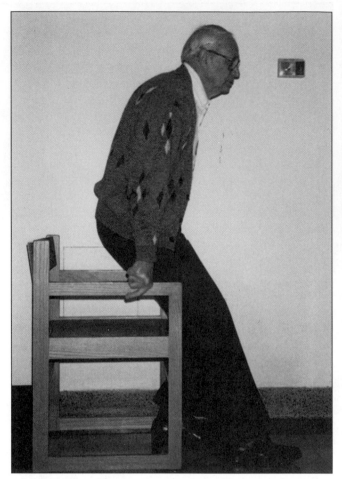

Figure 24-8. Carl standing up. (Reprinted from Ryan, S. E. [1993]. *Practice issues in OT: Intraprofessional team building.* Thorofare, NJ: SLACK Incorporated.)

1. Rearrange commonly used items to avoid excessive bending and reaching.
2. Remove clutter, cords, and scatter rugs to prevent tripping and falls.
3. Rest periodically and whenever needed to avoid fatigue.
4. Sit on a firm, sturdy armchair.
5. Use assistive devices as required.
6. Observe all precautions and limitations when engaging in daily living activities.

At the conclusion of the afternoon treatment session, Carl, his wife, and the OTA agreed to meet the next day to review the treatment activities and procedures and to answer questions. The OTA summarized and reported Carl's progress to the supervising OT who determined that his program would be discontinued on the next day if dressing goals were met and the patient demonstrated a thorough understanding of the precautions and limitations.

The next day, the OTA saw Carl in his room. He was able to demonstrate lower extremity dressing techniques and the effective use of assistive devices. He was able to verbally list the precautions and limitations that he must observe and related them to specific tasks and activities. Carl had several questions that the OTA answered and several that she helped Carl to answer for himself. Upon completion of this session, the OTA verified treatment and documentation with the OT, who co-signed the note, and placed the note in Carl's medical chart.

Program Discontinuation

Treatment was discontinued after Carl met the established treatment goals. The OT and OTA met with Carl and his wife and again stressed the importance of following THA precautions and limitations discussed in OT, as well as those addressed by physical therapy, nursing personnel, and his physician. The OTA suggested that they refer to the precautions handout when in doubt of performance techniques for activity. She also indicated that both she and the OT were available by phone if they needed assistance with unanticipated problems. The OT Orthopaedic Rehabilitation Discharge Note shown in

Patient: _____   Date of initial contact: _____

Diagnosis: _____   Today's date: _____

Physician: _____   MR #: _____

Living situation: _____

ADL status: Homemaking:_____

               Bathing: _____

               Dressing: _____

               Bathtub and toilet transfers: _____

Instruction in work simplification and energy conservation techniques completed: _____

Precautions reviewed: _____

Adaptive equipment reviewed: _____

               Provided:_____

Assistance available during recovery: _____

Additional comments: _____

_____

_____

Figure 24-9. Discharge note form. (Reprinted from Ryan, S. E. [1993]. *Practice issues in OT: Intraprofessional team building.* Thorofare, NJ: SLACK Incorporated.)

Figure 24-9 was completed and entered in the medical chart.

Six months after his surgery, Carl was able to complete minor plumbing jobs independently for friends and family members. He had also achieved his main objective of playing golf without pain, something that he had not been able to do for years. His only regret was that he had not had the surgery several years earlier when it had been first discussed.

CONCLUSION

This case study discussed the treatment given to a patient after a THA. There are a variety of factors to consider in the treatment of THA, including the type of surgical procedure performed and the individual situation of the patient. Although treatment precautions and protocols are similar, it is imperative to follow the physician's orders for each individual's unique situation regarding weight-bearing, hip mobility, and positioning. Precautions apply to participation in all performance areas.

Once a OTA has demonstrated service competency working with this type of patient and treatment protocol, the OTA can usually implement the treatment program with minimum general supervision. The entry-level OTA requires closer supervision from the OT. In all cases, consultation should take place with the supervising OT after reviewing the medical chart and in preparation for discharge.

CLINICAL PROBLEM-SOLVING

Frequently, a secondary diagnosis or other factors will affect the patient's ability to perform or follow routine THA treatment. Clinical reasoning is required to problem solve and adapt treatment to meet the unique needs and abilities of each individual. The following cases require such adaptations.

Read each scenario, identify "other" factors and resulting limitations, and use problem-solving strategies to identify ways to adapt or grade treatment. Remember to consider performance areas, performance components, and performance context.

- Maria is 73 years old and will return to the nursing home where she has lived for the past year. Following surgery, Maria is exhibiting increased confusion.

- Bill is an 80-year-old man who lives alone in his own home. Following surgery, Bill will go to a long-term care facility for a period of 1 to 3 months, with the expectation of returning home as soon as he is able to safely function independently.

- Gary is 56 years old, is employed full-time, and lives at home with his wife. Due to extreme bilateral hip pain and decreasing mobility, Gary is having both hips replaced at the same time. Gary will be returning home following surgery and is concerned about his sexual relationship with his wife.

- Elsie is 75 years old and has severe arthritic deformities in her hands that limit her functional upper extremity mobility and strength. She will return to her own home and is having difficulty in using adaptive equipment presented to her.

ACKNOWLEDGMENTS

The authors would like to acknowledge the following individuals for their contributions and assistance: Mr. and Mrs. Carl Eisenach, Joel A. Zamzow, MD, Carol Herman, OTR, CHT, and Cheryl Esala, OTR.

REFERENCES

American Academy of Orthopaedic Surgeons (1996). *Public information: Total joint replacement* (on-line service). (Available Internet).

Brashear, H. B., & Rainey, R. B. (1978). Shand's Handbook of Orthopedic Surgery (9th ed.). St. Louis, MO: CV Mosby.

Health Answers. (1999). http://www.healthanswers.com.

Pedretti, L. W. (1996). *OT: Practice skills for physical dysfunction* (4th ed.). St. Louis, MO: C. V. Mosby.

Wheeless III, C. R. (1996). *Wheeless' textbook of orthopaedics: Pre-op planning for total hip replacement* (on-line service). http://wheeless.belgianorthoweb.be/Welcome.html.

A Senior Homemaker with Substance Abuse

Chapter 25

Denise Rotert, MA, OTR/L
Frank Gainer, MHS, OTR/L

INTRODUCTION

Abuse of and dependence on substances is an issue seen in virtually all areas of OT practice. Traditionally, it has been thought of as a mental health issue, and OT personnel working in mental health settings may have patients with psychiatric as well as substance use diagnoses. The use/abuse of substances may also emerge as a treatment issue in acute physical disabilities treatment, rehabilitation, long-term care, or home health, for example (Stoffel & Moyers, 1997).

Substance use disorders have been identified by the *Diagnostic and Statistical Manual of Mental Disorders* (4th ed.), also referred to as DSM-IV (American Psychiatric Association, 1994). They are viewed as diseases that are chronic, progressive, and fatal, but can be halted through abstinence from abused substances. DSM-IV also distinguishes between substance abuse and dependence.

For a diagnosis of substance dependence, an essential feature is a cluster of cognitive, behavioral, and physiologic symptoms of which an individual must present with a minimum of three (of seven) symptoms within the same 12-month period. The symptoms as stated in DSM-IV are:

- Tolerance—The need for increased amounts of the drug to obtain the same effect or diminished effect with continued use of the same amount.
- Withdrawal—A characteristic withdrawal syndrome or the use of the substance to relieve or avoid the withdrawal syndrome.
- Taking the substance in larger amounts or over a longer time period than was intended.
- A persistent desire or unsuccessful efforts to cut down or control the substance use.
- Time spent in obtaining or using the substance or recovering from the effects of substance use.
- The giving up or reduction of important social, occupational, and recreational activities.
- The continuation of substance use despite knowledge of having recurrent physical or psychological

KEY CONCEPTS

- Substance abuse treatment: An interdisciplinary program that helps individuals establish a personal plan for sobriety.
- Lifestyle management: Process of choosing and engaging in daily activities that support alcohol-free living.
- Twelve-step programs: Base recovery on total abstinence from substances, following steps that have been outlined, a sharing of personal stories, and participating in the fellowship of the program.

problems caused or exacerbated by the substance (American Psychiatric Association, 1994).

Substance abuse includes the essential feature of a maladaptive pattern of use occurring within a 12-month period that is characterized by recurrent and significant adverse consequences including:

- Repeated failure to fulfill major role obligations at work, school, or home.
- Use of the substance despite obvious physical hazards.
- Use of the substance despite obvious social or interpersonal problems.
- Recurrent substance-related legal problems (American Psychiatric Association, 1994).

Polysubstance dependence is characterized by using at least three groups of substances (in the same 12-month period) but a single substance does not predominate. Dependence criteria needs to be met for substances as a group but not for any specific substance. Using substances (including illicit drugs, alcohol, and/or prescription drugs) in combination or as alternates if the drug of choice is not available is a pattern of use that is frequently seen. Generally, once a problem with alcohol or another drug arises, there is an increased vulnerability to substance dependence problems of all kinds (Rotert & Gainer, 1993).

The process of regaining important life roles, developing healthy relationships with others, and establishing healthy daily routines, all of which support abstinence and sobriety, is termed recovery. Detoxification is the process of removing the substance from the person's system and is frequently done under the management of a physician. Abstinence is a period of alcohol and drug-free living. Sobriety is used to describe a new way of living without alcohol and drugs (Stoffel & Moyers, 1997).

Twelve-step programs have developed to meet the needs of individuals with a desire to recover from the negative effects of substance use. Alcoholics Anonymous (AA) was the first 12-step program. Twelve-step programs base recovery on total abstinence from substances, following the steps that have been outlined, a sharing of personal stories including use of substances and sobriety, and participating in the fellowship of the program which is based on recovering individuals assisting individuals who are new to the program (Alcoholics Anonymous Fact File at www.alcoholics-anonymous.org). Examples of other 12-step programs that address specific needs include Narcotics Anonymous (NA) for persons abusing narcotics, and Alanon for anyone in a significant relationship with a substance abuser. AA describes the progression of the disease from spiritual to emotional to physical. Recovery is from physical to emotional to spiritual.

Individuals with substance use disorders have some common characteristics. As the disease progresses, the various areas of an individual's lifestyle performance will deteriorate. Leisure time is the prime time for individuals to use/abuse substances and work time gets protected. It is speculated that one of the reasons that work time is protected is as a source of revenue. The healthy activities and behaviors associated with leisure and work performance also show signs of decreasing as the use of substances increases. Role performance problems develop as the disease progresses. Relationships frequently take on attributes that enable the user to continue using. ADLs tend to show a decline in skill, the amount of time, and the energy that are dedicated to related tasks. The spectrum of interests, ideas, and activities in the lifestyle of the substance user/abuser becomes constricted (Rotert, 1993).

FRAMES OF REFERENCE

Sobriety is used to describe a new way of living without alcohol and drugs. It is more than abstinence and includes development of coping skills to prevent future alcohol/drug use (Stoffel & Moyers, 1997). OT's purpose can be described as guiding patients in the development of a lifestyle that is supportive of sobriety. The sober lifestyle is organized around temporal adaptation, role performance, and competency behaviors that are the components of occupational behavior.

The function of OT is to view the individual needs of the alcoholic patients, to establish a treatment plan based on those individual needs, and to provide intervention opportunities. The overall goal is to assist the patient in development of an alcohol-free lifestyle. Short-term goals will support the overall goal and will be directed at specific deficit areas of occupational behavior. OT teaches patients a functional, practical approach to living sober. (Rotert, 1993)

The evaluation includes assessment of performance areas, performance components, and context factors (AOTA, 1994). The general areas to be addressed will include ADLs, work, and leisure. Cognitive, psychological, or social deficits must be addressed and can be either contributing factors or the result of heavy, chronic use/abuse of substances. The context of the individual plays a role in the development of a substance abuse problem as well as contributing to a successful recovery program. In order to complete a thorough evaluation, the full spectrum of skills, abilities, and needs must be included.

Evaluation of the "occupations" of individuals will provide OT personnel with the basis for an OT treatment plan. Some examples of performance areas of concern in the evaluation and treatment of the individual with substance use/abuse issues include: self-care and personal hygiene, support system, interpersonal relationships, money management, work activities, nutrition and meal preparation, safety, and engagement in leisure activities of interest. Some examples of performance component areas of concern include body scheme, perceptual processing, endurance, coordination, attention span, problem solving, self-concept, interpersonal skills, time management, coping skills, and skills for competent role performance. And finally, some examples of context areas of concern include age and stage of development and the physical, social, and cultural environment. While each evaluation needs to be individually determined, the clinical reasoning skills of the OT and OTA will be utilized to choose the specific assessment tools needed for each individual patient/client.

When a patient/client or caregiver uses or abuses substances, it can have an adverse effect on engagement in any other treatment. If a recipient of OT services has problems in performance areas, components, or contexts, those problems must be addressed.

CASE STUDY

Mrs. Nancy Jarvis, a 65-year-old white female, was referred to OT for rehabilitation of her right dominant hand after she had sustained a distal radial/ulnar fracture. She was admitted to the hospital and surgery was done the following wee, which consisted of an open reduction internal fixation (ORIF) of the distal radius/ulna. She was placed in an external fixator for 12 weeks. Mrs. Jarvis was instructed on proper care of the pin sites and on ROM exercises for the fingers and thumb. She was given follow-up appointments with the surgeon for every 2 weeks.

Mrs. Jarvis has been a widow for the past 2 years. Her husband passed away after a 5-year bout with cancer. She has two children, both of whom live out of the area. She has infrequent contact with them. Mrs. Jarvis lives alone in a large three-story home. Since her husband passed away, she has limited contact with their mutual friends. She used to enjoy playing cards, going out to lunch with friends, and being active with a local community organization. She used to attend church on a regular basis but now attends only on special occasions. She has one good friend whose health has been failing. She talks to her friend daily by phone and sees her about once every other week.

Mrs. Jarvis has had difficulty making her orthopedic surgeon appointments. Her excuses have been that she has forgotten them or she has not been feeling well enough. She has had difficulty getting out of bed, getting herself cleaned and dressed, and taking a taxi to the doctor's office. The only time she would consistently make her follow-up appointments was when she needed a pain medication refill. The surgeon initially referred her to an OT for ROM exercises after 4 weeks in the external fixator. However, Mrs. Jarvis never followed through with scheduling the OT evaluation.

After 12 weeks, the surgeon removed the external fixator. Mrs. Jarvis presented with very stiff and swollen fingers. The surgeon inquired about her OT treatment and she admitted that she never followed through with making the evaluation appointment. She stated that she thought stiff and swollen fingers were normal when you had an external fixator and that it would become automatically better once you removed the fixator. The surgeon's secretary scheduled Mrs. Jarvis for her OT evaluation for that afternoon.

Mrs. Jarvis presented to the OT holding her right hand close to her chest in a very protective position. The initial evaluation consisted of:

- Medical background data
- ROM measurements
- Fine motor coordination test
- Edema measurements
- Sensation testing
- Discussion of home set-up

The OT was concerned about Mrs. Jarvis' personal hygiene. She appeared unkempt and did not seem to have bathed for several days. In addition, there seemed to be an odor of alcohol on her breath. She also seemed to have an unusual dependence on her pain medication for someone who was over 12 weeks from her original date of injury. Finally, she appeared lethargic and did not seem to be overly concerned about the status of her dominant hand and the significant loss of function that was evident. The OT suspected that Mrs. Jarvis might be depressed and was using alcohol and her pain medication as a way of self-medicating. Due to the questionable pattern of substance use, both alcohol and pain medications, it was decided to include as part of the initial evaluation the following:

- ADL evaluation
- A complete social history to include support systems
- Leisure interests inventory
- Time management assessment to include the structure of a typical day

In order to begin to address the psychosocial issues that were occurring with Mrs. Jarvis, the OT had a very frank conversation with her to discuss her personal hygiene, the consistent odor of alcohol, and her seeming over-dependence on pain medication. She was counseled that all of this would have a negative impact on her realizing the best improvement she possibly could for her hand. Mrs. Jarvis related that since her injury, she was withdrawing even further from her previous interests. She was encouraged to complete a leisure interest and social history questionnaire (Figure 25-1). In addition, she was given a time clock (Figure 25-2). This allowed the OT and OTA to see how Mrs. Jarvis was structuring a typical

Occupational Therapy Questionnaire

Name: _____

Age: _____   Sex: Male / Female

Home address: _____

Work Background

Current paid job(s):_____

Have you ever been fired from a job? Yes / No   If yes, why? _____
_____

Other job(s): _____

Volunteer job(s): _____

What do/did you like about your job(s)? _____

What do/did you dislike about your job(s)? _____

How did you get along with others at work? _____

What are your responsibilities at home? _____

Educational Background

What is the highest grade that you completed in school?_____

Do you have diplomas, certificates, or degrees? (Describe) _____
_____

What do you like to study? _____

Leisure Interests

What do you do to have fun? _____

List those activities that you usually do by yourself: _____
_____

List those activities that you usually do with others: _____
_____

What clubs/organizations do you participate in? _____

How would you describe your skills or talents? _____

List those activities you used to participate in but no longer do: _____

Social History

Do you find it easy to do the following:

Socialize with others?_____   Why or why not? _____

Start conversations? _____   Why or why not? _____

Share feelings and emotions? _____   Why or why not? _____

Describe your strongest points:_____

Describe your weakest points: _____

What are your goals for the future? _____

What effects has substance abuse had on your life? _____

Do you want to get and stay sober? _____

What would you like to change about yourself or your life to help you be sober? _____
_____

Figure 25-1. OT questionnaire.

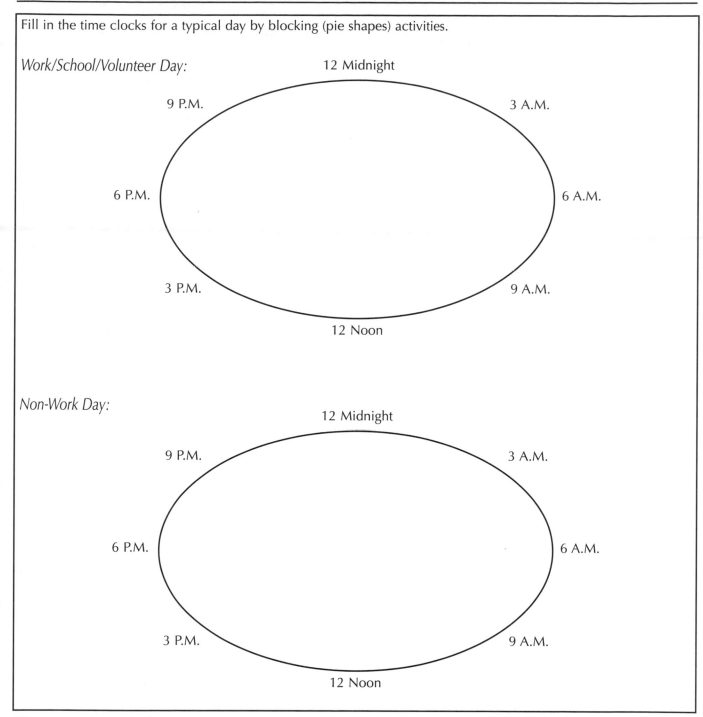

Fill in the time clocks for a typical day by blocking (pie shapes) activities.

Work/School/Volunteer Day:

12 Midnight
9 P.M.   3 A.M.
6 P.M.   6 A.M.
3 P.M.   9 A.M.
12 Noon

Non-Work Day:

12 Midnight
9 P.M.   3 A.M.
6 P.M.   6 A.M.
3 P.M.   9 A.M.
12 Noon

Figure 25-2. Time clocks.

day. They could then assess whether a certain time of the day was more problematic than another.

The OTA was responsible for completing the ADL evaluation and assessment of leisure interests and time management. The OT completed the neuromusculoskeletal evaluation as well as the social history and the assessment of substance use. Goals for Mrs. Jarvis' OT treatment program were collaborated.

General Goals

Goals included:
1. Independence in ADLs, which is supported by:
   - ROM, strength, and fine motor coordination of right dominant hand within functional limits
   - Edema of right upper extremity within functional limits

2. Pursuit of identified leisure or other interests, which is supported by ability to structure her day so she is up and active during the majority of the day.

3. Identification of an appropriate support system.

Initially, treatment sessions were scheduled for 3 days a week, and each session was 1 hour in length. The OT and OTA worked together in treating Mrs. Jarvis. The first 20 minutes of each session consisted of using a heat modality, in this case fluidotherapy, which provides a dry heat maximizing functional activities. This was followed by a combination of exercises (active and passive ROM) and functional activities that required her to use her right hand for sustained periods of time. In addition, the patient was provided with an edema glove to wear throughout the day and at night to assist in reducing the swelling. She was also given a home program that consisted of retrograde massage, ROM exercises, and education about using routine, daily, home activities to increase her competence in performance of her chosen occupations.

Mrs. Jarvis was receptive to the inquiries about her psychosocial issues, as she felt that she was losing control of her life and no longer found a lot of meaning and satisfaction in the few activities she still participated in. She was concerned about her friend's failing health and how unbearable her life would be if something were to happen to her friend. The OT and OTA developed a plan of action with Mrs. Jarvis. It was decided that she would:

1. Abstain from using alcohol and after consulting with her physician, would take one pain pill an hour before every OT treatment session.

2. Make a commitment to attend an AA meeting once a week for the next 6 weeks. She was directed to a group that consisted primarily of people in her age group so that she would be able to better relate to their issues.

3. Resume attending mass once every week to try and regain the spirituality that she felt was missing.

4. Make a commitment to visit her friend at least once a week and try to go to an outside activity with her.

5. Commit to attending her monthly civic organization meeting.

6. Contact her son and daughter a minimum of every 2 weeks for the next 6 weeks to try and reconcile her relationship with them.

7. Finally, that for the next 4 weeks she would call an old friend each week and make an effort to get together and participate in some type of community activity.

CLINICAL PROBLEM-SOLVING

Each patient who presents with substance abuse/dependence issues also has other factors that may need to be addressed as part of his or her OT treatment. Those factors may be physical or psychosocial or a combination of both. The following are some mini cases that demonstrate some of those complicating factors. How many possibilities can you identify? How would you evaluate those factors presented? What treatment techniques might you use to reach your treatment goals?

- Nate, a retired veteran diagnosed with alcohol dependence and diabetes, has had bilateral lower extremity amputations and uses a wheelchair full-time. His friends brought a bottle when they picked him up after his discharge, and they all sat outside the hospital and got drunk. Nate comes to an outpatient OT appointment for assistance with retirement planning but comes at the wrong time and on the wrong day and does not seem to recognize you.

- Susan, an 18-year-old methamphetamine abuser who has sustained a gun shot wound to her right elbow in a domestic fight after she told her boyfriend that she is pregnant.

- Joe, a Native American male who is returning to the reservation and has tried numerous times to get clean and sober with traditional AA. Joe's wife is also alcohol dependent and drank alcohol and smoked cigarettes throughout her pregnancy with their son who is now 5 years old and showing signs of fetal alcohol syndrome.

- Evie is a 29-year-old intravenous drug user diagnosed with AIDS. Evie requests evening appointments so that she can keep everything a secret from her employer, who thinks she was hospitalized for acute pneumonia and has fully recovered.

REFERENCES

American Psychiatric Association. (1994). *Diagnostic and statistical manual for mental disorders* (4th ed.). Washington, DC: Author.

AOTA. (1994). Uniform terminology for occupational therapy (3rd ed.). *Am J Occup Ther, 48,* 1047-1054.

Rotert, D. A. (1993). OT in alcoholism. *OT Practice, 4,* 1-11.

Rotert, D. A., & Gainer, F. E. (1993). The adolescent with chemical dependency. In S. Ryan (Ed.), *Practice issues in OT: Intraprofessional team building.* Thorofare, NJ: SLACK Incorporated.

Stoffel, V., & Moyers, P. (1997). *OT practice guidelines for substance use disorders.* Bethesda, MD: AOTA.

1) Focus for evaluation & treatment (effects on occupational performance, evaluation methods & tools, general tx goals, tx methods/interventions, etc.)

1 year old

A Businessman with a Stroke

Martha Logigian, MS, OTR/L

INTRODUCTION

Stroke is the third leading cause of death and disability in the United States. Approximately 500,000 adults have a stroke each year. It is a rapid onset of neurological deficits that persists for at least 24 hours as a result of intracerebral hemorrhage, thrombosis, embolism, or vascular insufficiency leading to the infarction of brain tissue. Eighty-five percent of strokes are due to brain infarctions, while intracerebral and subarachnoid hemorrhages account for about 15%. Strokes occur at any age, but the incidence dramatically increases with age (Acquaviva, 1996). A stroke, which is a lesion in a hemisphere of the brain, produces motor impairment or hemiparesis of the contralateral side of the body. For example, a stroke (brain attack or cerebral vascular accident [CVA]) in the left cerebral hemisphere is referred to as a left CVA with resulting hemiparesis on the right side of the body. Due to this weakness or lack of motion on one side of the body, the patient will experience difficulty with most ADLs including self-care tasks, ambulation, and homemaking. In addition, depending on the location in the brain of the stroke, the patient may have sensory, cognitive, language, and visual deficits as well as confusion. Table 26-1 defines a variety of these impairments.

Many stroke survivors with impairments such as these will benefit from rehabilitation. In one study, patients who received rehabilitation achieved greater and more rapid gains in physical function than those who did not receive rehabilitation (Kelly-Hayes & Paige, 1995). Most recovery takes place within the first 3 months, and in this era of cost containment, shorter lengths of stay in the hospital and rehab setting are the norm. Thus, short-term functional gains are the focus of the OT program (Van Dyck, 1999).

FRAME OF REFERENCE

OT for stroke rehabilitation uses several frames of reference. Many frames of reference address specific ADLs through a focus on mobility, dressing, grooming, and homemaking. They are typically approached from a learning theory perspective in which specific tasks are learned. In

KEY CONCEPTS

- Stroke rehabilitation: A program to restore functional independence of a person after a cerebral vascular insufficiency led to the infarction of brain tissue.
- Subacute rehabilitation: An organized setting for stroke rehabilitation. Multiple disciplines provide intensive treatment for clients.
- Adaptive equipment: Devices designed to make tasks easier and safer.
- One-handed techniques: Methods of performing activities using one hand/arm to accomplish the task.

ESSENTIAL VOCABULARY

Dysarthria: A disorder of articulation due to muscle weakness that is often manifested as slurred speech.

Facilitation techniques: Manual methods used to encourage movement and sensory awareness.

Flaccid: Inability to move an extremity due to loss of motor control.

Hemiparesis: Weakness on one side of the body.

Shoulder subluxation: The downward dislocation of the humerus.

Visual field deficit or hemianopia: Blindness in one-half of the field of vision in one or both eyes.

Table 26-1

Possible Impairments Following a Stroke

Visual field deficit: The patient experiences a hemianopia or blindness in one-half of the field of vision of one or both eyes.

Limited attention span: The patient is unable to attend to a specific stimulus without being distracted by extraneous environmental stimuli.

Memory loss: The patient is unable to store new experiences or perceptions for later recall.

Cognitive deficits: These can include difficulty with problem-solving, sequencing patterns, and completing math problems.

Perceptual impairments: Often seen when the lesion is in the right hemisphere; these can include visual spatial neglect (the failure to register stimuli from one side of the body), impairment in spatial relations (the inability to perceive the position of an object in relation to other objects), and visual agnosia (the lack of recognition of familiar objects).

Aphasia: Often seen when the lesion is in the left hemisphere, it is the inability to use and understand spoken and written language.

Dysarthria: A motor speech disorder leading to difficulty with speech articulation.

Apraxia: The inability to perform purposeful movements despite the presence of intact mobility, sensation, coordination, and comprehension.

(Adapted from Logigian, M. K. (1982). Adult rehabilitation: A team approach for therapists. Boston, MA: Little, Brown and Co.)

---

this chapter, ADLs are addressed via a neurodevelopmental treatment frame of reference. A coping frame of reference is also utilized through personal adaptations to respond to the needs and demands of the situation. Lastly, an occupational behavior frame of reference is used in this section for the adult in the case study. The client's avocation as a chef and host is a meaningful role in his life.

CASE STUDY

Mr. Callahan is a 65-year-old businessman who experienced a sudden onset of weakness on the left side of his body with slurred speech. He lives in a large, single-story home with his wife, and he has three married sons who live in the area. He was brought from home by ambulance to the hospital emergency room where the neurologist diagnosed a right middle cerebral artery infarct. He began treatment in the emergency room and was transferred to a patient care unit in the hospital. In the acute phase of illness, the patient's medical condition is evolving with stabilization of accompanying neurological symptoms and the beginning stages of recovery. During these critical days in the acute care hospital, upper extremity ROM, bed mobility, and positioning are the primary concerns of the OT program. On day 2 of hospitalization, the OT was asked by the physical therapist to see Mr. Callahan at bedside, as his left hand and arm were flaccid and swollen. In addition, his arm had impaired sensation. He was unable to complete any self-care activities, and he had difficulty articulating his responses to the OT screening as he was dysarthric.

Mr. Callahan could move in bed from side to side, although he was uncomfortable doing so, as his arm became tangled in the sheets. He was usually found slipped down in bed and unable to regain a comfortable position. Mr. Callahan transferred bed to chair with the maximum assistance of the OT. He used a wheelchair to get to the bathroom, although he was unable to independently move the wheelchair. With maximum assistance of the OT, he was able to transfer onto the toilet. Mr. Callahan could feed himself if all of the food on the tray was set up, cut up, and opened. He could wash his face during a bed bath but was unable to bathe the rest of his body, dress, or shave.

It was anticipated that Mr. Callahan would remain in the acute care hospital for 2 more days. Due to the limited time, the OT program focused on upper extremity ROM, positioning while in bed, bed mobility, and bed to chair transfers. ROM exercises for the left upper extremity were demonstrated to Mr. Callahan, although he had difficulty doing them. His son, who was in attendance during the treatment session, learned to do the ROM exercises, and the therapist suggested that he do them daily for his father. The OT demonstrated positioning (Figures 26-1 through 26-3) and bed mobility (Figures 26-4 through 26-7) to the nurses caring for Mr. Callahan, to ensure he was comfortable in bed. Mr. Callahan's son was instructed in bed to chair transfers (Figures 26-8 and 26-9). The OT checked back with Mr. Callahan on day 3

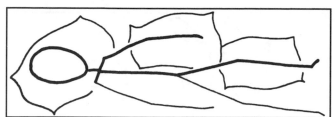

Figure 26-1. Supine position. When the patient is totally dependent, position with pillows under head and under shoulder for protraction; under extended arm and hand, with hand elevated if edematous; under calf with some knee flexion and no pressure on heel. Trunk should be aligned. (Reprinted with permission from Logigian, M. K. (1982). *Adult rehabilitation: A team approach for therapists.* Boston, MA: Little, Brown and Co.)

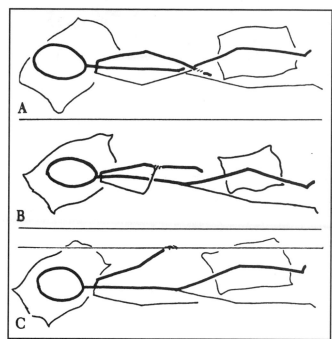

Figure 26-2. When the patient is more independent, use fewer pillows with A. Arms extended, hands clasped together, resting on abdomen. B. Involved arm extended by side, in supination if possible, with sound hand keeping involved elbow extended. C. Involved hand on side rail, legs extended, pillow under the calf with some knee flexion, and no pressure on heel. (Reprinted with permission from Logigian, M. K. (1982). *Adult rehabilitation: A team approach for therapists.* Boston, MA: Little, Brown and Co.)

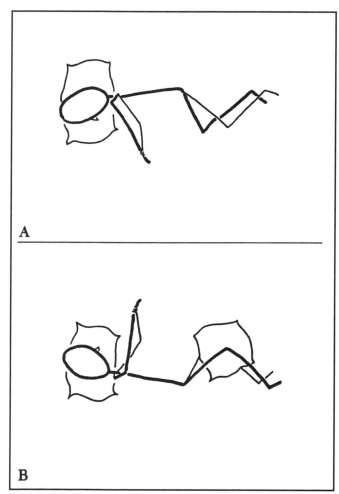

Figure 26-3. Side-lying. When the patient lies on either side (A and B), position with scapula protracted, arms extended with hands clasped together, or sound hand holding involved wrist; or knees and hips flexed, pillow between legs if necessary to keep bony prominences apart. Elevate hand on pillow if it is edematous (not shown). (Reprinted with permission from Logigian, M. K. (1982). *Adult rehabilitation: A team approach for therapists.* Boston, MA: Little, Brown and Co.)

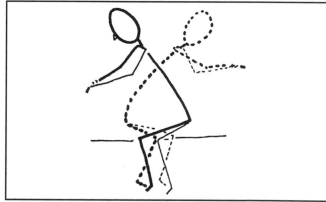

Figure 26-4. Shifting and sitting. The patient transfers all weight to feet, and lifts and moves hips to one side and sits gently on that side. The patient continues moving down one side of the mat or bed by lifting and shifting weight, repositioning feet each time, with assistance as needed. Reverse directions; keeping involved foot behind sound foot, maintain sitting balance and move slowly with control. (Reprinted with permission from Logigian, M. K. (1982). *Adult rehabilitation: A team approach for therapists.* Boston, MA: Little, Brown and Co.)

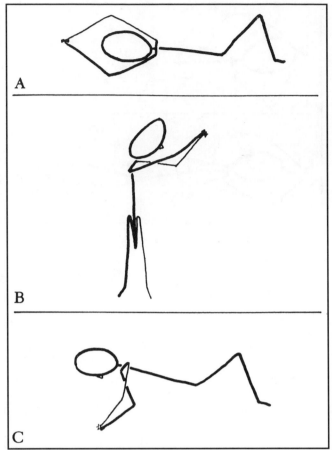

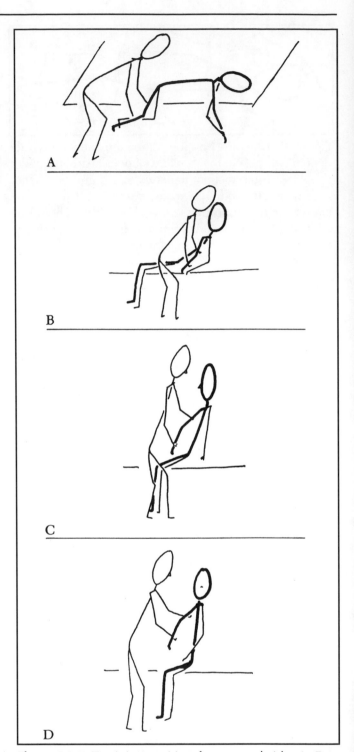

Figure 26-5. Rolling. A. With legs to one side, hold, then roll to other side, upper body relaxed. B. Arms and head to one side, hold, then to other side, lower body relaxed. C. Combine first two motions in opposite directions. Resist or assist patient as needed. Practice separately and together. Combine motions in same direction (one segment at a time) for rolling sequence. (Reprinted with permission from Logigian, M. K. (1982). *Adult rehabilitation: A team approach for therapists*. Boston, MA: Little, Brown and Co.)

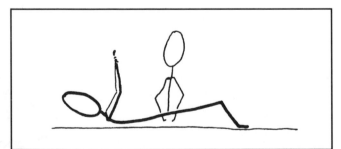

Figure 26-6. Bridging. Raise hips up, hold, lower. Keep knees together and weight evenly distributed. Repeat with knees in more flexion. Use resistance and joint compression. Hold up position and shift weight to left and right, keeping knees upright. Hold up position and abduct and adduct knees evenly. (Reprinted with permission from Logigian, M. K. (1982). *Adult rehabilitation: A team approach for therapists*. Boston, MA: Little, Brown and Co.)

Figure 26-7. To sitting position from sound side. A. Feet over edge, sound foot involved as necessary. Hands clasped together, arms extended. B. Prop up onto sound elbow with head turned toward involved side. Hands are still clasped, if possible, or therapist holds arm extended and scapula protracted. C. Push up onto sound hand, elbow extended. Hands are still clasped, if possible, or therapist holds extended. D. Come to full sitting position, hands in lap, feet flat on the floor. Therapist assists balance as needed. (Reprinted with permission from Logigian, M. K. (1982). *Adult rehabilitation: A team approach for therapists*. Boston, MA: Little, Brown and Co.)

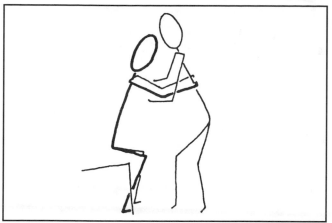

Figure 26-8. Sitting to standing. The therapist's hands are under the patient's elbow, patient's hands are around therapist's waist or elbows extended, hands are clasped together. The patient leans forward so some weight is shifted forward onto the legs, increasing the amount of leaning and weight-shifting as tolerated. Involved foot is positioned slightly behind sound foot. Lean forward so weight is transferred more on involved leg as the patient leans forward. (Reprinted with permission from Logigian, M. K. (1982). *Adult rehabilitation: A team approach for therapists.* Boston, MA: Little, Brown and Co.)

and found that he was comfortable and his son was carrying out the ROM program.

It was decided that Mr. Callahan had excellent rehabilitation potential, and the plan was that as soon as his neurological symptoms stabilized he would be transferred to a subacute care rehabilitation unit with the long-term goal of return to home. On day 4, the OT wrote a discharge summary that included a statement on the program he participated in while in the acute care hospital. He was transferred to the subacute program later in the day.

The following morning, the OT at the subacute program began a complete assessment of Mr. Callahan following a review of his medical record. During the record review, medical issues are identified including age, general health, vital signs, medications, and precautions. The assessment included sensation and motor status of the involved upper extremity such as muscle tone, edema, and hand use; hand dominance; perception; vision status (e.g., are glasses worn); visual field; praxis; cognition; and ADLs. In addition, through discussion with Mr. Callahan and his family, information was gained concerning his level of function, work, and leisure activity (Chang & Hasselkus, 1998) prior to the stroke. Their goals and expectations and plan for discharge from the subacute program were discussed. The family provided information on Mr. Callahan's home environment, as return to

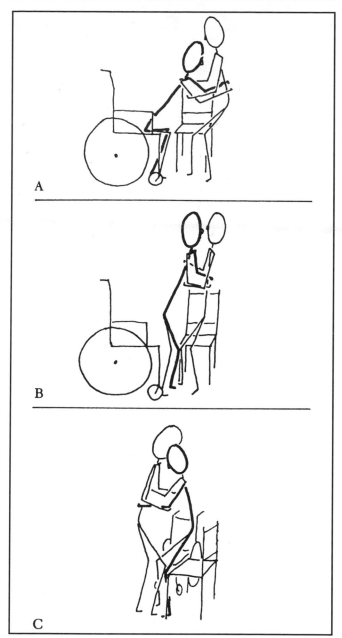

Figure 26-9. Moderate to maximum assistance toward involved side. A. Patient transfers all weight to feet, B. pivots toward involved side, and C. sits by leaning forward. Therapist assists to maintain knee extension and to keep trunk forward, as needed. (Reprinted with permission from Logigian, M. K. (1982). *Adult rehabilitation: A team approach for therapists.* Boston, MA: Little, Brown and Co.)

home was part of the plan. The OT reviewed the findings with the OTA and a plan of care was developed.

The results of the assessment indicated that Mr. Callahan was in good health prior to his stroke. He worked 4 days a week in the construction business he had established, which his sons now managed. He lived with his wife in a large, ranch-style home in the suburbs. He has a ranch-style

Table 26-2

Scales to Measure Functional Performance

Total assistance: The need for 100% assistance by one or more persons to perform all physical activities and/or cognitive assistance to elicit a functional response to an external stimulation.

Maximum assistance: The need for 75% assistance by one person to physically perform any part of a functional activity and/or cognitive assistance to perform gross motor actions in response to direction.

Moderate assistance: The need for 50% assistance by one person to perform physical activities or provide cognitive assistance to sustain/complete simple, repetitive activities safely.

Minimum assistance: The need for 25% assistance by one person for physical activities and/or periodic, cognitive assistance to perform functional activities safely.

Standby assistance: The need for supervision by one person for the patient to perform new activity procedures that were adapted by the therapist for safe and effective performance. A patient requires standby assistance when errors and the need for safety precautions are not always anticipated by the patient.

Independent status: No physical or cognitive assistance is required to perform functional activities. Patients at this level are able to implement the selected courses of action, consider potential errors, and anticipate safety hazards in familiar and new situations.

Adapted from Health Care Financing Administration. (1996). Medicare intermediary manual, Publication 13, Section 3906.4. Washington, DC: U.S. Government Printing Office, 21-21.

---

vacation home on the ocean, which is where he spends every weekend year round. At the vacation home, he had been doing all the cooking, his specialty being Italian cuisine. Although his wife enjoyed this home, she preferred to remain in the suburban home, and Mr. Callahan frequently went to the vacation home alone or with friends.

Mr. Callahan had a flaccid left upper extremity with shoulder subluxation, although slight movement and sensation was noted in the fingers. The shoulder was painful when passively moved and his hand was swollen. Shoulder subluxation is the downward dislocation of the humerus and a common problem for a patient with a flaccid or weak upper extremity. In the flaccid extremity, the supraspinatus, part of the rotator cuff muscles, along with all the other scapular and humeral muscles, can no longer hold the humerus in place, as they are weak or paralyzed. The upward motion of the glenoid fossa is no longer maintained as gravity, the weight of the arm, spasticity, or a tendency to lean toward the weak side bring the scapula into a downward position. Prolonged subluxation can be extremely painful.

Mr. Callahan had good trunk mobility and was able to move in bed with minimal assistance (Table 26-2). He could transfer bed to chair and chair to toilet with moderate assistance of one. At present, he was using a wheelchair for mobility, although he needed assistance to move it any distance. The physical therapist planned to have him ambulating with a quad cane. The speech pathologist was consulted and provided the team with suggestions for dealing with Mr. Callahan's dysarthria.

On the ADL index, he was found to have difficulty in bathing, dressing, and personnel hygiene due to left side weakness and neglect. He required moderate assistance to sponge bathe in bed and don/doff his shirt. He needed maximum assistance of one to don/doff his underwear and pants. He was able to shave himself although he had frequent cuts, as he insisted on using his single blade razor. He was able to feed himself if the food had been set up on the tray (e.g., cartons and packages opened, meat cut, and rolls buttered). He exhibited neglect of his left visual field, yet in all areas of perception, praxis, and cognition he was within the norm.

The plan of care included the following long-term goals:

1. Mr. Callahan will return home with his family.
2. Mr. Callahan will be independent in ADLs, including bathing, dressing, toileting, shaving, brushing teeth, and feeding.
3. Mr. Callahan will be independent and safe in kitchen activities with the use of adaptive equipment for food preparation.

Short-term goals (within 2 weeks) are:

1. Mr. Callahan will be independent in upper extremity dressing and require minimal assistance in lower extremity dressing.
2. Mr. Callahan will be independent in feeding, brushing teeth, and shaving with the use of compensatory techniques.

3. Mr. Callahan will maintain appropriate positioning of his upper extremity while in bed, chair, and standing.

4. Mr. Callahan will prepare a simple snack in the kitchen using adaptive equipment and one-handed techniques.

Although daily notes are written by the OT and OTA following each treatment session, a progress note is written every 2 weeks. At this time, short-term goals are reviewed and updated or, if needed, new goals established. The OT discussed the assessment and plan with Mr. Callahan and his wife, and they were in agreement with it.

All records are kept in the patient's medical record so that team members have access to the information. In addition, the results of the assessment and treatment plan were presented at the weekly patient care team meeting to ensure consistency.

The OT and OTA worked as a team to initiate the program to improve Mr. Callahan's left upper extremity function, ADL ability, and kitchen skills. Initially, the OT sought to eliminate Mr. Callahan's subluxation with manual support and mobilization of the humerus in the glenoid fossa. With support, the force of gravity is reduced, articular surfaces are in place, and pain diminished. An arm sling is one means of support, and it was decided that it would be tried due to his arm pain. Whatever type of sling is utilized, it must be evaluated routinely with special attention given to its effectiveness in eliminating subluxation, ease of use, and ability to control pain. It is not intended for 24-hour use. It is most useful when worn during standing, ambulation, and transfer activities. The hand must be positioned within the sling, maintaining wrist and finger extension. The elbow should be at 80 degrees of flexion and the strap fit comfortably on the back and neck.

A lap tray was found to be useful when Mr. Callahan was in his wheelchair, and pillows continued to be helpful while he was in bed. The lap tray and pillows are used for scapula support and normal alignment (Figure 26-10). A therapy program of scapular mobilization was initiated by the OT. It focused on the scapular upward rotators and supraspinatus portions of the rotator cuff muscles (Figures 26-11 through 26-15). Although the therapist anticipated that Mr. Callahan would need to learn one-handed techniques to accomplish self-care and daily living tasks, mobility techniques were a part of Mr. Callahan's program to enable maximum mobility of his left side. Mr. Callahan hoped that he would regain normal movement of his left arm and hand.

In addition, PROM (passive range of motion) to the shoulder, elbow, and wrist as well as active motion of the fingers were continued daily by Mr. Callahan's son. The OTA taught Mr. Callahan how to put on the sling and position his arm and monitored the use of the sling. The assistant also provided joint mobilization through PROM, ultimately teaching Mr. Callahan how to do the exercises.

The OT program also addressed Mr. Callahan's ability with self-care activities. The OTA saw Mr. Callahan each morning for 30 minutes for bathing, grooming, and dressing/undressing. She suggested that Mr. Callahan use an electric razor for shaving and an electric toothbrush for cleaning his teeth. He completed these tasks while seated at the sink. The OTA reinforced that Mr. Callahan look to the right and left of his face while shaving, cleaning teeth, and brushing hair. Balancing safety and Mr. Callahan's wishes, it was agreed that he would use a straight razor when his son was able to help him shave.

He preferred a shower to a bed bath, so the OTA arranged for him to shower each morning while seated on a shower chair. He was instructed in one-handed methods for bathing and dressing. A long-handled bath sponge and shoe horn were provided by the OTA to enable independence in bathing and lower extremity dressing. Within 2 weeks, he was independent in bathing and upper extremity dressing but required minimal assistance with lower extremity dressing. A new short-term goal was established to address the issue with lower extremity dressing. One week later, Mr. Callahan was independent in dressing and undressing, and the morning session with the OTA was discontinued.

During the first few days of treatment, the OTA stopped by at lunch time to demonstrate one-handed techniques for self-feeding. She also reinforced compensatory techniques for his left side visual neglect during feeding. By reminding him to turn his head to look at and feel the entire edge of the tray, Mr. Callahan quickly learned not to neglect items in his left visual field.

The OT made arrangements for Mr. Callahan to be loaned a wheelchair with hand controls on the right side, thus making it easier for him to manipulate it independently. Each afternoon, the OTA accompanied Mr. Callahan to the therapeutic kitchen. During the trip to the kitchen, Mr. Callahan was able to wheel the wheelchair independently. Initially, Mr. Callahan had to do all kitchen activities seated, but after 2 weeks he was able to stand using a quad cane for support. During this half-hour session, Mr. Callahan practiced simple kitchen activities incorporating one-handed techniques and adaptive equipment. He began with preparing a cup of tea, and by the end of 2 weeks he was able to complete a snack of cheese and crackers. He used a cutting board to secure the cheese and Fiskar scissors to cut open packaged goods. By the third week he was able to prepare pasta, yet needed to use a bottled sauce, opening it with the help of a jar opener. He was disappointed about this, as his specialty was marinara sauce. The OTA used counseling techniques to address his initial disappointments.

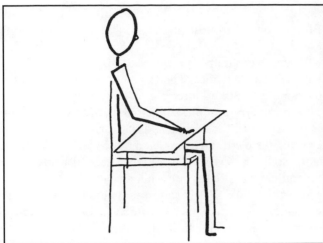

Figure 26-10. When sitting in a wheelchair or standard chair, the patient is positioned with head in midline (may need head support), trunk aligned with pillows or side supports, buttocks with special cushion to protect skin and provide comfort, thighs parallel to floor, weight evenly distributed along thighs, knees with 90 degree flexion, if possible. Feet are flat, with weight evenly distributed on both feet, foot rests, or floor; seat belt is used as indicated. Arms are extended in front and supported on a pillow, rolled-up blanket, lapboard, arm board, or table. If legs are elevated, put cushion under calves, heels free and ankles dorsiflexed. (Reprinted with permission from Logigian, M. K. (1982). *Adult rehabilitation: A team approach for therapists.* Boston, MA: Little, Brown and Co.)

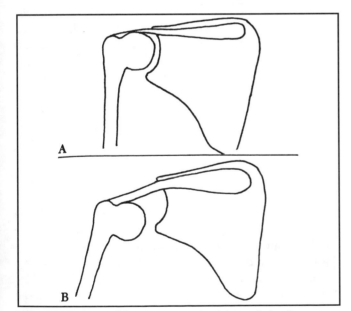

Figure 26-11. Subluxation. A. Position of the humerus in the glenoid fossa and the supraspinatus muscle in the locking mechanism. B. Position of the humerus and scapula during subluxation. Note downward rotation of the scapula and horizontal motion of the humerus. (Reprinted with permission from Logigian, M. K. (1982). *Adult rehabilitation: A team approach for therapists.* Boston, MA: Little, Brown and Co.)

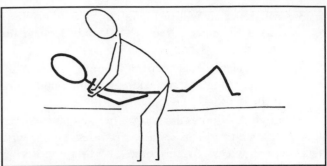

Figure 26-12. Scapular mobilization. The therapist moves the scapula through ROM by placing a hand over it, fingers on the medial border. The humerus is kept approximated in fossa so it works with the scapula as one unit. Supine. With a hand on the scapula and one under the axilla, the patient's arm relaxed by side, hand on abdomen, and keeping humerus and scapula together, passively 1. elevate and rotate upward, then depress and rotate scapula downward. 2. Protract and retract scapula by pulling and pushing on the medial border. (Reprinted with permission from Logigian, M. K. (1982). *Adult rehabilitation: A team approach for therapists.* Boston, MA: Little, Brown and Co.)

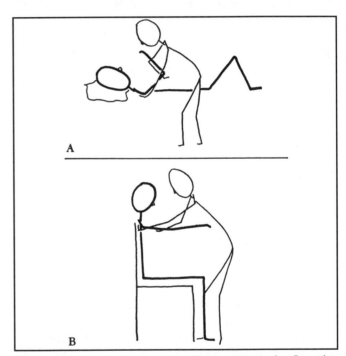

Figure 26-13. A. Supine. B. Sitting. Passively flex the humerus, staying in the pain-free range. Elbow may remain flexed or be extended. Mobilize the scapula through the following ranges: 1. Protraction and retraction using hand on the medial border while passively pulling the humerus and scapula together, forward, and back. 2. Rotate upward using a hand on the medial border and inferior angle of the scapula and increasing flexion of the humerus (it is important for humerus and scapula to work together). 3. With the humerus in abduction, rotate upward, retract and protract the scapula. Increase humeral range as tolerated. (Reprinted with permission from Logigian, M. K. (1982). *Adult rehabilitation: A team approach for therapists.* Boston, MA: Little, Brown and Co.)

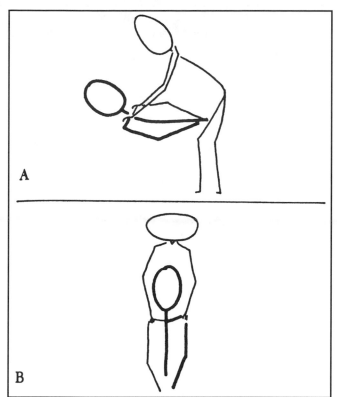

Figure 26-14. Scapula elevation (shrugging). A. Supine. B. Sitting. Active assistance to elevation; tapping on the upper trapezius; resistance to active elevation; quick stretch of the upper trapezius; associated reactions by resisting the sound side; combinations of above. (Reprinted with permission from Logigian, M. K. (1982). *Adult rehabilitation: A team approach for therapists.* Boston, MA: Little, Brown and Co.)

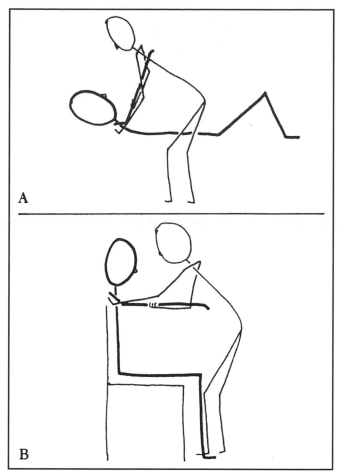

Figure 26-15. Scapula protraction and upward rotation. A. Supine. B. Sitting. With scapula placed in protracted position, the patient is asked to "hold," "reach arm forward," or "make arm longer"; quick stretch to scapula protractors then actively assisted through protraction (feel for catching reaction), giving resistance to protraction. (Reprinted with permission from Logigian, M. K. (1982). *Adult rehabilitation: A team approach for therapists.* Boston, MA: Little, Brown and Co.)

The OT saw Mr. Callahan daily for 30 minutes to provide an upper extremity mobilization program that included facilitation techniques to encourage movement and sensory awareness of the left side. Mr. Callahan demonstrated a reduction of shoulder subluxation and improvement in scapular and humeral motion. As a result, it was decided that Mr. Callahan would discontinue using a sling when ambulating.

Although Mr. Callahan was making progress in his OT program and he and his wife were anxious for him to return home, he was extremely concerned about his ability to return to his weekends at his oceanside home. These concerns were shared with the OTA while working in the kitchen with Mr. Callahan. The OTA discussed this with the OT, and it was decided that a family team conference be held to develop a plan. At the conference, which was attended by Mr. Callahan and his family, as well as all team members, it was decided that the OTA would make a home visit to the vacation home with Mr. Callahan to determine accessibility. The social worker would investigate the option of having an aide go with Mr. Callahan to the vacation home each weekend. As Mr. Callahan was not able to drive a car due to his visual deficits, the aide would need to drive them to the ocean home.

The home visit was useful, as an exact layout of the kitchen and living area was determined that enabled suggestions to be made for several environmental changes to enable maximum mobility. The house had only one step into it and one step up from the kitchen to the living room. A railing was recommended for the entrance to the house and living room. The master bedroom and bath were near the living room and kitchen. Toilet rails and a shower chair were recommended for the bathroom. The kitchen was spacious and had adequate counters to allow Mr. Callahan to slide objects from the refrigerator to the stove. All of the adaptive equipment Mr. Callahan had been using was suggested for installation in the kitchen.

Following the home visit, the team and family decided that Mr. Callahan would be discharged by the end of his fourth week in the subacute program. Thus, during this final week, Mr. Callahan spent 1 hour each day in the kitchen practicing his one-handed techniques in final preparation for making his famous sauce. Two days prior to discharge, he invited the OTA, OT, and his wife to the OT kitchen for a pasta feast with his homemade sauce. He took great pride in preparing it independently.

Mr. Callahan was discharged home with his wife at the time anticipated by the team. He was able to arrange for an aide to accompany him to his vacation home on weekends and resumed his cooking activities on a regular basis. The OT note at discharge included a statement on the progress he made, as well as indicators for follow-up care. It was suggested that Mr. Callahan continue his upper extremity mobilization program twice a week for 6 weeks as he was continuing to make gains in this area. A follow-up phone call 1 week after discharge found that Mr. Callahan was receiving a mobilization program at an outpatient ambulatory clinic near his suburban home.

CLINICAL PROBLEM-SOLVING

If Mr. Callahan had been younger, he would need to return to work to support his family. If this had been the case, what would you have done to assist him with this situation?

A work site visit would be useful to make suggestions for modifications. One-handed techniques for office activities, such as a telephone holder and use of a computer for written communication, can make return to work easier. In addition, the OTA could suggest office modifications to enhance accessibility, such as removal of carpets and positioning of a desk and chair to allow ease of movement.

Mr. Callahan had a great deal of difficulty accepting that his left arm was non-functional. What would have happened if he had refused to accomplish his ADLs utilizing one-handed techniques and adaptive equipment? A family team conference could be useful to discuss the situation with all involved, making compromises about what activities Mr. Callahan would accomplish independently with devices and those for which the family agreed to provide assistance. For example, a clean, neat shave was important to Mr. Callahan and no matter how hard he tried he could not accomplish it to his satisfaction. Perhaps his son could shave him with the understanding that Mr. Callahan would bathe and dress himself.

REFERENCES

Acquaviva, J. (1996). *OT practice guidelines for adults with stroke.* Bethesda, MD: AOTA.

Chang, L. H., & Hasselkus, B. R. (1998). OTs' expectations in rehabilitation following stroke: Sources of satisfaction and dissatisfaction. *Am J Occup Ther, 52*(8), 629-637.

Health Care Financing Administration. (1996). *Medicare intermediary manual, Publication 13, Section 3906.4.* Washington, DC: U.S. Government Printing Office, 21-21.

Kelly-Hayes, M., & Paige, C. (1995). Assessment and psychologic factors in stroke rehabilitation. *Neurology, 45*(Suppl. 1), S29-S32.

Logigian, M. K. (1982). *Adult rehabilitation: A team approach for therapists.* Boston, MA: Little, Brown and Co.

Van Dyck, W. R. (1999). Integrating treatment of the hemiplegic shoulder with self-care. *OT Practice, 4*(1), 32-37.

A Homemaker and Volunteer with Parkinson's Disease

Chapter 27

Kathryn Melin Eberhardt, MAEd, COTA/L, ROH

INTRODUCTION

Parkinson's Disease (PD) was first described in 1817 by James Parkinson, a British physician who published a paper on what he called "the shaky palsy." In the early 1960s, researchers identified a fundamental brain defect that is a hallmark of the disease: the loss of brain cells that produce a chemical called dopamine, which helps direct muscle activity. The four primary symptoms are:

1. Tremors of the arms, legs, jaw, and face
2. Rigidity or stiffness of the limbs and trunk
3. Bradykinesia or slowness of movement
4. Postural instability or impaired balance and coordination

PD occurs when certain nerve cells, or neurons, in the substantia nigra die or become impaired. Normally, these neurons produce a brain chemical known as dopamine. Dopamine is a chemical messenger responsible for transmitting signals between the substantia nigra and the next "relay station" of the brain—the corpus striatum—to produce smooth, purposeful muscle activity. Loss of dopamine causes the nerve cells of the striatum to fire out of control, leaving patients unable to direct or control their movements in a normal manner. Individuals who have PD have a loss of 80% or more of dopamine-producing cells in the substantia nigra. The cause of this cell death or impairment is not known. This disease is both chronic, meaning it persists over time, and progressive, meaning its symptoms grow worse over time. PD is a disease of late middle age, usually affecting people over the age of 50. The average age of onset is 60 years. However, physicians have been reporting more cases of "early-onset" PD in the past several years, and some have estimated that 5% to 10% of patients are under the age of 40.

KEY CONCEPTS

- Etiology of Parkinson's disease (PD): All factors involved in PD, including nature and course of the disease.
- Instrumental activities of daily living (IADLs): Home management, community living, health management, safety management, and environmental hardware.
- Proprioceptive neuromuscular facilitation (PNF): Therapeutic technique that helps initiate a proprioceptive response.
- Considerations for exercise and activity: Use of exercises and activities unique to the symptoms of persons who have PD.
- Home program: Exercises and activities to be completed at home, usually after discharge from OT treatment.

ESSENTIAL VOCABULARY

Akinesia: An abnormal state of motor hypoactivity or muscular paralysis.

Bradykinesia: General loss of spontaneous movement.

Dopamine: A chemical messenger, deficient in the brains of patients who have PD.

Dysarthria: Difficult and poorly articulated speech, due to poor muscle control.

Festination: A symptom characterized by small, quick forward steps.

Micrographia: Abnormally small writing.

Postural instability: Impaired balance and coordination.

Progressive resistive exercises (PRE): Increases the strength of a weak muscle by gradually increasing the resistance against which the muscle works.

Proprioceptive neuromuscular facilitation (PNF): Therapeutic technique that helps initiate a proprioceptive response.

Substantia nigra: Movement control center in the brain where loss of dopamine-producing nerve cells triggers symptoms of PD.

There are many theories about the cause of PD. Researchers have reported families with apparently inherited PD. Until recently, however, the prevailing theory held that one or more environmental factors caused the disease. Severe Parkinson's-like symptoms have been described in people who took an illegal drug contaminated with the chemical MPTP and in people who suffered a particularly severe form of influenza during an epidemic in the early 1990s. Studies of twins and families where PD is common have suggested that some people have an inherited susceptibility to the disease that may be influenced by environmental factors (Miller & Keane, 1992; National Institutes of Health, 1998; National Parkinson Foundation, 1998).

In 1997, the National Human Genome Research Institute (NHGRI) reported strong evidence that a gene on chromosome 4 can lead to PD in some families. The NHGRI research suspects that the abnormal gene may account for only a small portion of the total number of PD cases. The researchers also say that PD may be one of a group of neurodegenerative disorders in which the body's normal cell mechanisms for breaking down protein go awry. This deficit then leads to the accumulation of debris that clogs brain cells, eventually becoming severely disabling and ultimately deadly to these cells. Another possibility may be some kind of environmental insult or toxin that twists the protein into an abnormal shape and blocks normal protein breakdown (National Institutes of Health, 1998; National Institute of Neurological Disorders and Stroke, 1998).

SIGNS AND SYMPTOMS OF PD

PD affects about 50,000 Americans each year, with more than half a million Americans affected at one time. PD strikes men and women in almost equal numbers and it knows no social, economic, or geographic boundaries. PD does not affect everyone in the same way. The disease can progress quickly in some patients and is more insidious in others (National Institutes of Health, 1998; National Parkinson Foundation, 1998).

PD has been characterized in three common stages. In stage 1, the disease is mild with signs of slowing and tremor. The duration of this stage is from onset to 4 years. In stage 2, the disease is moderately severe. The duration of this stage is 5 to 10 years from onset. By stage 3, the disease has exceeded 10 years from its onset and has become severely involved (Lazaruk, 1994). Tremors are one of the major symptoms of PD, however, many other symptoms are just as troublesome. The following are the major symptoms associated with PD.

- Tremor—The tremor typically takes the form of a rhythmic back-and-forth motion of the thumb and forefinger at three beats per second. This is some-

times called "pill-rolling." Tremors usually begin in the hands and are most obvious at rest, especially during the first stage; this may also be described as non-intention tremors. The tremors often disappear during sleep and improve with intentional movement (Miller & Keane, 1992).

- Rigidity—In PD, rigidity is apparent in response to signals from the brain; the delicate balance of opposing muscles is disturbed. The muscles remain constantly tensed and contracted so that the person aches, feels stiff, and/or weak. The rigidity can be classified as ratchet-like, jerky movements called "cogwheel" rigidity or no movement, called "lead-pipe" rigidity (Miller & Keane, 1992).

- Bradykinesia—The slowing down of movements, which causes a slowness of initiating and executing movements. Fine motor deficits and difficulty in performing repetitive movements are common problems with this symptom (Miller & Keane, 1992).

- Postural instability—Impaired balance and coordination causes the individual with PD to develop a forward or backward lean and to fall easily. When balance is disturbed from the front or when starting to walk, the patient with a backward lean has a tendency to step backward, which is known as retropulsion. This deficit can cause stooped posture in which the head is bowed and the shoulders droop (Miller & Keane, 1992).

- Festination—Walking in rapid, short, shuffling steps. This symptom is also a leading cause of falls with persons who have PD (Miller & Keane, 1992).

- Akinesia—The term given to impaired ability to initiate voluntary and spontaneous motor responses. It is characterized by the interruption of performance of an ongoing movement or "freezing" when attention is distracted (Miller & Keane, 1992).

Other symptoms observed in some persons with PD can include:

- Small, cramped handwriting (micrographia)
- Lack of arm swing
- Decreased facial expression (hypomimia)
- Lowered voice volume (dysarthria)
- Feelings of depression or anxiety
- Episodes of feeling "stuck in place" when initiating a step ("freezing in place")
- Slight foot drag
- Increase in dandruff or oily skin
- Less frequent blinking

- Urinary problems or constipation
- Sleep problems
- Difficulty with swallowing and chewing

MEDICAL MANAGEMENT

At present, there is no cure for PD. However, a variety of medications and treatments are available to provide dramatic relief from the symptoms. Levodopa (L-Dopa) is the most commonly prescribed medication for relief of the symptoms of PD. Levodopa helps to replace the missing dopamine levels in the brain. In persons who are very severely affected, various kinds of brain surgery have been effective in reducing symptoms. These include pallidotomy (excision or destruction of the globus pallidus) and implantation of an electrical stimulator to counteract the effects of the loss of dopamine-producing cells. Another surgical procedure is the transplantation of healthy dopamine-producing tissue into the brain (National Institute of Neurological Disorders and Stroke, 1998; National Parkinson Foundation, 1998).

Rehabilitation management by a treatment team consisting of the physician as well as the occupational, physical, and speech therapists can do much to assist the individual who has PD to achieve maximum occupational performance.

FRAME OF REFERENCE

Rigidity and akinesia produce a stiff individual who is limited in active movement. Proprioceptive neuromuscular facilitation, or PNF, techniques such as chopping, lifting, and unilateral diagonal patterns may assist in improving trunk mobility, which will assist in overall functional movement. Since PNF techniques lend themselves to functional tasks, they allow the individual with PD to complete the performance skills necessary to be independent and at the same time assist with the difficult mobility problems that affect these persons. Rapid, rhythmical movements are most appropriate for remediation of the mobility deficits seen in this diagnosis. PNF patterns could be set to music to assist in fluency of movement and create more automatic and purposeful smooth movements. Rhythmic initiation is used to improve the ability to initiate movement. This technique involves passive rhythmic motion, followed by active motion. Once again this technique is used during functional activities to assist in fluid movement and to allow for independence in various performance components (Newman, Echevarria, & Digman, 1995).

CASE STUDY

Elizabeth is a 65-year-old woman who has been admitted to a skilled nursing facility from the local hospital after being admitted for medication adjustment for the treatment of PD. Elizabeth is married with two grown children and two grandchildren. She is a full-time homemaker who volunteered at the local hospital gift shop 2 days a week. She was diagnosed with PD 5 years ago and was well-managed up until the past 2 months, when her symptoms became much more intense and she was unable to function independently at home. She was admitted to the hospital to re-evaluate her medication and is now responding well to the new regimen, but has suffered setbacks due to her immobility for the past several months. Elizabeth demonstrates a moderate resting tremor with consistent cogwheel rigidity. She requires moderate assist for all self-care activities and mobility due to her fair standing balance with symptoms of akinesia. Elizabeth's active movement is limited due to her rigidity, and her coordination skills are fair due to her resting tremors. She expresses great concern regarding her personal self-care and has verbalized how depressed she feels that her husband must assist her in her personal self-care skills. Her goal is to return home with her husband and to be able to take care of her own needs. Elizabeth lives in a raised ranch home with a two-step entrance to the home. Her husband and children are very supportive and are willing to assist her as necessary. Elizabeth was referred to OT by her attending neurologist, who prescribed evaluation and treatment as needed.

OT Evaluation and Assessment

Evaluation

The evaluation process must focus on the performance deficits seen in the individual who has PD. The OT determines the performance deficits that the person exhibits and then chooses the evaluative procedure for each deficit. Commonly used evaluations include ROM, muscle tone, righting reactions and other automatic postural movements, speed and accuracy of voluntary movements, coordination, cognitive skills, and functional performance in daily living tasks. Other areas of concern may be addressed based on the individual and possible multiple diagnoses. The OT performs the evaluation(s) and, after demonstrating service competency, the OTA may assist in the assessment process. Various standardized assessments are available to determine performance deficits and the OT/OTA team together will decide which assessments are necessary and who will be performing them. State regulations may dictate the role of the OTA in the evaluation process. The OTA must be aware of the legislation that pertains to his or her practice and adhere to those standards (AOTA, 1995).

In Elizabeth's case, the evaluation began with a initial interview. During the initial interview, the OTA explained the role of OT to Elizabeth and began obtaining some information that was identified on the standard evaluation form for the facility. The OTA asked about the architecture of her home, emphasizing the stairs, kitchen, and bathroom layout, as well as the characteristics of other rooms. The OTA inquired about what type of assistance she has at home for the performance areas of shopping, laundry, and heavy cleaning. Other questions focused on her goals, knowledge of her disability, and awareness of her prognosis. After the initial screening, the OTA organized all of the data and reported back to the supervising OT. The OT then analyzed the screening data to determine the appropriate assessment to be completed and conferred with the OTA as to the delineation of the assessments. In this case, the OT identified the following areas of evaluation: ADL and IADLs, sensorimotor components, and psychosocial components. Before conducting the evaluations, the OT discussed her concerns with the OTA and explained the other areas in which she wanted the OTA to focus, such as using her observational skills during the evaluation to further assess Elizabeth's functional motor skills. Because the OTA had demonstrated service competency, the OT felt comfortable delegating the following assessments: ADL and IADL skills, upper and lower extremity status, fine and gross motor coordination, and strength and endurance during the ADL/IADL assessment.

OTA Assessment

The OTA began by having Elizabeth fill out a structured interview form that gathered additional data about her family history, self-care abilities, school and work history, and her leisure interests and experiences. The OTA performed the assessments in the following areas:

ADLs:
- Grooming
- Head/neck and oral hygiene
- Dressing: Upper and lower extremity
- Functional mobility: Transfer skills (bed, toilet, tub)
- Functional communication skills: Telephone and writing skills
- Balance and endurance while sitting and standing related to ADL skills

Upper and lower extremity status:
- Observation of A/PROM (active/passive) in functional ADL activities
- Testing of gross and fine motor coordination with standardized assessments

- Observation of strength and endurance during functional activities

After completing her evaluation, the OTA summarized the data and reported the findings to the OT. Together they discussed the OTA's findings and determined what additional assessment would be needed.

OT Assessment

The OT assessed Elizabeth's neuromuscular status, concentrating on A/PROM and the quality of movement to include tremors and rigidity. The OT performed a manual muscle test and noted that Elizabeth was not experiencing any pain or discomfort. When all the assessments were completed, the OT analyzed the data collected, documented the findings, and made recommendations regarding course of treatment. It was determined that Elizabeth was experiencing decreased AROM in the upper extremities, problems with gait, balance, and tremors that led to her lack of independence in ADL skills. Both the OT and OTA found Elizabeth to be motivated toward OT treatment and willing to work on her deficits. These findings were shared with Elizabeth, priorities were set, and a treatment plan was developed based on the overall OT findings and Elizabeth's needs.

General Goals

Upon completion of the formal evaluation, the OT and the OTA will confer and develop a problem list. This list must include the goals of the patient and/or significant others and the identified occupational role to which the individual will be returning or adapting. In general, the goals for individuals who have PD are as follows:

1. To increase mobility and prevent deformity
2. To improve initiation of movement and to increase the fluency of movement
3. To improve psychosocial status
4. To improve or maintain independent performance of daily life tasks
5. Improve ability to participate in leisure activities
6. Provide education and support to the patient and family (Ber, 1998; Newman et al., 1995)

In the case of Elizabeth, the OT and OTA began to develop long-term and short-term goals for a program of treatment to be carried out by the OTA. The main areas of concentration in treatment included the improvement of ADL skills, motor proficiency, improvement in general mobility and balance skills, investigate leisure opportunities, and education and adjustment to her disability. During this process, a discussion regarding Elizabeth's IADL skills should take place. These areas may not be applicable until Elizabeth has developed improved postural stability, increased mobility, and improved motor proficiency. However, Elizabeth's priority was to return to her former occupational role as a homemaker, so treatment activities should focus on these areas. In addition, goals regarding an ongoing home program should be addressed during the treatment planning process.

Treatment Precautions

One of the more dangerous symptoms of PD is the lack of postural stability. Ten to 15% of individuals who have PD also exhibit hypotension, usually caused by the medication Levadopa. The combination of poor postural stability and hypotension leads to a significant risk of falls. This must be taken into account during all mobility activities (Ber, 1998).

Treatment Activities/Techniques

The OT treatment for the individual who has PD is often developed on a trial-and-error basis. Since PD is unique to each individual and the response to medications vary for each individual, the course of treatment is dependent on the deficits of each individual and a combination of techniques to remediate the performance deficits. The maintenance of normal muscle tone and function is an important aspect of the treatment of PD. In part, the medication for this disease achieves this goal. However, to realize the full benefit of the medication, daily exercises and activity are essential. The following are suggestions based on the frame of reference noted earlier and common techniques that have worked with many individuals who suffer from PD. Each individual may react differently to these suggestions (Ber, 1998; National Parkinson Foundation, 1998; Newman et al., 1995).

Increase Mobility and Prevent Deformities

Rigidity and akinesia put an individual with PD at great risk of developing contractures and becoming deconditioned. A daily self-ROM program that includes rhythmical exercises is recommended. This program should be continued upon discharge from OT services. Family and/or significant others should be instructed in the home program as well as in the techniques of passive stretch if the individual has difficulty with completing the ROM exercises independently. Verbal cues and written instructions may be necessary for improved follow-through. PNF techniques, such as chopping, lifting, and unilateral diagonal patterns, may be beneficial for improving trunk mobility. These activities lend themselves to functional activities and should be incorporated in ADL and IADL tasks. Auditory commands, counting out loud, and music may be beneficial in improving the fluency of movement and assist with difficult mobility tasks, such as transfer training. Anticipatory activities such as balloon volleyball or catch are excellent activities

that can improve strength as well as postural stability and general mobility (Ber, 1998; National Parkinson Foundation; 1998, Newman et al., 1995). The Schenkman model suggests a progression of treatment within the treatment session and over time. The model is as follows (Christiansen & Baum, 1991):

1. Relaxation
2. Breathing exercises
3. Passive muscle stretching and positioning
4. AROM and postural alignment
5. Weight shifting
6. Balance response
7. Gait activities
8. Home exercises

Activities of Daily Living

Akinesia presents great challenges for the individual who has PD to complete occupational performance tasks. Issues of postural instability greatly interfere with ADL and IADL success. The use of adaptive equipment such as long-handled shoe horns, reachers, sock aids, and a dressing stick are helpful to eliminate bending for individuals who have poor balance. Feeding devices, such as built-up handles, weighted utensils and cups, scoop dishes, or plate guards, may assist in independent feeding for individuals with tremors and decreased hand function. Zipper pulls, button hooks, and Velcro closures can assist in dressing tasks for individuals with poor coordination and/or tremors. Safety issues must be addressed when dealing with bathroom considerations. Due to the high incidence of falls among individuals with PD, bathroom safety equipment will be most essential. The use of a tub bench or seat, non-skid mats rather than throw rugs, toilet frames, and possibly a raised toilet seat are most helpful. Individuals should be cautioned not to use towel bars, soap dishes, or sinks as mobility aids and should have grab bars professionally installed to ensure they are anchored in the wall studs. The use of toilet frames and tub grab bars can be commercially obtained without having to install grab bars on the wall. Family and/or significant others should also be instructed in the use of adaptive devices and equipment to ensure safety with all ADL skills at home (Ber, 1998; National Parkinson Foundation, 1998; Newman et al., 1995).

Communication

Individuals who have PD often have problems with dysarthria. The symptoms are usually described as a monotone voice and low speech volume. This is often due to poor vital capacity and postural difficulties. The OT intervention used most often is to teach deep breathing and postural control exercises. Also, counting out loud during all exercises or reading out loud has been successful in increasing communication skills. Singing is another activity that incorporates the rhythmical component of treatment as well as improving overall volume of speech. Because of the indication of micrographia, handwriting exercises encouraging large letter formation are helpful; if the individual becomes fatigued or the letter formation becomes significantly smaller, the activity should be discontinued. Use of built-up pens, markers, or felt-tip pens can assist with this deficit. Telephones with automatic dialing and large buttons may also assist communication for the individual with poor hand skills (Ber, 1998; National Parkinson Foundation, 1998; Newman et al., 1995).

Psychosocial Status

The individual who has PD faces several difficult issues regarding psychosocial skills. The absence of facial expressions, incidents of depression, impaired communication skills, and mobility deficits all contribute to social isolation. Lack of facial expressions and slowness of movement is often misunderstood for the individual not being interested in a conversation or being lazy. These misunderstandings can lead to continued social isolation especially if the individual has severely impaired communication and mobility. Family and/or significant others' education is key to avoiding these misunderstandings. Support groups for both the individual who has PD and for his or her family are paramount in battling stereotypes and misinformation. The National Parkinson Foundation offers support groups, literature, a web site, advice, and education regarding issues related to PD. The individual who has PD may also benefit from adult day treatment programs and group counseling. Providing an emotional outlet will assist the individual who has PD to successfully adjust to his or her disability (Ber, 1998; National Parkinson Foundation, 1998; Newman et al., 1995).

Leisure Skills

The disease process of PD often makes it difficult for individuals to participate in leisure skills. Adaptive devices such as card holders, craft frames, and adaptive board games are available to assist individuals with limited mobility and hand function. Exercise groups offered by local Parkinson Foundation support groups can become a new leisure opportunity. Local exercise activities, such as swimming and walking clubs, may also be helpful (Ber, 1998; National Parkinson Foundation, 1998).

Home Evaluation

A home evaluation is an extremely important component of the overall treatment program for an individual who has PD. The home evaluation is critical for safety because of the incidence of increased falls among these individuals. Individuals who demonstrate impaired mobility often have a shuffling gait, which prevents the individual from picking up his or her feet upon ambulation. This impairment can lead to significant safety concerns if the individual has carpeting and/or rugs in the home. It is imperative that scatter or throw rugs be removed and any carpeting that is loose should be removed or tacked down. Doorway thresholds may also be a problem and should be removed or altered to be flush with the floor surface on each side of the threshold. As mentioned earlier in this chapter, the use of adaptive bathroom equipment is recommended for safety. A firm mattress, chair, and sofa are necessary to assist with transfers. This furniture may be adapted by using a solid surface under the cushions. Also, the height of the furniture may need to be increased by putting blocks under the legs of the furniture. This will also assist in safe and efficient transfer skills. In the kitchen, the individual should consider the items used most often and place those items in easy-to-reach areas. Incorporating a push cart or purchasing a walker basket will assist in homemaking activities (Ber, 1998; National Parkinson Foundation, 1998).

Home Program

PD is known to be a progressive disorder and, as stated earlier, every individual responds to treatment differently. For these reasons a home program is essential to the maintenance of function. The home program should be initiated while the individual is receiving therapy services. The individual and family and/or significant others must understand the importance of continuing to remain active. These activities should be practiced during the treatment session with the family and/or significant others present. Written materials and possibly audio or visual tapes should be given to reinforce the home program. The home program should include exercises to maintain ROM, mobility, and postural stability. It may also contain suggestions for leisure skills, outside exercise activities, video list of appropriate exercise tapes, support group names and numbers, and any other information that would assist the individual to maintain his or her present status. The National Parkinson Foundation offers pamphlets regarding exercises and suggestions for several problems seen in PD (Ber, 1998; National Parkinson Foundation, 1998).

Treatment Implementation for Elizabeth

The following is a brief overview of Elizabeth's treatment program utilizing the theories and treatment techniques discussed in this chapter. The treatment plan was implemented by the OTA. Elizabeth was scheduled for the OT morning dressing program as well as two additional treatment times during the day. During the morning dressing program, the OTA focused on the use of a reacher, sock aid, and built-up handles for hygiene activities.

Elizabeth was successful with the use of the equipment and was also able to successfully manage her personal hygiene by utilizing a wash mitt and soap on a rope. The OTA also had Elizabeth complete a shower in the OT mock apartment. She was able to utilize a tub bench, extended shower hose, soap on a rope, and a long-handled bath brush. Elizabeth's husband was also trained in the supervision of Elizabeth and the appropriate equipment to install in their home prior to Elizabeth's return home. During the morning and afternoon treatment sessions, Elizabeth participated in ROM exercises, coordination activities, mobility/balance activities, and group discussions with other residents. Elizabeth was taught to complete self-ROM exercises and was given directions to begin her home exercise program. PNF patterns of chopping and lifting were incorporated into homemaking activities, such as filling and emptying the dishwasher, putting away groceries, and light meal preparation. Work simplification and energy conservation techniques were also incorporated into the homemaking activities. Elizabeth was given several worksheets to practice handwriting skills starting with shapes, progressing to printing, and then to cursive skills. This activity was also added to Elizabeth's home program. Elizabeth participated in group exercise programs, which included several anticipatory activities, such as balloon volleyball, football fling, and catch. During these activities, Elizabeth was encouraged to count out loud and each treatment session began and ended with deep breathing exercises. Elizabeth was exhibiting difficulty in using a standard cup for drinking due to her tremors. The OTA suggested a weighted cup and practiced with Elizabeth, who found it very beneficial.

Elizabeth also participated in a leisure skills discussion group in which she identified her leisure interests. During a treatment session, the OTA assisted Elizabeth in finding solutions to assist her in returning to her desired leisure skills. Elizabeth also discussed with the OTA her concerns regarding other individuals' reactions to her disability. The OTA suggested that a community outing may be helpful in practicing and anticipating how others would react to her. Elizabeth agreed and participated in a group outing. A follow-up discussion was helpful to Elizabeth and the other group members to discuss their feelings about issues related to architectural barriers, stereotypes of persons with disabilities, and other issues related to social interaction.

A home visit was completed 2 weeks prior to Elizabeth's anticipated discharge date. The OT, OTA, PT, social worker, Elizabeth, Elizabeth's husband, and her son were all participants in this visit. Elizabeth demonstrated her mobility skills by getting into and out of bed, a kitchen chair, the living room sofa, and the bathtub. Elizabeth's husband and son were directed in the type of supervision that was needed for Elizabeth and the home

program was discussed. Elizabeth also demonstrated her ability to prepare a light meal utilizing her utility cart and the skills learned in OT treatment. During this evaluation, it was noted that Elizabeth's sofa and bed were too soft, which made it difficult to be independent in mobility skills. Elizabeth's husband and son were given suggestions on how to remediate this problem. Architectural barriers were also discussed with Elizabeth and her family regarding the entranceway, discarding the throw rugs, and removing the carpet runners. Upon returning to the skilled nursing facility, Elizabeth continued to refine her mobility skills, coordination activities, ADL training, and homemaking activities. Elizabeth also continues to work on her home program daily.

Discharge Planning

Because of the progressive nature of this diagnosis, it is imperative that individuals with PD continue a regimen of exercise and movement. Referrals to the Parkinson's Association support groups, respite care, service agencies that provide attendant care and home management assistance, and local adult day care facilities are essential. In the case of Elizabeth, she began to attend support group meetings while in the skilled nursing facilities, and intends to continue going with her husband. Elizabeth's husband was given information regarding respite care and homemaker services. Both Elizabeth and her husband were instructed in the home exercise program and appear motivated to follow through with the activities. A written home program with diagrams and pictures was given to Elizabeth upon discharge, as well as several pamphlets from the National Parkinson Foundation.

CLINICAL PROBLEM-SOLVING

Taking the case of Elizabeth, what accommodations or additions to her treatment plan would you include in the following situations?

1. Elizabeth will be returning home alone, with minimal supervision from an elderly neighbor. What services could you recommend to assist Elizabeth? Where would you find these services? Who might you talk to first regarding these issues?

2. Elizabeth's husband is working full-time and is not available during the day to assist her. What community assistance is available during the day to assist Elizabeth and her husband?

3. Elizabeth is a 40-year-old female who is working full-time when she becomes unable to function without assistance. She has two teenagers and a husband who works full-time. What services may be helpful to Elizabeth? What would be your focus of treatment? What is Elizabeth's occupa-

tional role, and how would you assist her in returning to that role?

4. What recommendations/suggestions would you give to Elizabeth and her family regarding the process of aging and how it affects this disease? What should they expect? What is normal?

ACKNOWLEDGMENTS

This chapter was originally co-authored with Jovan E. Walker Jr., MA, OTR. His endless encouragement and dedication to the role of the OTA will never be forgotten. To my students, I give much thanks; they have always been a never-ending source of inspiration to me. Additional appreciation is offered to Jennifer Myler, MPH, OTR/L, for her endless support and encouragement and her editorial suggestions and modifications.

REFERENCES

AOTA (1995). Guide for supervision of occupational therapy personnel. *Am J Occup Ther, 49,* 1027-1028.

Ber, P. (1998). Degenerative diseases of the central nervous system. In M. B. Early (Ed.), *Physical dysfunction skills for the OTA* (pp. 481-484). St. Louis, MO: Mosby.

Christiansen, C., & Baum, C. (1991). *OT: Overcoming human performance deficits.* Thorofare, NJ: SLACK Incorporated.

Lazaruk, L. (1994). Visuospatial impairment in persons with idiopathic Parkinson's disease: A literature review. *Physical and Occupational Therapy in Geriatrics, 12*(2), 37-38.

Miller, B. F., & Keane, C. B. (1992). *Encyclopedia and dictionary of medicine, nursing, and allied health* (5th ed.). Philadelphia, PA: W. B. Saunders.

National Institutes of Health. (1998). *NIH researchers find Parkinson's disease gene.* Bethesda, MD: Author.

National Institute of Neurological Disorders and Stroke. (1998). *Parkinson's disease: Hope through research.* Bethesda, MD: National Institute of Neurological Disorders and Stroke.

National Parkinson Foundation. (1998). *The Parkinson handbook.* Miami, FL: Author.

Newman, E. M., Echevarria, M. E., & Digman, G. (1995). Degenerative diseases. In L. W. Pedretti (Ed.), *OT for physical dysfunction* (4th ed., pp. 745-747). Baltimore, MD: Williams and Wilkins.

A Retired Librarian with Sensory Deficits

Chapter 28

Paula W. Jamison, PhD, OTR

INTRODUCTION

Sensory Loss and Normal Aging

Vision loss related to aging is one of the most common disabling conditions affecting the elderly, ranking third after arthritis and heart disease (Warren, 1998). It often goes unmanaged, in part because it is often difficult to distinguish from the gradual sensory loss that accompanies the normal aging process. Natural changes most noticeably affect what have been called the distance senses—vision and hearing. The ability to see and hear makes it possible to explore and survey the world from afar, to scan a crowd for a friend's face, or hear an oncoming car on a dark street. Even partial loss of these abilities can have a profound effect on a person's sense of independence, restricting mobility both at home and in the community. Gradual disturbances in sight and hearing can also affect interpersonal relationships: it may become impossible to recognize a familiar face or hear a conversation. These impairments can have a significant impact on the quality of function in the older adult, who may additionally be suffering from other chronic or acute conditions. The OT and OTA working with older people need to be particularly alert to problems posed by vision and hearing loss.

Beginning in midlife, many individuals begin to experience visual impairments and deficits in hearing. During natural aging, the eye's ability to receive and process visual input is affected as the lens becomes less clear and the photoreceptor cells in the retina—the actual visual sensory receptors—decline in number. The eye also loses its ability to accommodate, or adjust its focus, as it moves from objects at a distance to those close at hand, such as reading material. This age-related deterioration of close-up vision is called presbyopia and occurs in most people (Schumer, 1997). By the ages of 50 to 60, most individuals require corrective lenses, at least for reading, and people who have worn glasses or contact lenses for years may now require bifocals.

Nighttime vision also becomes less reliable, as the eye no longer accommodates as well to dim light or glare. Even for otherwise healthy individuals, activities such as driving and reading may require special

ESSENTIAL VOCABULARY

Accommodation: Shifting focus between close and distant objects.

Cataracts: Clouding of the eye's lens; occurs naturally with aging.

Center vision: The central part of what one sees when looking straight at an object.

Continuous reading: Reading long passages, such as a book or magazine.

Diabetic retinopathy: Vision disorder associated with diabetes; can cause total vision loss if not controlled.

Glaucoma: Causes loss of vision when fluid pressure in the eye damages the optic nerve.

Macular degeneration: Incurable eye disorder; affects ability to see objects in center vision.

Ophthalmologist: Medical doctor specializing in the eye.

Optometrist: Medical professional specializing in the correction of vision.

Presbyopia: Loss of ability to see details at close range due to aging.

Scotoma: "Blind spots"; often occurs as a result of disease or injury.

Spot reading: Reading a few words at a time, such as a sign or label.

Visual fields: Areas/angles of vision that are seen without moving head or eyes.

KEY CONCEPTS

- Blindness: Refers to the eye's total inability to perceive light.
- Legal blindness: Legal, not functional, definition of vision problems developed to determine qualification for services.
- Low vision: A variety of conditions in which vision loss affects the ability to carry out daily activities.
- Vision rehabilitation: Refers to programs of training/adaptation to vision loss.
- Visual impairments: Any type of reduction in the ability to see.

adjustment; older adults may prefer not to drive in low-lighted conditions, such as on rural roads at night, or they may find that there is too much glare to read a magazine with glossy pages. Moreover, because their reaction times have slowed, joints are stiffer, and balance has become impaired, many older adults find themselves at increased risk of falling. As a result, they may also experience increased fear and anxiety about venturing out into the community, leading to a sense of isolation. Formerly pleasurable leisure activities such as reading or television may no longer be as satisfying.

Vision Loss

Older adults undergoing normal changes in vision and hearing are usually able to adapt to these losses, and in many cases corrective lenses or hearing aids may drastically improve their quality of life. However, more severe vision loss is also common among older people. In 1995, it was reported that over 16% of people 45 years of age noted moderate to severe visual impairments. Among adults who had reached the age of 75 or beyond, 25% stated they suffered from such problems (Warren, 1998). While OT practitioners have not traditionally reported serving large numbers of individuals with vision problems, vision loss touches the lives of approximately half of middle-aged and older adults, either directly or through a friend or family member (Warren, 1995).

Despite these large numbers, older persons with vision loss have been an underserved population. Many reasons contribute to this. First of all, for many people, vision deteriorates slowly, and changes in the ability to see are often difficult to pinpoint. One may have the perception that ability is still present. Because the eyes function together, and changes in one eye can often be compensated for by the other eye; people may become habituated to dimmer and fuzzier images on the television, for example. In addition, since most individuals began to experience changes in vision as a result of normal aging, many people—including health care professionals—fail to distinguish between normal, age-related visual impairments and disease-related vision loss.

It has been estimated that most older adults wait 5 to 7 years between the onset of vision problems and seeking rehabilitation (Warren, 1995). Delayed intervention means increasing possibilities for social isolation and such mental health issues as anxiety and depression, as well as needless loss of dependence. When vision loss is complicated by additional chronic medical problems, it is often overlooked or considered to be a factor that interferes with recovery or adaptation to new circumstances. Finally, while a variety of techniques and assistive technology devices are available to assist older adults in maintaining as independent a life as possible, the general public is largely unaware of available options.

How Vision Problems Are Defined

Specialists describe and measure vision in a number of different ways. Standardized terms have come into use to help everyone understand the varying degrees of vision loss. This type of uniform terminology is useful in helping professionals and lay people alike to understand levels of function and dysfunction, as well as to understand the standards applied that determine eligibility for services. For example, visual impairment refers to decreased visual ability as it impacts on daily activities and applies to a range of impairments, from total blindness at one extreme to partial vision at the other (Colenbrander & Fletcher, 1995). Table 28-1 lists the common classification of degrees of vision loss, along with accompanying problems with activities.

Low vision is a term used when an individual retains some amount of usable vision but is unable to carry out desired tasks because of impaired visual functioning. It is a broad term that refers to a wide range of disability. It has been estimated that approximately two-thirds of the people over 65 who suffer from low vision have at least one other chronic condition that interferes with function (Orr, 1992). However, even with the additional limitations in function resulting from low vision, most older adults with visual deficits continue to reside in their own homes and to live alone.

One measurable quality of vision is acuity, or the eye's ability to see details with clarity. Acuity is measured with a Snellen chart, the familiar eye chart that contains rows of letters or figures of decreasing size. Results are given in the form of a fraction. For example, an individual with 20/40 vision is able to see at a distance of 20 feet what a normal individual could see at 40 feet (Schumer, 1997). Low vision is defined as visual acuity of 20/70 in the better eye with the best possible correction. In addition, specialists also refer to the visual field, a term that refers to the area that the eye is able to see while remaining focused. People with low vision may also have a reduced visual field. Low vision may occur throughout the lifespan and does not necessarily lead to total vision loss or blindness (Colenbrander & Fletcher, 1995).

The individual with low vision still has some usable sight; however, he or she may require training in compensatory strategies or the use of adaptive equipment to function independently. Some forms of low vision, such as macular degeneration, may affect the individual's central or center vision (i.e., the ability to see objects straight on) (Mogk & Mogk, 1999). Other forms may affect peripheral or side vision. In addition to reduced visual acuity, low vision may cause problems with discerning contrasting images, impaired depth perception, difficulties with color vision, or the development of blind spots (scotomas) and field cuts that limit the angle of vision (Colenbrander & Fletcher, 1995). Other forms of low vision may be the

Table 28-1

Visual Impairment in Terms of Visual Acuity

Normal Vision	*(Snellen Chart)*
Range of Normal Vision	20/12
• Normal reading distance	20/20
• Normal reading performance	20/25
Near Normal Vision	20/30
• Normal reading using shorter	to
reading distance	20/60
Low Vision	*(Snellen Chart)*
Moderate Low Vision	20/80
• Near normal performance using	to
magnifiers, other aids	20/160
Severe Low Vision	20/200
• Slower than normal, with aids	to
• "Legal blindness," in the U.S.	20/400
Profound Low Vision	20/500
• Limited reading with aids	to
• Problems with orientation and mobility	20/1000
Near Blindness	*(Snellen Chart)*
Near Blindness	20/1250
• Vision unreliable	to
	20/2500
Total Blindness	No light perception (NLP)
• No vision	

(Adapted from Colenbrander & Fletcher, 1995)

result of cataracts, scarring of the cornea or retina, and cause overall blurred or distorted vision. However, the individual still has some ability to perceive light and may—depending on the services available—other contributing illnesses, and family and social support, be able to successfully adapt to this major loss (Warren, 1995). While low vision can affect people of any age, the older adult faces special challenges and conditions.

It is important not to confuse low vision with legal blindness, another phrase often used to describe persons with visual impairments. "Legal blindness" is used by the federal government to determine eligibility for government and agency services and benefits. A person who is legally blind has at best a corrected vision of 20/200 in the better eye or a visual field of 20 degrees or less

(Colenbrander & Fletcher, 1995; Mogk & Mogk, 1999). Often, individuals who experience low vision are not classified as legally blind. Until 1990, when Medicare guidelines were changed to include low vision as a physical impairment appropriate for rehabilitation, many individuals with vision loss did not meet the criteria of legal blindness and found it difficult to receive services (Warren, 1995).

THE FUNCTIONAL IMPACT OF LOW VISION

If normal vision loss requires management and adaptation on the part of the individual, low vision poses additional problems that require skilled intervention. At any age, vision loss can occur because of congenital, hereditary, or acquired medical conditions. Disabling conditions associated with aging, such as diabetes or stroke, contribute greatly to the incidence of low vision among the aging population. For example, each year thousands of adults become visually impaired as the result of strokes. It has been estimated that between 40% to 75% of persons who have suffered some type of neurological damage, either through stroke or injury, experience visual impairments that are serious enough to require special rehabilitation (Warren, 1995). Visual impairments often persist long after motor and cognitive function have been recovered and can continue to have a major impact on function (Warren, 1995).

Since most older adults have enjoyed normal or correctable vision throughout their lives, the changes they now experience may be a source of anxiety and frustration. Applying makeup or picking out matching socks becomes difficult, and finding lost objects, such as a dropped coin or bottle cap, no longer seems worth the bother. Previously enjoyable activities—playing cards, visiting with friends, reading, or sewing—become next to impossible. Friends and loved ones may respond with anger or concern because the person with low vision appears to ignore them by failing to greet them. It may become difficult to walk safely in low-lighted areas, such as restaurants, or to see the edge of a chair when the carpet beneath it is of similar color. It becomes increasingly challenging to see low lying tables and scatter rugs, and while it is still possible to move through familiar surroundings, venturing into the street or a shopping mall becomes difficult and anxiety-provoking.

With some conditions, the individual's ability to see may vary widely from day to day. On a good day, he or she may be able to read without difficulty or recognize a friend's face. The following day, these activities may be difficult or impossible, leading to acute feelings of frustration and problematic social interactions. Family and friends may find the older person's behaviors puzzling, and their reactions may further aggravate feelings of isolation or anger.

COMMON CAUSES OF LOW VISION IN THE ELDERLY

The most common causes of low vision in the elderly are cataracts, macular degeneration, glaucoma, and diabetic retinopathy. Strokes and injuries to the brain may also result in damage to vision.

Cataracts are the result of a continued clouding of the lens that may eventually make it impossible to see at all. Cataracts grow slowly and in most cases may be surgically removed and the lens replaced. Surgical techniques using lasers have made cataract removal a relatively simple and common procedure. Once the most common cause of blindness in the elderly, cataracts are now medically manageable for most people.

Age-related macular degeneration (ARMD) is an extremely widespread but as yet little understood degenerative condition causing scarring in the area in the center of the retina known as the macula. The result is the progressive loss of central vision. There is no cure, and vision losses of this type cannot be corrected. Individuals with ARMD experience problems with reading small print or seeing details, such as facial features, and find that their center vision becomes increasingly blurred. They may have trouble distinguishing between similar colors. Glare may pose a problem, due to the eye's inability to adjust to higher light levels, and night vision deteriorates. In addition, about 10% to 40% of individuals diagnosed with ARMD complain of what has been called "phantom vision," in which they see objects such as patterns of flowers that they know are not actually there (Mogk & Mogk, 1999). In cases of ARMD, however, the individual retains use of peripheral vision, and thus is able to detect objects on the edge of the visual field. Although ARMD is extremely distressing to the people who suffer from it, it does not lead to total loss of vision. Indeed, many times people with ARMD can learn to use eccentric viewing techniques, in which they use their peripheral vision to compensate for lost center vision. However, if the individual does not learn how to adapt, the results are limitations in the ability to perform ADLs, work, and leisure activities, which in turn have an impact on the individual's sense of independence and relationships with others.

Despite the fact that ARMD is the most widespread cause of low vision in the elderly, it is relatively little known. The reason for this lies in part with the gradual and painless onset of the condition. ARMD usually begins in one eye, and most people do not notice any troubling symptoms for a long time. Not only does the unaffected eye compensate for the loss, it is easy to make simple adaptations without noticing them, for example, by turning on an extra lamp because light levels no longer seem sufficient. Thus, an individual who has not had regular eye check-ups may not notice any changes in vision until the condition has progressed significantly. Sadly, one of the contributing factors to recognizing ARMD, as with other types of low vision, is hearing loss. People who have spontaneously used auditory cues, such as listening for a friend's voice, and lose this aid as their hearing deteriorates, may suddenly be confronted with the realization that they may have to learn to rely on other ways of interacting with friends and loved ones.

Diabetic retinopathy is a condition caused by diabetes, a disease that if left untreated has a profound effect on the body's circulatory system. The tissues of the retina become swollen and abnormal blood vessels develop, which can bleed or constrict, or lead to a detached retina. If detected in its early stages, and the underlying diabetes is controlled, laser surgery may be successful in repairing the damaged tissue.

Unlike ARMD, which affects only the center, or macula, of the retina, diabetic retinopathy can affect the entire retinal surface. Vision losses associated with diabetic retinopathy may disrupt both center and peripheral vision. If the underlying diabetes is not managed, diabetic retinopathy can lead to blindness. Vision may also fluctuate according to blood sugar levels if medication and diet have not been properly adjusted. In addition to blurred center vision, individuals with diabetic retinopathy may have difficulty in shifting focus from near to distance vision, and may experience a decrease in their color vision.

Glaucoma has been termed the most feared disease of vision. At the same time, it is the most preventable. Glaucoma is characterized by an increase in the pressure of the internal fluid of the eye, which can then damage the optic nerve, resulting in blindness. In the acute stage, it may be painful as a result of the increased intraocular pressure (IOP); however, the chronic state is usually painless. Regular eye examinations using a pressure test can provide early detection, and medication in the form of eye drops is successful in keeping the IOP under control. Individuals who have required frequent prescription changes to correct their vision, who complain of seeing halos around lights or mild headaches, or who find that their eyes have problems adapting to darkness may be experiencing symptoms of glaucoma and should be seen by an eye care professional immediately.

Vision loss due to neurological damage from strokes and head trauma can cause a wide range of impairments. Most common among these are diplopia, or double vision, and visual field cuts, such as homonymous hemianopsia, in which the temporal and nasal aspects of each visual field no longer appear to the individual. In addition, other visual impairments may be the result of brain lesions affecting the oculomotor nerves; as a result, for example, it may become difficult or impossible for a person to read because the ability to visually track, or follow a written line with the eyes without moving the head, has been lost.

OCCUPATIONAL THERAPY INTERVENTIONS

Service-Delivery Models

Older adults with vision problems can benefit from the skills provided by an OT and OTA. Traditionally, services for individuals with visual impairments are provided through the blind rehabilitation model. This includes government and community agencies established to help the blind or those with severe visual impairments. It was for this purpose that the term "legally blind" was adopted. Individuals whose impairments meet the specifications are eligible to receive training in such areas as orientation and mobility, which focuses on techniques and the use of equipment (e.g., the familiar white cane) or aids (e.g., guide animals) to determine position and move in familiar and unfamiliar environments. Training is also offered in communication skills, including, but not limited to, teaching the use of the Braille, a tactile system based on a grouping of six raised dots arranged in various ways to represent letters, numbers, and abbreviations. The overall goal of such programs has traditionally centered on providing the severely visually impaired with vocational skills and enough education to be self-supporting, independently functioning members of the community.

Programs devoted specifically to blind rehabilitation are found throughout the world. They include specialists who provide comprehensive rehabilitation and training and play a key role in helping countless numbers of individuals with severe visual impairments to live independently in a "sighted" world. In addition, service clubs and special organizations, such as the Lions Club and Lighthouse for the Blind, have dedicated their efforts toward fundraising and community-based activities to provide services for those who qualify.

The traditional blind rehabilitation model for service delivery has been of less immediate help to many of the elderly suffering from low vision (Warren, 1995). There are a number of reasons for this. First, in order to qualify for services, one has to be identified as legally blind. Many elderly who are experiencing gradual deterioration of their sight have severe functional limitations even though they do not qualify. Second, since the focus of blind rehabilitation services has been to prepare people for vocational and educational performance, older individuals, who may be retired, already disabled due to other conditions, or who are preparing to leave the workforce are a lower priority for services. Third, specialized blind rehabilitation programs are centralized. Many people living in small towns or rural areas find it impossible to travel the distances needed to participate in these programs.

Vision specialists in the health care field include ophthalmologists, who are physicians who treat diseases of the eye, and optometrists, who usually specialize in correcting vision with glasses and lenses. Until recently, these professionals primarily focused on treating correctable vision problems. Lately, increasing numbers of optometrists in particular have begun to turn their attention to providing assistance to individuals with low vision (Mogk & Mogk, 1999). They provide an important resource in communities without specifically defined vision rehabilitation programs. Increased help for elderly adults with low vision became available in 1990, when the Medicare guidelines changed to include visual impairment as a category eligible for rehabilitation services.

Services specially targeted at helping people with low vision are available from OTs and OTAs working in the medical model and now, increasingly, in community-based practice. As a result, OTs and OTAs have the opportunity to become more active in servicing clients with low vision. Their contributions are particularly valuable in teaching techniques for increasing functional performance of ADLs, such as grooming, dressing, feeding, home and money management, leisure activities, and community mobility.

OTs and OTAs who wish to devise and deliver a full spectrum of services to the person with low vision, particularly to teach reading and orientation skills, require specific training (Riddering, 1999). However, the skills that OTs and OTAs have in clinical observation, combined with their abilities to grade and adapt activities, make them uniquely suited to helping individuals adapt to vision and other sensory loss. As a general rule, OTs and OTAs working with older people should be especially aware of the potential for sensory problems in the aging population, even if these problems have not been formally diagnosed.

Frames of Reference

Professionals in the field of low vision specialize in vision rehabilitation. Like any other type of rehabilitation, vision rehabilitation focuses on developing an individualized strategy to teach the individual ways to compensate for his or her impairment (Watson, 1996). Vision rehabilitation can be a key component of the services provided to a person suffering from other chronic conditions, such as arthritis, heart or pulmonary disease, or diabetes. As in other forms of rehabilitation, the individual's needs and personal desires must be evaluated prior to treatment by means of a thorough assessment of his or her current abilities, along with problems with functional skills. Particularly when low vision is suspected, a home-site evaluation, ideally followed by training in the home, is crucial to understand and then make it possible for the patient to learn key strategies for adapting to the specific characteristics of the home environment.

Once the assessment has been completed, vision rehabilitation focuses on training individuals with low vision to use their remaining vision. The emphasis may be on ADLs, mobility, leisure, or vocational interests. Vision rehabilitation can also include adapting the patient's home environment, through the use of lighting, the removal of clutter, or providing high color contrast between furniture and carpeting to permit higher visibility. Vision rehabilitation may also include helping the client select appropriate household appliances, such as talking thermometers, or special adaptive equipment, such as special professionally fitted magnifiers or high-powered lenses for reading, and then offering training in their use (Watson, 1996).

The illnesses and dysfunctions associated with aging are often accompanied by other losses. People who are struggling with changes in their accustomed mobility, familiar leisure activities, work roles that may have to be abandoned, or the companionship of friends due to an inability to drive are responding to both physical and psychological stressors. Depression in particular is a risk. When an ongoing rehabilitation program focuses on the needs of the whole person, the regular one-on-one contact provided during OT allows OTs and OTAs opportunities to monitor crucial shifts in the patient's emotional state as well as changing physical abilities. In some communities, counseling and support groups especially designed to meet the needs of people with low vision are available. In addition to providing important local resources and encouragement to help people cope with the frustrations of learning new ways of carrying out familiar tasks, these groups offer emotional support and may help counteract the feeling of isolation so often experienced.

Other frames of reference that are particularly useful to the OTA who is treating an individual with low vision focus on the importance of occupation and its role in helping individuals adjust to the major life changes brought about by any physical, cognitive, or emotional dysfunction. The Model of Human Occupation stresses the creation of an environment in which it is possible for the client to regain feelings of competence and mastery. This model offers OTs and OTAs alike a way of organizing and grading meaningful activities, all the while keeping the patient's goals in mind. The professional also serves as a problem-solver and offers counseling, as client and professional cooperate to find the most workable solutions to problems in carrying out accustomed roles and activities. Likewise, although it has a slightly different emphasis, the Occupational Adaptation frame of reference looks at the client's interactions with his or her environment. Here the focus is on the client's adaptive responses. OT evaluation and treatment is aimed at fostering the achievement of a sense of mastery over these environmental challenges. In short, all of these frames of reference provide a way in which the client's unique personality, life history, and strengths and weaknesses can be taken into account in order to create a personalized plan of client-centered treatment. Overall goals focus on ensuring the safe performance of daily activities, including mobility, and either increasing or maintaining the ability to perform ADLs, leisure activities, and vocational tasks (Table 28-2).

Table 28-2

Principles of Low Vision Management of Older Adults

- Distinguish the effects of normal aging from the effects of disease

- View the older individual as a whole person

- Use teamwork: employ a multidisciplinary team approach

- Develop interventions that focus on the person's goals

- Improve quality of life by facilitating independence and meaningful activity

(Adapted from Watson, 1996)

TREATMENT PRINCIPLES

A wide range of adaptations have been devised to assist persons with low vision (for the following and other examples, see especially Mogk and Mogk, 1999; Riddering, 1999; and Warren, 1998). Some of the general principles that have found to be useful for individuals with little or no vision can be useful to people with low vision. For example, since people with low vision rely more on memory than fully sighted individuals, it is important to make the environment as predictable and uncluttered as possible. Organizing shelves with toiletries or medications in a logical way and always returning items to the same place makes self-care activities manageable. Keeping pathways clear inside the house decreases the risk of falling. For people with severely impaired vision, mobility techniques such as memorizing the number of steps into the house or the bus stops between home and one's destination can be useful. In addition, being able to locate landmarks using other senses, such as the smell of a bakery, may make it possible to move independently in the community.

Other principles of adapting to low vision focus on utilizing the patient's remaining vision to the maximum possible. Light levels must either be raised or adjusted to provide sufficient brightness but avoid glare. High contrasting colors can be used to make it possible to distinguish between the edge of a table, for example, and the floor beneath it. Printed materials can be magnified into a larger format, or optical magnifiers can be used. Adaptations that permit the user to employ tactile cues, such as folding money into different sizes according to denomination, are also useful (Table 28-3).

Specific Problems and Adaptations

A variety of techniques and equipment are available to permit individuals with low vision to maintain or increase their level of independence in the performance of self-care, home management, and money management tasks, to name a few. These can often be further adapted for individuals with special needs, which can vary according to the nature and degree of visual impairment. In addition, individual preferences and the presence of other chronic or acute conditions affect the selection of suitable, usable equipment. Older adults may be less receptive to high technology alternatives or unable to afford extensive outlays for new equipment, for example.

Self-Care

Many individuals with vision loss experience difficulties with once-simple tasks, such as seeing in the mirror to comb their hair, apply makeup, or shave. For people with moderate vision loss, changing the lighting may be sufficient. It is important to consider the possibility that glare is a factor; both brightness and the position of the lighting may need to be adjusted. It may also be necessary to position the patient's face closer to the mirror. Magnifying mirrors, sometimes with lighted frames, may also be useful. Tasks such as shaving, combing hair, or applying toothpaste to a toothbrush can be performed using tactile cues rather than relying on vision. Bathing can be made easier by using a wash mitt instead of a washcloth, and using soap on a rope may make it easier for the person to keep track of that slippery item. For safety in tub transfers, tub or shower areas should have non-skid surfaces, and bath mats should be either non-skid or eliminated.

Table 28-3

Resources for the Person with Low Vision

National Organizations
The following is a partial list of organizations serving individuals with low vision. Many national organizations also have local chapters.

- The Lighthouse, Inc. Information and Resource Caller Service. 1-800-829-0500.
- Foundation Fighting Blindness. 1-800-683-5551.
- National Association for the Visually Handicapped. 1-800-677-9965.
- U.S. Department of Veteran Affairs, Blind Rehab Services. 1-202-535-7637. (Also, contact the local VA hospital and ask for a Blind Liaison.)
- Association for Macular Diseases. 1-212-605-3719.
- Glaucoma Foundation. 1-800-832-3826.
- National Society to Prevent Blindness. 1-800-221-3004.
- United States Association of Blind Athletes. 1-719-630-0422.

Reading Materials, Audiotapes, etc.
- Library of Congress Talking Book Program. Free audiotapes of books, magazines, descriptive videos, and large print books. Contact local library or 1-800-424-8567.
- Choice Magazine Listening. Selected readings, free if person is registered with the Library of Congress. 1-515-883-8280.
- The Bibles Alliance. Free Bible on audiocassette. Several languages are available. 1-941-748-3031.

In addition, the American Printing House for the Blind offers free cassette tapes of *Reader's Digest* and *Newsweek* articles on tape. 1-800-223-1839. Many publishers have large type formats, and both books and newspapers, such as *The New York Times,* can be found on tape.

(Adapted from Riddering, 1999)

In keeping with the general principle of predictability, self-care products and medicines should be organized. Items should also be clearly marked, either with high-contrast, easy-to-read labels or with tactile cues, such as rubber bands, tape, or Velcro strips. For individuals who have learned simple Braille, labels can be produced either using a special stylus designed for that purpose or made on a computer using a special Braille printer. Avoiding clutter and using trays with built-in compartments can do much to make important items easier to find and use.

Eating and Food Preparation

Kitchen and eating areas should be assessed for sufficient lighting and be free of glare. It is helpful to have simple, unbreakable dishware in both white and dark colors to make it easier to see foods of different colors. Using the principles of high contrast is helpful. Plates and kitchenware should contrast with the surface underneath them, and this principle applies to serving food as well. It can be very difficult to see mashed potatoes served on a white plate, for example. Pouring milk into a dark mug may help avoid spills. When pouring cool or cold liquids, a finger can be placed inside the container to determine liquid levels; liquid level indicators are also available that beep when the cup or bowl is full. Liquids should always be poured over the sink or kitchen counter to avoid spills on the floor. Persons with extremely low vision may find it helpful to organize their plate using a clockface as a guide: peas are at 2:00, meat loaf at 6:00, etc.

Cutting should be done with care. Cutting boards should be available in white and dark surfaces to contrast with food. Many items are now available pre-chopped. Stoves and appliance settings can be marked with large print or tactile labels (using velcro dots, for example, on commonly used settings). Oven mitts should be used instead of potholders, as they provide better protection against burns. So-called spatter screens made of mesh that can be placed over cooking pots are available at most stores that sell household goods. Again, it is important to organize and label shelves. Salt shakers can be distinguished from pepper shakers by wrapping a rubber band around the salt shaker. Tactile cues are helpful when spreading margarine or mayonnaise on bread.

Clothing and Laundry

Many people with low vision experience difficulties seeing subtle variations in color and find selecting clothes difficult. Whenever possible, increase the lighting in closets, which again should be free of clutter and organized in an understandable and easy-to-use fashion. For example, clothes can be arranged so that like colors are hung together or outfits can be hung together on a hanger to prevent confusion. Safety pins placed on tags to color code clothing is another helpful idea. Using tactile cues can also be helpful in identifying items (e.g., socks of like colors can be marked with thread made into one or two knots near the top). Limiting one's wardrobe to two or three basic colors can also eliminate the need for much marking, guessing, and rearranging.

If laundering is done at home, efforts should be made to spot clothing immediately after a spill; stain remover sticks are useful for this purpose and are readily available at the grocery store. One way to check for stains is to use a scanning technique. This task should be carried out in a well-lighted area. To do this, the person mentally divides up the area of clothing being examined, then, just as one would mow a lawn strip by strip, makes a tactile or visual search (perhaps using a magnifying device) until the entire area has been covered (Watson, 1996). This is also a useful technique to use when looking for an item that has been dropped. The laundry area should be lighted and kept clean. Commonly used settings on the washer and dryer can also be marked with high contrast labels or tactile markings. Small hand-held magnifiers can also be used for reading dials and placed in a pocket when not in use.

Appliances and Safety Devices

Today, many simple and useful adaptations of common household items are available, often at local stores. Telephones may be purchased with large buttons and can be programmed to make dialing frequently used numbers simple and accurate. Thermostats embossed or printed with large, bold, and easy-to-read numbers can be found at large home supply stores. Clocks are available with faces printed in many sizes: digital displays may be difficult to read, however, as there is often insufficient contrast. Alarm clocks with alarms that can be adjusted to variable pitches or that have a vibration setting may be helpful for people who also have hearing loss. Alarms can also be connected to a lamp, to turn on the lights.

Reading and Writing

People who are adjusting to low vision may experience significant problems when reading. Professionals distinguish between spot reading, in which small amounts of information need to be visually processed, and continuous reading, where more lengthy amounts of text are read. Spot reading is necessary for reading labels, addresses, dials, pill bottles, or restaurant menus. For these short bursts of reading, hand-held magnifiers can be useful, as they can be easily adjusted for distance and do not need to be held for long periods of time. For continuous reading, which takes more time, stand magnifiers that rest on the page and can cover a whole line may be more practical. For people whose vision is less than 20/400, video magnifiers or closed circuit televisions (CCTVs) may be most useful for both spot and continuous reading.

As mentioned previously, individuals with severe visual impairment may also be trained to read simple Braille, which is useful for labeling medicines or storage bins, for example. High contrast labels made with felt markers can also be used for people with more moderate impairments.

Leisure

A number of adaptations and pieces of equipment can be used to make handwriting easier and more legible. Contrast between ink and paper should be maximized, which can most easily be done by writing with a black felt-tip pen on white paper. Dark lined paper or a dark guide sheet can be used as a guide for handwriting. In addition, big-print check registers, checks, calendars, and date books are all available. For those who use computers, some adjustment to the monitor may be all that is necessary to make items on the screen more visible. Purchasing a larger monitor will increase the text size by up to 40%. Otherwise, software programs are available that can enlarge the text on the screen up to 16 times the normal size. Before suggesting the purchase of any new hardware or software, however, make sure that the software is compatible with the computer in use and that there is enough space on the hard drive and enough memory (RAM) to store the program. Often the state's commission for the blind or department of rehabilitation offer advice to consumers and even opportunities for computer demonstrations and training.

As many older people are likely to be retired, leisure pursuits are important. Many of the principles mentioned in the earlier sections also apply to leisure. For example, cooking or reading may be a hobby, as well as an ADL. Transportation may be an issue for the older adult with sensory deficits, and the OTA should have a complete understanding of the activities the person finds meaningful in both ADLs and leisure. Connecting the client to town services such as Dial-a-Ride or senior citizen transportation services may be appropriate. If the client prefers not to use transportation services outside the family, then the OTA should investigate leisure interests that keep the older person connected to friends and family.

OTHER SENSORY LOSS

In the United States, approximately 25% to 40% of the population over age 65 is estimated to have a hearing impairment (Strouse, DeChicchis, & Bess, 1997). While the joint occurrence of severe visual and hearing loss is relatively rare, older people with visual impairments are also susceptible to hearing losses brought about by the normal aging process. Sensitivity to high frequencies normally begins to diminish in midlife, affecting the ability to detect higher pitched sounds. As a result, it may become difficult for individuals to hear women's voices yet still be able to hear the ranges of a male voice. Individuals who may benefit from using "talking" books and products should order them with male voices, as these may be more easy to hear and understand.

Not all types of hearing loss can be corrected with hearing aids. Moreover, these devices, while extremely useful to some individuals, do not restore "normal" hearing. It is usually necessary to learn how to screen out normal background or ambient noise, as all sounds are amplified to the same degree. Without proper fitting and training, many older adults abandon their hearing aids or turn them off, finding the noise level confusing and unhelpful. Moreover, in situations with large amounts or high levels of background noise, many hearing aids are not practical. Newer, more expensive models now may contain gain controls, which automatically dampen the amplification level when noise reaches a certain volume or can even selectively amplify the frequency levels (pitches) where losses have occurred. However, even users of such devices may have to go through an adjustment period to learn how to use the device properly.

Many people with hearing loss related to nerve damage are unable to be satisfactorily fitted with a hearing aid (Weinstein, 1997). Compensatory strategies can be useful in preventing social isolation and other loss of function. When communicating with individuals with residual hearing loss, the following strategies can be useful:

- Eliminating competing background noise makes it possible to focus on what is being said.
- Pitch may be as important as volume: lower pitches are generally more easily heard than higher frequencies.
- If more than one speaker is present, speak in turn.
- Speak slowly and clearly, and avoid unfamiliar words.

Devices to ensure safety in the home for individuals who are experiencing the loss of both vision and hearing are particularly important. Alarm systems, such as smoke detectors, may have to be modified to set off a flashing light, such as a lamp. Telephones for the hearing impaired are also available; telephone devices for the deaf (TDD) are systems requiring a special device that holds the receiver and transmits and receives typed messages. If an individual is able to read using a magnification system, these adaptations can be useful. Appliances and equipment that provide auditory cues can sometimes be adapted by varying the pitch and volume. Additionally, people who experience loss of both vision and hearing must rely increasingly on the so-called near senses—touch, movement, taste, and smell.

When older people are away from home, explicit identification is an important safety precaution. Persons with visual impairments may require a white cane, typically associated with low vision, as an aid to navigation as well as a means of identifying them to others. Carrying a laminated card with important information, including blood type, known allergies, and emergency contact information can be vital in providing needed attention in case of an accident or illness. Elderly persons with specific impairments or physical conditions (e.g., diabetes, heart conditions, or allergies) may wish to wear Med-Alert bracelets or pendants containing this information. Furthermore, monitoring systems are available for use in the home. These range from devices that permit the monitoring of health conditions, such as respiratory failure, sleep disorders, cardiovascular function, or falling, to simple push-button pendants that can be used to notify designated friends or neighbors in case of an emergency.

CASE STUDY

Louise is a 76-year-old former librarian who has a history of falling, cardiac disease, and hypertension. She is taking several medications and uses at least two inhalers for asthma and bronchial problems. Her husband died a year ago, and she is currently living alone in the house that they shared for more than 40 years. Her oldest daughter lives in the area and has been concerned because she believes that her mother is losing her ability to take care of herself—her personal hygiene appears to have deteriorated and the house is increasingly untidy and dark. The daughter also states that her mother has been withdrawn, frightened, and unwilling to communicate— "She doesn't seem her old self. She's not getting Alzheimer's, is she?"

Two weeks ago Louise fell again and fractured her right hip. She has made a good physical recovery, but the medical team has expressed concern about Louise being able to manage on her own. However, since her daughter has offered to stay with Louise, she is being discharged to her home from inpatient rehab. She will receive home health visits from physical therapy and OT, and the OTA will be providing most of the OT treatments.

The OT evaluation included assessments of ADLs and cognitive abilities as well as clinical observations and functional testing. Results confirmed the health care team's suspicion that Louise was having difficulties with center vision, even with her glasses, and that she demonstrated some hearing loss as well. Based on this information, the physician recommended a vision check, which revealed ARMD in her right eye. This condition, which had been undetected (it had been 6 years since Louise had been to the eye doctor), had progressed to the point that Louise was unable to read, watch television, or go outside the house safely alone. A hearing exam revealed that Louise had moderate loss in the higher frequency ranges. Louise's cognition was within normal limits for her age; however, Louise was prescribed an antidepressant to reduce symptoms of anxiety and social withdrawal.

While the OTA working with Louise had begun by reviewing techniques for lower extremity dressing and reinforcing hip precautions during tub transfers, it became clear that in the morning Louise was unable to identify clothing and self-care items by sight. She was also having difficulties identifying and managing her medications, especially the inhalers that she used for her asthma.

The OTA assisted Louise in developing a system to sort her clothing by colors and attach identifying markers that Louise could use. All of her blue outfits were coded by putting two small safety pins on the labels, green had one. Using a simple eccentric viewing technique, Louise was able to read very large print; her medications were labeled and stored where she could see them more easily. Because she used the inhalers so often, they were distinguished by winding several layers of tape around the one she used most frequently, so she could easily determine it by touch. With the assistance of Louise's daughter, brighter lighting was brought into the house, in most cases by choosing lightbulbs with higher wattage. Simple white and black plastic dishware replaced the pastel floral pattern Louise had used before, to make it possible for her to see what she was eating. Louise qualified for Meals on Wheels, which meant that her need to prepare her own meals was kept to a minimum, and her daughter took care of the laundry.

In addition to removing all scatter rugs, Louise's daughter put bright yellow tape on the edges of all the chairs she used, which provided a contrast with her dark green carpeting. Although Louise began to demonstrate increasing ability to dress herself and move through the house safely, she continued to voice concerns about her loneliness and fears of falling. OT sessions began to focus on improving Louise's leisure skills and encouraging her

to be in touch with friends. Card games with large format playing cards were attempted, but Louise, who had been receptive at first to the idea, was clearly bored. Although Louise had loved to read, she was frustrated trying to use a magnifier, and on more than one occasion threw the book across the room. The OTA had suggested that Louise's daughter check out talking books from the library, but Louise resisted the idea, saying she could not concentrate. She insisted on keeping the television on but did not seem to be paying any attention to it. Neither Louise nor her daughter followed up on any recommendations for local support groups or to take part in activities at the local senior center. Louise was able to meet her goals for independence in upper and lower extremity dressing, bathing, and grooming. However, she was unable to adapt her old leisure skills to her reduced level of vision and hearing.

CLINICAL PROBLEM-SOLVING

Despite her expressed concerns about loneliness, she resisted participating in activities that took her outside of the house or placed her in contact with other people of her age group. What are some other ideas you could use to address Louise's problems with her leisure activities?

As you work with Louise, it becomes clear to you that she is having difficulties hearing you. What are some techniques that you could use to communicate with Louise? How would you change her treatment activities? Considering leisure, other than the magnifier, which Louise has difficulty using, are there any kinds of adaptive or specialized equipment that she might use?

Based on her response to treatment, do you think Louise is still depressed? Why or why not? What is your role as an OTA in addressing this problem? You notice the smell of alcohol on Louise's breath one day when you are working together and are concerned that she may be drinking too much. What would you do?

After spending part of a treatment session with Louise in the kitchen, you have concerns because she leaves the gas burner on after removing the tea kettle. How do you respond? How can you explain her behavior when her cognitive performance was within normal limits on her assessment?

SUMMARY

People who suffer from low vision find that their lives are affected in multiple ways. OTAs play a crucial role by providing skilled interventions that make it possible to regain a lost sense of independence and dignity or maintain current levels of functioning. For the older adult, the adaptation process may be particularly difficult. Cognitive changes, such as the onset of mild dementia, may interfere with the learning of new habits or the ability to use memory and other mental organization techniques. Even in cases where independent function cannot be achieved, however, the use of adaptations for low vision—such as tactile cues or large-print formats—can enable the older client to take part in self-care activities and make communication easier. These interventions can help diminish the sense of isolation and helplessness that often intensifies the pain of coping with the chronic and progressive conditions that may accompany aging. It is important to remember, however, that like any other rehabilitation process, adapting to low vision and hearing loss requires a great deal of energy and concentration on the part of the elderly client. Successful adaptations are most likely to occur when the client is able to focus on his or her personal goals and not those of family members, peers, or even clinicians.

REFERENCES

Colenbrander, A., & Fletcher, D. C. (1995). Basic concepts and terms for low vision rehabilitation. *Am J Occup Ther, 49,* 865-869.

Mogk, L. G., & Mogk, M. (1999). *Macular degeneration: The complete guide to saving and maximizing your sight.* New York, NY: Ballantine Books.

Orr, A. L. (1992). Aging and blindness: Toward a systems approach to service delivery. In A. L. Orr (Ed.), *Vision and aging: Crossroads for service delivery* (pp. 3-31). New York, NY: American Foundation for the Blind.

Riddering, A. T. (1999). *Low vision rehabilitation: An introduction.* Paper presented at the meeting of the Michigan Occupational Therapy Association, Mackinaw Island, MI.

Schumer, R. A. (1997). Changes in vision and aging. In J. Higginbotham, & R. Lubinski (Eds), *Communication technologies for the elderly: Vision, hearing, and speech* (pp. 41-70). San Diego, CA: Singular Publishing Group.

Strouse, A. L., DeChicchis, A. R., & Bess, F. H. (1997). Changes in hearing with aging. In J. Higginbotham, & R. Lubinski (Eds.), *Communication technologies for the elderly: Vision, hearing, and speech* (pp. 103-128). San Diego, CA: Singular Publishing Group.

Warren, M. (1995). Providing low vision rehabilitation services with OT and ophthalmology: A program description. *Am J Occup Ther, 49,* 877- 884.

Warren, M. (1998). *OT practice guidelines for adults with low vision.* Bethesda, MD: AOTA.

Watson, G. R. (1996). Older adults with low vision. In A. L. Corn, & A. J. Koenig (Eds.), *Foundations of low vision: Clinical and functional perspectives* (pp. 363-394). New York, NY: American Foundation for the Blind.

Weinstein, B. E. (1997). Hearing aids and older adults. In J. Higginbotham, & R. Lubinski (Eds.), *Communication technologies for the elderly: Vision, hearing, and speech* (pp. 129-159). San Diego, CA: Singular Publishing Group.

A Married Couple Dealing with Alzheimer's Disease

Chapter 29

Carolyn M. Baum, PhD, OTR/C, FAOTA

INTRODUCTION

Alzheimer's disease robs the mind of its capacity to make decisions and carry out activities that define the individual. OT offers a client-centered, occupational performance-oriented approach to the person and family as they build the strategies to live their lives. This chapter will provide information for the OTA to employ with persons with cognitive loss, and although it will focus on Alzheimer's disease, the strategies presented will be helpful in interacting with clients or patients who are experiencing cognitive problems or cognitive decline (e.g., multiple sclerosis, Parkinson's disease, stroke, head injury, schizophrenia, and learning disabilities).

Dementia of the Alzheimer's type (DAT) is a progressive, degenerative, and devastating disease for which there is no cure. *The Diagnostic and Statistical Manual of Mental Disorders* (DSM-IV) (American Psychiatric Association, 1994) characterizes DAT by memory loss, impaired abstract thought and judgment, and abnormalities in higher cortical function with resulting personality changes. As it progresses, the disease increases impairment in cognitive function, reflected in deterioration of the ability of the individual to perform tasks and interact socially with family and others.

For centuries, senility was viewed as an inevitable consequence of old age. Only within the past 20 years have doctors applied the medical diagnosis of DAT (Ramsdell et al., 1990). The search for a cure has spurred families overwhelmed by the consequences of the disease to demand action from Congress, which responded by allocating monies for research and services (Fox, 1989). Currently, 7.5% of the population over 65 have DAT (Gurland, 1985).

KEY CONCEPTS

- Brain functions: In Alzheimer's disease, the brain atrophies and loses functional connections, which impairs the nervous system's ability to process the sensory information it receives from the environment.

- Brain dysfunction: An individual with Alzheimer's disease becomes unable to process information, access memory, utilize language, and perform motor acts.

- Function and behavior: Baum (1993) found that individuals who remained engaged in activities displayed less difficulty with dressing, feeding, bathing, and grooming and had fewer occurrences of disruptive behaviors.

- Caregiver roles: For individuals to remain engaged in activities as the disease progresses, it is necessary for the caregiver to compensate for the planning and organizational deficit and memory loss. Family members derive satisfaction from providing care when the caregiving activities are predictable and controllable (Kinney & Stephens, 1989).

ESSENTIAL VOCABULARY

Agnosia: The inability to recognize objects and/or people.

Aphasia: Absence/impairment of the ability to communicate through speech, writing, or signs.

Apraxia: Form of brain damage that results in a motor planning deficit.

Clinical dementia rating: Staging instrument that categorizes the level of the disease experienced by the patient.

Declarative memory: Memory for general knowledge.

Episodic memory: Memory for personal episodes or events that have contextual reference.

Occupation: Meets the individual's needs for self-maintenance, expression, and fulfillment. (See Figure 29-1.)

Procedural memory: Knowing how to perform an activity.

Prospective memory: Difficulty remembering what to do.

Semantic memory: Memory of facts.

Short-term memory: Working memory, holds recent events.

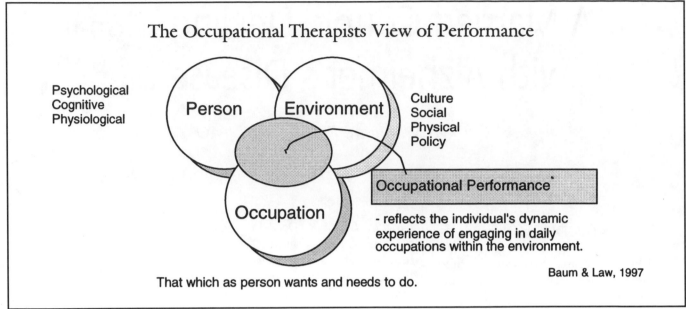

Figure 29-1. Conceptual framework. (Modified from Christiansen and Baum 1991,1997; Law, Cooper, et al. 1996.)

The prevalence rises to over 20% in individuals over the age of 80 (Magaziner, 1989). These percentages apply to the current elderly population of 34.9 million, rising to 65.6 million by the year 2030 (American Association of Retired Persons, 1988), and establishes DAT as a major societal problem.

The family, as the primary caregiver, is faced with the functional, behavioral, and neurological problems of the person with DAT, often without having access to treatment because DAT is not a diagnosis that requires acute medical intervention, therefore, they and their families are not given access to many institutional-based rehabilitative services. Community programs must emerge to help families learn to manage the problems associated with neurological deficits.

Cognitively impaired persons experience anxiety and display disrupting behaviors that may be related to their diminished ability to process information to perform instrumental, self-care, and social activities. Such behaviors may be indications that the person with cognitive loss is bored or not able to do what he or she wants or needs to do. It can be posited that if the caregiver can set up and support the environment to keep the impaired person engaged in a routine of activities, the effort could potentially minimize the disruptive behaviors of his or her loved one and reduce his or her stress.

OTs and OTAs play a critical role in helping families acquire the knowledge and skills to support their loved one's behavior as they strive to maintain dignity and engage in activities. There is consensus that activity is important to maintain cognitive and physical health (Almli, 1992; Christiansen, 1991; Fidler & Fidler, 1963; Kielhofner, 1992; Lawton, 1990).

ALZHEIMER'S DISEASE AND ITS FUNCTIONAL PROGRESSION

The brain processes information and organizes behavior. In DAT, the brain atrophies and loses functional connections, which impairs the nervous system's ability to process the sensory information it receives from the environment. Persons with DAT often have primary sensory impairments (visual, olfactory, gustatory, auditory), as the key centers of the brain that interpret information do not allow the person to create appropriate responses. This means that his or her vision, taste, smell, and hearing may be impaired, complicating his or her ability to participate with others.

Cognition is the process by which sensory input is transformed, reduced, elaborated, stored, recovered, and used (Duchek, 1991). Since behavior is dependent on sensory input, DAT interferes with the individual's performance. As the disease progresses, the individual with DAT becomes unable to process information. People experience losses in the their ability to access memory, use language, and perform motor acts (Baum et al., 1988). The loss is demonstrated when the person has trouble carrying out tasks of daily living and interacting socially. He or she also has difficulty in solving problems (Baum et al., 1993; Edwards & Baum, 1990).

DAT has been thought to be a deficit of memory. Memory is a problem, however, and individuals can exhibit many different neurological deficits. These deficits are not always present, and if they are present, they may be displayed differently in different stages of the disease. This means that a person with DAT requires accurate assessment to determine the extent of the deficit and how it contributes to the person's occupational performance.

People with Alzheimer's disease may display the following:

- They may not be able to discriminate facial expression or voice tone qualities (Allender & Kaszniak, 1989; Eslinger & Damasio, 1986). This can explain why people have difficulty recognizing staff and family. If someone were to change his or her glasses or hair color or style, the person with DAT would not be able to recognize him or her.

- Aphasia may limit or obscure the person's ability to comprehend or express language (Faber-Langendoen et al., 1988). Just because someone cannot speak, it does not mean he or she cannot communicate. A speech pathologist can help identify successful strategies, such as having the person read—some people have difficulty initiating speech, and sometimes just starting a story will help them speak.

- Agnosia is an even greater difficulty for families as a person's inability to recognize objects and/or people is impaired (Mendez et al., 1990). People who cannot recognize objects need labels on the items and need a helper to be sure they have the right tool for the task they are trying to accomplish.

- Organized or purposeful movements are often difficult due to apraxia (Edwards et al., 1991). Families have great difficulty with apraxia, not understanding how the person can do some things and not others. Families sometimes think persons with apraxia are willful and difficult until they understand that the inability to move is a brain deficit.

- Impairment also exists in problem-solving, judgment, organization, and sequencing due to frontal and temporal lobe damage (Baum & Edwards, 1993; Sullivan et al., 1989). These functions are basic to people who are able to engage in activities. When these deficits exist, the person needs a caregiver who can get them started on tasks.

- Memory is affected in persons with DAT. Short-term memory is the memory that holds recent events prior to the event being stored. Persons with DAT cannot retain items in short-term memory. This is why you never want to ask a person with DAT "What did you have for breakfast?", "Was your daughter here this morning?", or "What did the announcer say about the weather?"

- Long-term memory is more complex; it can also be used if you can figure out strategies to tap it. Episodic memory is memory for personal episodes or events that have contextual reference. You can often trigger episodic memory with stories, pictures, and smells. Semantic memory is the memory for facts. It is difficult to tap semantic memory unless the person has extensively used information in their daily life. Some persons retain information about birds or flowers, or other categories of knowledge. Declarative memory is memory for general knowledge and is not often preserved. Prospective memory is the memory that we use to remember *what* to do. This is impaired in DAT, yet it is amenable to adaptive strategies and cues. The final type of long-term memory is procedural memory. This type of memory is knowing *how* to do something. We most often think of procedural memory when we think about how we know how to ride a bike, even though we have not done it since childhood. If we know what the person has done in the past, we can tap their procedural memory to perform tasks and activities that he or she could not do if it required new learning.

A FRAMEWORK FOR ASSESSMENT

Occupational Therapy Evaluation

Information to frame treatment must be collected from both the person with the impairment and the caregiver. Because treatment involves training of the caregiver to construct opportunities for the person to stay engaged in occupational tasks, it is important to have a clear picture of the pattern of the person's deficits, a history of interests and activities, and the expectations and skills of the caregiver. Figure 29-2 presents a model to guide the assessment process. Each of the instruments included in the model is described below.

The Kitchen Task Assessment (KTA) (Baum & Edwards, 1993) requires the person with DAT to make a cooked pudding from a mix. It allows the clinician to administer a standardized measure without employing an artificial task. The KTA is a valid and reliable measure that can be used as a clinical as well as a research tool because it discriminates the performance of individuals across all stages of the disease. It records changes in the person's performance in initiation, organization, sequencing, incorporation of all steps, safety and judgment, and task completion. The information gained from the administration of the KTA can be used by the clinician to train the caregiver to assist the impaired individual in daily living tasks. The person must be directly observed in the performance of the task. The test takes approximately 15 minutes.

The Functional Behavior Profile (FBP) (Baum et al., 1993) is a reliable and valid assessment that documents the caregiver's observation of the task, social, and problem-solving behaviors of a person with DAT. The FBP can help the caregiver focus on the presence of productive behaviors useful in managing the impaired person. When used with the KTA, it helps the clinician understand how the caregiver sees the capabilities of the person with the impairment and how that might differ from the responses that the therapist can elicit from the impaired person with the appropriate level of cueing. It can be completed in checklist or interview format.

The Activity Card Sort (ACS) (Baum, 1993) is a card sort of 61 activities including 13 instrumental, 36 leisure, and 12 social activities identified by older adults as activities they typically do. Using this assessment, it is possible to calculate the person's previous and current level of engagement in activities from the information provided by the caregiver. The ACS gives the clinician information about the interests, activities, and hobbies of persons to use in planning care. It can be completed in card sort or checklist format.

The Memory and Behavior Problem Checklist (MBPC) (Zarit & Anthony, 1986) reports the problems identified by the caregiver in managing the person with cognitive impairment. The instrument has two sections: one documenting the presence of the behavior and the second documenting the caregiver's tolerance for the behavior, if it is observed. In addition to recording the presence of disturbing behaviors, such as wandering, rudeness, losing things, and not recognizing others, it also reports the help needed to perform basic and instrumental tasks of daily living. The instrument can be completed in interview or checklist format by the caregiver and provides information that can help the clinician help the caregiver.

The Zarit Burden Interview (Zarit & Anthony, 1986) reports the burden experienced by the caregiver in managing the person with cognitive impairment. It includes questions that address both demand and emotion-focused stress. Demand stress involves issues such as time for self, dependency, access to resources, and social life. Emotion-focused stress addresses issues such as guilt, anger, fear, and embarrassment. The instrument is completed in interview or checklist format by the caregiver.

A FRAMEWORK FOR INTERVENTION

Baum (1993) found that individuals with DAT who remained engaged in activities displayed less difficulty with dressing, feeding, bathing, and grooming and had fewer occurrences of disruptive behaviors. Some have suggested that caregivers should be given formal or informal support with tasks such as bathing and dressing (Miller, McFall, & Montgomery, 1991; Vitaliano et al., 1986). Help with the self-care tasks alone would not alleviate the caregiver's stress, as the stress is related to the disturbing behaviors, not the frequency with which help

The Occupational Performance Assessment	
Person Factors	The Kitchen Task Assessment (Baum & Edwards, 1993)
	The Functional Behavior Profile (Baum & Edwards, 2000) (Baum, Edwards, et al. 1993)
Environment Factors	The Memory Behavior Problems Checklist ((Zarit & Anthony, 1986)
	The Zarit Burden Interview (Zarit, Reever, et al. 1980)
Occupation Factors	The Activity Card Sort (Baum 1995, Baum & Edwards, in press)

Figure 29-2. Model to guide the assessment process.

is required in self-care. Some disturbing behaviors may surface during dressing and bathing tasks, particularly if the tasks are presented at a level beyond the impaired person's capability. Figure 29-3 describes relationships that can guide OT intervention.

For individuals to remain engaged in activities as the disease progresses, it is necessary for the caregiver to compensate for the planning and organizational deficit and memory loss. The caregiver must be taught how to provide the organizational strategies and memory supports that the person with the impairment can no longer provide for him- or herself. Productive behaviors in the form of instrumental, leisure, and social tasks become the mechanism to minimize the disturbing behaviors. To minimize disturbing behaviors, activities important and meaningful to the person must be organized into routines that are consistent from day to day.

Family members derive satisfaction from providing care when the caregiving activities are predictable and controllable (Kinney & Stephens, 1989). Using this explanation, the caregiver would not be stressed by the actual tasks of caring, but by the unpredictability of the occurrence of disturbing behaviors.

The following is a description of the changes that occur in the individual's performance as the disease progresses. The following is also a summary of the performance reported by the caregiver on the FBP (Baum et al., 1993) and staged using the Clinical Dementia Rating (Berg, 1988).

During the earliest stage of the disease, the individuals usually are appropriate in activities and can do what they

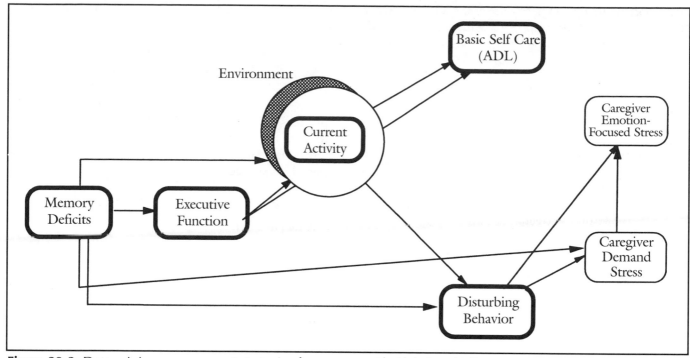

Figure 29-3. Determining management strategies for persons with Alzheimer's disease.

are asked to do if the instructions are simple. They usually perform activities without frustration and in a reasonable time frame. They may need encouragement to begin a task. It is impossible for persons to learn a new complex activity, but they can perform complex tasks that are over-learned without assistance. The caregivers begin to face problems at this level. One problem concerns the person's ability to drive. Additional problems involve the ability to manage money and maintain relationships.

In the mild stage of the disease, individuals remain appropriate in activities and independent in grooming and hygiene. They can independently do a simple task; however, they often need encouragement to begin the activity and will do better if the tools and supplies they need are placed at the point of use. They need assistance in doing more complex tasks (those with multiple steps).

The next stage of the disease (moderate) is very problematic for the caregiver, as the impaired person can no longer perform any activity without either verbal or physical assistance, meaning that the person cannot be left alone. Impaired persons can still identify familiar persons, and their behaviors are usually appropriate.

In the severe stage, persons cannot do anything for themselves. Often individuals are in nursing homes but for many reasons (costs ranging from $24,000 to $40,000 per year being just one), a substantial number remain at home. Individuals in this stage can still carry out a response to a one-step command. However, the request must take into consideration their physical capabilities. Specific verbal guidance must be provided to

elicit every movement. If you were feeding a person with DAT, you would have to say, "Here, hold this bread. Put it to your mouth. Open your mouth. Take a bite. Chew." The important thing to remember is even though the person appears quite disabled, he or she still has a social need to be part of his or her family social unit and enjoys being a part of interactions (Baum et al., 1993).

Cognitively impaired persons experience anxiety and display disrupting behaviors that may be related to their diminished ability to process information to perform instrumental, self-care, and social activities. Disruptive behaviors include aggressiveness, outbursts, assaultiveness, wandering, disturbed sleep, incontinence, agitation, insecurity, decreased responsiveness, decreased cheerfulness, irritability, selfishness, crudeness, sexually inappropriate behavior, suspiciousness, the hiding of objects, and repetitive actions (Buckwalter, 1990; Rabins, Mace, & Lucas, 1982; Sinha et al., 1992; Swearer et al., 1988). Such behaviors may be indications that the person with cognitive loss is bored or not able to do what he or she wants or needs to do. It can be posited that if the caregiver can set up and support the environment to keep the impaired person engaged in a routine of activities, the effort could potentially minimize the disruptive behaviors of his or her loved one and reduce his or her stress.

OTs and OTAs play a critical role in helping families acquire the knowledge and skills to support their loved one's behavior as they strive to maintain dignity and engage them in activities. There is consensus that activity is important to maintain cognitive and physical health (Almli, 1993; Christiansen, 1991; Fidler & Fidler, 1963; Kielhofner, 1992; Lawton, 1990).

OCCUPATIONAL THERAPY PRINCIPLES GUIDING TREATMENT

OT offers guiding principles that are basic to developing and implementing a client-centered program for people with cognitive loss.

- An individual's performance results from the relationship between that individual and the specific environment in which the activity occurs (Bronfenbrenner, 1979; Christiansen, 1991).
- Engagement in activity makes it possible for individuals to influence their own physical and cognitive well-being (Csikszentmihalyi, 1988; Fidler & Fidler, 1963).
- There is a dynamic interaction among the biological, social, and environmental factors that underlies the individual's capacity for performance in instrumental, leisure, and social activities (Almli, 1993; Kielhofner, 1992; Lawton, 1990).
- Individuals whose activity is within their capabilities do not demonstrate anxiety or boredom related to the task (Csikszentmihalyi, 1988).

Problems Experienced by Individuals with Cognitive Deficits

Most individuals with cognitive impairment have predictable behaviors associated with their deficits. The following are common, however, nothing should substitute for assessments that focus on the client's and the caregiver's needs as a treatment plan is developed.

- Difficulty with awareness—They have difficulty making insightful statements, and it is particularly difficult to modify behavior..
- Poor impulse control—They have difficulty thinking before acting.
- Poor short-term memory, although long-term memory is well-preserved.
- Perseveration—They often display inappropriate and repetitious behaviors.
- Difficulty initiating and organizing tasks.
- Difficulty recognizing objects, people, and sounds.
- They present safety problems for family and themselves.
- Changes in their sensory systems limit vision, they do not smell as well, and they do not have

the same level of taste, making food not as appetizing.

TREATMENT STRATEGIES

The social science and occupational science literature provides guidance to practitioners with general strategies to teach the family members of the person with the cognitive loss. The strategies in Table 29-1 have been determined to be effective.

General Strategies to Support Occupation

The following specific strategies can be used by the OTA to help the family member acquire the understanding and skills to help his or her loved one maintain independence.

- Build a consistent schedule, build routines around activities he or she has previously enjoyed.
- Do not expect new learning; perform activities that have been previously overlearned.
- Speak with the person about issues that he or she will hold in long-term memory, as he or she will not be able to store more recent events (e.g., Did you have a nice visit with your daughter yesterday? What did you have for breakfast?)
- Play music from the person's era, not current music.
- Use strong lighting.
- Create contrast on surfaces.
- Avoid distractions, work in a quiet environment.
- Alter recipes to give them more spice or herb flavor.
- Engage the family in care so they can learn cueing skills and see their loved one perform successfully.
- Find activities that couples can do together.
- Do not expect caregivers to do things for which they need skills.
- Talk openly about the issues of driving and refer the family member to resources.

Environmental Strategies

- Organize daily activities (occupations) into a consistent pattern.
- Build a message center in the home. Post a weekly schedule and specific daily schedule at the center.
- Provide choices in menu items, activities, and clothing.
- Construct memory books, and ask for the help of the children and grandchildren.

Table 29-1
Treatment Strategies

Strengthen remaining capacity of person with impairment	Averbuch & Katz, 1992; Baum & Edwards, 1993
Keep them active & involved	Burns & Bruell, 1990; Corcoran, 1994; Dougherty & Radomski, 1993; Oakley, 1993; Zarit & Anthony,1986
Practical advice to carer	Baum & Edwards, 1991, 1993; Cohen et al., 1984; Corcoran, 1994; Vitaliano et al., 1986; Dougherty & Radomski, 1993; Haley et al., 1987; Oakley, 1993; Quayhagen & Quayhagen, 1988
Organization of a schedule	Baum, 1993; Cohen et al., 1984; Corcoran, 1994; Dougherty & Radomski, 1993; Oakley, 1993
Organization of the environment	Baum, 1992; Dougherty & Radomski,1993; Oakley, 1993; Toglia, 1992; Zarit & Anthony, 1986
Exercise	Baum, 1992; Quayhagen & Quayhagen, 1988
Maintenance of interpersonal relationships	Cohen et al, 1984; Corcoran, 1994; McDonald, 1978; Motenko, 1989
Family included in care plan	Clipp & George, 1990; Cohen et al, 1984; Corcoran, 1994; Dougherty & Radomski, 1993; Quayhagen & Quayhagen, 1988
Training in communication skills	Bourgeois, 1993; Quayhagen & Quayhagen, 1988; Rabins et al., 1982

- Pets are great companions and offer a temporal aspect to the day.
- Keep patterns of church attendance or visiting with friends.
- Go to the same restaurant to maintain familiarity with surroundings and menu.
- Continue walking or exercise programs.
- Build a work station. Create a stable environment with tools and items needed to do a task.
- Lay out clothes or items that will be used in a task.
- Continue activities that offer socialization.
- Enroll in a support group (for both the client and caregiver).
- Attend a work-oriented day program.
- Teach the family to engage the person in activities even if he or she is not capable of interacting.
- Help the family choose activities to do together so that socialization is maintained.

Some individuals in the early stage of the disease are able to use self-instruction strategies. These are suggested by Sholberg and Mateer (1989).

- Verbalize out loud each move and the reason for the move before and during execution of the task.
- Whisper rather than verbalize out loud.
- Talk to yourself during the task.
- Switch tasks and repeat the preceding steps.

Note: Generalizations occur only after direct extended training using real-life situations. With an individual with DAT, only activities that have been previously performed can be used, as the potential for new learning is very limited.

Self-Instruction Interventions

- Make lists (gauge improvement on the completeness of the list).
- Proceed with verbalization sequence (above).
- Time management training (Sholberg & Mateer, 1989).
- Time estimation—estimate time it will take as part of planning.
- Creating time schedules, generate a plan for the activities to be accomplished.

- Execute a plan within scheduled time constraints.
- Calendar, day planner.
- Schedule, have a schedule center in home.
- Post-it notes.

Most persons with DAT require compensatory interventions. Usually the compensatory strategy is provided by the caregiver, aides, and attendants who often fulfill that role and require training. Interventions that are compensatory include:

- Person directed by another person (Luria, 1963).
- Organize the setting.
- Build a daily schedule to foster daily routines.
- Help families learn why their loved ones have difficulty initiating and organizing tasks and activities, and teach them how to cue and organize environments for successful interactions.

Individuals with DAT have lives to live (some live 15 years from the time of diagnosis), as do those who are providing care. The OTA is a key professional to help families learn how to manage their loved one, and how to manage without disrupting the lives of the family.

The ideas presented in this chapter seem intuitive and simple. They are not. Families who are experiencing the behavioral changes of their loved one have a hard time recognizing the behaviors as a neurological problem. Deficits such as agnosia, apraxia, and memory are complex neurological problems, and families have no context to understand them. They know their loved ones are acting differently and making demands on them. The OTA can have a major role in helping them understand that their loved one's behavior in not willful but a plea for help to make sense out of experiences that are too complex or too fast for them to process.

The following case is presented to highlight how effective strategies can help family members manage their loved one with mild stage DAT. A person in the mild stage of the disease was chosen because OT intervention can make a difference in helping the family manage these individuals at home.

CASE STUDY

Meet Mr. and Mrs. Johnson

For several years, Mr. Johnson, age 63, had been having difficulties that his family found out of character. He misplaced things, would miss appointments with his plumbing clients, became lost when driving and got frustrated, and frequently lost his keys. He had always been responsible for keeping his company books. Mrs. Johnson took him to the geriatric clinic after the bank talked to her son-in-law about problems with the business account.

On medical examination, there appeared to be no other medical explanation for the symptoms. There was no evidence of hypothyroidism, vitamin B-12 deficiency, or other potentially reversible causes of dementia, such as severe hypertension, stroke, kidney, or heart disease. Additionally, there was no evidence of drug abuse or psychiatric illness. The physician gave the Johnsons the diagnosis of probable Alzheimer's disease and referred them to the social worker and OT. Additionally, she gave them a packet of information about services available through the Alzheimer's Disease and Related Disorders Association.

Social History

The Johnsons have a strong marriage. Each had their own interests and together they shared their family, church, bowling, and camping interests. They raised three children, two of whom lived within six blocks of their parents. Mr. Johnson finished high school and completed an apprenticeship as a plumber. He worked for a company for 35 years before it closed. For the past 10 years, he managed a small plumbing company with his son-in-law. His wife is a secretary in the chemistry department at a small private college. She is 61 years old and in relatively good health. Since she began a low fat, sugar-free diet and a daily walking program, she had brought her blood sugar under control and lost 25 pounds.

Occupational Therapy Assessment Results

Mr. Johnson displayed no evidence of apraxia, and previous neuropsychological testing had not revealed aphasia nor agnosia. He did have some facial masking which made it difficult for family to read his emotional status. The physician team had identified his level of impairment as CDR (Clinical Dementia Rating) 1 (mild Alzheimer's disease). Characteristics of mild DAT include moderate memory loss, especially for recent events; deficits that interfere with everyday activities; and moderate difficulty with time relationships. These characteristics were descriptive of Mr. Johnson.

From the KTA, Mr. Johnson's executive skills were impaired. He required verbal cues to initiate, organize, perform all steps, and sequence the kitchen task. He also needed verbal assistance in managing the stove and pouring the hot liquid. He did recognize that the task was finished. He was capable of performing all aspects of the task but needed the presence of a person to verbally cue him throughout the task.

From the FBP: Mrs. Johnson reported that her husband was able to concentrate for long periods of time as evidenced by his daily activity of continuing with plumbing tasks around the house. (She had encouraged him to continue with his plumbing at home after he no longer went to work.) He usually finished tasks that he started (when he had done them in the past), performed his work neatly, and had no trouble using tools or manipulating small items like buttons on clothing. He did need help with his razor, so Mrs. Johnson got him an electric razor, which he could manage. His activities were usually appropriate to the time of day, however, lately he had been waking at night and going to the kitchen to get something to eat. He continued to make decisions concerning what to wear and what to eat, but Mrs. Johnson found that he was better at this when he was given choices. He continued to bathe and groom with only a little encouragement. He really enjoyed getting out to church activities and being with the children and grandchildren. However, Mrs. Johnson reported that he did not want to stay at events as long as she did. He continued to recognize family and most friends, however, friends helped by saying their name when they greeted him. He rarely initiated conversation but conversed when others started the conversation. Family and friends prompted him when he got lost in a story. Rarely did he know what day it was and he could no longer make independent decisions or problem-solve.

From the ACS, Mr. Johnson gave up the tasks of managing personal finances, investments, and general car maintenance. He continued to do home repairs and frequently drove on familiar routes in the neighborhood. He managed the telephone, as his wife had programmed and labeled the frequently called numbers. He read the newspaper and watched sports on TV.

He had given up his church committee activities, however, he still enjoyed going to church. He and Mrs. Johnson went bowling each week in a couples' league and went dancing with friends at least two times a month. They did less family visiting and went out to eat less frequently than 1 year ago. He had given up fishing and hunting, but still did woodworking, camping, and gardening, although less frequently than before because he needed to find time when his son or son-in-law could help him. He had always taken a Sunday afternoon ride in the country.

He watched birds in the back yard but could no longer name them all, and he tended his flowers, but not carefully. He needed help to get started and move from task to task. He had given up reading the Bible and reading in general.

Mrs. Johnson still worked full-time and worried how she would finish the year so she could collect her early retirement from Social Security. She had help from the daughter and son and their families, but all of them worked so she had limited assistance during the day. Mr. Johnson had worked alongside his son-in-law until 6 weeks ago. Mrs. Johnson reported that the future was frightening to her.

From the Zarit Behavior Problem Checklist, Mrs. Johnson reported that Mr. Johnson occasionally had got-

ten lost, and she thought it was time to take away the car. She reported that he asks repetitive questions and that it was beginning to get on her nerves. She also indicated that he was misplacing things. She reported that he did not destroy things or do things that could be dangerous to himself or others. However, she said he was frustrated frequently, as evidenced by his yelling at her and the dog; and recently she had found him wandering about the neighborhood. She did not recall that he had reported hearing voices or having hallucinations. If she laid out his clothing, he could dress himself. She indicated that he did not have difficulty with self-care tasks, however, she did have to help him with money. She had programmed the telephone so he could get in touch with her during the day. She admitted that he called her frequently and her office seemed to understand, but she felt that it would be a problem soon. She reported being very committed to providing care for him. She reported that they have had a good marriage and that she continued to feel very close to him.

Intervention

Strategies suggested by the OT based upon information obtained from the assessment interview and preferences stated by the Johnsons included:

General Strategies

- Mrs. Johnson was helped to build a consistent schedule. She filled out daily schedules for several weeks until she realized that a consistent schedule had been constructed. She noticed an improvement in Mr. Johnson's behavior when he functioned in a routine.

- Mrs. Johnson was taught to deliver cognitive support. Mr. Johnson mostly required verbal cues and functioned fairly independently when the environment was organized to cue him. It was important to help Mrs. Johnson understand that Mr. Johnson needed help in getting started (initiation) with an activity and also required assistance in getting the task organized. She learned that his difficulty with initiation was not due to stubbornness, but due to the related neurological deficit.

- The family was introduced to cueing strategies, and they chose activities that each of them would be able to do with their father/grandfather including taking walks, growing flowers, playing with the dog, watching birds, managing house plants, and bowling. Mrs. Johnson integrated these activities into the weekly schedule.

- The family was taught about the related neurological deficits. Because Mr. Johnson displayed some facial masking, it was important for the family to learn to look beyond his facial expression when he was expressing feelings and emotions.

Strategies to Support Behavior in the Absence of Ability to Solve Problems

- The family built a message center in the home so that Mr. Johnson would have a place to go to find out where Mrs. Johnson was, even if she was in the yard. The weekly schedule and specific daily schedule was posted at the center. The children learned to use the center when they were in the home.
- Mrs. Johnson found that when she gave Mr. Johnson choices in menu items that he eats better. He loves French fries and rather than let him choose them daily, she includes them as a menu choice two times a week. He had never been one to help with dinner preparation, but Mrs. Johnson found that he preferred to be with her and that he would do simple tasks like tearing lettuce or stirring a pot of soup or stew. He can do most any task when she chooses to guide him verbally through the task.

Strategies to Support Socialization

- A memory book was constructed with the help of the children and grandchildren. This book was to be used to engage Mr. Johnson in conversation and help him remember familiar people and important past events. A special section on birds were included so that he could keep up with his bird watching.
- Bowling and dancing have been an important part of their routine, so Mrs. Johnson is trying to keep them going. His attention span is decreased but he enjoys the socialization that they offer.
- Mr. Johnson is very fond of his dog. The dog actually cues him to let him out and feed him. They are great companions. The dog is always by his side when he is working in the garage. The problem is the dog is old, so the therapist suggested that a younger dog might be a good investment to maintain the companionship in the future.
- Mr. Johnson no longer can manage Sunday School, but he does sit patiently through church. Mrs. Johnson noted that he does better when they go consistently.
- Mrs. Johnson wanted Mr. Johnson to have a process to express his frustrations and concerns, so she enrolled him in the group for persons with mild DAT sponsored by the local Alzheimer's Disease and Related Disorders Association. He goes to the group weekly. While he is there, Mrs. Johnson can run errands or meet with the other spouses.

- The Johnsons had always enjoyed going out to dinner. They always go to the same restaurant so that Mr. Johnson can manage the menu and visit with the staff and friends that frequent the restaurant.

Strategies to Support the Performance of Tasks

- Mr. Johnson began a work-oriented day program where he could use his handyman skills to make toys for underprivileged children.
- A plumbing work station was built in the garage where Mr. Johnson could safely work with his tools and keep busy while at home. His time in this task gave Mrs. Johnson time to do her activities at home.
- He continues to dress himself when she places the clothes in the same order each day.
- Mr. Johnson's driving skills were evaluated by an OT in an on-the-road assessment. It was determined that it was no longer safe for him to drive. Mrs. Johnson takes him to day care on her way to work and picks him up after work. Because Mr. Johnson always liked to see the hills in the country, either his son or son-in-law takes him for a weekly drive to keep him in touch with nature.
- Mrs. Johnson continued with her walking program but included Mr. Johnson. In good weather they used the college track; in inclement weather they walked in the mall.
- The entire family came to understand how important a stable environment was to support Mr. Johnson's function. The grandchildren have learned why his paper should be in the same place, why his tools should not be moved. The family marked their father's bathroom door with a picture of him shaving. A card labeling the TV stations with news (Channel) 4, sports (Channel) 2, etc., was pasted on the back of the remote control so that he could watch his shows. The power button was painted white. The remote is always in a basket on the table by his chair.

When Mr. Johnson stays involved in activities that are important to him, he does not exhibit as many disturbing behaviors as when he is bored or anxious. He particularly enjoys working in his garage workshop. Mr. Johnson's memory has not improved, but the modifications that the family has made is providing an environment that maximizes his function and keeps him active and engaged. Mrs. Johnson reports that she is able to continue working, which is an important goal for both of their long-term security.

Discussion

Mrs. Johnson was a caregiver with a mission: to maintain a purposeful relationship with her husband, to be a successful caregiver, and to remain at work. She was meeting and continues to meet those goals. Of course there were difficult days, but she had a sense of humor, a very supportive family, and a friendship network at home and at work to help her. She was particularly happy when the Family Leave Bill passed, knowing that she had the resources to manage problems as they arrive and can take some time off if it is necessary.

An adaptive approach was the treatment of choice, not only because it makes good clinical sense, but it was what the family wanted and needed. They were willing to take on their role of caring, they just needed the skills to be successful.

REFERENCES

Allender, J., & Kaszniak, A. W. (1989). Processing of emotional cues in patients with dementia of the Alzheimer's type. *International Journal of Neurosciences, 146*, 3-4, 147-155.

Almli, C. R. (1993). *Abstract: Motor system, development, and neuroplasticity: Implications of theory and practice in OT.* AOTF Research Colloquium, Seattle, WA, June, 1993.

American Association of Retired Persons. (1988). *A profile of older Americans.* Long Beach, CA: Author.

American Psychiatric Association. (1994). *Diagnostic and statistical manual of mental disorders* (4th ed.). Washington, DC: Author.

Averbuch, S., & Katz, N. (1992). Cognitive rehabilitation: A retraining approach for brain-injured adults. In N. Katz (Ed.), *Cognitive rehabilitation: Models for intervention in OT* (pp. 219-239). Boston, MA: Andover Medical Publishers.

Baum, C. M. (1993). *The effects of occupation on behaviors of persons with senile dementia of the Alzheimer's type and their caregivers.* Dissertation. George Warren Brown School of Social Work, Washington University, St. Louis, MO.

Baum, C. M. (1995). The contribution of occupation to function in persons with Alzheimer's disease. *Journal of Occupational Science, 2,* 59-67.

Baum, C. M., & Edwards, D. F. (1993). Cognitive performance in senile dementia of the Alzheimer's type: The Kitchen Task Assessment. *Am J Occup Ther, 47*(5), 431-436.

Baum, C. M., & Edwards, D. (2000). Documenting productive behaviors: Using the functional behavior profile to plan discharge following stroke. *Journal of Gerontological Nursing.*

Baum, C. M., & Edwards, D. F. (in press). *The Washington University Activity Card Sort.* St. Louis, MO: Penultimate Publications.

Baum, C. M., Edwards, D. F., Leavitt, C., Grant, B., & Deuel, R. M. (1988). Performance components in senile dementia of the Alzheimer's type. *OT Journal of Research, 8,* 356-364.

Baum, C. M., Edwards, D. F., & Morrow-Howell, N. (1993). Identification and measurement of productive behaviors in senile dementia of the Alzheimer type. *The Gerontologist, 33*(3), 403-408.

Berg, L. (1988). Clinical dementia rating (CDR). *Psychopharmacology Bulletin, 24*(4), 637-638.

Bourgeois, M. S. (1993). Using memory aids to stimulate conversation and reinforce accurate memories. In *Gerontology Special Interest Section Newsletter* (pp. 1-3). Rockville, MD: AOTA.

Bronfenbrenner, U. (1979). Purpose and perspective. In U. Bronfenbrenner (Ed.), *The Ecology of Human Development* (pp. 1-15). Cambridge, MA: Harvard University Press.

Buckwalter, K. C. (1990). *Alzheimer's disease: Supportive interventions at home and in the institution.* Recent Advances in Alzheimer's Disease: Conference Proceedings. University of Kentucky.

Burns, T., & Buell, J. (1990). The effectiveness of work programming with an Alzheimer population. *OT Practice, 1*(2), 64-73.

Christiansen, C. (1991). OT: Intervention for life performance. In C. Christiansen & C. M. Baum (Eds.), *OT: Overcoming Human performance deficits* (pp. 4-43). Thorofare, NJ: SLACK Incorporated.

Christiansen, C., & Baum, C. M. (Eds.). (1991). *OT: Overcoming human performance deficits.* Thorofare, NJ: SLACK Incor-porated.

Christiansen, C., & Baum, C. M. (Eds.). (1997). *OT: Enabling Function and Well-Being.* Thorofare, NJ: SLACK Incorporated.

Clipp, E. C., & George, L. K. (1990). Caregiver needs and patterns of social support. *Journal of Gerontology, 45*(3), S102-S111.

Cohen, D., Kennedy, G., & Eisforder, C. (1984). Phase of change in the patient with Alzheimer's dementia: A conceptual dimension for defining health care management. *Journal of the American Geriatrics Society, 32*(1), 11-15.

Corcoran, M. A. (1994). Management decision made by caregiver spouses of persons with Alzheimer's disease. *Am J Occup Ther, 48*(1), 38-45.

Csikszentmihalyi, M. (1988). A theoretical model for enjoyment. In M. Csikszentmihalyi (Ed.), *Beyond boredom and anxiety* (pp. 35-54). San Francisco, CA: Jossey-Bass.

Dougherty, P. M., & Radomski, M. V. (1993). *The dynamic assessment approach for adults with brain injury: The cognitive rehabilitation workbook.* Gaithersburg, MD: Aspen Publications.

Duchek, J. (1991). Cognitive dimensions of performance. In C. Christiansen & C. M. Baum (Eds.), *OT: Overcoming human performance deficits* (pp. 284-303). Thorofare, NJ: SLACK Incorporated.

Edwards, D. F., & Baum, C. M. (1990). Caregiver burden across stage of dementia. *OT Practice, 2*(1), 17-31.

Edwards, D. F., Baum, C. M., & Deuel, R. M. (1991). Constructional apraxia in senile dementia: Contributions to functional loss. *Physical and Occupational therapy in Geriatrics, 9*(3), 53-68.

Eslinger, P. J., & Damasio, A. R. (1986). Preserved motor learning in Alzheimer's disease: Implications for anatomy and behavior. *Journal of Neuroscience, 6*(10), 3006-3009.

Faber-Langendoen, K., Morris, J. C., Knesevich, J. W., LaBarge, E., Miller, J. P., & Berg, L. (1988). Aphasia in senile dementia of the Alzheimer type. *Annuals of Neurology, 23*(4), 365-370.

Fidler, G., & Fidler, J. (1963). *OT: A communication process in psychiatry.* New York, NY: Macmillan.

Fox, P. (1989). From senility to Alzheimer's disease: The risk of the Alzheimer's disease movement. *Milbank Quarterly, 67*(1), 58-102.

Gurland, B. J. (1985). Public health aspects of Alzheimer's disease and related dementias. In Kelly (Ed.), *Alzheimer's disease and related disorders: Research* (pp. 146-158). Springfield, IL: Charles C. Thomas.

Haley, W. E., Levine, E. G., Brown, S. L., Berry, J. W., & Hughes, G. H. (1987). Psychological, social, and health consequences of caring for a relative with senile dementia. *Journal American Geriatric Society, 35*(5), 405-411.

Kielhofner, G. (1992). *Conceptual foundations of OT.* Philadelphia, PA: F. A. Davis.

Kinney, J. M., & Stephens, M. A. (1989). Hassles and uplifts of giving care to a family member with dementia. *Psychology of Aging, 4*(4), 402-408.

Law, M., Cooper, B., Strong, S., Rigby, P., & Letts, L. (1996). The person-environment-occupation model: A transactive approach to occupational performance. *CJOT, 63,* 9-23.

Lawton, M. P. (1990). Environmental approaches to research and treatment of Alzheimer's disease. In E. Light & B. D. Lebowitz (Eds.), *Alzheimer's disease treatment and family stress: Directions for research* (pp. 340-362). New York, NY: Hemisphere Publications Co.

Luria, A. R. (1963). *Restoration of function after brain injury.* New York, NY: Oxford University Press.

MacDonald, M. L. (1978). Environmental programming for the socially isolated aging. *Gerontologist, 18,* 350-354.

Magaziner, J. (1989). Demographic and epidemiologic considerations for developing preventative strategies in the elderly. *Maryland Medical Journal, 38*(2), 115-120.

Mendez, M. F., Mendez, M. A., Martin, R., Smyth, K. A., & Whitehouse, P. J. (1990). Complex visual disturbances in Alzheimer's disease. *Neurology, 40*(3), 439-443.

Miller, B., McFall, S., & Montgomery, A. (1991). The impact of elder health, caregiver involvement and global stress on two dimensions of caregiver burden. *Journal of Gerontology, Social Sciences, 46*(1), S9-S19.

Motenko, A. K. (1989). The frustrations, gratification and well-being of dementia caregivers. *Gerontologist, 29*(2), 166-172.

Oakley, F. (1993). *Understanding the ABC's of Alzheimer's disease: A guide for caregivers.* Rockville, MD: AOTA.

Quayhagen, M. P., & Quayhagen, M. (1988). Alzheimer's stress: Coping with the caregiving role. *Gerontologist, 28,* 391-396.

Rabins, P., Mace, H. L., & Lucas, M. J. (1982). The impact of dementia on the family. *Journal of the American Medical Association, 248,* 333-335.

Ramsdell, J. W., Rothrock, J. F., Ward, H. W., & Volk, D. M. (1990). Evaluation of cognitive impairment in the elderly. *Journal of General Internal Medicine, 5,* 55-64.

Sholberg M. M., & Mateer, C. A. (1989). *Introduction to cognitive rehabilitation: Theory and practice.* New York, NY: The Guilford Press.

Sinha, D., Zemian, F. P., Nelson, S., et al. (1992). A new scale for assessing behavioral agitation in dementia. *Psychiatry Research, 41,* 73-88.

Sullivan, E. V., Sagar, H. J., Gabrieli, J. D., Corkin, S., & Growdon, J. H. (1989). Different cognitive profiles on standard behavioral tests in Parkinson's disease and Alzheimer's disease. *Journal Clinical Experimental Neuropsychology, 11*(6), 799-820.

Swearer, J. M., Drachman, D. A., O'Donnell, B. F., & Mitchell, A. L. (1988). Troublesome and disruptive behaviors in dementia. Relationships to diagnosis and disease severity. *Journal of the American Geriatric Society, 36*(9), 784-790.

Toglia, J. P. (1992). A dynamic interactional approach to cognitive rehabilitation. In N. Katz (Ed.), *Cognitive rehabilitation: Models for intervention in OT* (pp. 104-143). Boston, MA: Andover Medical Publishers.

Vitaliano, P. P., Russo, J., Breen, A. R., Vitiello, M. V., & Prinz, P. N. (1986). Functional decline in the early stages of Alzheimer's disease. *Psychology of Aging, 1*(1), 41-46.

Zarit, S. H., & Anthony, C. R. (1986). Interventions with demential patients and their families. In M. L. M. Gilhooly, S. H. Zarit, & J. E. Biren (Eds.), *The dementias: Policy and management.* Englewood Cliffs, NJ: Prentice Hall, 66-92.

Zarit, S., Reever, K., et al. (1980). Relatives of the impaired elderly, correlates of feeling of burden. *The Gerontologist, 20*(6), 649-655.

Treatment Techniques, Procedures, and Concepts

Applied Group Dynamics and Therapeutic Use of Self

Chapter 30

Roseanna Tufano, LMFT, OTR/L

INTRODUCTION

The group model has its roots in anthropology, sociology, communication theory, and psychology. In the 1920s, OT originally included treating patients in groups for the sole purpose of working on projects or performing activities. The therapeutic value of the group experience was not fully recognized at that time, however.

During the 1940s, a social psychologist named Kurt Lewin founded the first training for human relations group, also known as T-groups (Yalom, 1995). His research was to have significant impact on the development of group theory principles. The state of Connecticut had passed a Fair Employment Practices Act and Lewin was asked to train group leaders who could effectively deal with individual tensions regarding racial issues evident in social groups at that time. The goal of these groups was to change the racial attitudes of the public. These discussion groups were held in a unique way. Observers recorded the behavioral interactions of the group members while the therapy process was occurring in a room. Although not part of the original plan, eventually group participants, group leaders, and group observers met together to analyze and discuss the interactions that took place within the group experience. These discussion meetings reflected the concept of experiential learning, a term that has come to be associated with Kurt Lewin and this research project. When used in a group setting, the concept of *experiential learning*

ESSENTIAL VOCABULARY

Consensual validation: Comparing one's personal perceptions with others in a group experience.

Content: Actual words spoken or used within a group.

"Here and now": Pertaining to only what is experienced in the present.

Interpersonal: Occurring between oneself and others.

Intrapersonal: Occurring within oneself.

Norms: Codes or rules for behavior.

Ontogeny: Normal course of development.

Process: Nature of relationships within a group.

Projection: A defense mechanism; taking the unacceptable parts of oneself and forwarding them onto the environment.

Roles: Expected social behavior or position.

Task: An activity or process with a tangible end product.

Therapeutic communication: Verbal and nonverbal interaction that occurs within a therapeutic relationship.

KEY CONCEPTS

- Experiential learning: Learning by doing.
- Therapeutic use of self: A complex concept used by therapists who form a therapeutic relationship with clients and actively use their own intrapersonal and interpersonal knowledge to foster change in their clients.
- Group dynamics: Conscious and unconscious forces within a group.
- Group process: Deliberate reflection on the interactive patterns between group members following a group experience.
- Social microcosm: Enactment of one's typical interpersonal style.
- Interpersonal learning: Yalom's therapeutic factor describing a complex process that leads to therapeutic change within groups.
- Cohesiveness: Stage of group development in which members feel bonded to each other, share mutual identification, and can tolerate conflict among themselves.
- Seven-step process for activity groups: Format for an OT group to develop interpersonal communication skills but can also be adapted for lower functioning needs.

describes a unique way to instruct members about their behaviors. Simply stated, experiential learning is learning from your personal experiences. As an intervention, observations are made about a person's behavior and feedback is given immediately to this member during the group process, just like Lewin's T-groups. Observations can be made by the group leader and participating group members. This feedback is offered to assist a person in learning how one's behavior influences him- or herself and others.

Experiential learning is an effective way to increase one's awareness of interpersonal relationships and/or social skills and is an integral part of OT interventions. Therapeutic observations are given most effectively when the OT practitioner makes clear statements and shows respect for the person, regardless of his or her behavior. Therapeutic communication is a learned skill that is different from our everyday, personal style of interaction. It takes practice to learn how to give constructive feedback in a nonjudgmental way, especially when a client shows a different set of values and behaviors from the practitioner. Giving constructive feedback is an art that enhances group process.

An OT practitioner who uses group models as a form of intervention should have knowledge of group theory and be skilled at effective communication. Therapeutic communication refers to the ways that practitioners and clients exchange information, thoughts, and ideas (Tufano, 1997). An essential component of group work is to establish trust and rapport with the members, which can be enhanced by both nonverbal and verbal interactions. A competent practitioner is self-aware of his or her own strengths and limitations and continuously works at developing a style that is therapeutic and conducive to the various needs of clients.

The purpose of this chapter is to discuss various components of group intervention and group dynamics typically used in OT domains of practice. The reader will find:

- A brief history of the origins of group activities that have influenced OT, including a selection of OTs who have made significant contributions with a brief description of their group model.
- An overview of group theory and the process of therapeutic communication; developmental stages of groups.
- Leadership styles and membership roles.
- A format for creating an integrative communication group.

It is this author's intention that the reader will grasp general concepts of group theory, OT practice models, and basic therapeutic communication to assist him or her in the development of a therapeutic sense of self and the successful achievement of client functional outcomes.

OCCUPATIONAL THERAPY ORIGINS AND ACTIVITY GROUPS

During the early 1900s, many large hospitals, such as Sheppard-Pratt in Maryland, McLean Hospital in Massachusetts, and Bloomingdale Hospital in New York, developed occupation programs for their patients with mental illness. Significant contributors of this time included Dr. William Rush Dunton, Jr., who has also been referred to as the "father of OT." Dr. Dunton was among the first to recognize that crafts provided a positive distraction for persons with mental illness. He was highly influenced by the work of Dr. Adolph Meyer, a psychiatrist who founded the psychobiological approach to psychiatry. Dr. Meyer believed that mental illness was composed of physical and psychological causes. Dr. Dunton noted how occupations helped patients become healthier, and he proposed that research be conducted to understand why "occupation therapy" worked. So began a long-standing professional relationship between Eleanor Clark Slagle, who was a social worker, and Dr. Dunton. This relationship eventually led to the founding of the AOTA (Quiroga, 1995) (See Chapter 1).

OT continues to promote the role of occupation and its significance for healthy functioning. In its origins, activities were used for diversion, to decrease boredom, and as a productive way to keep patients active. In the 1920s, patients worked on activity projects that included crafts, basketry, and work-related activities. Patients worked in parallel fashion, side-by-side, on their own individual projects without specific treatment goals or a clear therapeutic focus. There was no emphasis on their socialization and interpersonal skills (Quiroga, 1995).

In the 1950s, significant contributions were made to group process by OTs. The Azimas (1959) recognized the therapeutic value of creative activities such as art, music, poetry, drama, dance, and clay/sculpting. These activities are also referred to as projective media. The purpose of projective media groups is to increase self-awareness and promote self-understanding to encourage *intrapersonal* change. The Azimas were influenced by psychodynamic concepts, including Freud's psychoanalytic theory. OT practitioners who use the psychoanalytic frame of reference as a theory base for activity groups believe that unconscious conflicts and unresolved issues from one's past influence one's personality development. The goal of projective groups is to increase a person's self-awareness by uncovering conflicts buried within one's unconscious. Groups like art therapy and music/dance therapy, activities like journal writing and poetry, projects like sculpting and pottery, all provide an opportunity for clients to freely express feelings in a symbolic way. An OT practitioner who leads projective groups reminds the clients that there are no "rights or wrongs" and that it does not matter whether one has had art, music, or dance lessons. The activity process itself becomes significant. Once a client can express his or her internalized conflicts, which are triggered by projective arts media, he or she is now free to change these identified feelings and behaviors. The energy that was once used to repress these conflicts and bury them into one's unconscious is now freed up and available to use again. A healthy person is free to love, work, and play in ways that are satisfying to oneself and society, in other words, to engage in productive and meaningful occupations (Stein & Cutler, 1998).

While the Azimas were influenced by psychodynamic theories and focused on a client's intrapersonal change process, Kurt Lewin (1945) took another therapeutic path. He believed that behavior is an outcome of one's personality traits plus one's interaction with the social environment. This blending of one's personality and interpersonal experiences comprise our "life space." According to Lewin, "life space" is in a state of constant change since it is influenced considerably by one's social environment. Lewin concentrated his research on group process and how social behaviors develop and change among persons. Along with the development of the notion of experiential learning, he also defined another significant concept pertaining to group process. *Group dynamics* (Edelson, 1964) are the forces within a group that encourage social interaction between members. Lewin recognized how powerful and influential these forces, or dynamics, are toward a person's change process. Examples of dynamics include group process, development, and norms, as well as leadership and membership roles. OT practitioners recognize the various group dynamics that are found in every group and use them to promote healthy functioning in members.

FIDLER'S TASK-ORIENTED GROUP MODEL

An OT who was influenced by both psychodynamic theory and Lewin's experiential learning is Gail Fidler (1969). Fidler founded the *task-oriented group*, which she developed from her research at New York State Psychiatric Institute and her work with male patients who were diagnosed with schizophrenia. According to Fidler (1969), "task" is defined as any activity or process that results in an end product or demonstrable service. Examples of task groups include arts and crafts, cooking, horticulture, work/vocational activities, and volunteer or charity projects, such as participating in a soup kitchen or collecting toys for tots. Gail Fidler believed that the purpose of a task-oriented group was to create a working and sharing environment where a client's productive and non-productive behaviors could be observed as he or she

attempts to complete an end product. It is assumed that clients will naturally show their abilities and dysfunctional patterns in the OT group similar to what they do in their own social environments. She recognized how the process of completing a task allowed the group leader and fellow members an opportunity to observe the relationship between one's feelings, thoughts, and behaviors (Fidler, 1969).

The task-oriented group emphasizes how a person functions in such areas as decision-making, problem-solving, task initiation and engagement, cause and effect, sharing and cooperation with others, reality testing, and task accomplishment. Emphasis is not on the end product or task. According to Fidler, the task becomes the driving force in which healthy, productive behaviors can be learned and eventually transferred into the client's everyday life. An OT practitioner constantly notices how a client's feelings, thoughts, and behaviors impact the completion of a task. The group leader shows concern for the client's feelings about the group process, encouraging appropriate expression and self-understanding. The task group provides an excellent opportunity for experiential learning to take place because feedback about one's performance and feelings are immediately given by the group leader and members. The client is encouraged to experiment with new, more productive behaviors in the group process (Fidler, 1969).

The OT practitioner also identifies how the behaviors of a client, represented in the "here and now" of the group activity, influences his or her functioning ability to complete meaningful activities. Clients are encouraged to transfer their learning from the OT task group into their own natural environments. The group leader encourages and guides the therapy process without taking responsibility for the task. Sometimes we learn more effectively from our mistakes, although it is hard for practitioners to sometimes let clients experience the natural consequences of their behavior. It is not the job of the OT practitioner to make the end product successful, but to encourage and teach productive behaviors that the client could use now and in his or her future. The OT practitioner is also concerned with the client's feelings about the group process and encourages appropriate expression and self-understanding. The reader is encouraged to consult Gail Fidler's (1969) article, "The Task-Oriented Group as a Context for Treatment" for further details and knowledge about this significant OT group model.

MOSEY'S DEVELOPMENTAL GROUP MODEL

Another significant contributor to OT group models is Anne Cronin Mosey (1970). Mosey was influenced by

Fidler's task-oriented group. However, her frame of reference was different from the psychodynamic origins of Fidler. Mosey attempted to apply a developmental approach to OT group treatment. She believed that treatment should be a "recapitulation of ontogeny." In other words, OT should repeat the normal course of development (Jacobs, 1999).

According to Mosey (1970), developmental groups are non-familial, task-oriented groups that imitate common experiences in normal development. They were specifically designed to address *group interaction skills* described by Mosey as "...the ability to engage in a variety of primary groups." A person's ability to successfully participate and live in one's community is dependent on group interaction skill formation. OT practitioners give positive reinforcement in a step-by-step and graded fashion, encouraging success and a feeling of social accomplishment.

Mosey (1970) identified five stages of developmental groups, which occur in sequential order. They are called parallel, project, egocentric-cooperative, cooperative, and mature. Here is a brief description of each level.

- Parallel group—This is the most basic level of group interaction, typically occurring in children ages 18 months to 2 years of age. Clients are involved in their own individual tasks with little required interaction between members. The group leader helps with task accomplishment and takes major responsibility for meeting the social-emotional needs of each client.

- Project group—This level of group participation is typically shown in children ages 2 to 4 years of age. Clients are involved in short-term tasks with the main emphasis on task accomplishment. There is some group interaction required, such as sharing of tools. Cooperation between members is encouraged, as it relates to the completion of the task. The group leader once again responds to the social-emotional needs of group members.

- Egocentric-cooperative group—Participation at this level is typical of children ages 4 to 9 years of age. Members select, implement, and execute their tasks, which may be moderately long-term and requiring some social-emotional satisfaction from each other. The group leader provides any needed support and guidance for group members to achieve task accomplishment and continues to supply emotional need satisfaction.

- Cooperative group—This level of social interaction is typically accomplished between 9 to 12 years of age. This group experience includes a very supportive atmosphere where both task accomplishment and social-emotional needs are met by fellow members. The group leader is often an advisor and may not be present at all group meetings.

- Mature group—This is the highest level of group interaction skill typically seen in adolescents between the ages of 15 to 18 years old. All task accomplishment needs and social-emotional needs are met by members. The group leader acts as a co-equal.

The reader is encouraged to consult Anne Cronin Mosey's (1970) article titled "The Concept and Use of Developmental Groups" for further clarification and understanding of this group model.

KAPLAN'S DIRECTIVE GROUP

Kathy Kaplan (1988) is also an OT who designed a group for acutely ill and minimally functioning clients. Similar to Fidler and Mosey, Kaplan's *directive group* is a structured experience, suited for persons in an inpatient unit who are often not appropriate for verbal psychotherapy groups. Clients who are referred to this group often show chronic functional impairments such as decreased verbal communication, limited self-initiative, and poor judgment. Kaplan used group dynamic principles and the Model of Human Occupation frame of reference as foundation theories for this model.

The directive group is designed to provide a consistent and structured experience as a way to increase the adaptive functioning level of clients. Kaplan suggests that the group be offered daily, at the same time and place, for a duration of 45 minutes. There is a predictable sequence of events that should take place in every group. The group sequence includes:

1. Reality orientation
2. Introduction of the group members
3. A warm-up activity
4. An activity experience
5. A wrap-up/summary

The OT practitioner acts as a role model who readily supports and guides clients to meet their cognitive, social, and emotional needs (Kaplan, 1988).

There are four main goals to the directive group: to increase participation, interaction, attention span, and initiation. The group leader documents daily on each client, using a directive group progress sheet. This progress sheet is a type of grid with a numbered rating scale beginning at level 1 (lack of skill) and progressing to level 5 (skill adequately demonstrated for 45 minutes). The OT practitioner notes a client's daily progress and/or regression by using this progress sheet and comparing the scores. Clients are discharged from the directive group when they demonstrate readiness to engage in other OT experiences, such as a task-oriented group or communication group.

The reader is encouraged to consult Kaplan's (1988) book titled *Directive Group Therapy: Innovative Mental Health Treatment* for further group description and explanation, as well as examples of suitable activities designed for clients with low level functioning.

ROSS' INTEGRATIVE GROUP

Mildred Ross (1997) created a unique OT group experience that is composed of five steps or stages. Similar to Kaplan, Ross designed a group model that is highly structured, predictable, and consistent in its format. It is best suited for persons who show limitations in sensorimotor development and who require stimulation and cueing to engage with their environment in meaningful ways. While it can be used with all age groups, the *integrative group* is designed for persons with developmental disabilities, mental retardation, chronic mental illness, and cognitive disorders due to dementia, stroke, head trauma, etc.

Ross (1997) based her integrative group on concepts from neurophysiology and sensory integration principles. The OT practitioner selects various activities that provide sensory stimulation in meaningful ways to each client. The goal of this group is to facilitate organized sensory, motor, affective, and/or cognitive responses. There are five specific, organized sequences to every group format. Activities are selected to provide sensory stimulation, movement, visual motor responses, and cognitive reasoning. They may be selected to provide alerting or calming responses based on the needs of the clients. The desired outcome goal of each group is to acquire calm alertness, which increases one's ability to interact in an organized and adaptive fashion. A benefit of this group experience is to enhance the quality of a client's life, even if it is for a brief period of time. The reader is encouraged to consult Mildred Ross' (1997) book *Integrative Group Therapy* for further information and examples of sensorimotor activities.

There are many other group models and methods that have been designed by OTs. The reader may want to further explore some of the following examples. Claudia Allen (1985), who designed cognitive disabilities theory, believes that function is an outcome of one's cognitive level. In her *Cognitive Disabilities Groups*, she proposes that in order to change one's behavior, a client's thinking process must change. Lorna Jean King pioneered the use of sensory integration approaches, originally researched by Jean Ayres, to the treatment of persons with mental illness. King's (1974) *Gross Motor Activities* are designed to stimulate the sensory processing systems, particularly of persons with schizophrenia. Over the many years since the profession's origins, OT practitioners have developed various other group methods. For example: self-awareness groups, reality-oriented groups, role-oriented groups, social skills training groups, prevocational groups, ADL groups, arts and crafts groups, psychoeducational groups, leisure skills groups, assertiveness training groups, stress management groups, values clarification groups, etc. While this list may appear overwhelming to the novice practitioner, it verifies that OT practice is an ever-evolving and changing profession.

GROUP PROCESS

The reader has now been introduced to a brief history of the origins of OT group treatment and various group models that influence our profession. It is evident that activity groups are an inherent and significant form of intervention in OT practice. The following sections of this chapter will review group theory principles, including a discussion of various dynamics that are used in OT group intervention.

A paramount notion that acts as a basis for all group therapy is a concept called *social microcosm* (Yalom, 1995). Members who are allowed to freely interact in a group, with minimal structural restrictions, will naturally show their interpersonal style. Regardless of the frame of reference used by the group leader, group members will eventually show more and more of their typical social behaviors, for better and for worse. Both adaptive and maladaptive patterns of behavior will be evident. In relation to the emergence of social microcosm, the group leader can also observe triggers of one's behaviors and come to understand the meaningfulness of one's actions.

Consider the following example. John, a group member, becomes anxious because the OT group leader is 15 minutes late for group. He begins to fear that something catastrophic has occurred and that the leader is seriously injured. His anxiety is high and John begins to have signs of a panic attack. As the group leader arrives, she apologizes and describes how she got stuck in traffic for 1 hour. John is so nervous that he is unable to listen. The OT practitioner recognizes that John's response is an overreaction to this particular situation. In the course of discussion, John reveals that he was abandoned by his mother at an early age. To this day, he struggles with anxiety attacks when he fears that someone of significance may leave him.

Another significant dynamic, common to all groups, is that each client will have a unique and different reaction to the same event. Using the above example describing the arrival of the late therapist, an effective group leader would consult with other members of the group to seek their views of what happened. Did everyone panic? Did everyone think that a catastrophic accident occurred to the therapist? The concept of comparing one's thoughts and feelings with others is called *consensual validation* (Fidler, 1969). A benefit to using consensual validation is that a client will hopefully change his or her distorted thinking and formulate an adaptive response that he or she may have learned from others in the group. The OT practitioner asks other members to comment on how they feel about the same situation. This inquiry can be done so easily in groups because there are several members who are present and hearing the same information at the same time. John will hopefully hear that other members may have been concerned about the "missing therapist," but not panicked. John can come to understand that his reaction was different and out of proportion in relation to others. The client can be encouraged to understand that "waiting for someone" may be a trigger for feelings of abandonment, which leads to feelings of intense anxiety and panic. The skilled OT practitioner can appreciate differences and allow each member to express his or her opinion appropriately.

In order to promote "interpersonal learning," a group leader must guide a group to understand its *process*. According to Yalom, a well-known psychiatrist who has researched group psychotherapy and written several books, the term *process* refers to the "nature of the relationship between interacting individuals" (1995, p. 130). Process is different from content in client discussions. The *content* refers to the actual words or topics used by the speaker. Content can be described by quotes. For example: John said to the OT group leader as she arrived late to group, "Where have you been? I was beginning to panic. I thought that you were dead." Group leaders who are process oriented are concerned with why a client says what he or she did, at a certain time, in a certain manner, and to a certain person (Yalom, 1995). Focusing on the process is a main component of experiential learning and experiential groups.

Another significant aspect to encouraging interpersonal learning through experiential groups is giving and receiving feedback about the various behaviors that are being shown during the group process (Yalom, 1995). The skill of giving feedback is challenging for all group leaders and members. It often takes practice to become a good observer and then to figure out how to verbally express these observations in a therapeutic and nonjudgmental way. An effective group leader continues to develop his or her therapeutic sense of self and efficient communication techniques.

When giving feedback, there are three steps or levels that an OT practitioner should follow (Yalom, 1995). These steps should occur in sequence because each statement builds upon the other. You will also notice that each step gets deeper into a client's emotions and behaviors. You do not have to use all three levels each time you give feedback. The art of running a therapeutic group includes having a good sense of timing and knowing when a client is ready to hear and accept feedback from others.

Step 1 involves giving information about how a client's behavior is being noticed and understood by others. It includes making observations about a client's verbal and nonverbal behaviors. These statements are often concrete and very specific. They often begin with "I see...", "I notice...", or "I hear..." An example of such a statement is: "John, I notice that you have tears in your eyes while you are talking about how worried you became when I did not arrive for group on time." Notice that the OT practitioner does not make any interpretations about the client's behavior at this step. It is now up to the client to affirm or deny what is being stated and observed.

Step 2 involves more depth and understanding on the group leader's part. This level of feedback can be made when the OT practitioner has established a rapport with a client and has come to understand patterns of behavior. In step 2, a group leader comments on how a client's behavior reflects his or her self-image to others. This feedback is an attempt at interpreting what a person's behavior says about him or her. In keeping with the example above, the following statement could be made as part of step 2: "John, you appear frightened and panicked about the possibility of being left or abandoned." Notice how this statement is different from the first one. The OT practitioner is commenting on how the client's self-image is reflected by both the verbal and nonverbal behaviors observed in group.

Step 3 includes statements about how a client's behavior impacts the group leader and/or fellow members of a group. The purpose of this feedback is to offer perspectives on how one's behavior is affecting other people in the environment. It provides information about the consequences of a client's behaviors. For example, one group member may respond to John in this way: "When I saw you crying and feeling scared, I wanted to comfort you and tell you that everything is going to be all right." Another member of the group may have a different perspective to offer: "I find that it is hard to be around you because you are so anxious and high strung. I get nervous just from being around you." These different responses allow John to understand how people may respond to him both in group as well as socially in the community. Remember, the group becomes a social microcosm of the real world. John has gained some awareness as to how his behaviors may draw some people closer to him and push others away. The client should be encouraged by the group leader to respond to these statements and discuss what, if any, changes he would like to make about his behavior. Remember, a benefit for using an experiential approach is to encourage immediate behavioral change.

OT groups can provide the opportunity to use experiential learning and processing. Some examples of group activities include self-awareness, communication, task, social skills, self-esteem, self-management, and projective arts. In general, clients who are suited for these group experiences have adequate motivation, verbal skills, and the ability to reflect and explore the meaning of their behaviors. The group leader is often a facilitator who probes members about their behaviors, provides feedback, and supports the group to take risks and experiment with new behaviors.

On the other hand, there are also OT groups whose therapeutic value is in the experience of an activity. Examples include: developmental groups, sensory integrative groups, directive groups, and psychoeducational groups that teach basic ADL skills such as cooking, budgeting, doing laundry, etc. Clients suited for these interventions are often nonverbal, have low motivation and self-awareness, with chronic maladaptive behavioral patterns and illness. The group leader is active and provides varying degrees of structure to maintain both physical and emotional safety.

An effective OT practitioner is knowledgeable of various types of groups that are suited for a range of functioning levels. It takes both experience and knowledge of group dynamics theory and competent therapeutic communication to become a skilled leader. The reader is encouraged to consult Tufano's (1997) chapter titled "Therapeutic Communication" in *OT Student Primer*, a book edited by Karen Sladyk.

GROUP NORMS

A dynamic that influences group process is group norms (Yalom, 1995). Norms may be described as the rules of behaviors or expectations within a group. They can be stated verbally or implied nonverbally. The group leader has a basic responsibility to guide the development of norms. The leader's influence is significant in setting up rules of both acceptable and non-acceptable behaviors, similar to how parents establish expectations within a family. An example of a positive group norm is confidentiality, which is usually discussed during a first session. A group leader typically initiates conversation about confidentiality and explains its purpose for increasing a feeling of emotional safety within the group. Other examples of positive norms include arriving on time for group, remaining for the entire duration of group, giving constructive feedback, supporting members in non-judgmental ways, and disclosing one's thoughts and feelings. Sometimes members are asked to sign a contract that states they are in agreement with the group norms and commit to following those rules.

Norms evolve within every group with which we partake within our society (Yalom, 1995). For example, a norm within a classroom is that students raise their hand to get their teacher's attention before speaking. These rules are often set early in the group experience and are often difficult to change. Norms are expressed in both direct and non-direct ways, otherwise called explicit or implicit norms (Yalom, 1995). An explicit norm may be the verbal decision of group members to attend every group unless there is an emergency. The norm will be discussed explicitly and directly in group while members decide together what constitutes an emergency and what is an acceptable absence. On the other hand, indirect or implicit norms get unconsciously set by factors such as imitating the behaviors of others and social reinforcement. For example, a group member begins to cry and the group leader extends a tissue to her. This act of support is a nonverbal and implicit way of giving the member permission to cry and nonverbally "stating" that it is acceptable to express sad feelings in this group.

Norms have both a positive and negative influence on group process (Yalom, 1995). Examples of non-productive norms are interrupting others when one is talking, subgrouping, avoiding topics, criticizing and/or blaming others, talking through the group leader rather than directly to each other, and talking about members outside of group. Negative norms create dissension rather than cohesiveness and trust. An effective leader will address both the positive and negative norms of group, inviting members to discuss and take responsibility for their own actions. Sometimes, there are serious consequences for breaking group rules, and a member may be asked to leave a group. An effective way to address inappropriate behavior in a group is to give the member a choice—he or she could either comply with the group expectations and rules or choose to leave. This technique should be used after various attempts have been made to discuss the problem behavior. In a cohesive group, members are willing to negotiate and compromise their needs for the benefit of the whole group. The group leader should role model behaviors and values, such as respect and concern for others, while also standing up for group principles and setting limits on inappropriate behaviors, especially those that violate others. Asking a member to leave a group should be used as a last resort because it creates tension between members and the leader. A natural response for other members is to wonder if they will also be asked to leave the group by this leader, and they may begin to question the level of trust and balance of control within the group.

GROUP DEVELOPMENT

There is a sequential set of stages that often occur as part of group development. Several theorists have researched the phases of group process and have titled these stages in different ways. Regardless of the theorist, there is overall agreement about the typical patterns, themes, and dynamics that occur within any therapy group.

According to Yalom (1995), a group passes through a beginning phase of *orientation,* whereby members are looking for direction, structure, goals, and behavioral expectations (norms) from the leader. This stage is similar to early childhood development, where we are dependent on our parents for nurturance and support, eventually feeling ready to distinguish ourselves and become more independent. The catalyst of this stage is the search for individual purpose and meaning, and to establish a significant role within the group.

The second phase (Yalom, 1995) includes an individual's awareness of differences and *conflicts* among others in the group. A common group tension is that members both desire approval and closeness from the group, yet strive to keep self-control and independence. This stage resembles adolescence and can therefore be challenging and confusing for both the leader and members as they try to balance the formation of both a personal identity as well as a group identity. The group leader will likely be confronted during this stage and must be able to discriminate between an attack on one's person vs. an attack of one's role. An effective group leader will demonstrate the ability to understand differences and conflict and appreciate that a member's rebellion is a way to try and reclaim some personal control. A confident and secure leader will respond, negotiate, and compromise the various themes and issues that are presented in group without trying to control or dominate the members. A leader who implicitly or explicitly supports suppression of anger and conflict will create other group problems. Members will remain inhibited and therefore unable to fully express who they are or what they want from the therapy experience. Another dynamic that is evident of group suppression is the emergence of a scapegoat. Members will displace anger felt toward the leader onto a "safe" member, one who is willing to become the sacrificial lamb for the group. It is the responsibility of the group leader to point this out and redirect the anger toward him- or herself in order to preserve group functioning.

Yalom's (1995) third stage is called *cohesiveness*. During this phase, members report feeling close, trusting, and supportive of each other. Self-disclosure is heightened, with a desire for mutual acceptance and positive group spirit. True cohesiveness cannot be reached without members working through the conflict stage. This phase resembles early adulthood, when children healthily return to their families as adults with their own separate identity, and feel proud to be part of the family unit recognizing both its strengths and limits.

It is worth noting other theorists who have researched and labeled the stages of group development. Schutz (1958) focused on the interpersonal needs of group members, believing that groups follow a similar sequence to normal child development. He called these phases inclusion, control, and affection. Bion (1961) focused his research on task accomplishment within corporations rather than interpersonal development. He called his stages flight, fight, and unite. Lastly, Tuckman (1965) believed that there are four consistent stages of group regardless of whether they are short- or long-term based. He called his stages forming, storming, norming, and performing.

The OT practitioner must have an understanding of group development to support healthy, productive occupations and functioning among members. Within this social microcosm, the practitioner becomes a role model for ways to manage both effective and non-effective communication patterns and working through dependent vs. independent functioning.

LEADERSHIP STYLES

The OT practitioner must decide what style of leadership will complement his or her own personality and the functioning level of group members. Your style of leadership is an example of how you incorporate your therapeutic use of self. Practitioners who are self-confident with good self-esteem will model a positive, accepting regard for clients because they accept who they are in real life. This means that the practitioner accepts both the positive and negative parts of him- or herself without self-degradation. In turn, the OT leader can provide non-judgmental and unconditional positive regard for every person in treatment, aside from their diagnosis, labels, or history.

In general, clients with low functioning abilities will need more direction and structure from the leader, which requires an active, attentive leader. Examples include Mosey's (1970) parallel and project level groups and Ross' (1997) integrative group approach. When members have high cognitive functioning, demonstrated by their ability to communicate with good insight and judgment, the group leader acts as a facilitator of group process. Sometimes, the leader can even act as a fellow member. For example, Mosey's egocentric-cooperative level group requires that an OT practitioner facilitate the process, while Mosey's mature level group allows the leader to act like a member or peer.

According to Yalom (1995), the effective group leader guides the group through an experience and then encourages members to reflect and learn about the process. OT practitioners must decide what style of leadership is best suited to guide both the experiential and processing aspects of group. Levels of control and direction must match the needs of clients and suit the type of group model that is selected for intervention.

Kurt Lewin and his colleague (1938) identified three main styles of leadership: autocratic, democratic, and laissez-faire. Autocratic leadership reflects complete control, similar to a dictatorship. There is no input or feedback sought from the members. It is hard to imagine that an OT practitioner would use such a leadership style. Even under extraordinary circumstances, where one may be giving passive ROM to a client who is comatose, the practitioner is always monitoring the potential response of the client. A more humane, acceptable approach that is suited for low functioning clients is the directive style of leadership. A group leader who is directive will recognize that clients may have impairment in communication, judgment, and reasoning; therefore, the practitioner will set goals, determine group structure, set limits on inappropriate and unsafe behaviors, and closely monitor the social-emotional needs of clients. It is common for OT practitioners to use the directive style of leadership because we provide many group interventions for clients with impaired cognitive abilities.

A democratic style of leadership allows for feedback to be exchanged between the group leader and group members. Freedom and choices, expression of wants and needs, and personal self-disclosure are all encouraged by the OT practitioner who uses this approach. Lewin and Lippitt (1938) believed that a group is most likely to become cohesive if the leader is democratic. Another way to define this level of leadership is facilitative. A facilitator guides the group to accomplish its goals and reach its highest level of functioning by empowering members to take risks and make good decisions. This style of leadership is suited for persons who have adequate self-awareness and the verbal ability to express personal wants, desires, and needs.

A group leader who uses a laissez-faire approach appears passive and non-directive. All goal setting, decision-making, and problem-solving is accomplished by group members without any influence from the leader (Lewin & Lippitt, 1938). The group's functioning is the total responsibility of its members. This approach can be used with a mature and high functioning group where members are capable of leading and processing their own group experience without any direction or guidance from the leader. An OT practitioner who is laissez-faire deliberately refrains from interfering in the process, a different role from acting like a fellow member or advisor. An example of a positive group experience that is run with minimal guidance from a leader is a community meeting. Members hold office (president, vice president, secretary, and treasurer) and independently conduct daily or weekly informational meetings with both fellow clients and staff present.

GROUP MEMBERSHIP ROLES

As discussed, the OT practitioner can have significant impact on group development and process by his or her leadership role. Another important influence that greatly impacts group functioning is the membership roles. In 1948, two researchers, Kenneth Benne and Paul Sheats, defined three categories of membership roles. In general, they defined group roles as predictable behavioral patterns that will emerge in every group experience regardless of who participates in them. Roles are interchangeable and assumed by various members who re-enact their interpersonal style in the social microcosm experience. A healthy-functioning individual can assume many roles and accommodate the needs of the group by relating to others in a variety of ways. A goal for every OT practitioner is to develop as many healthy, productive roles as possible. A group leader can enhance group functioning and development by supporting and role modeling an assortment of roles.

Benne and Sheats (1978) defined three categories of group roles from their research at the National Training Lab in Group Development. They are:

1. Task roles
2. Group building and maintenance roles
3. Individual roles

The following is a brief summary of these descriptions.

Group task roles describe behaviors that contribute to how work gets done and how solutions can be reached. These roles impact discussions and problem-solving, evident within the content of group. There are 12 roles.

1. Initiator contributor—Provides ideas and new perspectives.
2. Information seeker—Seeks clarification and factual information.
3. Opinion seeker—Wants clarification of values and attitudes.
4. Information giver—Readily provides facts as needed.
5. Opinion giver—Offers values and attitudes to others.
6. Elaborator—Expands on suggestions.
7. Coordinator—Assembles/organizes ideas.
8. Orienter—Reminds the group of its intent and purpose.
9. Evaluator critic—Offers standards used to measure accomplishments.
10. Energizer—Motivates the group to decide and/or take action.
11. Procedural technician—Takes on various duties and jobs.
12. Recorder—Keeps notes on group and recalls information.

Group building and maintenance roles are those that promote a relationship between members and sustain functioning within the group. These roles are identified by exploring the group process. There are seven supportive roles.

1. Encourager—Supports others in positive ways.
2. Harmonizer—Attempts to mediate differences of opinions.
3. Compromiser—Will accommodate and trade off own position for good of the whole.
4. Gatekeeper and expediter—Keeps lines of communication open and flowing.
5. Standard setter—Sets expectations and ideals for the group.
6. Group observer and commentator—Shares views and interpretations.
7. Follower—Passively goes along with members.

Individual roles describe behaviors that serve personal needs rather than group needs. They distract a group from becoming cohesive because they have a negative impact on group development and interfere with group functioning rather than encourage it. There are eight individual roles.

1. Aggressor—Demeans and attacks the status of others by expressing negativity.
2. Blocker—Resists group progress.
3. Recognition seeker—Attracts attention to self.
4. Self-confessor—Attracts attention by inappropriate disclosures.
5. Playboy—Uses joking and provocative behavior to distract attention onto self.
6. Dominator—Shows inappropriate authority by monopolizing others.
7. Help seeker—Appears needy; seeks pity.
8. Special interest pleader—Disguises own prejudices through social positions.

A productive and healthy functioning group exhibits a balance of task and group building/maintenance roles and shows a scarcity of individual roles. The reader is encouraged to complete the Role Analysis worksheet on pages 46 to 48 from Cole's *Group Dynamics in OT* (2nd ed.) (1998) as an experiential exercise to increase understanding and application of these concepts.

CREATION AND DESIGN OF AN ACTIVITY GROUP

Now that the reader has come to understand basic components of group dynamics, this next section will focus on a group format, designed by Marli Cole (1998), which will encourage group process and the integration of experiential learning. Cole adapted her "seven step process for activity groups" from Pfeiffer and Jones' *Reference Guide to Handbooks and Annuals* (1973, 1977).

While this group format is easily suited for high functioning groups with good cognitive ability, it can be adapted to meet the goals of any group. The following is a summary of the seven sequential steps (Cole, 1998).

1. Introduction—In this step, both the leader and members introduce themselves to each other. The purpose of this step is to acknowledge every person in group and to begin the process of building trust and rapport among members. Within this step, the OT practitioner must include the following components:
   - Warm-up.
   - Expectations/norms of the group.
   - Explanation of purpose and goals reflecting OT domains of practice.
   - Brief outline of the group structure, including the time frame.

2. Activity—This step includes the experience portion of the group. The OT practitioner explains the directions of the activity in ways that can be optimally understood by members. For example, the group leader may give directions verbally, in writing, and/or through demonstration. Depending on the cognitive level, directions may be provided in a step-by-step fashion or in a series of steps. Inherent in this step, the OT practitioner must have adequately considered the therapeutic goals and desired outcome of the activity, physical and mental capacities of the members, knowledge and skill of the leader, and grading needs and adaptation of the activity to the clinical setting.

3. Sharing—Each member is asked to share his or her experience with others. The group leader models effective verbal and nonverbal communication such as listening, attending, asking open questions, and conveying empathy. Members should once again be acknowledged for their participation and self-expression. It is important not to exclude anyone in the group, therefore, every member should be invited to participate in the experience.

4. Processing—This is the most challenging aspect of group. It is where interpersonal learning (Yalom's therapeutic factor) can occur between members. In this step, the members are guided by the leader to reflect on what they have learned from the experience or activity. An OT practitioner who is knowledgeable about group dynamics will incorporate this understanding, asking members to discuss norms, developmental stages, leadership, and membership role functioning, as they all reflect the interaction patterns of members. A group leader will encourage expression of feelings and the

development of self-awareness about both intrapersonal and interpersonal aspects.

5.   Generalizing—The group leader in this step addresses the cognitive learning aspects of the group. Principles are highlighted and discussed in preparation for the next phase of group.

6.   Application—Here, members are asked to consider how they will transfer what they learned during this group into their own lives. The meaning and/or significance of the group activity is discussed and members are encouraged to think about how this group reflects issues and concerns that are part of their everyday relationships outside of groups. In other words, this is where members explore the social microcosm experience and apply it to their own individual lives.

7.   Summary—This is the final step of group. The most important learning principles of the experience are reviewed and summarized. It is also highly effective for the group leader to remind the group of its original purpose and goals and discuss what goals have and have not been reached. Members are asked to define goals for their future and summarize what other learning they would like to accomplish outside of this group. Each member is thanked for his or her contribution.

The reader is encouraged to consult Cole's *Group Dynamics in OT* (2nd ed.) (1998) for further explanation of this group format, including other factors that contribute to a successful group experience.

SUMMARY

The profession of OT began in the 1920s as a group-oriented approach for the treatment of persons with mental illness. "Occupation therapists" observed how purposeful occupations increased the adaptive functioning of their patients, although they did not understand the reasons why. With the ascent of further research from various theorists representing different schools of thought about clinical practice, pathology, and group theory, OTs began to adapt these concepts into their practice. As a result, significant contributions were made to group development by OTs from a variety of theoretical orientations. Some well-known contributors include the Azimas, Fidler, Mosey, King, Kaplan, Allen, Ross, and Cole.

An effective OT practitioner must have comprehensive knowledge about the various group models, their foundation constructs, and the applicable domains of practice areas that are best suited for treatment intervention. Upon the determination of a client's clinical needs, the practitioner must select an appropriate group intervention. The OT practitioner also needs to understand basic group dynamic principles to appreciate how the group model can be used for experiential learning and the achievement of positive functional outcomes in members. Social microcosm theory is a basic assumption that underlies all group work. Other significant components of group intervention include the formation of norms, stages of development, interpersonal learning, development of cohesiveness, group process, leadership style, and membership roles.

Even though the OT practitioner may understand group dynamics, he or she must develop a communication style that fosters a therapeutic relationship with the members. Therapeutic communication is different from the typical ways of interacting and socializing with people in our natural environments. Practitioners who exemplify a proficient therapeutic use of self demonstrate core qualities such as respect for others, genuine and unselfish concern for others, authentic expression of attitudes and behaviors, and dignity in valuing the uniqueness of every individual. Practitioners who are self-aware and self-accepting will naturally model ways to encourage the formation of intrapersonal and interpersonal aspects of oneself.

OT practitioners who are knowledgeable about group theory, possess a repertoire of group models for practice, and manifest proficient therapeutic communication are likely to become competent group leaders. They can create, design, and adapt any therapy group to suit a variety of performance areas and components within the designated domains of OT practice.

REFERENCES

Allen, C. K. (1985). *OT for psychiatric diseases: Measurement and management of cognitive disabilities.* Boston, MA: Little, Brown, & Co.

Azima, H., & Azima, F. (1959). The therapeutic use of self. *Am J Occup Ther, 12,* 215-225.

Benne, K., & Sheats, P. (1978). Functional roles of group members. In L. Bradford (Ed.), *Group development* (2nd ed.). La Jolla, CA: University Associates.

Bion, W. (1961). *Experiences in groups and other papers.* New York, NY: Basic Books.

Cole, M. B. (1998). *Group dynamics in OT. The theoretical basis and practice application of group treatment* (2nd ed.). Thorofare, NJ: SLACK Incorporated.

Edelson, M. (1964). *Ego psychology, group dynamics, and the therapeutic community.* New York, NY: Grune & Stratton.

Fidler, G. (1969). The task-oriented group as a context for treatment. *Am J Occup Ther, 23*(1), 43-48.

Jacobs, K. (1999). *Quick reference dictionary for OT* (2nd ed). Thorofare, NJ: SLACK Incorporated.

Kaplan, K. (1988). *Directive group therapy.* Thorofare, NJ: SLACK Incorporated.

King, L. J. (1974). A sensory integrative approach to schizophrenia. *Am J Occup Ther, 28*(9), 529-536.

Lewin, K. (1945). *Dynamic theory of personality.* New York, NY: McGraw Hill.

Lewin, K., & Lippitt, R. (1938). An experimental approach to the study of autocracy and democracy: A preliminary note. *Sociometry, I,* 292-300.

Mosey, A. (1970). The concept and use of developmental groups. *Am J Occup Ther, 24*(4), 272-275.

Pfeiffer, J., & Jones, J. (1973). *Reference guide to handbooks and annuals.* La Jolla, CA: University Associates.

Pfeiffer, J., & Jones, J. (1977). *Reference guide to handbooks and annuals* (2nd ed.). La Jolla, CA: University Associates.

Quiroga, V. A. M. (1995). *OT: The first 30 years 1900 to 1930.* Bethesda, MD: AOTA.

Ross, M. (1997). *Integrative group therapy: The structured five-stage approach.* (2nd ed.). Bethesda, MD: AOTA.

Schutz, W. (1958). The interpersonal underworld. *Harvard Business Review. 36*(4), 123-135.

Stein, F., & Cutler, S. K. (1998). *Psychosocial OT. A holistic approach.* San Diego, CA: Singular Publishing Group.

Tuckman, B. (1965). Developmental sequence in small groups. *Psychological Bulletin, 63*(6), 384-399.

Tufano, R. (1997). Therapeutic communication. In K. Sladyk (Ed.), *OT student primer. A guide to college success.* Thorofare, NJ: SLACK Incorporated.

Yalom, I. D. (1995). *The theory and practice of group psychotherapy.* New York, NY: Basic Books.

Arts and Crafts as Occupation

Chapter 31

Margaret Drake, PhD, OTR/L, ATR-BC, CPAT, FAOTA

INTRODUCTION

Crafts are occupations using special skills such as manual arts. They are part of our OT legacy from founders and professional elders. Despite the fact that the world has changed so that computer technology and information management occupy a good part of many peoples' work lives, crafts continue to engage our creative impulses. The proliferation of craft supply stores and craft departments in super stores attests to this. In the early part of the 20th century, industrialization removed workers from direct contact with the materials they were shaping into objects. Assembly lines removed the opportunity for workers to put their individual mark on their work. The parallel development of the craft movement provided this connection with creative hands-on construction that had previously been an integral part of many workers' lives. As crafts came to be thought of as leisure activities, they were no longer as worthwhile in our culture, a culture in which work is a central value. Crafts were no longer considered work (Drake, 1999).

Though crafts are no longer the main treatment modality in OT, more than half of OT clinics still use some crafts. This is not reflected in our textbooks and journals (Drake, 1999). It may be likened to the way that cleanliness was an early and integral value for nurses, and while nurses are still taught techniques of cleanliness even as they learn the newer technologies, they have not abandoned this central practice of their profession. The nursing journals and books have little about cleanliness, just as our literature has little about crafts and arts.

DO THEORIES INFLUENCE HOW CRAFTS ARE USED?

Theories are ideas about why things work the way they do. In OT, theories and ideas continue to change. OT practitioners call their theories models. Each model listed below has some central concepts. Each has an example of how a paper weaving craft might be used.

- The neuromotor behavior model concept is that dysfunction comes from chemical or structural prob-

---

KEY CONCEPTS

- Crafts and OT: A historic legacy in OT.
- Crafts and frames of reference: Different theories emphasize different uses for crafts, and there is a vast variety of crafts available for use with clients and patients.
- Crafts and occupation: How someone does a craft is an example of how he or she lives his or her life.

ESSENTIAL VOCABULARY

Art: A skilled way of decorating or illustrating.

Craft: An object usually made by hand using tools and skill.

Kits: Pre-prepared materials for a craft project.

Theory: An explanation of why the world is the way it is and why things work the way they do.

lems in the nervous system. Problems can be remedied by restructuring the nervous system or compensating for chemical imbalance with medication. A craft would be used to overcome a brain dysfunction by stimulating activity that would cause chemical changes or would enhance neuron restructuring in the brain. An OTA might choose paper weaving because it has repetitive features that cause a person's neurological system to produce more or less of a chemical or reroute information in the brain around the damaged pathways.

- The learning/cognitive disabilities model believes task performance shows the level of cognitive function or ability to learn. Levels of conscious awareness are given numerical values. The type of craft used would be on the level the patient can do without too much challenge and stress. The OTA might choose paper weaving because it is the right amount of challenge for a person functioning at a lower level.

- The developmental/spatiotemporal model views human life as a series of stages. Dysfunction is the failure to pass through the appropriate life stages and to achieve certain milestones. A craft would be expected to assist the person to grow toward the next life stage of development. The OTA might choose paper weaving to help the person to learn a lesson that will help him or her grow mentally so he or she can do the things expected at the next life stage.

- The lifestyle/adaptive performance model is based on the idea that a person has four domains. Each domain includes needs that each human must satisfy in order to function in a healthy way. The domains are interpersonal relationships, welfare of others, self-care, and intrinsic gratification. A craft would be expected to assist the person to satisfy the needs of his or her four basic domains. The OTA might help the patient make a paper weaving gift to satisfy an interpersonal need or to gain intrinsic gratification from creating something attractive.

- The rehabilitation model emphasizes the team approach in which continued challenge is part of a patient's treatment. The therapist is considered a teacher. A craft would be used to challenge the individual to learn new skills. The OTA might choose paper weaving in order to challenge a patient who needs to improve fine motor control and dexterity.

- The Model of Human Occupation is based on the idea that all things are connected. The mind, brain, and body cannot be separated in therapy. There are three subsystems that deal with level of motivation, habitual learning, and functional performance of the combined mind-brain-body. The craft would be used to integrate skills and learned behavior with understanding of one's own values, motivations, and acceptance of personal responsibility for his or her life. The OTA might offer paper weaving as a choice with some other crafts to assist the individual in increasing responsibility in decision-making and personal choice.

- The occupational adaptation model deals with how individuals adapt to changing conditions in their life. Crafts would be used to assist individuals to experiment with adapting to changes in life by adapting to changes in projects and materials. The OTA might use paper weaving to assist the person in adapting him- or herself to the simple paper materials available.

An OTA may work in a situation in which one theory is used, however, it is more usual to combine theories in using crafts with patients. The best therapists are able to use whatever model most thoroughly explains why a patient needs the craft activity. Such a therapist is an eclectic thinker. Eclectic means to use whatever best fits the situation (Drake, 1999).

WHEN ARE CRAFTS THERAPEUTIC?

Most people feel more capable when they are able to prove to themselves that they can complete a craft. Some crafts are also associated with self-care (e.g., mending and sewing to maintain clothing, cooking to provide adequate nutrition). While these crafts apply to almost everyone, there are specific crafts that fit a specific dysfunction better than other crafts. The best way to assess whether or not a craft will be therapeutic is to look at the OT treatment goals for that person. Will the craft help achieve either the short-term objectives or the long-term goals? Can the craft be finished in the time the patient is expected to be receiving OT treatment? Is the craft likely to make the person feel good about him- or herself, his or her work, and his or her relationship to other people? Does it fit with the patient's interests? If the answer to these questions is yes, the craft is probably therapeutic.

Not all people respond well to craft occupations. They may have had little experience working with their hands, or little experience in creatively expressing themselves. For them, a craft may not be therapeutic. It may make them feel inadequate or frustrated.

UNIFORM TERMINOLOGY HELPS IN ACTIVITY/OCCUPATION ANALYSIS

Uniform Terminology is OT's way of organizing its knowledge. The performance areas into which most crafts can be categorized are play or leisure exploration or play or leisure performance. It is possible that craftwork could fall into several other performance area categories, such as safety procedures, meal preparation, or perhaps vocational exploration if a person plans to make crafts for profit (AOTA, 1994).

Performance components include all the different categories of human response upon which OT practitioners may focus their treatment (AOTA, 1994). A craft such as assembling a wooden birdhouse kit could involve 30 components all in the same activity. The components provide a way for OT practitioners to sort out the complexity of human behavior into more manageable chunks.

The performance contexts (AOTA, 1994) assist in choosing the right craft for each patient. They guide OT practitioners to focus on the person's age, progress through the lifespan, restrictions placed upon him or her by the disability, the place in which he or she lives and works, the people around him or her, and cultural considerations. These contexts offer guidance in being appropriate in craft choices for individuals (See Chapter 6).

WHICH IS ART AND WHICH IS CRAFT?

Crafts have often been thought of as lesser than arts. The problem of distinguishing art from craft is an old one. Both craftspeople and artists have felt undervalued by Western cultures, as their pay was never equivalent with hourly pay of other workers. Some think of art, such as drawing and painting, as more skilled than craftwork, such as ceramics and woodworking. Almost every craft requires the use of some skill from art. In some art shows, work that has been judged to be a craft rather than art has been rejected. This may have to do with pricing, as the prices of art are often much higher than craft. Those who judge work by its monetary value may adhere to the idea that art is higher than craft. OT practitioners and art therapists seldom make those distinctions because therapists know that all personal expressions have value and meaning.

KITS: THE MODERN EQUIVALENT OF A CAKE MIX

OT practitioners have traditionally prepared their materials in large quantities for efficiency sake. Some therapists are more skilled in using raw materials than

others. The modern health care environment does not encourage therapists to use their time in materials preparation, as the time we spend with patients is billable. The time we spend preparing craft materials is not billable. Even non-profit hospitals want their therapists to pay for themselves through their work. Consequently, therapists are encouraged to use kits because they can spend most of their time with patients and be paid for it, rather than preparing materials and not being paid for it. Nonetheless, it is still a valuable skill for an OTA to know how to prepare and use raw materials. Sometimes kits are not readily available, but the OTA can still utilize crafts if raw materials are available in the same way that a modern cook may have to fall back on baking a cake from scratch if a cake mix is not available. Kits take up less space in the modern clinic than raw materials, just as a cake mix takes up less space than a canister of flour, a canister of sugar, a can of shortening, and a can of baking powder. The eggs and milk are raw materials that must be kept separate and refrigerated for both the cake and the cake mix. A wooden birdhouse requires that the finishes be kept separate whether it is made from a kit or cut from boards.

COOKING

"...Cooking is the most commonly practiced craft in all OT clinics" (Drake, 1999, p. 157). Cooking is a craft media that appeals to childhood memories. Food fills needs of nutrition, symbolizes love, and provides opportunities for creative expression. Food appeals to everybody. Each culture has food that has special meaning. It is important to explore these meanings with clients before actually cooking. Some cultures and religions have foods that are prohibited. For example, pork is prohibited in both Judaic and Islamic religions. Some patients have food restrictions that are part of their treatment regime. For example, persons with diabetes have dietary guidelines they must follow as do people with eating disorders, high blood pressure, and cholesterolemia. These are all considerations the OTA must resolve before cooking with patients.

Cooking is an activity that lends itself to group cooperation. Each person can be responsible for one small piece of the cooking activity in the same way that potlucks offer the opportunity to be part of a larger production that gives pleasure to many.

WOODWORKING

Crafts made with wood can range from something as simple as assembling a kit to complex projects such as designing furniture. Woodworking has a special mystique as traditionally it involved skills and knowledge not easily acquired. The feel of the smooth finish on wood products has been called sensual. Wood products remind us that we, too, are a part of nature. Woodworking has the classic features of constructive/destructive materials. While creating something with it, we are also destroying its previous state. This is the constructive/destructive feature.

In the past, many clinics had big floor tools, powered either by electricity or foot pedals. Modern clinics are more apt to have one cupboard with hand tools purchased at a hardware store. Some use kits, which require only sandpaper, glue, and a hammer. Wood carving on soft wood, such as balsa, still offers the opportunity to whittle like our ancestors did.

Woodworking was traditionally identified as man's work. Currently, it is considered appropriate for women, men, children, and the elderly. Age or gender is not a qualification for woodworking. Strength, endurance, and awareness of safety measures are important qualifications in this craft. Because so many woodworking tools are capable of inflicting wounds, therapists in psychiatric settings need to be especially careful to prevent their use as weapons, for self-mutilation, or as safety hazards for the cognitively impaired.

LEATHERWORK

Few of us live our lives without leather clothes, games, or tools. While many mammals and reptiles produce leather, most therapists use cowhide, which comes in several thicknesses. Cowhide is readily available and most leather kits are made of this.

Leatherwork offers a spectrum of crafts from very difficult to extremely simple. Examples are a complex leather briefcase to a keychain. Leather can be easily graded. It can be tooled in intricate designs by higher functioning patients. Stamping tools provide quick, uncomplicated patterns for lower functioning patients. Plastic templates can be used to press pre-drawn pictures unto the leather. Leather can be colored with stains and paint. There are a variety of kinds of lace and lacing for piecing leather together.

Few younger children are able to benefit from leatherwork. Adolescent and older children may enjoy it. Since hand strength is so important in leatherwork, leather craft is a challenge for many elderly (Drake, 1999).

NEEDLE CRAFTS

One out of five OT clinics uses needlework at least one time per week in patient treatment (Drake, 1999). Sewing and needlework are among the easiest and most controllable crafts for very sick patients. Needlework includes simple sewing of clothing and home furnishings;

quilting; and surface decorations such as embroidery, needlepoint, knitting, and crocheting. These crafts traditionally have been considered women's work. For this reason, it may be difficult to motivate males to try them, although many famous male athletes have used needlework to improve fine motor skills. Small children may not know about the gender stereotyping of needlework and be eager to try sewing. For them, sewing can be just another way to make a picture.

Most movement in sewing is in the hands and arms. It is good for improving dexterity but can cause repetitive motion injuries in some patients. Sewing can be adapted for patients with vision problems by using contrasting threads, such as dark thread on light-colored cloth. Tools such as left-handed scissors make this craft accessible to almost everyone. Those with immune disorders and poor circulation, such as diabetes, need extra precautions when using needles to avoid infection in a needle-prick wound. Many sewing tools are capable of inflicting wounds. Therapists in mental health facilities need to be especially careful to prevent their use as weapons, for self-mutilation, or as safety hazards for the cognitively impaired.

METAL CRAFTS

Metalworking is a skill that few people learn before they experience it in OT. Shaping a flat piece of metal, such as in copper tooling, is one method. Piercing metal in a pattern is another. More sophisticated metal treatments include soldering, etching, enameling, and riveting. All of these methods require extra safety precautions. Grading of metalwork can start with simple plastic template copper tooling to a sophisticated metal sculpture.

All metal work requires good strength, eye hand coordination, and sensory awareness. The simplest techniques require few supplies or tools and can be done at bedside with therapists completing in the clinic what cannot be done in the patient's room. Almost complete assurance of a pleasing outcome makes cooper tooling an ideal project for patients who need immediate gratification. Children can use simple tools and materials, such as piercing copper or aluminum foil with a toothpick. For the elderly with cognitive impairment, copper tooling or piercing does not challenge their capabilities, while still providing a pleasing outcome.

MOSAICS

Mosaic is an ageless craft in which colored pieces of material, such as tile, are assembled to make a picture or design. One-third of clinics have mosaics as a treatment occupation (Drake, 1999). This craft is part of several formal OT assessments because it is able to determine color discrimination, spatial awareness, dexterity, and praxis. A client can complete a tile trivet in two sessions, which appeals to therapists whose patients stay only a few days. It can be done by bed patients, by one-handed patients, by low functioning mental health patients, and the elderly. The attention span of children is usually not long enough to do traditional mosaics; however, there are ways to hasten the process to adapt to short attention spans, such as mosaics made with paper "tiles."

FIBER CRAFTS

Fiber crafts include things made from reeds, grasses, paper, yarn, cord, and string. It is basically the same process for all fiber crafts—intermingling one strand of fibers with another strand of fibers. In weaving, the warp and weft fibers cross each other at square angles. Macramé and tatting are special forms of knotting fibers. Rug hooking involves special knots through a coarse cloth to make a nap on one side. In Turkish knotting, special knots are tied around two warp strands. While needlework was often the responsibility of females, in some cultures, males had the responsibility for fiber crafts. Men learned how to make special nautical knots and nets as well as weaving carpets. Currently, some clinics use these crafts for fine motor strengthening as well as to increase bilateral dexterity.

CERAMICS

While whole buildings can be built of fired ceramic clay, for the purposes of OT, small projects are best. The clay used in ceramics has special properties that make it harden in the intense heat of the ceramic oven, called a kiln. Many newer manufactured materials have appeared that mimic ceramics. Some of these imitators are very adaptable to the clinic. They can be baked in the clinic kitchen oven (Dierks, 1994), and they can be painted to look like ceramic glaze. However, traditional ceramic clay pieces are more durable and impervious to water.

One in three therapists uses clay or one of its imitators in therapy. In psychiatry, it is often used as part of a battery of assessments for patients. Because of its malleability, clay helps therapists understand how patients deal with structure and control. Wet clay allows a person to reshape his or her mistakes without penalty. The pottery wheel is seldom used in clinics now because it requires advanced skills not acquired in short hospital stays. It also requires upper body strength, which many sick people do not have. Most ceramics currently used in treatment is hand built or slip cast, which is liquid clay poured into a plaster mold and allowed to harden.

Clay imitators, called therapy putties, are used daily in physical rehabilitation for strengthening, increasing ROM, and developing coordination. The visually impaired respond to the tactile quality of clay. Some psychiatric patients use clay as a method of expressing ideas that are difficult to verbalize. Children find clay a natural toy, which they manipulate in a way developmentally parallel to drawing—first the head, then the body, and so on. Elderly have sensory losses that can be both enhanced or cause endangerment through clay work. Ceramic clay is inexpensive, however, the kiln, kiln wiring, and kiln furniture to hold pieces being fired can be major expenses (Drake, 1999).

COMPUTER CRAFTS

Most new computers come already equipped with a graphics drawing program. Graphics programs come in all levels of complexity. Some are for people who like to draw freehand. Others are pre-drawn images assembled like a collage. Computer crafts are especially helpful for those patients whose self-image is tied to the age of information technology. Journal writing, poetry writing, and other forms of expressive language are easy on the computer. There are programs for music composition and programs for assisting children to create stories. If scanners are available, computers can be used in conjunction with photography. Many skills can be the focus of treatment while using a mouse or a joystick to control the pictures.

FOUND MATERIALS

In many situations, therapists are called upon to improvise with available non-commercial materials that were not intended for crafts. These could include household items like empty containers, natural materials such as pinecones, scraps of cloth, paper, or small metal items. These found items can be assembled into wall decorations, sculptures, mobiles, puppets, or decorated containers. The possibilities are limited only by the creativity of the therapist and patient and availability of glue, staples, string, and tape. Therapists have always resorted to found materials when their budget did not provide for more expensive supplies. The capability to see possibilities in the humblest materials is the skill of a superior therapist.

OTHER CRAFTS

Some departments have a category of crafts called "minor media." This usually includes decorative processes not included in the above categories. Some of these are printing, which includes silkscreen, linoleum blocks, and vegetable prints; decoupage, in which pictures are glued to wooden plaques; suncatchers, which are small transparent window decorations; and other specialty crafts. This by no means covers all the craft possibilities. New products are developed constantly. An alert therapist keeps his or her eyes open for such new treatment options for patients. Some places to look for these new ideas are in home magazines, the craft book section of bookstores, craft catalogs, home decorating programs on television, and from other therapists.

MISCELLANEOUS MEDIA

Therapists have often used creative media, some of which are called crafts, to elicit from patients their own creative impulses. Some of these crafts are face-painting, clowning, pantomime, and magic. Another kind of media that encourages creativity is non-competitive games, which get people to think in new cooperative ways about how to solve problems. Some of these games can be played on the playground and some are board games. These games help people have fun without the pressure to win. All these media help people approach their problems in new ways.

SUMMARY

Crafts continue to offer patients the opportunity to see their work behavior as a microcosm of their way of being in the world. When patients hold up a completed project and proclaim, "I did this," therapists are able to give real praise for a job well done. If the craft project is not well done, the therapist can use it as a teaching opportunity to discuss how the experience of working on the craft mirrors the patient's experiences in life. The "doing" of crafts is a sample of the "doing" in life. To learn more about these benefits, read *Crafts in Therapy and Rehabilitation (2nd ed.)* (Drake, 1999).

REFERENCES

AOTA. (1994). Uniform terminology for OT (3rd ed.). *Am J Occup Ther, 48,* 1047-1054.

Dierks, L. (1994). *Creative clay jewelry: Designs to make from polymer clay.* Ashville, NC: Lark Books.

Drake, M. L. (1999). *Crafts in therapy and rehabilitation* (2nd ed.). Thorofare, NJ: SLACK Incorporated.

Assistive Technology and Adaptive Equipment

Chapter 32

Mary Kathryn Cowan, MA, OTR, FAOTA

INTRODUCTION

The term *adaptive equipment* has been used throughout the course of OT and rehabilitation history to describe assistive devices, aids, or equipment that allow a person with a handicap to perform an occupational activity that otherwise would have been difficult or impossible. Although a variety of equipment is available for purchase, time constraints, budget limitations, reimbursement problems, and/or the uniqueness of a specific participation problem may require the construction of special devices to suit a particular situation.

Adaptive equipment is selected or designed and constructed when an individual cannot perform a life task without some form of assistance. Appropriate aids are needed when problems with postural control, reaching, grasping, or accessing materials interfere with active participation in meaningful occupational activities. Many individuals whose treatment plan includes the possible use of adaptive devices may also have goals to improve the very abilities that interfere with performance as well. Either on a temporary or long-term basis, change in component abilities that underlie the occupational performance may not be extensive enough to allow independence in some activities. Adaptive equipment may then fill the need for this individual. By increasing the individual's independence in important life tasks (activities that must be accomplished for successful living throughout the life span) and roles through use of adaptive devices, a sense of achievement and satisfaction can be realized.

Individually constructed equipment may be as simple as using a waxed paper container to hold playing cards ("low tech") or as complex as the design and use of computerized environmental control systems ("high tech"). Whether simple or complex, the focus of this chapter is to acquaint the reader with principles of selection, design, and construction that usually guide a therapist in solving a functional problem with the use of adaptive equipment.

HISTORICAL USES

The earliest forms of adaptive equipment in OT included page turners, card

ESSENTIAL VOCABULARY

Adaptive equipment: Devices used to allow performance of a functional task.

Bolsters: Soft therapeutic equipment that provides support under a child's axilla in the prone position.

Clinical reasoning process: A type of thinking used in clinical work.

Cost-effective: Equipment that is worthwhile to make considering the therapist's time and materials involved.

Cowan stabilizing pillow: An example of an adaptive device that assists a child's balance or stability when sitting.

Half-lapboard: An example of an adaptive device that provides support to a patient's or client's hemiplegic arm.

Life tasks: Daily activities.

Specific needs: Activities the patient or client requires in daily life.

Trial use: An established period of time when equipment may be applied and evaluated as to its effectiveness.

KEY CONCEPTS

- Equipment clinical reasoning: Thinking that evaluates equipment procedurally, interactively, and conditionally.
- Precautions: Factors that consider safety first.
- Characteristics of good construction: Solid design, ease of use, comfort, acceptable to user.
- Equipment design process: Steps involved in developing new adaptive equipment.
- Presentation and follow-up: Education and review of equipment use.

holders, and nailboards, which allowed the person with a handicap to read a book without using his or her hands, to play cards with only one hand, and to peel a fruit or vegetable when the person did not have use of a stabilizing hand, respectively. Although adaptive equipment was originally developed to provide improved ability to perform ADLs and participate in leisure pursuits, it also became commonly used as a term to apply to therapy equipment that is used to develop a person's abilities or skills in therapy. Eventually balance boards, bolsters, standing tables, prone boards, and related equipment were designed and used by one or several therapists before they became standard pieces of therapy equipment.

Therapist-made equipment was a necessity for many years and only in recent OT history have many of these innovations been mass produced, marketed through catalogs, and readily available to OT personnel. When suitable equipment is available commercially, the device must still be carefully selected. This availability of equipment from catalogs does not rule out the need for individually constructed equipment. The unique needs of the individual may require the design and construction of a device that is not commercially available or is too costly to purchase. These situations require the OT or OTA to use problem-solving skills to determine the relationship between the individual's motor skill problem and the life task that needs to be accomplished, then design and construct a helpful tool to make participation possible. These skills include studying the situation that presents uncertainty or doubt and arriving at the most appropriate solution. The process involves definition, selection of a plan, organizing steps, implementing the plan, and evaluating the results.

Occupational Therapy Personnel Roles

The *OT Roles* paper (AOTA, 1999) describes the OTA's role in program planning as dependent upon establishing service competency by the OT. Designing and constructing a positioning device for a child with cerebral palsy based on the theoretical principles of neurodevelopmental treatment is an example in which OT supervision is required. A therapist with this specialized training should decide if the design and the final product do indeed fulfill the principles and intent of this therapeutic approach. A neonatal positioner that is based on such principles as well as use in a complex therapeutic environment (the neonatal intensive care unit) is another example of adaptive equipment selection or construction that requires close supervision by the OT (Monfort & Case-Smith, 1997). Frequently, the OTA who works closely with an OT in a complex treatment setting may be

the individual with the most knowledge of tools and equipment and, therefore, the one who will actually construct the needed equipment once the OT/OTA team has determined the need and type of equipment required. Equipment developed in these situations requires that the OT establish the OTA's service competency, as the performance components involved need "ongoing interpretation."

The OTA working in a setting where chronic conditions are prevalent is continually dealing with recurring functional problems that may not require the OT's clinical involvement in the adaptive equipment decision-making process. The selection, design, and construction of card holders, book holders, and built-up handles on recreational games for people with physical handicaps are examples of situations in which the OTA would not require close supervision. This type of equipment may be part of a generally accepted routine.

Selecting, designing, and constructing adaptive equipment at various levels can be a collaborative effort between the OTA and the OT, but it must also be emphasized that the patient or client is the third partner in this collaboration. The individual receiving treatment will often exhibit or describe a problem that creates a need for adaptive equipment. The user gives the OT or OTA feedback on fit and comfort. Finally, the user determines the ultimate effectiveness and usefulness of the item by his or her choice to use it or not.

Selection of Adaptive Equipment— Clinical Reasoning Process

A study by Gitlin and Burgh (1995) involved focus groups of OTs who decided on client needs for adaptive equipment in order to determine the methods of clinical reasoning used by OTs. It was determined that the methods used were *procedural* (concrete steps and procedures implemented by the therapist), *interactive* (interacting with the patient to individualize the treatment), and *conditional reasoning* (developing a comprehensive understanding of patient's situation and potential for change). The following steps were used by therapists in this study when selecting adaptive equipment.

1. Selecting a device—Involved consideration of many factors, which were either (Figure 32-1):
   - *Patient-focused* (patient status and characteristics, role history, activity level, and performance goals)
   - *External* (physical and emotional environmental support factors)
2. Fitting a device to an activity—Issuing a device involved selecting an activity that had meaning to the individual or would match the patient's cogni-

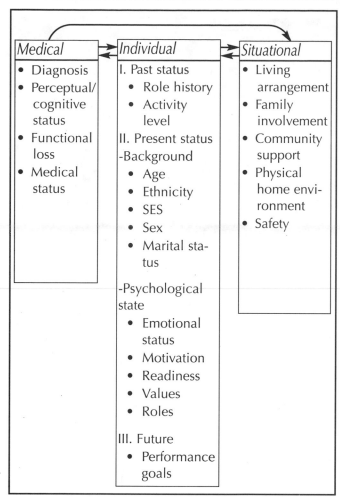

Medical	Individual	Situational

• Diagnosis
• Perceptual/
  cognitive
  status
• Functional
  loss
• Medical
  status
	I. Past status
	  • Role history
	  • Activity
	    level
	II. Present status
	-Background
	  • Age
	  • Ethnicity
	  • SES
	  • Sex
	  • Marital sta-
	    tus
	
	-Psychological
	state
	  • Emotional
	    status
	  • Motivation
	  • Readiness
	  • Values
	  • Roles
	III. Future
	  • Performance
	    goals
		• Living
		  arrangement
		• Family
		  involvement
		• Community
		  support
		• Physical
		  home envi-
		  ronment
		• Safety

Figure 32-1. Twenty-two factors that therapists considered in selecting and training patients in adaptive equipment (SES=Socioeconomic status). (Reprinted with permission from Gitlin, L. N., & Burgh, D. [1995] Issuing assistive devices to older patients in rehabilitation: An exploratory study. *Am J Occup Ther, 49*(10), 996.)

tive and functional abilities in order to ensure the success of the device and its acceptance.

3. Determining the best time to introduce a device—Often decided based on the stability of the patient's condition, the patient's readiness to accept the use of a device, and the future involvement of the patient in rehabilitation services after leaving their facility.

4. Choice of an instructional site—Depends on the activity selected (a device used for independence in dressing might be demonstrated on the ward instead of the clinic area). Consideration for the individual's privacy in trying a new piece of equipment was often made.

5. Instruction in use—Approaches to instruction might include describing the use of the device by other individuals with similar problems, use of group training, role modeling by another patient, verbal instruction, and inclusion of a family member in instruction. An exploratory study of elderly patients who were taught to use bathing and dressing devices showed that those patients "most satisfied" with the device had greater knowledge of its use (Schemm & Gitlin, 1998). Lack of knowledge about a device or inadequate instruction can be reasons patients do not continue to use a device (Finlayson & Havixbeck, 1992, Neville-Jan, et al., 1993).

6. Reinforcement of device use—Included providing opportunities for independent use, convincing staff in the rehabilitation setting of its location and importance, and educating the family (Gitlin & Burgh, 1995).

Whether a piece of adaptive equipment is temporary or permanent, it should meet a specific need for the individual. Unnecessary use of specialized equipment has the potential for making any person feel additionally or visibly "handicapped." Therefore, it is important for the OTA/OT team to ascertain that the individual meets the following criteria:

1. Unable to complete the task without the use of an aid.

2. Understands the need for additional equipment.

3. Is agreeable to trial or long-term use of the needed equipment.

CONSTRUCTING ADAPTIVE EQUIPMENT—PRECAUTIONS

Whether a device is commercially available or constructed by the OTA/OT team, safety is a constant and essential concern. When the equipment is not available commercially and must be constructed, safety is determined during three stages of the process of development:

1. Design

2. Construction

3. Use

When designing equipment, safety must be considered so that time in construction is not wasted on a piece of equipment rendered useless later when it is discovered to be unsafe. In this context, safety refers specifically to the employment of measures necessary to prevent the occurrence of injury or loss of function. Some questions the OT or OTA should ask during the design phase are:

• Will a breakdown of materials from ordinary wear cause discomfort or injury?

• Will the shape of the equipment interfere with safe use of any other equipment regularly used, such as a wheelchair or crutches?

When constructing adaptive equipment, safety problems can be anticipated by eliminating rough finishes on wood, metal, or plastic and by sanding all surfaces, edges, and corners smoothly to prevent splinters, cuts, and bruises. It is also important to use non-toxic finishes, particularly for equipment used with children who might be likely to mouth or chew objects.

Instructing the client, family, and caretakers in safe usage of equipment is the final step in making safe equipment. Observing the individual using the equipment and discussing with him or her where, when, and how to use it properly alerts the person to any possible misuse, and therefore unsafe use, of equipment made by OT personnel.

CHARACTERISTICS OF WELL-CONSTRUCTED ADAPTIVE EQUIPMENT

Simplicity in Design

A simple design facilitates the construction of the device and increases the likelihood of it being used more frequently. An example is provided in Figure 32-2, the Cowan stabilizing pillow, an adaptive pillow for children who have balance problems when sitting on the floor (Cowan, 1988). The design's simplicity (eight sections of cloth, sewing of simple seams, filling with Styrofoam pellets) makes it possible for other such as therapists, assistants, volunteers, teachers, or parents to make more pillows when recommended for other children (Figure 32-3). The chance of the next item being made improperly is also reduced by having a simple design. Because a small, soft pillow is easily transported and easily stored in a corner of the classroom, both children and teachers will be more likely to use it. If the stabilizing seat had been made from a more complicated design (e.g., a metal and leather seat with a backrest), it would be more difficult to make, move, store, and use.

Controlling the Size of Equipment

It is important that the size of equipment be limited so that it does not become awkward or cumbersome to use. An example of this might be carrying devices for wheelchairs, such as lapboards or trays, armrests, and back pockets. Although anyone in a wheelchair may want to carry large items occasionally, making the tray or pocket too large may make daily use of the wheelchair cumbersome. The half-lapboard for patients with hemiplegia, shown in Figure 32-4, demonstrates this principle by having a surface large enough to support the person's hemiplegic arm without having the surface extending out to either side (Walsh, 1987). This thoughtful consideration allows the person in the

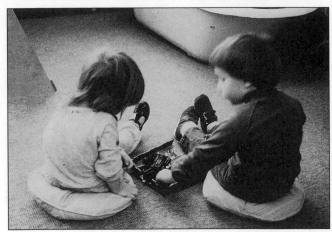

Figure 32-2. Cowan stabilizing pillow. (Reprinted from Ryan, S. E. [1993]. *The certified occupational therapy assistant: Principles, concepts, and techniques.* 2nd ed. Thorofare, NJ: SLACK Incorporated.)

wheelchair to avoid bumping into objects and people with extra or unnecessary tray extensions, and also allows adequate space to transfer in and out of the chair. (See Walsh [1987] for specific information on how to construct this equipment.) Another example of this principle is the calf board in Figure 32-5 (Chandler & Knackert, 1997) designed to keep elderly nursing home residents' feet and legs from slipping off their wheelchair foot rests and thus causing poor position as well as skin tears on feet and ankles from rubbing against the metal edges of the foot rests. The calf board clips on to the vertical supports of the foot rests with just enough soft surface to support and maintain the legs and feet in correct position, in this way preventing foot slippage backward. (See Chandler and Knackert [1997] for specific information on how to construct this equipment.)

Consideration of Cost of Materials and Construction Time

If a piece of adaptive equipment requires expensive materials, or if it takes a long time to make, the item is no longer *cost-effective.* The hourly wages of the OT and OTA, as well as the cost of the materials, must be considered. Many hours of therapy time spent constructing one piece of equipment may increase the cost of that equipment to such a point that purchasing a similar item may prove less expensive, as well as a better use of valuable clinic time.

The inexpensive *bolsters* shown in Figure 32-6 are designed for use with children under 3 years and demonstrate the use of economical materials. Mary Clarke, a COTA in Portland, OR, uses vinyl or oilcloth

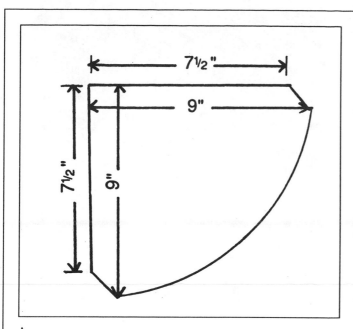

A.

Basic Materials

- 1¼ yards washable upholstery fabric
- Small Styrofoam pellets
- Heavy-duty sewing thread
- Graph paper, pencil and ruler for pattern making
- Pins, scissors and sewing machine

Instructions

1. Using paper, pencil and ruler, make a pattern as shown in Figure A.
2. Cut eight pieces of fabric to pattern specifications.
3. Using heavy-duty thread and a sewing machine, sew four pieces of fabric together to form a circle; repeat with remaining four pieces, as shown in Figure B.
4. Sew the two large circles together, leaving an opening of about four inches.
5. Reverse the pillow so that the finished outside is visible.
6. Stuff the pillow with Styrofoam pellets until it is approximately one-third to one-half filled (this makes it possible for the child to fit snugly into a "nest" of pellets).
7. Top-stitch around the edge of the pillow to finish and close the opening.

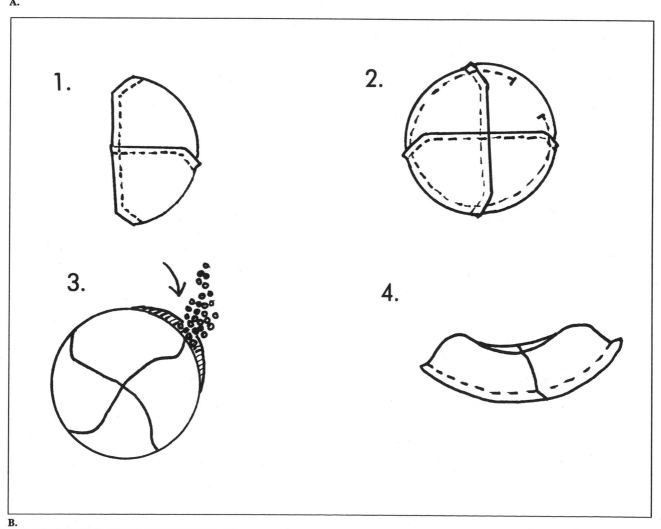

B.

Figure 32-3. Instructions for constructing a Cowan stabilizing pillow. (Reprinted from Ryan, S. E. [1993]. *The certified occupational therapy assistant: Principles, concepts, and techniques.* 2nd ed. Thorofare, NJ: SLACK Incorporated.)

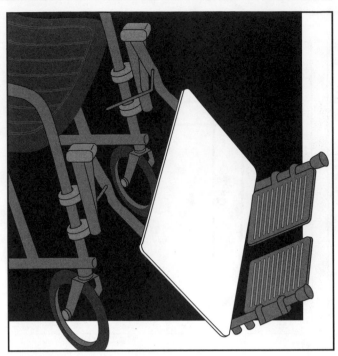

Figure 32-5. Calf board. (Adapted from Chandler & Knackert, 1997).

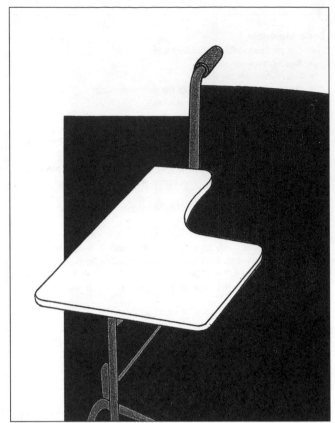

Figure 32-4. Wheelchair half-lapboard. Adapted from Walsh, 1987. (Reprinted from Ryan, S. E. [1993]. *The certified occupational therapy assistant: Principles, concepts, and techniques* [2nd ed.]. Thorofare, NJ: SLACK Incorporated.)

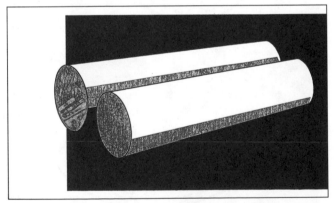

Figure 32-6. Bolsters. Adapted from Clark, 1990. (Reprinted from Ryan, S. E. [1993]. *The certified occupational therapy assistant: Principles, concepts, and techniques* [2nd ed.]. Thorofare, NJ: SLACK Incorporated.)

for the covering and lightly rolled newspapers for the interior (Clark, 1990). The seam on the outside is closed with cloth tape. Larger bolsters can be made by taping empty 3-pound coffee cans together, covering them with 1-inch foam, and then adding an outside cover of vinyl (Clark, 1990). She has also used large cardboard tubes from carpet rolls to provide the inner shape of the bolster, adding a layer of foam followed by a vinyl covering to create the finished equipment (Clark, 1990). All of these bolsters involve the use of economical materials and require very reasonable construction time. Because the bolsters are inexpensive, they can be provided to many families. In this way, it is possible to leave adaptive equipment in a home, a practice that is often not possible when similar commercially made but more expensive bolsters are used.

Attractive Appearance

An unattractive piece of equipment, no matter how useful, can interfere with its potential use. People do not like to use equipment that is roughly made, battered from use, or that has unappealing surfaces. For example, a waxpaper box makes a quick and easy piece of adaptive equipment for the one-handed card player. By covering the box with attractive vinyl shelf paper or other washable, durable material, it is not only useful but pleasant to look at.

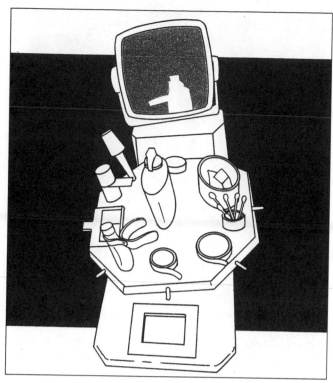

Figure 32-7. Make-up board. Adapted from Hague, 1988. (Reprinted from Ryan, S. E. [1993]. *The certified occupational therapy assistant: Principles, concepts, and techniques* [2nd ed.]. Thorofare, NJ: SLACK Incorporated.)

Figure 32-7 shows an example of a make-up board designed for use by women with quadriplegia (Hague, 1988). It is simple in design and attractive without being medical or therapeutic in appearance and would be a natural addition to a woman's bedroom. (See Hague, 1988 for specific instructions on how to make this equipment.)

Safety in Use

Although safety as a principle has already been addressed, it is an essential characteristic of well-constructed adaptive equipment that cannot be overemphasized. For example, if a stabilizer for a bowl or a pan used on the stove is not predictably stable (i.e., it can become easily detached from the surface), it can cause spilling of hot liquids onto the homemaker. Although the equipment may serve a purpose for the individual with the use of only one hand, it can create a danger that could be avoided by more careful design and construction.

Comfort in Use

The comfort of the user is affected by the placement of the equipment when it is used, materials that touch the user's body in some way, and a comfortable fit when the item is worn by the user. A handle that requires the fit of

a hand grasp or a situation in which the body or extremities are resting on the equipment are examples that illustrate the need to consider user comfort. An example of this principle is the foam positioning device shown in Figure 32-8 (von Funk, 1989). Because it uses soft foam as a basic material, it appears to be comfortable for long periods of contact with the skin, particularly when the person is immobile. (See von Funk, 1989 for specific instructions on how to make this equipment.) Possible allergy to any substance used in making equipment for a specific individual or groups of individuals should be checked. Children with spina bifida, for example, are known to have allergies to latex materials, which should not be used in any of their adaptive devices (Scoggin & Parks, 1997).

Ease in Application and Use

The ultimate test of the ease in application and usage principle is to determine if the patient can apply the device to him- or herself independently. If this is not the case, the individual(s) responsible for assisting the patient must be familiar with its proper positioning and use. The knitting device designed for use by a bilateral upper extremity amputee shown in Figure 32-9 is a good example (Duncan, 1986). The piece of equipment requires the use of a C-clamp and wing nuts (both of which the patient can manage with the bilateral prosthesis) to attach the device to the table and tighten or loosen the tension on the yarn. (See Duncan, 1986 for specific information about how to construct this equipment.)

Ease in Maintenance and Cleaning

Simplicity in the design and choice of materials for any device makes it easier to maintain and clean. A simple design eliminates corners, holes, and crevices that collect debris that is difficult to remove. If the equipment is to be used with people who have infections or are highly susceptible to infection, the construction materials must withstand the intense steam or hot water required for adequate removal of bacteria. Most clinics or schools require that all equipment be washed or cleaned periodically to promote normal infection control. Nonporous surfaces such as plastic and metal are less likely to retain dirt or agents that cause infection and heavier, porous fabrics that can be washed easily (e.g., upholstery fabric) are recommended.

DESIGNING ADAPTIVE EQUIPMENT

A Problem-Solving Process

The design of every adaptive device begins with a therapist, assistant, and the patient facing a deficit in function

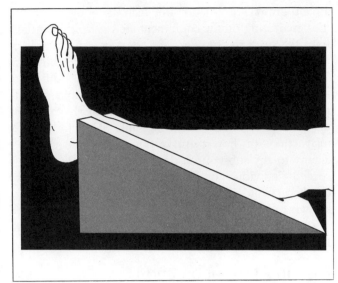

Figure 32-8. Foam positioning device. Adapted from von Funk, 1989. (Reprinted from Ryan, S. E. [1993]. *The certified occupational therapy assistant: Principles, concepts, and techniques* [2nd ed.]. Thorofare, NJ: SLACK Incorporated.)

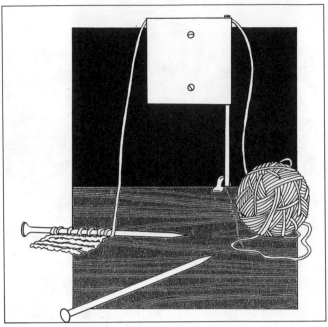

Figure 32-9. Knitting device for amputees. Adapted from Duncan, 1985. (Reprinted from Ryan, S. E. [1993]. *The certified occupational therapy assistant: Principles, concepts, and techniques* [2nd ed.]. Thorofare, NJ: SLACK Incorporated.)

together in a thoughtful, problem-solving process. If the patient is unable to participate in an activity or attain the position necessary for optimal work or task completion, new methods are tried and catalogs are perused for available equipment likely to alleviate the problem. In some instances, the problem will be solved only by designing a new piece of equipment.

Use of Patterns

Very early in the process of designing equipment, a pattern can be developed to guide the construction process. The Cowan stabilizing pillow (see Figure 32-2) provides a useful example. One-quarter of one surface of the pillow was drawn on graph paper to establish the necessary size and shape. The paper pattern was then checked in relation to the patient's body or body part, and any necessary adjustments were made. All of the other examples shown in various figures in this chapter required a basic pattern for construction. Making a pattern is an important step in the problem-solving process, as it guides the OT or OTA in estimating size and shape of the piece of adaptive equipment. Errors in the construction phase will be reduced, thus increasing efficiency and reducing the cost of production.

Constructing a Model

Once a pattern has been developed, the next step is to construct the first model or prototype of the device. This step allows the patient and the OT or OTA to discuss and experiment with changes in the design. This first model

should be viewed as flexible and malleable, as well as experimental. At this point, the shape of the pattern can be changed, new materials can be tried, and dimensions can be altered.

Redesign After Trials

After any necessary redesign, the patient begins to use the piece of equipment. Some new problems may arise at this stage, which inform the patient and OT personnel of changes that may need to be made. Only through a longer period of trial use can all of the patient's needs in regard to use of an adaptive device become completely clear. In trial use, a piece of equipment is repeatedly used in order to ensure its effectiveness.

FABRICATING ADAPTIVE EQUIPMENT

Materials

This chapter does not present a complete list of materials and their characteristics for use in fabricating adaptive equipment; however, the following characteristics are examples of those that should be considered when evaluating or selecting materials.

- Softness and pliability of shape—Necessary for pillows, slings, positioning equipment. Use cloth, canvas, or webbing; lamb's wool or "moleskin" for surface coverage; Styrofoam pellets, cotton baton, foam rubber, or polyfoam for fillers.

- Resilience and pliability of shape—Needed for positioning devices. Use splinting materials such as Orthoplast, tri-wall, acetate film, leather, rubber, or vinyl.
- Strength, solidity, and weight—Needed for laptrays, wheelchair arm supports, stabilizing equipment. Use wood, metal, hard plastics, or Formica.

Tools

The materials chosen will determine the tools required to fabricate any piece of equipment. For example, cloth requires scissors and a sewing machine; splinting materials require scissors and a heating device; and the use of wood, metal, or plastic requires hand tools or power shop equipment during the construction process. The availability of tools and the OT's or OTA's skill in using tools contributes to the quality of the finished product.

Finishing

The final step in the construction of equipment is finishing. This step is of primary importance when one considers the emotional impact of equipment use for some patients. Rough or sharp surfaces and edges need to be sanded and rounded. Extraneous threads and uneven seams need to be trimmed and repaired. Finishes such as polyurethane varnish or nontoxic paint need to be applied to wooden objects. Colors selected may be neutral to de-emphasize the equipment or bright and colorful to make equipment more attractive. The work of finishing adaptive equipment, like making furniture for a home, merits fine workmanship with attention to important details so that the product is both professional and attractive.

PRESENTATION OF CONSTRUCTED EQUIPMENT

Whether or not the use of the designed and constructed adaptive equipment has been part of the collaboration process, when it is completed the OT or OTA should review the following information with the patient:

- Purpose
- Uses
- Limitations
- Care and maintenance
- Any precautions

Even a young child needs to know that the stabilizing pillow "helps you sit better or longer" (see Figure 32-2). The adult should know that the half-lapboard shown in Figure 32-4 places his or her affected arm in view to

improve body awareness, control swelling, and prevent injury to an arm that lacks sensation. This review of the purposes of the equipment encourages proper use and, therefore, greater likelihood of its success. If the adaptive device is to be applied by another individual (nurse, aide, teacher, or parent), the details of proper application and positioning must be presented to avoid any discomfort to the patient and to ensure safe use. On hospital and rehabilitation center wards, in classrooms, and in other community settings where several people assist the individual with equipment use, the placement of a diagram or picture of the equipment properly set up can be attached to the device as a helpful reference.

DOCUMENTATION OF EFFECTIVENESS OF DESIGN

The final step when constructing adaptive equipment is to follow-up, checking with the modification of the equipment or improvement of its design for optimal function. If a particular device is used by many people, all of them should be followed and the fulfillment of the original purpose of the equipment validated with every individual. Questions such as the following can then be asked:

- How many individuals have used the equipment?
- For what length of time?
- How successfully did it fulfill its purpose?
- Should any modifications be made?

Compilation of this information will inform the OTA and OT who design and construct adaptive equipment whether the equipment's purpose is confirmed. If the equipment is also accepted and used by several patients, it may be timely to share this information with other OTs and OTAs through professional publication in journals and newsletters, as the examples provided in this chapter demonstrate. It is even possible to consider pursuing presentation to companies who manufacture adaptive equipment, so that it becomes easily and commercially available.

SUMMARY

Construction of adaptive equipment is addressed within the whole continuum of selection, design, and construction that is a part of the OT process of problem-solving and clinical reasoning. A definition of adaptive equipment is given, together with significant historical uses of such devices. The role of the OTA/OT team was presented to inform the reader of the areas of supervision, collaboration, and independent work. Principles are delineated for determining need, selecting, designing, fabricating, presenting the device to the user, and follow-up.

Important precautions and safety measures are stressed. Examples of well-constructed adaptive equipment are used to illustrate important considerations.

REFERENCES

AOTA. (1999). *OT roles*. Bethesda, MD: Author.

Chandler, D., & Knackert, B. (1997). Positioners for wheelchairs in long-term care facilities. *Am J Occup Ther, 51,* 921-924.

Clark, M. (1990, September). Unpublished material and personal correspondence.

Cowan, M. K. (1988). Pillow helps keep young OT clients "stabilized." *OT Week, 2*(19), 5.

Duncan, S. (1986). Brief or new: Knitting device for bilateral upper extremity amputee. *Am J Occup Ther, 40,* 637-638.

Finlayson, M., & Havixbeck, K. (1992). A post-discharge study on the use of assistive devices. *Canadian Journal of OT, 59,* 201-207.

Gitlin, L. N., & Burgh, D. (1995). Issuing assistive devices to older patients in rehabilitation: An exploratory study. *Am J Occup Ther, 49,* 994-1000.

Hague, G. (1988). Brief or new: Makeup board for women with quadriplegia. *Am J Occup Ther, 42,* 253-255.

Monfort, K. & Case-Smith, J. (1997). The effects of a neonatal positioner on scapular rotation. *Am J Occup Ther, 51,* 378-384.

Neville-Jan, A., Piersol, C. V., Kielhofner, G., & Davis, K. (1993). Adaptive equipment: A study of utilization after discharge. *OT in Health Care, 8*(4), 3-18.

Schemm, R. L., & Gitlin, L. N. (1998). How OTs teach older patients to use bathing devices in rehabilitation. *Am J Occup Ther, 52,* 276-282.

Scoggin, A. E., & Parks, K. M. (1997). Latex sensitivity in children with spina bifida: Implications for occupational therapy practitioners. *Am J Occup Ther, 51,* 608-611.

Von Funk, M. (1989). Positioning devie has multiple benefits for patients. *Advance for Occupational Therapists, 13,* 13.

Walsh, M. (1987). Brief or new: Half-lapboard for hemiplegic patients. *Am J Occup Ther, 41,* 533-535.

Basic Splinting

Chapter 33

Jaclyn West-Frasier, MA, OTR

INTRODUCTION

The human hand is an amazing tool that sets us apart from other animals on this planet. We use our hands while still in the womb and continue throughout our lifespan. Our hands allow us to explore the environment, communicate through gestures and touch, and create through such forms as art and architecture. Our hands are powerful enough to grasp a 100-pound barbell but gentle enough to wipe a tear from a child's cheek. On any given day an individual may use his or her hands to comb his or her hair, communicate by keyboard, greet someone with a handshake, or turn the pages of a novel.

OT practitioners are concerned with the individual's ability to successfully perform ADLs, work activities, and leisure or play activities. The human hand plays an integral role in occupational performance and any impairment of the hand will affect function. OTs use the technology of upper extremity splinting as one of the methods to restore or improve hand function. This chapter will provide basic information on hand splinting, including history, description of splints, principles of splinting, assessment, techniques of fabrication, and special considerations.

HISTORY

Splinting is a technology that has been used by OT practitioners for decades. The theoretical basis for splinting is derived from the biomechanical model of practice. OT practitioners apply the biomechanical model to those individuals who have limitations in movement, strength, and endurance that interfere with successful

---

KEY CONCEPTS

- Biomechanical model of practice: The treatment approach that deals with increasing strength, endurance, and range of motion.
- Purpose and type of splints: The classification of splints according to their design and intended outcome.
- Biomechanical and anatomical principles of splinting: Use of splints to improve strength, ROM, and function of the hand through selective application of force.
- Assessment: The process to determine if the client is a good candidate for a splint and what type of splint is appropriate for his or her particular problem.
- Fabrication techniques: Steps in splint construction.
- Client education: Process to ensure that the client understands the purpose of the splint, wearing schedule, and precautions.
- Follow-up procedures: Scheduled appointment to determine if splint program is satisfactory.

performance of occupational tasks. Biomechanical components of functional movement include joint ROM, muscle strength, and endurance. Intervention through this model can be described by three approaches.

1. Prevention of deformity through programs of ROM and positioning, which may include the use of static splints.

2. Restoration of lost function through programs that gradually increase the demand for movement, strength, and endurance until the desired level of function is achieved.

3. Compensation for permanent or prolonged limitations through programs that involve altering procedures or methods to accomplish desired tasks, or using devices attached to the body or placed in the environment to assist with task performance (Kielhofner, 1992).

Splinting is a valuable tool the OT may use to help prevent or minimize deformity, correct impairment, and restore or improve function in the upper extremities. The process of splinting does require an in-depth understanding of normal hand function, pathologies that can limit hand function, and the biomechanical principles involved in splint design. Incorrect use of splinting principles can have a negative impact on the final outcome and actually create additional deformities and further loss of function. To develop basic splinting skills, the OTA should work closely with the OT. As the OTA grows in expertise, he or she can work more independently in the design and fabrication of splints. OTAs with a desire to become proficient in splinting should also participate in continuing education opportunities.

BASIC CONCEPTS

Purpose of Splints

Splints are external devices that are applied to treat upper and lower extremity problems that result from injury, disease processes, birth defects, or the aging process (Fess & Kiel, 1998). Splints may serve one or more of the following functions:

- Promote healing through support, restriction of movement, or immobilization
- Correct or prevent deformity
- Provide or assist motion
- Base upon which to attach an assistive device

The ultimate goal of a splinting program is to improve or restore upper extremity function, which allows the individual to regain independence in daily activities and resume occupational roles (Fess & Kiel, 1998). Samples of splint functions are presented in the following examples.

A surgeon may refer a patient to OT for splinting after carpal tunnel repair. The OT may provide a rigid lightweight splint that immobilizes the wrist but allows finger movement. The wrist splint protects the hand during the healing process but allows the individual to perform low stress activities. An individual with hemiplegia from a cerebrovascular accident may be provided with a resting hand splint to prevent loss of ROM and formation of contractures. The same splint may serve to protect the hand from injury if sensory loss occurred as a result of the stroke. An individual with weak extensors of the fingers after an injury may be provided with a splint that uses springs to assist the fingers to straighten after he or she releases an object. This splint will allow the individual to effectively use the hand during daily activities and at the same time maintain ROM and strengthen the finger extensors. An individual with a spinal cord injury may wear a positioning hand splint that also allows for the attachment of assistive devices such as eating utensils or hygiene implements. He or she is not able to grasp an object due to loss of muscle function, but the splint attachment allows him or her to independently feed him- or herself and perform hygiene activities.

Types of Splints

The materials used for splint construction have increased in variety. In the early years, OTs used plaster cast material or high temperature plastic to construct their splints. The use of high temperature plastics involved the creation of a plaster of Paris mold of the client's extremity. The splint material was heated in an oven to reach moldable consistency and then draped to conform to the mold of the individual's body part. This process was expensive, time-consuming, and hazardous to the therapist who had to work with the highly heated material.

Low temperature plastics were introduced several decades ago. The therapist heats the material in hot water to soften, then cools it to a temperature tolerated by the client. The material is then draped and molded directly to the client's extremity. Today, therapists may select from a wide assortment of materials and splint designs. Therapists are able to create custom splints by creating a pattern and fabricating the piece with materials of their choice. Splints can be ordered already pre-cut in common patterns that can be heated and molded to the individual patient. Pre-fabricated or ready-made splints can be ordered through a catalog. Pre-fabricated splints are made from a variety of materials such as high temperature plastic, low temperature plastic, and fabric such as neoprene, cotton duck, and knit elastics. The therapist measures the client and orders the proper size splint (Fess & Kiel, 1998).

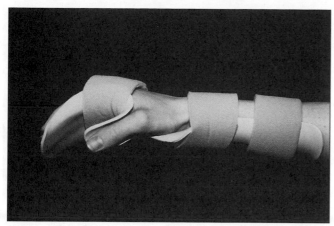

Figure 33-1. Resting hand splint. (Reprinted from Ryan, S. E. [1993]. *The certified occupational therapy assistant: Principles, concepts, and techniques* [2nd ed.]. Thorofare, NJ: SLACK Incorporated.)

The types of splints can be categorized as follows:

1. A *static splint* immobilizes a joint or part of the extremity. The purpose of a static splint is to rest or protect during healing, reduce pain, or prevent contracture. An example of a static splint is a resting pan splint (Figure 33-1).

2. A *dynamic splint* provides one or more of the following: increases PROM, assists with AROM, or substitutes for lost motion. A dynamic splint usually has a static base upon which a moveable component has been added. The moveable component may consist of elastic, rubber bands, or springs (Belkin & English, 1996). An example of a dynamic splint is a dynamic MP flexion splint (Figure 33-2).

PRINCIPLES OF SPLINTING

Hand Function

Hand function is dependent upon the interplay between bony structures, muscles and ligaments, blood supply, nerve supply, and mobility of the skin. The hand and wrist complex contains 27 bones. There are 19 bones distal to the carpals and 19 joints that make up the hand complex. The hand consists of five digits—four fingers and a thumb. Each digit has a carpometacarpal (CMC) joint and a metacarpophalangeal (MCP) joint. The fingers also have two interphalangeal (IP) joints, while the thumb has one. The function of the CMC joints of the fingers is to allow cupping of the palm. The palmar arches allow the hand to conform to the shape of the object being held. The MCP joints, carpal joints, and associated

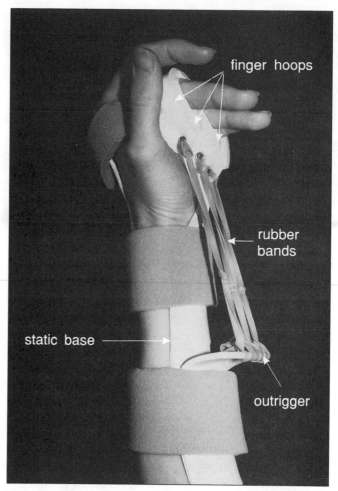

Figure 33-2. Dynamic MP flexion splint. (Reprinted from Ryan, S. E. [1993]. *The certified occupational therapy assistant: Principles, concepts, and techniques* [2nd ed.]. Thorofare, NJ: SLACK Incorporated.)

muscles and ligaments form the palmar arches. They can be visualized across the width of the palm and down the length of the palm (Figure 33-3). The palmar arches also allow the fingers to be positioned for prehension activities (Norkin & Levangie, 1992).

Prehension involves the grasping or holding of an object between any two surfaces of the hand. There are infinite grip combinations but research has identified classifications for various grips. A simple way to conceptualize grips is to consider either a power grip or precision handling (Norkin & Levangie, 1992). Power grip is a strong forceful flexion of all fingers to hold an object securely. An example of a strong power grip is holding tightly to a rope during a tug-of-war game. Precision handling is the placement of an object between fingers or finger and thumb. Picking up a raisin with the thumb and index finger is an example of precision handling.

Placement of the hand for grasp activities is dependent upon intact wrist function. The optimal position of the wrist and fingers for effective hand function is referred to

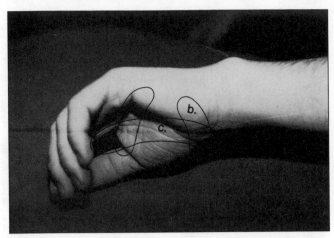

Figure 33-3. Arches of the hand. A. Distal transverse arch. B. Proximal transverse arch. C. Longitudinal arch. (Reprinted from Ryan, S. E. [1993]. *The certified occupational therapy assistant: Principles, concepts, and techniques* [2nd ed.]. Thorofare, NJ: SLACK Incorporated.)

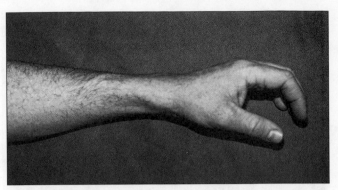

Figure 33-4. Functional position of the hand. (Reprinted from Ryan, S. E. [1993]. *The certified occupational therapy assistant: Principles, concepts, and techniques* [2nd ed.]. Thorofare, NJ: SLACK Incorporated.)

as the functional position (Figure 33-4). The functional position is:

1. Wrist in 20 degrees of extension and 10 degrees of ulnar deviation
2. Fingers flexed 45 degrees at the MCPs, 30 degrees at PIPs, and 20 degrees at DIPs
3. Thumb abducted

In this position, finger flexion occurs with the least amount of effort and the muscle tension in the hand is balanced (Fess & Kiel, 1998). When a resting hand splint is constructed, the therapist often chooses to splint the hand in the functional position.

Mechanical Principles

Mechanics deals with the effect of force. Muscles supply force in the hand. That force is transmitted to the ligaments and joints, which produces motion. Splints also apply force, which means they provide a degree of stress to structures they contact. Force from the splint should be sufficient to prevent contracture and increase ROM but not cause damage. Undesirable effects of too much force from a splint may be damage to skin or underlying structures of ligaments, muscles, and joints. The amount of force to prevent contracture should be just enough to hold the joints in the end of range position (Belkin & English, 1996). Force applied through dynamic splints must be carefully calibrated. A gauge is available to measure the force applied through elastic. Rubberbands and springs need to be checked frequently and adjusted to apply the desired amount of force and direction of pull to the joint. A well-designed, well-contoured splint will minimize stress from pressure and be tolerated much better by the client.

Design Principles

Before deciding which splint to make for the individual, several factors need to be considered. Consideration must be given toward the design of a splint program that is practical for the individual but also meets the specific needs of his or her condition. The therapist should try to answer the following questions before making a final decision on splint design.

*   Does the client understand his or her condition and how he or she may benefit from a splint program?
*   Is the individual likely to comply with the program?
*   Will he or she perceive that the splint program interferes with his or her independence or ability to participate in daily activities?
*   Is he or she self-conscious of being seen wearing a splint?
*   Is he or she motivated towards recovery?
*   Is he or she so motivated that he or she may overdo the specified program?
*   Is he or she able to apply and remove the splint?
*   If unable to do so, is there a motivated caregiver who can assist in this process?
*   Will he or she follow a splint schedule?
*   Does he or she have the cognitive abilities to fully understand and follow through with the program?
*   Will he or she leave the splint on too long and be at risk for skin irritation or edema?
*   Will he or she wear the splint long enough to produce desired results?
*   Does he or she have other conditions that place him or her at risk for injury, such as fragile skin or impaired sensation?

The therapist must consider the primary deficits of the hand and what splint type is most appropriate for treatment, taking into consideration the individual's characteristics of bony structures, scars, skin condition, any alterations in sensation, or other conditions (Fess & Kiel, 1998). The therapist will provide the most appropriate splint for the client's condition. However, if the therapist does not obtain answers to the above questions and fails to thoroughly educate the client on the benefits of the splint, the splint will not be worn and outcomes will not be achieved. The therapist should design an individualized splint program that incorporates the client's perception of his or her situation and his or her personal goals for recovery.

ASSESSMENT

Typically, the splint program is part of the client's overall treatment. The client may also be involved in a program of ROM, therapeutic exercise, and graded activities. He or she may be following through on a home program of ROM, exercises, and ADL tasks designed to improve hand function. The therapist's initial evaluation would have consisted of obtaining information on occupational roles and performance, the perceived impact of the injury or disease process on activity performance, and client's goals for recovery. Additional areas evaluated would be ROM, muscle strength, and upper extremity gross and fine motor coordination. The therapist would have obtained information on medical diagnoses, precautions, activity restrictions, and specific splint orders from the doctor, if issued. The OT will consider results of all assessments prior to making a final decision on splint design for the individual. Once the splint is fabricated, the OT will provide frequent reassessment to evaluate effectiveness of the program and to determine if revisions should be made to the splint or the program.

The OTA may contribute to the initial evaluation by obtaining measures of ROM, grip and pinch strength, and administering standardized evaluations such as the nine-hole peg test. The OTA may be the professional working most often with the client and will need to check with him or her for any problems or concerns with the personalized splint program. The OTA will provide information to the OT to assist with the reevaluation process. Under the supervision of the OT, the OTA may be making revisions to the splint or the splint program and monitoring the client's progress.

FABRICATION

Once a decision is made on splint design the therapist will either fabricate a custom splint or provide the indi-

vidual with the proper-fitting prefabricated splint. One of the easiest custom splints for the beginner to fabricate is the resting pan splint. Instructions on fabricating a resting pan splint will be given in the following sections. Much can be learned by observing an experienced therapist as he or she creates a splint. Not all of the details of the fabrication process can be represented in written form.

Materials

Organize the work area to promote efficiency as well as comfort for the client. The client should sit in a sturdy chair at a table so he or she can rest his or her forearms on the table surface. Assemble the following items on a nearby work surface:

- Electric fry pan with temperature control
- Splint heat gun with a funnel
- Curved blade scissors and straight blade scissors
- Clean towels
- Ace wrap
- 2-inch stockinette
- Paper and pencil for pattern
- Awl
- Tongs
- Soup ladle
- Sheet of thermoplastic splint material
- 1-inch sticky-back Velcro (Velcro USA Inc., Manchester, NH) hook
- Either one half-Velcro loop or similar strapping material such as Velfoam (WBC Industries, Westfield, NJ) (Figure 33-5)

Pattern

Use paper and pencil to trace a pattern for the client's hand. Paper towel works well, as it is flexible and thus easier to check the fit directly on the client's arm and hand. Trace around the contours of the hand, as shown in Figure 33-6, leaving extra margins so that the splint will fall midline along the arm and hand. It is better to err on the side of caution and have excess material that can be trimmed vs. creating a splint that is too small and not useable. Cut the pattern out and try it on the patient; this allows you to inspect the dimensions of the splint. A forearm-based splint should extend two-thirds of the way up the arm toward the elbow. The client should be able to bend his or her elbow unhampered by the splint. If the length of the splint is too short, pressure is not evenly distributed and pressure areas on the skin may be created. With the pattern placed on the client, you should make sure that it is long enough to extend partially beyond the end of the fingers and thumb, and evenly one-third to one-half up the sides of the forearm. Creating a correct

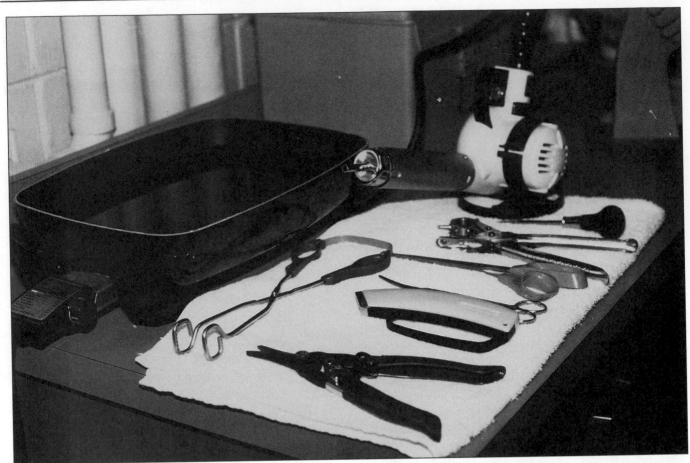

Figure 33-5. Splint construction tools. (Reprinted from Ryan, S. E. [1993]. *The certified occupational therapy assistant: Principles, concepts, and techniques* [2nd ed.]. Thorofare, NJ: SLACK Incorporated.)

paper pattern and sizing it on the client saves time and avoids errors during the fabrication process.

Preparing the Material for Fitting

A beginner should choose one of the more durable splint materials, such as Orthoplast (Sammons Preston, Bolingbrook, IL) or San-Splint (Smith+Nephew, Germantown, WI). Orthoplast can take heavy handling, will not become marked from fingerprints, and will not become over-stretched. It is a plastic material with a rubber component, which allows it to return to its former shape after being stretched. It can also be reheated if you are not satisfied with your first attempt. It can be easily spot heated to correct parts of the splint.

Take the paper pattern and trace the pattern onto the sheet of material using an awl (Figure 33-7). Some splint materials can be marked with a pencil or pen, but the pen marks cannot be removed and will affect the look of the final product. An awl will mark but not be obvious in the finished splint. Rough cut the pattern from the splint sheet. Rough cutting is cutting around the pattern but outside of the pattern lines using a blade or heavy duty splint scissors, as shown in Figure 33-8.

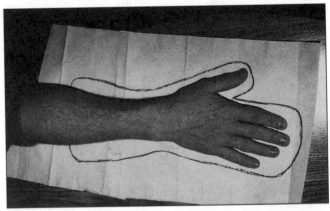

Figure 33-6. Making a pattern. (Reprinted from Ryan, S. E. [1993]. *The certified occupational therapy assistant: Principles, concepts, and techniques* [2nd ed.]. Thorofare, NJ: SLACK Incorporated.)

Heating the Material

Each material will have manufacturer instructions that will tell you at what temperature the material should be heated and how much working time you have before the material cools and resumes its rigid properties. Orthoplast

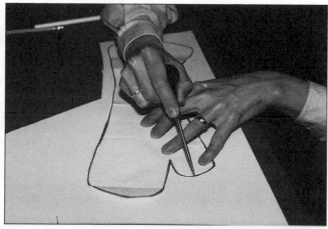

Figure 33-7. Tracing to the material. (Reprinted from Ryan, S. E. [1993]. *The certified occupational therapy assistant: Principles, concepts, and techniques* [2nd ed.]. Thorofare, NJ: SLACK Incorporated.)

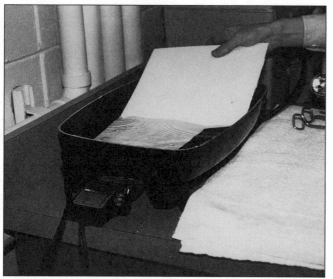

Figure 33-9. Heating the material. (Reprinted from Ryan, S. E. [1993]. *The certified occupational therapy assistant: Principles, concepts, and techniques* [2nd ed.]. Thorofare, NJ: SLACK Incorporated.)

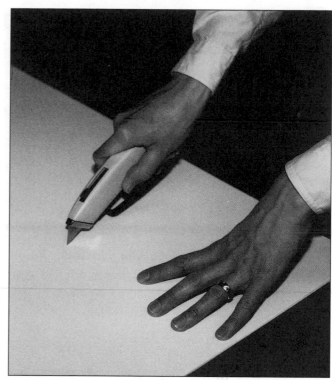

Figure 33-8. Rough cutting the splint. (Reprinted from Ryan, S. E. [1993]. *The certified occupational therapy assistant: Principles, concepts, and techniques* [2nd ed.]. Thorofare, NJ: SLACK Incorporated.)

a length of 2-inch stockinette and apply to the client's forearm, especially if he or she is unusually sensitive to heat. Have the client touch the splint material and let you know that it is a temperature he or she can tolerate. If you allow it to cool too much, it will limit the amount of time you have to mold the material.

As the material is cooling, have the client place his or her hand into the functional position. It may help to have him or her rest the arm on a pillow or place the elbow on a folded towel. It is important that he or she is comfortable and relaxed during this procedure so that you obtain an accurate fit. A beginner will do better to first place the material onto a supinated forearm and have the assistance of gravity help mold the material. First, make sure that the splint is lined up evenly on the forearm and that the material is correctly positioned in the web space (Figure 33-11). The next step is to use an ace wrap to secure the material to the contours of the forearm (Figure 33-12). If you are concerned with the client's ability to tolerate this procedure, you can speed up the setting of the material by using ace wrap dipped first in cold water. Once the forearm is wrapped, have the client pronate the arm. If you complete the splint with the forearm supinated, the fit will not be correct. Once pronated, realign the splint material if needed so that it comes up evenly on each side of the forearm. Check the wrist to make sure it is extend-

and San-Splint are both heated at 160°F and will take 1 to 2 minutes to soften and become moldable (Figure 33-9). Working time is approximately 3 to 5 minutes. Once the material has softened, use tongs to remove from the splint pan and place it on a clean towel. Lightly pat it to remove water. Use scissors to cut out the pattern on the lines (Figure 33-10). Make sure that all ends are rounded vs. angled. Curved blade scissors will help to neatly cut the web space in the pattern.

Forming to Client

Allow the material to cool so that it can be placed on the skin and tolerated by the client. It is advisable to take

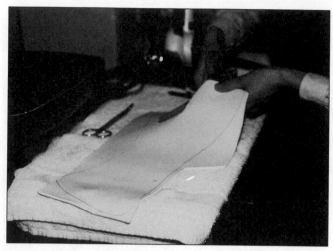

Figure 33-10. Cutting out the splint. (Reprinted from Ryan, S. E. [1993]. *The certified occupational therapy assistant: Principles, concepts, and techniques* [2nd ed.]. Thorofare, NJ: SLACK Incorporated.)

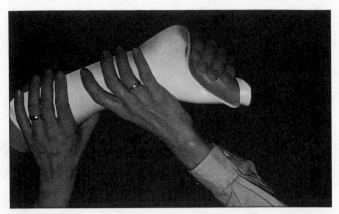

Figure 33-11. Placing the warmed material on the client. (Reprinted from Ryan, S. E. [1993]. *The certified occupational therapy assistant: Principles, concepts, and techniques* [2nd ed.]. Thorofare, NJ: SLACK Incorporated.)

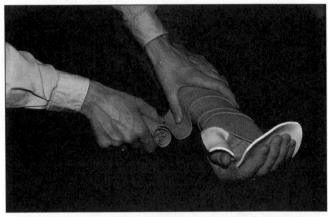

Figure 33-12. Wrapping with elastic bandage. (Reprinted from Ryan, S. E. [1993]. *The certified occupational therapy assistant: Principles, concepts, and techniques* [2nd ed.]. Thorofare, NJ: SLACK Incorporated.)

ed to 20 degrees and ulnarly deviated to 10 degrees. Check the web space for fit and then form the palmar aspect of the splint. With the client maintaining the functional position, gently press the material up into the palmar arches so that the palmar aspect of the splint replicates the arches of the hand. Finally, shape the material to flex the fingers and abduct the thumb. Once satisfied on basic fit, gently flare up the sides of the splint along the ulnar and radial aspects of the hand. Ask the client to maintain the functional position until the splint material has cooled.

Checking the Fit

Remove the ace wrap and check alignment of the splint a final time. While it is still slightly warm, some adjustments may be made. For instance, the splint may be too tight on the forearm edges due to pressure from the ace wrap. Gently stretch the splint away from the forearm. Also make sure that the splint is not placing pressure over the bony prominence of the wrist (Figure 33-13). Gently stretch the material away from the skin to create a bubble of material over the bony landmarks. Use a pencil or pen to mark areas of the splint that need further trimming (Figure 33-14). Gently remove the splint from the client's arm. To speed up the final set and not risk loosing the contours during handling, run the splint under cold water.

Final Adjustments

Check all edges of the splint for smoothness. If not smooth, the edges can create areas of pressure or irritation to the skin. Edges can be finished several ways. You can dip the edges of the splint in hot water to heat again to moldable consistency. It is difficult to heat the edges of the web space by dipping as you may loose the shape of the web space. Using a ladle or heat gun with nozzle will help apply heat only to the areas you need heated. Use sharp splint scissors to slightly trim edges. Orthoplast, if cut hot, will finish with a smooth edge. You can also roll your edges back slightly to create a rounded edge; this will also add to the stability of the splint. Roll back or slightly flare the proximal end of the forearm piece for added comfort for the wearer.

Try the splint on for a final fitting. Check for areas where the splint is too tight against the skin or bony prominence. Also make sure the splint does not fit loosely because it will slide or migrate on the arm and hand and cause friction irritation. Complete all necessary revisions before applying the strapping material.

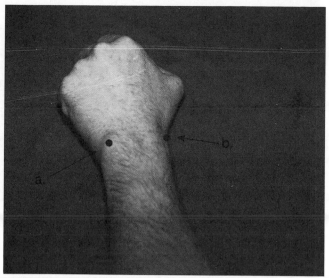

Figure 33-13. Bony prominences. A. Ulnar styloid. B. Radial styloid. (Reprinted from Ryan, S. E. [1993]. *The certified occupational therapy assistant: Principles, concepts, and techniques* [2nd ed.]. Thorofare, NJ: SLACK Incorporated.)

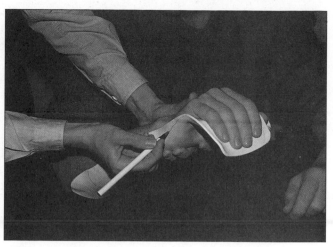

Figure 33-14. Marking the splint before trimming the excess. A. Ulnar styloid. B. Radial styloid. (Reprinted from Ryan, S. E. [1993]. *The certified occupational therapy assistant: Principles, concepts, and techniques* [2nd ed.]. Thorofare, NJ: SLACK Incorporated.)

Fasteners

Once you are satisfied with the fit, it is time to create the mechanism to fasten the splint to the extremity. Typically, a resting pan splint is fastened at three points: proximal forearm, wrist, and over the PIPs. This method of fastening will ensure that the splint will not migrate and that gentle pressure is applied to help maintain ROM. Strapping material can be purchased in rolls or pre-made straps may be purchased in packages.

Adhere the straps to the splint (Figure 33-15). This is commonly done using sticky-back Velcro hook. Trim the straps to fit and use your scissors to round the edges for comfort and to prevent fraying (Figure 33-16). For splints that require greater durability, the straps may be fastened with metal rivets.

Trial Wearing Period

It is highly recommended that you arrange to have the client wear the splint for the first time in your presence. After 10 to 15 minutes, check the client's perception of comfort and fit. Remove the splint and check for any reddened skin that indicates an area of pressure. Make necessary adjustments of the splint to eliminate those pressure areas. If significant areas of pressure are evident after the first wearing period, it is recommended that you repeat the trial after the adjustments and again check for pressure areas. Once you are satisfied that the splint fits properly, there is no evidence of pressure areas, and the client is satisfied with the comfort, you can issue the splint to the client (Figure 33-17).

Client Education

The client should understand the rationale for the splint program, be able to apply and remove the splint independently, and demonstrate understanding of the care of the splint and the wearing schedule. He or she should also be instructed on precautions. The client or client's caregiver needs to be able to monitor for pain, reddened areas, blisters, swelling, or rashes, and immediately report problems to the therapist. He or she should stop wearing the splint until the therapist corrects the cause of the problem. The client should be instructed verbally and be provided with written instructions on wearing schedule, care of splint, and precautions. The client or client's caregiver should demonstrate to the therapist the application and removal of the splint. He or she should be encouraged to report back to the therapist any problems or concerns with the splint program so that needed adjustments may be made. After providing a splint, the therapist should arrange a time for a follow-up appointment to review client's tolerance to the program.

Some minor suggestions to increase comfort include wearing a stockinette to absorb perspiration or lightly powdering the splint with cornstarch prior to application. If the client reports excess perspiration, a hole punch can be used to punch holes in the material to help with ventilation. It is helpful to provide the client with extra straps or stockinette should he or she misplace or lose these items.

Follow-Up

It is the responsibility of the OT to provide follow-up to a client who has received a splint and has been placed on a splint program. If the splint is one aspect of the ther-

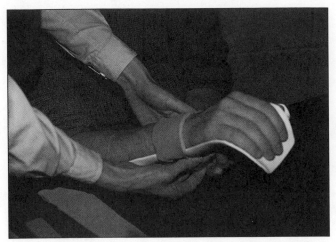

Figure 33-15. Adhering the straps to the splint. (Reprinted from Ryan, S. E. [1993]. *The certified occupational therapy assistant: Principles, concepts, and techniques* [2nd ed.]. Thorofare, NJ: SLACK Incorporated.)

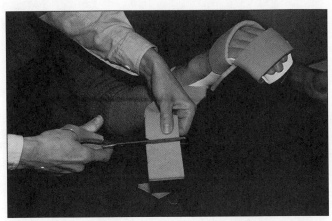

Figure 33-16. Trimming straps. (Reprinted from Ryan, S. E. [1993]. *The certified occupational therapy assistant: Principles, concepts, and techniques* [2nd ed.]. Thorofare, NJ: SLACK Incorporated.)

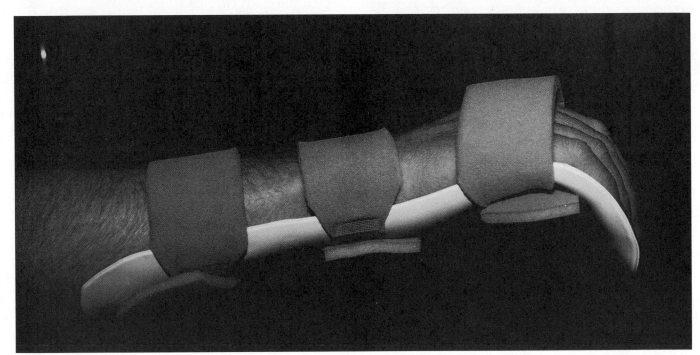

Figure 33-17. Completed resting splint. (Reprinted from Ryan, S. E. [1993]. *The certified occupational therapy assistant: Principles, concepts, and techniques* [2nd ed.]. Thorofare, NJ: SLACK Incorporated.)

apy program, follow-up can easily be incorporated into later treatment sessions. If the client was referred for the sole purpose of splinting, then formal appointments should be made for follow-up. The nature and severity of the condition and the individual needs of the client will determine the frequency of follow-up appointments and the interval between visits. The purpose of the visit is to check on fit of the splint, discuss any problems with the splint program, his or her success and compliance to the program, and to check for progress. The therapist may spend time problem-solving with the client on issues that

are affecting compliance. If fit and comfort is an issue, the therapist will make modifications to the splint and advise the client on further strategies to increase comfort. The therapist will also take time to review information on the splint program, exercise, graded activities, and the client's performance in occupational tasks. As the client demonstrates progress, the splint can be revised to obtain further gains and the exercise and activity program upgraded to obtain additional progress. The initial wearing schedule may need to be adjusted to accommodate to work schedules, self-care, and leisure activities. If the splint is interfering with performance of desired activities such as self-care, the therapist may be able to offer suggestions on adapting activities or the splint schedule to meet the activity needs of the client, as well as the rehabilitative needs of his or her upper extremity.

SUMMARY

This chapter presented basic information on splinting including purpose, biomechanical and anatomical principles, assessment, design, fabrication, and follow-up. The purpose of a splint is to maintain, improve, or restore function through the external application of force. The final outcome of a splint program is the improvement of upper extremity function to allow independent performance of daily activities and satisfactory execution of occupational roles.

The experienced OTA will be able to design and fabricate basic static splints, monitor effectiveness of the program, and perform needed revisions, all with minimal supervision from the OT. The OTA who is a novice splin-ter can gain experience through observing and assisting the OT. OTAs can develop advanced skills by attending relevant workshops, working with OTs who are experienced splinters or certified hand therapists, and working in a setting that provides frequent opportunities to splint.

REFERENCES

Belkin, J., & English, C. B. (1996). Hand splinting: Principles, practice, and decision making. In L. W. Pedretti (Ed.), *OT: Practice Skills for Physical Dysfunction* (4th ed., pp. 319-343). St. Louis, MO: Mosby.

Fess, E. E., & Kiel, J. H. (1998). Neuromuscular treatment: Upper extremity splinting. In M. E. Neistadt & E. B. Crepeau (Eds.), *OT* (9th ed., pp. 406-421). Philadelphia, PA: Lippincott.

Kielhofner, G. (1992). *Conceptual foundations of OT* (2nd ed.). Philadelphia, PA: F. A. Davis.

Norkin, C. C., & Levangie, P. K. (1992). *Joint structure and function: A comprehensive analysis* (2nd ed.). Philadelphia, PA: F. A. Davis.

Wellness and Health Promotion

Chapter 34

Karen Sladyk, PhD, OTR/L, FAOTA

INTRODUCTION

Not too many years ago, lack of information made it nearly impossible to choose healthy lifestyles. In television commercials of the 1950s, some medical doctors recommended smoking cigarettes as a way to reduce stress and lose weight. With today's overload of information on health, consumers have to wade through volumes of often conflicting information to find healthy lifestyles. OT can help with this process (Gourley, 2000).

The World Health Organization defines health as "a state of complete physical, mental, and social well-being" (1986). The National Wellness Association adds spiritual and intellectual components to the definition (Ratner, Johnson, & Jeffery, 1998). Health is not just the absence of sickness or disease. The concept of health becomes different for each individual, as the definition is inherently unique to different people and cultures.

OT is no longer just for those with a diagnosis. Health promotion is for those at risk of losing good health (Moyers, 1999). OT can provide a unique aspect to health promotion because of our understanding of occupation and daily living. Occupation is a nature format for health promotion because of its individuality. Health promotion is assisting ourselves and others in growth and development of sound body, mind, and spirit (Bowen, 1999). OT can use concepts of lifestyle redesign to assist clients individually, in groups, or whole communities in finding balance in their lives (Moyers, 1999).

Lifestyle redesign is a new concept in OT that involves customizing a person's routines of daily living to maximize health and satisfaction (Gourley, 2000). This process of redesign takes on many different facets and is specific to the needs of each individual. What might be identified as helpful to one person might be anxiety provoking to another. For example, computer ergonomics and managing the information highway is enjoyable to some, while expressing a talent in a craft is enjoyable to others. The key to lifestyle redesign is individual design.

The Department of Occupational Science and Occupational Therapy at the University of Southern California has

ESSENTIAL VOCABULARY

Americans with Disabilities Act of 1990: Public law that guarantees disabled citizens access to work and public services.

Ergonomics: Study of movement to accomplish tasks.

Lifestyle redesign: Assisting clients in examining how occupations contribute to healthy or unhealthy states and customizing change.

KEY CONCEPTS

- Health: A state of complete physical, mental, cognitive, and social wellness.
- Health promotion: Growth and development to foster soundness of body, mind, and spirit.

opened a Center for Occupation and Lifestyle Redesign that focuses on community-based practice, education, and research. Based on OT founder George Barton's 1914 Consolation House, this new community center of 6,000 square feet includes innovating programs for the people of the neighborhood including gardening, computer analysis, culturally focused activities, and crafts as occupation. Each program has a research component that allows faculty and students to study the importance of occupations on health (Gourley, 2000).

AREAS FOR HEALTH PROMOTION IN OCCUPATIONAL THERAPY

The concept of health promotion in practice is not new to OT practice. As OTAs, the well-being of the whole client has always been a focus of treatment. As people become more sophisticated about healthy lifestyles, opportunities for health promotion intervention have increased.

As this new and emerging area of practice is developing, new areas of practice are developing daily. This section introduces possible areas of practice for OT practitioners. Generally, the OTA would want to begin to integrate these areas into practice before specializing in health promotion. As community-based practice increases, so do the opportunities to include health promotion in practice.

Americans with Disabilities Act Consulting

The Americans with Disabilities Act (ADA) (1990) changed the face of the public's understanding of people with disabilities as productive, healthy people. Industries, businesses, public offices, and other services are eager to comply with the act in an effort to service all people in their community. OT practitioners are potential resources for ADA consulting because of their knowledge of occupation, adaptation, and activity analysis. Practitioners interested in this can begin with a copy of the ADA and read about specific issues in their state (Fontana, 1999). As this law is constantly refined and defined because of litigation, it is important for the practitioner to remain current on all aspects of the law.

Assisted Living

A new area of housing alternative for the older adult, assisted living provides people with independence and support in a warm community setting (Smith, 1999). Since assisted living programs are significantly lower in costs over skilled nursing facilities, this area of housing options is getting much attention lately. Regulation of this area is moving forward to ensure that these sites provide quality programs.

OT has not been automatically included in this arena but has great potential for helping people stay in assisted living programs. OT in assisted living centers can include fall prevention, energy conservation, health education, and social opportunities. OT practitioners must market themselves to assisted living administrators who generally have a business education instead of a health education (Smith, 1999). Practitioners interested in this area need to monitor state laws and regulations to ensure opportunities for OT. As a member benefit, AOTA monitors state laws and can assist in promoting OT in this new area (Smith, 1999).

Community Redesign

Community and business leaders are often confused in trying to meet the needs of citizens within their community. Opportunities exist for OT practitioners to improve community situations for well people. Moyers (2000) reported unique OTs who were employed to improve quality of life within whole communities. For example, an OT helped her community redesign the transit system to be less exhausting for senior citizens, and an OT worked with a packaging company to design packages that were easy to open. Other opportunities could include playground design or writing business manuals for homeowners.

Community Wellness Programs

Every community has some type of adult education program typically set up in the evenings at local schools or churches. These programs include computer training, crafts, exercise, and educational programs. Most of these programs are eager for new classes to be developed and openly invite potential teachers to develop new programs. As OT practitioners have training in teaching and learning, it is a logical progression that they could develop exciting programs for well people in the community. Opportunities include stress management, time management, role management, protecting your back and joints, helping your teen adjust to adult roles, and living with a person with a disability. The list of potential programs for community education is endless. Just look at the list of Uniform Terminology (AOTA, 1994) and you can begin to see the potential for health promotion in community education for both adults and children.

Ergonomics

The OT practitioner's understanding of anatomy, activity analysis, and movement provides the background for helping others utilize the workplace tools more effectively. Typically, ergonomics is an area that a practitioner enters after advanced training and work experience. Industry is particularly interested in specialists who can help their employees remain well and injury free (Fontana, 1999; O'Connor, 2000). Specialists in this area utilize the occupational performance areas of Uniform Terminology (1994) to facilitate success in the work performance area. As in the assisted living arena, ergonomics require the practitioner to advocate OT to business leaders. As with any consulting position, your employer might have different concerns and motivations for having ergonomic training available to employees. For example, rests from repetitive actions might reduce injuries but also slow production (O'Connor, 2000).

Home and Private Consultant

Several opportunities are available in the private sector. Often individual people are looking for guidance concerning specific issues in their home or work life (Jacobs, 2000). For example, evaluating a home for safety concerns for an elderly couple or job coaching a person who is up for a big promotion and nervous about the interview. Other opportunities exist such as consulting with a professional woman who is now on complete bed rest for the remainder of her pregnancy and missing her professional relationships from work or designing home gyms for specific families. Since OT is concerned with the job of living, consulting opportunities abound but are often untapped.

Spirituality and Hope

The depth of spirituality is in each activity we perform, for it adds richness to our lives (Peloquin, 1997). Acknowledging and understanding the role of spirituality in living a healthy life is currently of interest in OT (Christiansen, 1997). Spirituality can be used in health promotion as well as in rehabilitation. Spirituality work can be effective in both group and individual sessions. OT's role in spirituality is highlighted in different ways, including goal setting/attainment, occupational change, or life history (Spencer, Davidson, & White, 1997). First, practitioners can help clients utilize their spirituality by imagining the possibilities or evaluating the future through goal setting and goal attainment. Second, practitioners emphasize hope with the anticipated change over time. Third, the usefulness of narratives in telling life stories as therapy has been documented as an effective tool (Spencer, Davidson, & White, 1997).

GETTING STARTED

The first step in specializing in health promotion involves learning as much as possible about a specific problem and the need for service in that area. The OT practitioners may initially see health promotion opportunities as part of their regular work environment. Gaining experience in smaller health promotion opportunities will lead to confidence in large projects.

Initial opportunities in health promotion can include the following:

- Promote lifestyle redesign within your work environment during OT Month (April).

- Make a pamphlet for health promotion that addresses the specific needs of your current patient population. Design a second pamphlet that addresses needs of family and friends.

- Take a skill you are using in your current practice and bring it to a community adult education program. Teach a class in stress reduction at the local adult education program or teach a class on spirituality and healing at your church.

- Notify a local public school that you are willing to organize a health fair for the children. Design a class where you teach health promotion concepts to the children. Let the children design a poster on good health for the health fair.

- Offer to do free ergonomic evaluations for friends and family members. When your experience increases, offer the same service at work.

- Offer a class on fall prevention to a local senior citizen center. Repeat the class at an assisted living center. Invite administrators to attend the class.

Once the OT practitioner has experience, it may be time to consider an entrepreneurial business. This is not new to OT, as OTs and OTAs have been designing equipment, giving seminars, and consulting for years. Sorensen (1999) recommends developing business skills, being focused, and testing your ideas. OT practitioners are naturally good at developing and testing ideas because that is part of the OT process. Often lacking are the business skills. Taylor (1999) recommends beginning with the Internal Revenue Service (IRS) for information that clarifies employee relationships from independent contractors. Further assistance should be sought from business professionals familiar with national, state, and local laws.

REFERENCES

Americans with Disabilities Act. (1990). Public Law 101-336, 42 U.S.C. 12101.

AOTA. (1994). Uniform terminology for occupational therapy. *Am J Occup Ther, 48,* 1047-1054.

Bowen, J. E. (1999, December). Health promotion in the new millennium. *OT Practice, 20,* 14-18.

Christiansen, C. (1997). Acknowledging a spiritual dimension in OT practice. *Am J Occup Ther, 51,* 169-172.

Fontana, P. A. (1999, December). Pushing the envelope: Entering the industrial arena. *OT Practice, 20,* 20-22.

Gourley, M. (2000, May). Center for occupational therapy and lifestyle redesign. *OT Practice, 8,* 18-19.

Jacobs, K. (2000). *Under renovation: Incorporating change.* President's Keynote Address, 80th Annual AOTA Conference and Exposition, Seattle, WA; April 2.

Moyers, P. (1999). *The guide to occupational therapy practice.* Bethesda, MD: AOTA.

Moyers, P. (2000). *Promoting practice and the profession: Integrating the guide to OT practice.* NEOTEC Conference, University of Hartford, CT, June 14.

O'Connor, S. M. (2000, May). OTs and office ergonomics consulting. *OT Practice, 8,* 12-16.

Peloquin, S. (1997). The spiritual depth of occupation: Making worlds and making meaning. *Am J Occup Ther, 51,* 167-168.

Ratner, P., Johnson, J., & Jeffery, B. (1998). Examining emotional, physical, social, and spiritual health determinates of self-rated health status. *American Journal of Health Promotion, 12,* 275-282.

Smith, K. (1999, December). States move forward with assisted living regulation. *OT Practice, 20,* 8.

Sorensen, J. (1999). Entrepreneurs: The spirit of OT. *OT Practice, 4*(3), 27-29.

Spencer, J., Davidson, H., & White, V. (1997). Helping clients develop hopes for the future. *Am J Occup Ther, 51,* 191-198.

Taylor, L. D. (1999, December). Twenty tips for employees and independent contractors. *OT Practice, 20,* 12-13.

World Health Organization. (1986). A discussion document on the concept and principles of health promotion. *Health Promotion, 1,* 73-78.

Life Skills

Chapter 35

Denise Rotert, MA, OTR/L
Frank Gainer, MHS, OTR/L
Lisa Hindbjorgen, OTS

INTRODUCTION

Why is it that certain individuals cope with adverse circumstances better than others? It often seems like a mystery how some people can thrive under adversity. But it really is not a mystery. Many individuals bounce back from stressful life events when they are armed with appropriate life skills. Individuals with at-risk behaviors can become resistant to negative outcomes if OTs and OTAs address and incorporate a program that accentuates positive self-concept, competent performance of daily living skills, and effective interpersonal relationships. The goal is to empower individuals at risk to reshape and mold a new way of living through the teaching of life skills.

RESILIENCE

Resilience is showing up as a concept in diverse areas such as business, health care, sports, education, religion, and the public media. Researchers are demonstrating how the skills and abilities of resilient people will help them to be more productive, happier, and healthier when faced with change, stress, and the pressures of daily living.

Through a model called the "Circle of Courage," the acquisition of life skills will enable a person to transcend from "at-risk" to "resilient" (Brendtro, Brokenleg, & Van Bockern, 1990). This model is based on the Native American medicine wheel and is composed of four values: belonging, mastery, independence, and generosity. The Circle of Courage addresses empowerment and wholeness when the four values come together to close the circle.

Belonging

The value of belonging is a universal need. Many individuals lack the simple, yet significant, skills that promote belonging, including the following actions: saying hello, calling others by name, complimenting, touching, calling a friend, listening, and apologizing. (Curwin & Mendler, 1988). If the pursuit of belonging gets lost, alienation increases, along with withdrawal, guarded behaviors, loneliness, and distrust (Brendtro & Brokenleg, 1993). For example, a 14-year-old youth at risk,

---

KEY CONCEPTS

- Life skills program: An educationally based treatment program to help participants develop skills required for competent role performance.
- Stressful life event: An event that causes changes in and demands readjustment of an average person's normal routine.

ESSENTIAL VOCABULARY

Hardiness: Personal characteristics that function to resist succumbing to the negative effects of dealing with stressful life events.

Resilience: Characteristics and skills such as autonomy, competence, and problem-solving that help an individual bounce back from adverse situations.

named Paul, never received the appropriate supports to live a purposeful life. He was unwanted and unbonded. His unstable family consisted of a father who committed suicide and a mother who herself was without support or needed parenting skills (Brendtro, 1997). He formed attachments to nurturing teachers as a substitute, but lost those attachments and his dedication to being a student due to moving. As a result, he increasingly felt outcast, bullied, and alienated. He became labeled as a trouble-maker (Brendtro, 1997).

Mastery

The value of mastery is another component that will close part of the circle. Mastery is having the skills and the confidence in one's abilities in order to complete routine tasks (Larson, 1996). The drive for mastery will act as a motivator for behavior. The goals of the Circle of Courage are to "develop cognitive, physical, social, and spiritual competence" (Brendtro & Brokenleg, 1993, p. 8) which parallel the goals of OT. OT may enhance mastery within an individual by nurturing success, identifying achievements, highlighting the positive, and modeling basic social skills. The youth at risk, mentioned in the previous paragraph, illustrates how not feeling a sense of mastery can lead to detrimental consequences. His roles as student, son, or brother did not give him a sense of mastery and, as a result, at age 12, delinquent behavior began with stealing a piece of beef jerky from a store.

Independence

Individuals will be courageous if they develop a sense of independence. Independence can be referred to as personal power or autonomy and is characterized as the ability to recognize, decide on, and pursue a course of action by which one's life, happiness, and self-esteem can be based (Larson, 1996). OT may emphasize choice, problem-solving, mediation, and leadership in order to accentuate an internal locus of control in which individuals are influential in their destiny. Powerlessness or a lack of independence may lead to rebellious and aggressive behaviors. In the youth's case from above, the rebellious act of stealing a piece of beef jerky led to a crime that would change the course of his whole life. He and a 17-year-old friend kidnapped, robbed, and murdered a cab driver. His friend played the role of being the father Paul never had, which resulted in the youth's not learning to make prudent decisions. The deceptive older youth gave Paul a sense of belonging and, in turn, Paul made negative choices that resulted in living a life behind bars without the possibility of parole.

Generosity

The final component that makes a person resilient is the value termed generosity. "Unless the natural desire of children to help others is nourished, they fail to develop a sense of their own value and become absorbed in an empty, self-centered existence" (Brendtro & Brokenleg, 1993, p. 10). It is essential for OT personnel to give their clients an opportunity to show that they are needed and of value to other individuals. Through generosity, a life becomes purposeful. If it is not nurtured, one becomes a person at risk with a broken circle. Therapists may suggest volunteering to enhance responsibility, self-esteem, moral development, and commitment to democratic values (Brendtro & Brokenleg, 1993). The youth described above will be challenged to create ways he can exhibit generosity in prison, but hopefully he will still find purpose in his life. His story is an extreme example but illustrates that when the Circle of Courage is broken, feelings of alienation, inadequacy, and dependence result. The appropriate teaching and modeling of life skills may have resulted in this youth making positive choices to avoid prison and embrace a life full of freedom. His story can educate others that the human spirit is vulnerable.

HARDINESS

The term hardiness is used to describe individuals who do not develop and seem to be more resistant to the predicted illnesses that result from stressful life events (Kobasa, 1979). Hardiness is described as "a constellation of personality characteristics that function as a resistance resource in the encounter with stressful life events." (Kobasa, Maddi, & Kahn, 1982, p. 168). It is a difference that distinguishes persons who fall ill when they have a high degree of stress from those that experience similar levels of stress without falling ill. A life event is considered stressful if it causes an alteration, modification, or readjustment of an average person's normal routine (Kobasa, Maddi, & Kahn, 1982). In addition, Kobasa and colleagues (1982) related that stressful life events can provide opportunities for potential growth.

The concept of hardiness includes three characteristics which were common to and exhibited by a group of executives who had low incidents of stress-related illness. Those characteristics are commitment, control, and challenge (Kobasa, Maddi, & Kahn, 1982), which are described as:

- Commitment—"An ability to feel deeply involved in or committed to the activities of their lives" (Kobasa, 1979, p. 3). A feeling of commitment to work, play, socialization, and self-care will be the focus of interest by OT.
- Control—"The belief that they can control or influence the events of their experience" (Kobasa, 1979, p. 3). The purview of OT is to assist an individual to take charge of his or her life, actions, and decisions.

- Challenge—"The anticipation of change as an exciting challenge to further development" (Kobasa, 1979, p. 3). Change is stressful and OT can help individuals to be creative and manage their reactions to that change.

Woven within the three "Cs" of Kobasa and her colleagues is the idea of interpersonal relationships, which could be considered the fourth "C"—Connection: an involvement with others. OT has long addressed interpersonal relationships for social interaction, feedback, and a source of support.

Hardiness can be applied to the areas of performance of work, play, and self-care. An individual with high hardiness can solve problems, adapt, and be creative in order that life events that may be stressful do not necessarily result in illness.

LIFE SKILLS DEVELOPMENT GROUP

The life skills development groups were developed by two OTs in the U. S. Army in the 1970s. These groups were designed to treat acutely ill, psychiatric patients and included structured group tasks that were planned to assist the patient in development of adaptive behaviors. The life skills development groups were described as:

An educational approach to health development; however, the focus was not on what was taught but on the process of learning to satisfy one's needs in responsible ways. What the learner did was more important than what the teacher taught. (Thomes & Bajema, 1983, p. 40)

They were organized around three content areas, which included values clarification, competency training, and information classes. The groups started with values clarification since that was seen as a way to integrate group members quickly. Since the focus in the groups was on the tasks, members' participation was enhanced without the pressure seen in purely discussion groups. Competency training included the practice of skills related to work, play, socialization, and self-care (Thomes & Bajema, 1983, p. 35). Role playing was used within the group, the hospital setting, and the surrounding community. Information classes provided factual information furnished by the group facilitators or by speakers who may have been invited to speak on a specific area of expertise.

The life skills development groups were based on the idea that developing and practicing adaptive behaviors in "simulated, staged, or actual life settings" (Thomes & Bajema, 1983, p. 44) will help the patient take those behaviors from the hospital setting into other areas of life. A key element was modeling behaviors by the group facilitators. Thomes and Bajema (1983) described the focus of the group as an action, not a discussion, group.

Life Skills Program Description

A life skills program is an educationally based treatment program to help participants develop skills required for competent role performance. The program described here is based on the concepts of resilience, hardiness, and the life skills development group.

The life skills program can be used as a prevention or intervention tool. As a preventive measure, having a systematic approach to increase someone's hardiness and resilience and then to add an integration of skills/behaviors for healthy living will increase the likelihood that a person will not only survive but thrive through a variety of challenging life events. As an intervention tool, the elements of the life skills program can be used with substance abuse, rehabilitation, developmental disabilities, psychiatric—almost any age or diagnosis.

Participants in the life skills program are given the opportunity to practice adaptive behaviors, take risks in trying new behaviors, and receive constructive criticism. The program utilizes groups but can be modified for use with individuals and can be applied with residential or hospitalized patients or with individuals in outpatient or community-based treatment programs. The program is flexible in how it is structured and how the specific activities are selected to meet the needs of each participant as well as the group. It is experiential in nature, uses paper/pencil activities, and may also include community exploration, problem-solving, role playing, and interpersonal communication. Participants need to be active, organized, and boundaried in order to benefit from the program. The intent of the life skills program is not to provide answers but to give participants the tools to help them solve the problems of living (current and future).

Elements of the Program

- Stress management and relaxation—Seeking and trying new behaviors gives participants some adaptive skills for use in potential stress situations.
- Values clarification—Having an understanding of those things that are important will help the participants to have a better understanding of themselves.
- Goal-setting and future planning—Developing a systematic way to pursue future goals helps participants to focus on objectives and troubleshoot potential barriers.
- Decision-making and problem-solving—Identifying problem areas and looking at alternative solutions helps the participants to broaden their options.
- Leisure interests—Exploring activities that will tap participants' interests will support an adaptive lifestyle.

- Time management—Being able to schedule, plan, and effectively utilize time will encourage health and discourage stress.

- Social skills and interaction—Learning effective communications skills along with skills for interacting with others will give participants a better chance for establishing meaningful relationships.

- Assertiveness—Standing up for one's rights, values, and interests will increase the likelihood that one's needs will be met.

- Anger management—Learning to take charge of anger will prevent anger from getting out of control.

- Self-concept—Having a sense of self-identity and self-esteem will assist participants to take more risks and be more adaptive.

The educational sessions are sequenced to build one upon another or to stand alone depending upon the population to be served. The structure of the group can allow for an individual to enter the program at any point and then participate through the entire series of educational sessions. There are typically a couple of days between sessions to allow participants to carry out assignments or to seek outside information if needed.

The facilitators of the life skills groups should have experience and interest in group dynamics and leadership skills. The ideal leadership situation would be to have co-facilitator teams with an OT and an OTA.

CASE STUDY

John Rogers is a 21-year-old white male who is in his junior year at a midwestern college. He is currently working toward his bachelor's degree with a major in education and a minor in psychology. He has begun to experience some uncomfortable anxiety during the last several months. There have been a couple of things that have been weighing on his mind and have begun to affect his ability to concentrate. These things include:

- He is not sure about his major or minor and whether or not these subjects will allow him to find a fulfilling job after graduation.

- He has begun to question his sexual orientation. He is finding that he is attracted to other males, which frightens him because of the implications it will have on his future plans and the reaction of his family members.

John had planned out his life following graduation—he was going to go back to his small home town, get a job as a teacher, get married, and have a large family. This has been the expectation for as long as he can remember. He is the youngest of five children and his two older brothers and two older sisters are married, have children,

and all live within an hour of their parents. They all seem happy to him, but this does not seem to be the life that he finds meaningful.

John belongs to a fraternity and lives in the fraternity house. He is friends with all of the other guys in the house, and he has developed a close relationship with one guy in particular. They share many of their feelings and whenever the two of them are together there is an electricity between them that he cannot explain. John has never talked to his friend, Tim, about the feelings he has been experiencing about other men—especially him. John has been involved with females in the past, but those relationships never lasted more than several months.

All of these concerns have caused John to experience difficulty sleeping at night, a loss of his appetite, difficulty focusing on his assignments, and being somewhat short and curt with his friends. John did a recent student teaching practicum and he found himself easily irritated by some of the adolescent behavior.

Tim suggested that John might want to go to the student health center and talk to a professional about what was going on. John followed up on this suggestion and met with a counselor at the student health center. The counselor realized that what John was experiencing was something normal for his age group. He was not suicidal, did not need inpatient hospitalization, and did not require any psychotropic medications. The counselor referred John to the community mental health center, which includes a life skills program that allows individuals to focus on specific areas that are causing them anxiety or concern and to develop skills for living their lives.

The primary facilitator of the life skills program was an OT who has an OTA as a co-facilitator. The evaluation was directed at John's education/work history, family and other social support, current living environment, goal inventory, time inventory, and a self-assessment of problem areas. The OTA assisted by having John complete a pen and paper assessment in the form of a questionnaire which consisted of guiding questions on the above identified areas. The OT then reviewed the questionnaire, with John and asked probing questions that allowed John to expand on his written answers. The OT completed a comprehensive interview in order to evaluate the areas that John was having difficulty with in order to recommend the most appropriate therapeutic track.

It was agreed with John that he would benefit from addressing the following:

- Goal-setting and future planning to help him get a handle on what he wants to do with his life.

- Social skills and interaction to gain support and information with others who are questioning their sexual orientation and are in various stages of the process of coming out.

- Values clarification to assist him in identifying what is now important to him at this stage in his life.

- Stress management and relaxation in order to learn his response to stress and how he can cope with it in order to minimize the disruption caused to his life.

Treatment Implementation and Goals

John was placed into the following life skills program groups and the goals for each group were as follows:

Goal-Setting and Future Planning

- Goal: John will complete a vocational inventory assessment in order to identify possible career alternatives.
- Goal: John will identify personal goals and establish a plan of action for achievement of those goals.

Social Skills and Interaction

- Goal: John will discuss with his friend Tim the issues that are ongoing in his life in order to obtain the support of his best friend.

Values Clarification

- Goal: John will engage in a review of his values and what are the important aspects of his life in the areas of work/school, leisure, socialization, and self-care.
- Goal: John will attend the college's gay and lesbian student association weekly meetings in order to educate himself, further explore, and obtain support.

Stress Management and Relaxation

- Goal: John will complete a stress inventory and identify realistic coping mechanisms for his identified stressors.

John was involved in the life skills program for 8 weeks. He responded well to the groups and accomplished the following.

Goal-Setting and Future Planning

He completed a vocational inventory and found that his strongest interests were in a helping profession. Upon further exploration, he decided that he would complete his bachelor's degree in education with a minor in psychology and then pursue a master's degree in social work. He felt this would give him a variety of options when he graduates. He completed the goal-setting activity worksheet (Figure 35-1), which outlined the process for goal achievement.

Social Skills and Interaction

With the group's encouragement, John discussed the issues that he has been addressing with Tim. Tim stated that he was not gay, he wanted to remain John's best friend, and he was very supportive of John as he struggled to deal with these ongoing issues.

Values Clarification

John identified that it is important to him to share his news with his family, so he has begun to work on how and when to do that. In addition, he attended the weekly meetings of the college's gay and lesbian student association and has found them to be a great support system. He has begun dating one of the other members.

Stress Management and Relaxation

John completed a stress inventory and learned more about the physiological reaction that his body undergoes when he is under stress. He learned various coping mechanisms to include relaxation techniques.

John felt that he had benefited significantly from the various life skills program groups he was involved with. He found it very informative to hear what other people were experiencing and how they coped with various issues in their lives. He also found the education component helpful and the ideas generated could be carried over into his current situation.

CLINICAL PROBLEM-SOLVING

Since the principles and elements of the life skills program can be used with a diverse population (clients/patients) of virtually all ages and with a variety of needs, there is more than way to organize the experiential sessions. Following are some mini case studies which can be used to stimulate creative ways to address those needs. How might you plan a life skills program for each of these individuals? How would you facilitate a group with these individuals? What might be indicators that each one of these individuals is increasing his or her resilience, hardiness, and life skills?

- Allison was just promoted in an up and coming business. She is excited about the opportunity but would be required to relocate to a large city away from her family. This is the first time that she would not be close to her family members. She is worried that she cannot do it on her own. She is scared and wonders if the promotion is worth it.
- Leroy has been seen in OT for rehabilitation of his right dominant hand following laceration of his flexor tendons. He sustained the injury in a fight with his brother-in-law. He has a history of fighting and states that he is not able to control his anger.

Goal-Setting

Write down five (5) goals that you would like to accomplish within the next four (4) years:

1.
2.
3.
4.
5.

Copy the one that is the most important to you:

List three (3) barriers that might get in the way:

1.
2.
3.

List three (3) helpers that might help you get past the barriers:

1.
2.
3.

Write five (5) steps to get to your most important goal:

1.
2.
3.
4.
5.

Goal-Setting Facilitator Instructions

Objective: To help participants identify and plan for ways to reach their personal goals.

What facilitators do:
- Provide participants with worksheets to complete.
- Explain the task.
- Ensure that each participant understands the task. Provide examples if necessary.
- Assist participants in completion of the task by asking questions that might stimulate their thinking or formulate their goal statements.
- Encourage group discussion and feedback after participants have had time to complete the task.
- Model appropriate behaviors in writing goals, giving feedback, and discussing ideas.
- Ask questions that will help participants to clarify their own goals.

Materials needed:
- Goal-setting worksheets
- Pencils/pens

Figure 35-1. Goal-setting activity worksheet.

Decision-Making

Objective:

To identify a decision that needs to be made within the next 3 months.

Task instructions:

- Pass out a 3x5 card to each participant.
- On one side of the card, write a decision that you need to make within the next 3 months.
- On the opposite side of the card, list three possible alternative decisions.
- Each participant, in turn, will share his or her decision with the group along with the possible alternatives.
- Group members are asked to verbally vote for the best alternative and give the reason for their vote.

What facilitators do:

- Pass out a 3x5 card to each participant.
- Provide instructions for the task.
- Stimulate the discussion portion of the task.

Materials needed:

- 3x5 cards
- Pencils/pens

Figure 35-1 continued. Goal-setting activity worksheet.

- James knew his parents would eventually get divorced. During his second semester at college he received a phone call that his father was moving out. He contemplates how his life will change and hates the thought that his family life is unstable and uncertain.

- Madeline moved to town after her husband died, as she was clearly not able to continue managing the family farm. When she lived on the farm, she spent all of her time doing household chores in support of the workers such as cooking, cleaning, and washing. She identifies her only friends as her husband and the farmhands.

REFERENCES

Brendtro, L. (1997). Mending broken spirits of youth. Reclaiming children and youth. *Journal of Emotional and Behavioral Problems, 5*(4), 197-202.

Brendtro, L., & Brokenleg, M. (1993). Beyond the curriculum of control. Reclaiming children and youth. *Journal of Emotional and Behavioral Problems, 1*(4), 5-11.

Brendtro, L., Brokenleg, M., & Van Bockern, S. (1990). *Reclaiming youth at risk: Our hope for the future.* Bloomington, IN: National Education Service.

Curwin, R., & Mendler, A. (1988). *Discipline with dignity.* Alexandria, VA: Association for Supervision and Curriculum Development.

Kobasa, S. C. (1979). Stressful life events, personality, and health: An inquiry into hardiness. *Journal of Personality and Social Psychology, 37,* 1-11.

Kobasa, S. C., Maddi, S. R., & Kahn, S. (1982). Hardiness and health: A prospective study. *Journal of Personality and Social Psychology, 42,* 168-177.

Larson, S. (1996). Meeting needs of youthful offenders through the spiritual dimension. Reclaiming children and youth. *Journal of Emotional and Behavioral Problems, 5*(3), 167-172.

Thomes, L. J., & Bajema, S. L. (1983). The life skills development program: A history, overview and update. *OT in Mental Health, 3,* 35-48.

Activities of Daily Living

Chapter 36

Stanley Paul, PhD, OTR/L

INTRODUCTION

Activities of daily living (ADLs) are one of the three domains of OT. These domains are also referred to as occupational performance areas. The other two domains are work and play or leisure. According to AOTA's Uniform Terminology (1994), ADLs include grooming, oral hygiene, bathing or showering, toilet hygiene, personal device care, dressing, feeding/eating, medication routine, health maintenance, socialization, functional communication, functional mobility, community mobility, emergency response, and sexual expression. The role of OT in ADLs involves assessment of performance, identifying problems that interfere with the performance, developing treatment objectives, and providing training in order to increase the functional independence of the client. Under the supervision of an OT, an OTA can assist with evaluation, developing treatment goals, and program implementation. Both OTAs and OTs are referred to as OT practitioners in this chapter.

ADLs are categorized into two groups. They are basic activities of daily living (BADLs) and instrumental activities of daily living (IADLs) (Foti, Pedretti, & Lillie, 1996; Weiner et al., 1990). BADLs include activities of self-maintenance, which help an individual function in his or her immediate living environment. Activities that fall under this category are personal hygiene, bathing, dressing, feeding, functional mobility, and functional communication. IADLs include home management, health maintenance, and community living activities. The skills required for IADLs are more advanced in nature, such as problem-solving, social skills, safety management skills, and community and environmental interactions. See Table 36-1 for a list of BADL and IADL activities.

ACTIVITIES OF DAILY LIVING EVALUATION

Evaluation, planning, and intervention of ADL deficits should be the joint effort of the client, family, and the rehabilitation team. The rehabilitation team often consists of physician, nurse, physical therapist, OTR, speech pathologist, and social work-

KEY CONCEPTS

- Community living: Living in the community independently or with support services
- Environmental safety: Awareness of safety issues around a person
- Functional mobility: Minimum stregthand skills needed to move about

ESSENTIAL VOCABULARY

Environmental control units: Electronic aids designed to increase independence.

Hand-over-hand: Treatment technique where the OTA moves to assist the correct movement.

Verbal cues: Verbal hints given to the client by the OTA to trigger desired behaviors.

Table 36-1
Activities of Daily Living

Basic Activities of Daily Living	Instrumental Activities of Daily Living
Self-Care: Feeding Dressing Hygiene Grooming	**Home Management:** Meal preparation Shopping Cleaning Laundry Child care
Functional Mobility: Bed mobility Transfers Ambulation	**Community Living:** Money management Public transportation Driving
Communication: Writing Using telephone Computer and typing Communication devices	**Environmental Safety:** Fire safety Identifying dangerous situations Ability to call 911
Indoor Environmental Hardware: Light switches Faucets Windows/doors Keys	**Health Management:** Medication management Knowing health risks Ability to make appointment with physician
	Indoor Environmental Hardware: Handling electronic home appliances such as the stove/oven, vacuum cleaner, and microwave

er. In mental health settings, the rehabilitation team includes psychiatrist or psychologist. There are standardized and commercially available ADL evaluations on the market. Some of the known ADL evaluation scales include Barthel Index (Mahoney & Barthel, 1965), Functional Independence Measure (FIM) (Heineman et al., 1991), Kenny Self-Care Evaluation (Schoening et al., 1965), Klein-Bell ADL Scale (Klein & Bell, 1982), Katz Index of ADL (Katz et al., 1970), Kohlman Evaluation of Living Skills (KELS) (Kohlman-Thomson, 1993) and Milwaukee Evaluation of Daily Living Skills (MEDLS) (Leonardelli, 1988). However, most OT practice settings use their own homegrown evaluation tools, which are specific to their client population and service needs.

An OT evaluation of ADL performance should begin with an interview of the person, followed by a performance observation. Interview alone may not be sufficient since the client's performance may have been changed due to the health condition. Some clients may have cognitive deficits and may not remember their true performance level. Some may assume that they could perform daily activities without considering the recent changes in their health status. An interview cannot truly replace an observation of one's performance. The OT practitioner should observe the methods the client uses to complete the ADL tasks, determine the causes of performance deficits, and plan treatment accordingly. The causes of performance deficits could be due to low endurance, weakness, cognitive/psychosocial deficits, pain, incoordination, and limited ROM. A clear understanding of various causes of performance deficits could help a practitioner establish reasonable short- and long-term goals. It will also give a clear idea about the methods, assistive devices, and training regimens that may be needed to achieve the treatment goals.

A practitioner should be cognizant of cultural and privacy issues when doing the evaluation. For example, when doing toileting, dressing, and grooming evaluation, privacy should be considered. Sometimes the presence of a family member can help a shy person participate in the evaluation and training. In situations in which a young female client is uncomfortable about doing a dressing evaluation with a male OT practitioner, a female colleague could assist with the evaluation. Also, a male practitioner doing a dressing evaluation with a woman should have a female colleague present. When planning treatment, the goals should be set in collaboration with the client. Also, knowledge of the person's interests, occupational role history, and daily/weekly schedule can help OT practitioners plan treatment more effectively.

FACTORS INFLUENCING ACTIVITIES OF DAILY LIVING EVALUATION AND TRAINING

A thorough assessment of the client's performance components is necessary for ADL evaluation, treatment plan, and intervention. For example, the available muscle strength, ROM, sensory deficits, and cognitive skill level are important factors influencing the evaluation and training. Also important is an understanding of the client's present living environment or the environment the client will return to after discharge. Factors such as "Will the client live with a family member or live alone?" are important considerations. Will the client need assistance at home, and, if so, how much? These are all environmental factors that might influence ADL independence. Other factors that can assist an OT practitioner in service delivery include an understanding of the client's culture, personal values, interests, family assistance, and the sickness role of the person.

DOCUMENTATION OF EVALUATION RESULTS

Documentation of evaluation results, treatment goals, intervention, and progress is a way of communicating to the treatment team and third party payers the services rendered by OT (Robertson, 1998). ADL documentation might involve a separate ADL form or it may be part of a comprehensive evaluation. The documentation often involves a checklist with various areas of ADLs (Figure 36-1). Please note that this evaluation contains only the ADL portion of the OT evaluation. Self-care, mobility, home management, and information about home environment all need to be documented in a comprehensive manner. OTRs use various terms and descriptors in documenting the performance. For example, we use terms like maximal assistance and supervision. It is useful to

provide the rating guide in the evaluation form. OTRs and many other rehabilitation professionals use the following descriptors as a general guide during evaluation, planning, and intervention.

- Dependent—Requires total assistance or more than 75% of physical assistance to complete the activity due to any reasons, such as weakness, poor endurance, or cognitive deficits.
- Maximal assistance—Requires anywhere from 50% to 75% of physical assistance to complete the activity.
- Moderate assistance—Requires 25% to 50% of physical assistance with or without supervision, cueing, and assistive devices. Cueing generally includes verbal, visual, and/or tactile cueing.
- Minimal assistance—Requires supervision, cueing, and less than 25% of physical assistance.
- Supervision—Able to perform the activity but requires someone to be present due to safety issues such as occasional loss of balance and cognitive/psychosocial deficits.
- Independent—Able to perform the activity without any physical or verbal assistance and with or without the help of assistive devices (Hamilton et al., 1987).

INSTRUMENTAL ACTIVITIES OF DAILY LIVING

IADL tasks are evaluated in the same manner as the BADL tasks, starting with the interview followed by performance evaluation. However, observation of IADL performance evaluations may not be possible in many settings secondary to short stay and early discharge. When real performance evaluation is not possible, a thorough interview of the client and family should be carried out so that any immediate home management tasks can be incorporated into the OT treatment sessions before discharge. The IADL tasks include home management skills, health management, and community living skills. Home management skills include cooking or fixing a meal, managing household appliances, and safety management. If possible, a home evaluation and performance evaluation at home can provide valuable information for the treatment plan.

Evaluation of simple tasks such as cleaning the counter, taking things out of the refrigerator, and fixing a bowl of cereal should be tried before evaluating multi-step tasks, such as laundry, using the dishwasher, and vacuuming the house. Also considered are the tasks the client plans to do after returning home, such as shopping and carrying heavy objects. A cooking evaluation can be performed in the OT clinic's kitchen, and a shopping evaluation can be performed at the facility's mini store. Health maintenance and

Name _____

Address_____Age _____

Diagnosis _____Occupation _____

	Date	Needs Equipment	Needs Assistance	Needs Minimal Assistance	Needs No Assistance
Grooming					
Comb/brush hair					
Wash hair					
Set hair					
Shave					
Apply make-up					
Trim nails					
File nails					
Manage feminine hygiene					
Brush teeth					
Manage toothpaste or powder					
Bathing					
Shower					
Turn on/off faucet					
Bathe					
Dry self					
Dressing					
Over shirts					
Button shirt/blouse					
Ties					
Jacket/coats					
Hats/gloves					
Zipping					
Putting on shoes					
Tying shoes					
Lace shoes					
Putting on socks/hose					
Pants					
Skirts/slacks					
Dress					
Secure clothes from drawer					
Hang up clothing					
Communication					
Read book or magazine					
Write/type					
Speaks coherently					
Comprehends spoken words					
Transportation					
Bus					
Drive					
Walk					

Figure 36-1. Daily living skills evaluation. (Used with permission of Wayne County Community College OTA program.)

Name _____

Address _____ Age _____

Diagnosis _____ Occupation _____

	Date	Needs Equipment	Needs Assistance	Needs Minimal Assistance	Needs No Assistance
Cooking					
Peel					
Measure basic ingredients					
Mix					
Follow simple directions					
Follow complex directions					
Prepare cold meal					
Prepare hot meal					
Convenience foods					
Boxed					
Frozen					
Canned					
Clean-Up					
Wipe counters					
Sweep floors					
Scour sink					
Wash pots/pans					
Dishes/silver, glasses					
Put away supplies					
Dishes, bowls, spoons					
Find supplies (memory)					
Dusting					
Mop floor					
Make bed					
Change bed					
Wash clothes					
Vacuum					
Clean tub					
Clean toilet					
Windows					
Time Management					
Planning day					
Planning meals					
Coordinating schedules					
Manage watch					
Money Management					
Making change					
Checks					
Paying bills					

Figure 36-1 continued. Daily living skills evaluation. (Used with permission of Wayne County Community College OTA program.)

Name _____

Address_____Age _____

Diagnosis _____Occupation _____

	Date	Needs Equipment	Needs Assistance	Needs Minimal Assistance	Needs No Assistance
Eating					
Eat with fingers					
Pick up utensils					
Use fork/spoon					
Cut food					
Spread butter on bread					
Use salt and pepper					
Drink from glass/cup					
Open milk container					
Stir liquid					
Open screw-top bottles					
Mobility					
Sit balanced on edge of bed					
Get in/out of bed					
Turn over in bed					
Sit in straight chair					
Rise from straight chair					
Open doors					
Stand unsupported					
Walk					
Walk carying objects					
Pick up objects from floor					
Independent transfers					
Miscellaneous					
Manage keys					
Manage glasses					
Operate radio or TV					

Figure 36-1 continued. Daily living skills evaluation. (Used with permission of Wayne County Community College OTA program.)

safety evaluations can be performed in the OT clinic. Health management tasks include medication management, following emergency procedures such as dialing 911, being able to use a fire extinguisher, following fire evacuation procedures, and following safety precautions during all tasks at home and in the community. If a client plans to travel or take public transportation, transfer skills, safety while boarding the vehicle, and driving skills need to be addressed. These advanced skills are often not evaluated or treated in rehabilitation facilities. However, addressing these areas and referring to appropriate professionals or services are within the roles of an OT practitioner.

ACTIVITIES OF DAILY LIVING TRAINING: GENERAL CONSIDERATIONS

An evaluation helps the therapist to determine if ADL training is necessary, and the goal of ADL training is to help the client achieve a maximum level of independence in daily activities. ADL intervention follows two major approaches, restoration of impaired skills through skill retraining and adaptation of disability through environmental modifications or adaptive aids (Trombly, 1993). Independence means being able to perform the desired activity with or without the help of assistive devices and within a reasonable length of time. The concept of independence also varies depending on the person's diagnosis, needs, skills, values, interests, social support system, and financial resources. Short- and long-term goals will have to be developed following the evaluation. If a client has deficits across different areas, BADL training may be given immediate priority over IADL training since self-care often takes a higher priority over home and community management skills. The suggested sequence of BADL training includes feeding, grooming, transfers, toileting, dressing, and bathing. The above sequence is just a guide and not a rule. The functional abilities and diagnosis of the client should be taken into account when deciding on the sequence of ADL training. For example, a person with high-level quadriplegia may require assistance for most self-care ADLs but may have the potential to perform some IADLs, such as money management, communication, and travel in the community. In such instances, those skills should be trained rather than spending effort on areas in which the client may never become substantially independent.

APPROACHES TO ACTIVITIES OF DAILY LIVING TRAINING

Treatment approaches vary according to the skills and limitations of the client. A person with intact cognitive faculties would require a different approach than someone with cognitive deficits. The therapist must be able to adapt his or her approaches to suit the client needs. For example, a person with cognitive deficits might require concrete steps and directions. On the other hand, a person with T-10 paraplegia might be able to learn self-care tasks with just a few demonstrations. The different methods employed by the OT practitioners in ADL training include demonstration, verbal cues, or visual cues. For a person who requires more time to learn secondary to extensive physical and/or cognitive deficits, a step-by-step approach by gradually reducing the amount of assistance given might work well. This approach involves breaking down the tasks into smaller components. It may start with hand-on-hand physical assist to verbal cues with occasional physical assist to supervision and finally full independence. In the process of ADL training, tasks may be repeated a few times on each and every session or on a daily basis until the skill is mastered.

ADL training involves preparation. Before training a client, the practitioner should become thoroughly familiar with the specific ADL task and any adaptive equipment that may be used in the training. During the training, the practitioner presents the activity through demonstration along with verbal instructions. The client then performs the task either with the practitioner or separately while the practitioner supervises and provides additional cues or corrections. The process will be repeated until learning takes place. ADL training should be carried over from the clinic environment to the client's natural setting. For example, dressing training may start at the clinic, but once the client learns the task, it needs to be carried over in his or her room. In the same manner, transfers may be trained in the clinic followed by in his or her room, bathroom, and car.

A person's recovery phase involves different people, such as family members, nursing staff, and other members of the treatment team. Nursing staff, caretakers, and family members may have to be trained in proper ways of handling and reinforcing the learned skills. Learning has to be mastered to the maximum physical and cognitive potential of the client. The practitioner should monitor the adequacy of learning and carryover of performance to natural settings. There are specific ADL techniques used with specific client populations. However, it is important to remember that these techniques do not follow a cookbook approach to training but only serve as a guide to assist the therapist to utilize them in different combinations in accordance with the client's needs and abilities.

Role of Adaptive Equipment and Personal Assistance in Activities of Daily Living Training

ADL training might involve the use of adaptive devices. An adaptive device is any equipment that assists an individual to perform a task faster or more independently. Some, but not all, assistive and mobility devices are covered by the client's insurance. These devices may also be purchased from medical supply companies, large department stores, and pharmacies. Also, some practitioners construct simple adaptive devices specific to their clients' needs. A few common adaptive devices are illustrated in Figures 36-2 and 36-3. The role of OT also involves instructing the clients and caretakers on the proper use and maintenance of these devices. Some disabilities may require the assistance of another person for daily tasks. Family members or personal care attendants may be trained to assist these individuals in their home or work environments.

Condition-Specific Activities of Daily Living Techniques: General Principles

The intervention plan should include both short- and long-term goals. There is no one specific technique that will always work for a specific disability. The therapist should utilize different techniques or assistive devices as needed to meet specific client needs. A practitioner can also learn specific techniques from the clients themselves. Often times the clients have suggestions, which should be taken into account during the training process. Some general ADL principles specific to conditions requiring full-time wheelchair use, cerebrovascular accidents (CVAs), conditions affecting normal muscle strength, conditions affecting coordination, ROM limitations, and conditions with cognitive/psychosocial impairments are summarized below.

Activities of Daily Living Training for Wheelchair Users

A person who requires a wheelchair permanently will have to perform all activities from a seated position. This involves balancing the upper body and utilizing arm strength to perform daily activities. A person in a wheelchair has to face the world designed for people in an upright position. The difference in height of objects such as doorknobs and light switches must be considered during training. Carrying objects would be harder since the

person has to also operate the wheelchair simultaneously. A wheelchair user with intact upper extremity function, stable trunk mobility, and good upper extremity strength should be able to perform daily self-care activities independently with some training and familiarity.

Dressing, grooming, and hygiene can be performed either in a seated position or from the bed. Assistive devices such as long-handled shoehorn and reacher may be required to assist in dressing. When transferring to different surfaces, a wheelchair user has to get as close to the surface as possible. Toileting and bathing/showering might require the person to transfer to a tub bench and toilet seat. Often, desk arms and swing-away foot rests help a person get close to the work surface.

The wheelchair user should be aware of environmental barriers, such as doors opening toward them and reaching for objects at different heights. Work heights and adequacy of space for wheelchair maneuverability should be considered during training. Furniture rearrangement to accommodate wheelchair space, using reachers to reach objects, and environmental modifications might be needed for the individual to function independently at home and office. If a person also has upper extremity weakness, environmental control units (ECUs, also called electronic aids for daily living) might be required to enhance his or her independence. These individuals may also require powered wheelchairs for mobility. If a wheelchair user operates an automobile, special lifts may be required to transfer into the vehicle, and special controls may be required to operate the vehicle.

Activities of Daily Living Training for Cerebrovascular Accidents

CVAs, referred to as stroke, often result in loss of function or weakness to one side of the body. Persons who have suffered a CVA may have to relearn ADL skills using their intact upper extremity. Besides weakness and loss of function, these people may also have cognitive, perceptual, and speech deficits at varying degrees. Also, people with stroke may present with balance problems due to loss of function in the affected side. A person with normal cognitive skills can learn one-handed skills for performing ADLs.

Basic Activities of Daily Living

According to principles of one-handed dressing techniques, a person should begin with the affected extremities when donning and remove unaffected extremities first when doffing. Reachers and long-handled adaptive equipment may be useful for assistance with dressing. There are different techniques and methods available for learning specific skills. Since the purpose of this chapter is to give an introduction to ADLs, specific techniques are

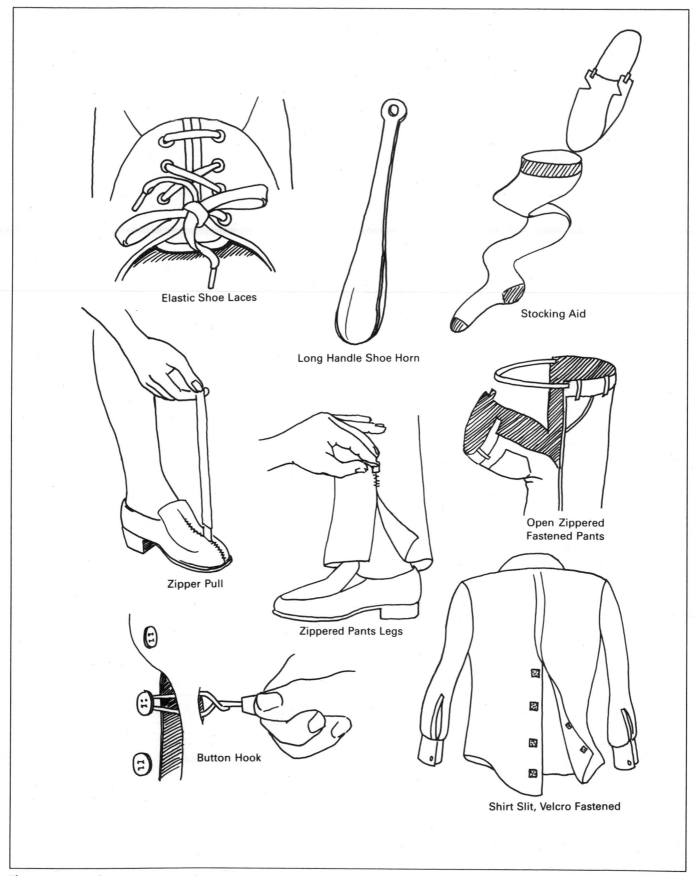

Figure 36-2. Adaptive/assistive dressing aids. (Reprinted from Ryan, S. E. [1993]. *The certified occupational therapy assistant: Principles, concepts, and techniques* [2nd ed.]. Thorofare, NJ: SLACK Incorporated.)

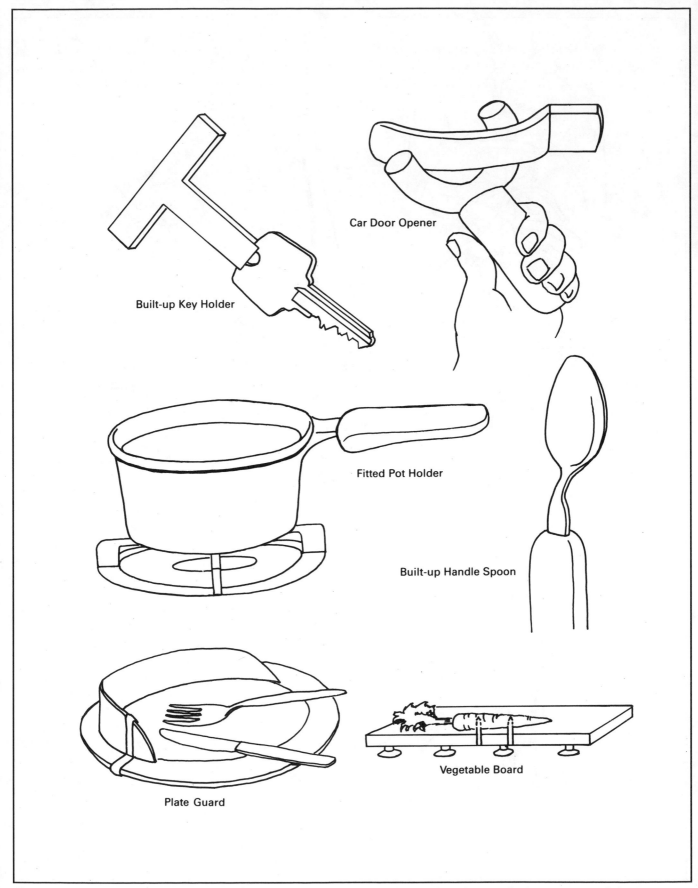

Figure 36-3. Adaptive/assistive devices. (Reprinted from Ryan, S. E. [1993]. *The certified occupational therapy assistant: Principles, concepts, and techniques* [2nd ed.]. Thorofare, NJ: SLACK Incorporated.)

not elaborated. Interested readers can refer to other OT books for details.

- Feeding—Cutting food may be a problem for these individuals. Adaptive eating utensils, such as a one-handed rocker knife, can be used to solve this problem.
- Communication—A person with dominant hand involvement can learn to write with the non-dominant hand. One-handed typing can be learned for communication purposes. A major problem faced by one-sided weakness is inability to stabilize paper when writing and difficulty with turning pages when reading. A clipboard or paperweight can help stabilize the paper and a book holder can eliminate the difficulty with turning pages while reading. A speaker phone or headset may be used to eliminate setting down the receiver to make a call.
- Mobility and transfers—People with stroke may need a wheelchair, walker, or cane for mobility. The need for adaptive aids is based on the level of involvement. The major problem is the weakness of the affected side, which may contribute to balance problems. Proper body mechanics, including positioning of the body, should be taught for safe transfer and mobility. Adaptive equipment, such as transfer boards and lifts, may be utilized if necessary.
- Home management—One-handed cooking and cleaning need to be learned in order for these individuals to perform home management tasks. There are various adaptive equipment, such as one-handed jar openers, pan holders, and electric mixers, which can assist an individual with these tasks. These devices can be purchased from adaptive tool catalogs, surgical supplies, large department stores, or pharmacies.

It is important to remember that using one hand to perform daily tasks compromises speed and dexterity. The OT practitioner should evaluate, advise, and train these individuals to conserve energy, pace time, and employ work simplification techniques to accomplish these tasks.

Activities of Daily Living Training for Muscle Weakness

The general principles guiding ADL performance for a person with muscle weakness are conserving energy and compensating for weakness. Adaptive equipment can be used to compensate for the loss of function resulting from the muscle weakness.

- Dressing—Front-opening garments, dressing sticks, Velcro openers, one-size-larger garments, long-handled shoehorn, and a reacher are some adaptive devices that can assist an individual to perform dressing.
- Feeding—Lightweight utensils, built-up utensils for weaker grip, universal cuffs, plate guards, and scoop dishes can assist with feeding tasks.
- Grooming—Adaptive aids and environmental adaptations, such as electric toothbrush, reacher, transfer tub bench, built-up faucets, and safety rails, may help these individuals perform these tasks.
- Communication—Writing aids, built-up handles for pen or pencil, book holders, key guards for computers, speaker phone, voice-activated phone, universal cuff, and a type stick can help accomplish communication tasks.
- Home management—Environmental adaptations, such as built-up doorknobs, faucets, safety rails, adapted scissors, and reachers, can all be used to assist with home management activities. Besides environmental adaptations and adaptive devices, energy conservation and work simplification techniques may be necessary to perform daily tasks.

Activities of Daily Living Training for Incoordination

Incoordination resulting from tremors is a symptom of many different disorders, such as Parkinson's disease and multiple sclerosis. The part of the body performing the activity needs to be stabilized. If not combined with muscle weakness, weighted devices such as eating utensils, pens, and cups can help stabilize the objects from excessive movement. Stabilizing bilateral upper extremities on the table while performing fine motor activities such as writing and typing can reduce incoordination.

- Dressing and grooming—Dressing can be performed in sitting position in order to avoid falls caused by poor balance. Aids such as large buttons, Velcro fasteners, front-opening garments, and clip-on ties could help with dressing. Weighted wrist cuffs could help reduce tremors. Non-skid mats inside the bathtub and non-skid floors can prevent accidents in the bathroom. A reacher, long-handled toothbrush, and bath brush could help compensate for bending and reaching. Items can be attached to a cord and hung on the wall or hung around the neck to prevent dropping. For example, soap and a toothbrush can be attached to a cord and hung around the neck while brushing or showering. A suction brush may be attached to the sink counter to assist with cleaning dentures and nail care.
- Feeding—To prevent spilling, stabilization of food by suction bases, plate guard, weighted utensils,

and weighted cups can help increase independence in feeding.

- Communication—Adaptations such as a telephone with large buttons, key guards for a computer to prevent slipping of fingers, book holders, and weighted pens can assist with reading, writing, and communication tasks.

- Transfers and mobility—Mobility aids may be used by clients depending on the severity of the condition. Severe incoordination may warrant a wheelchair to ensure safety. Walker, cane, or crutches may all be used if necessary. Non-skid floors, sliding objects instead of lifting, and using utility carts to transfer objects can assist in the safety and independence of ADL performance.

- Home management and environmental adaptations—Adaptations such as lever-type doorknobs, friction tapes on levers and faucets, speaker phone, key holders, and lamps with a wall switch instead of small buttons can all be helpful for independence in home management. The need for frequent cooking can be eliminated by pre-prepared food. Easy-to-open containers and electric jar openers can assist with handling containers. Non-skid mats can be used on work surfaces to prevent sliding of objects. Utensils made of unbreakable materials, weighted utensils, and built-up handles can assist with ease in cooking and home management. Also, holding and moving appliances with bilateral handles can increase stability while operation.

Activities of Daily Living Training for Range of Motion Limitation

People with ROM limitations have difficulty with reach and pain upon passive or active joint motion. Prolonged lack of full joint motion can lead to secondary muscle weakness. Compensatory techniques, joint protection principles, and adaptive devices can help these individuals attain varying degrees of independence in ADL tasks.

- Dressing, grooming, and hygiene—Reachers, long-handled shoehorn, long handle toothbrush, comb, dressing stick, sock aid, one-size-larger front-opening garments, Velcro or zipper fasteners, elastic shoe laces, and button hooks can assist with grooming and dressing. Devices that avoid the need for bending can be very helpful. For example, a hand-held shower, long-handled bath brush, and tub bench can be helpful during showering. A raised toilet seat can eliminate the need for sitting at a low level. Grab bars and tub rails can be installed to assist with transfers and increased safety. In case of limited grasp, spray

deodorants with spray-can adapters can be operated with more ease than regular deodorant stick.

- Feeding—Built-up lightweight utensils can help compensate for limited hand movements. Spoon-fork combinations and utensils with a swivel mechanism can accommodate for lack of forearm and wrist movement. A long straw can accommodate limited shoulder and neck movements.

- Transfer and mobility—If a person uses adaptive equipment, such as wheelchair, walker, or canes, built-up handles help accommodate limited grasp. Wheelchair, walker, and crutch bags can help a person carry objects with increased ease.

- Communication—A speaker phone, headset, or clip-type telephone holder can eliminate the need for holding the phone for a person with limited range of hand function. Built-up pens, writing aids, and book holders can assist with communication needs.

- Home maintenance and environmental adaptations—Items frequently used must be stored in shelves that can be reached most easily. For example, milk should be stored on the top shelf of the refrigerator. Using a high stool will eliminate the need for extreme joint ranges in the lower extremities. Electric appliances such as jar openers and mixers can eliminate the need for extreme hand movements required for mixing and opening cans. A cutting board with stainless steel nails and suction cups can stabilize the vegetables and meat for easy cutting. Long-handled mops and pans can assist with cleaning without the need for excessive bending. Built-up doorknobs and adapted key holders can help a person with limited hand movements.

Activities of Daily Living Training for Cognitive and Psychosocial Deficits

Cognitive and psychosocial deficits include psychiatric diagnosis, conditions with brain involvement, developmental disabilities, Alzheimer's disease, or a combination of physical and mental health disorders. People with CVA and traumatic brain injury often show cognitive/psychosocial deficits along with physical deficits. A thorough evaluation of the cognitive skills and abilities of the client will help the OT practitioner provide appropriate cues when necessary. People with cognitive deficits may still be able to learn some skills, but learning is often very slow and compensatory strategies may be needed to avoid injuries resulting from poor safety when performing daily tasks.

- Dressing, grooming, and hygiene—Verbal or visual cues may be needed for performing dressing, grooming, and hygiene activities. An activity can be broken down into smaller steps and learned in increments of complexity. Also, too many adaptive devices may confuse the person.

- Feeding—Safety should be taught in the proper use of sharp objects such as knifes. A fork-spoon combination can be used if a person has difficulty using different utensils appropriately.

- Transfer and mobility—A person with cognitive deficits may be susceptible to injury due to poor ADL safety. Walking aids and wheelchairs may be necessary if injury is warranted.

Instrumental Activities of Daily Living

- Home maintenance and environmental adaptations: If a person's prognosis is positive, cueing can be reduced as improvement occurs. On the other hand, if cognitive abilities decline progressively, appropriate cueing may be needed during various steps as the client starts to have difficulty.

In psychiatric settings, treatment may involve both individual and group sessions. Task-oriented groups are often used in the mental health setting to teach both self-care and IADL skills to these individuals.

RECORDING PERFORMANCE AND PROGRESS

The practitioner should monitor and document the changes in a client's performance on a regular basis. Any considerable improvements or decline in ADL status should be documented. The documentation should state short-term goals, goals achieved, goals not achieved, any modifications in ADL goals, long-term goals, family training, caregiver training, adaptive equipment used, client participation level, and any other pertinent information. Refer to the following case study for an example of an OT evaluation and treatment plan.

Case Study

Mrs. Bagel is a 68-year-old woman who sustained a right hip fracture due to a fall in her bathroom while trying to get out of her bathtub. She is widowed, and lives alone in a third-floor apartment complex, which is wheelchair-accessible. She was independent in all her daily activities, including shopping and visits to a senior center located 2 miles away twice a week. Mrs. Bagel did not drive but used the public transportation frequently for traveling. She enjoyed cooking, cleaning, and hosting her children and grandchildren, who lived in another part of the city. She has a son and a daughter. The son lives in a different state but the daughter lives just 5 miles away.

Mrs. Bagel has diabetes, which can be controlled by diet. Her daughter visits her once every 2 weeks to assist with financial matters and to make sure that her mother is following her diet restrictions. The daughter had noticed occasional forgetfulness in her mother for the past 3 months prior to the incident. She, however, dismissed her concern as part of the normal aging process for older people. Mrs. Bagel had Medicalert, a medical monitoring system for seniors, which was suggested by her son 6 months before the incident. At the time of her fall, she was wearing the Medicalert around her neck and managed to activate the button, which alerted the monitoring agency, which in turn called for emergency medical help. She was taken to a nearby hospital where she underwent surgery on her right hip and after 2 days was transferred to a subacute rehabilitation facility for further rehabilitation. After being seen by the physicians, she was referred to occupational therapy for evaluation and training in ADLs, safety, cognitive evaluation, and treatment.

OT Report

Mrs. Bagel had a diagnosis of right hip fracture and early Alzheimer's disease. Mrs. Bagel attended OT five times a week since admission into the facility. Evaluation revealed that she was independent in feeding and required minimal assistance for grooming and personal hygiene activities. Her mobility and transfers required moderate assistance due to her weightbearing as tolerated status. She had complained of pain, discomfort, and weakness in her right lower extremity. She had fear of falling and needed assurance while evaluating transfers and bed mobility. She required moderate assistance for transfers in the bathroom and lower extremity dressing. She showed signs of short-term memory deficits. However, on kitchen evaluation, she showed awareness of kitchen safety. OT short-term goals focused on her BADLs, such as bed mobility, transfers, dressing, and grooming. Her long-term goals focused on IADLs, such as simple cooking and cleaning activities.

SUMMARY

ADL tasks include both basic self-care tasks as well as instrumental tasks. ADLs are a major performance area assessed and treated by OT practitioners. Interview and observation of performance can help establish short- and long-term goals. OT treatment is aimed at increasing the person's independence in his or her daily tasks to his or her maximum potential. Different techniques and adaptive aids may be utilized in the treatment process. Appropriate documentation in checklist or summary format must be done in order to justify the need for continued OT services and to document the efficacy of our services.

References

AOTA. (1994). Uniform terminology for occupational therapy (3rd ed.). *Am J Occup Ther, 48,* 1047-1054.

Foti, D., Pedretti, L. W., & Lillie, S. (1996). ADLs. In L. W. Pedretti (Ed.), *OT practice skills for physical dysfunction* (pp. 463-506). St. Louis, MO: Mosby.

Hamilton, B. B., Granger, C. V., Sherwin, F. S., Zielezny, M., & Tashman, J. S. (1987). A uniform national data system for medical rehabilitation. In M. J. Fuhrer (Ed.), *Rehabilitation outcomes: Analysis and measurement* (pp. 115-150). Baltimore, MD: Brookes.

Heineman, A. W., Hamilton, B. B., Wright, B. D., Betts, H. B., Aguda, B., & Mamott, B. D. (1991). *Rating scale analysis of functional assessment measures.* Chicago, IL: Rehabilitation Institute of Chicago.

Katz, S., Downs, T. D., Cash, H. R., & Grotz, R. C. (1970). Progress in development of an index of ADL. *Gerontologist, 10,* 20-30.

Klein, R. M., & Bell, B. (1982). Self-care skills: Behavioral measurement with Klein-Bell ADL scale. *Archives of Physical Medicine and Rehabilitation, 63,* 335-338.

Kohlman-Thompson, L. (1993). *The Kohlman Evaluation of Living Skills* (3rd ed.). Rockville, MD: AOTA.

Leonardelli, C. A. (1988). *The Milwaukee evaluation of daily living skills: Evaluation in long-term psychiatric care.* Thorofare, NJ: SLACK Incorporated.

Mahoney, F. I., & Barthel, D. W. (1965). Functional evaluation: The Barthel Index. *Maryland State Medical Journal, 14,* 61-65.

Robertson, S. C. (1998). Why we document? In J. D. Acquaviva (Ed.), *Effective Documentation for OT* (2nd ed.). Baltimore, MD: AOTA.

Schoening, H. A., Anderegg, L., Bergstrom, D., Fonda, M., Steinke, N., & Ulrich, P. (1965). Numerical scoring of self-care status of patients. *Archives of Physical Medicine and Rehabilitation, 46,* 689-697.

Trombly, C. A. (1993). Anticipating the future: Assessment of occupational function. *Am J Occup Ther, 47,* 253-257.

Weiner, J. M., Hanley, R. J., Clark, R., & Van Nostrand, J. F. (1990). Measuring the activities of daily living: Comparisons across national surveys. *Journal of Gerontology: Social Sciences, 45,* S229-S237.

Work Injury Activities

Chapter 37

Barbara Larson, MA, OTR, FAOTA

Introduction

"Work 200 years ago was everyone's responsibility, a direct, positive effort to better one's lot in life and to improve the collective society" (Bing, 1989, p. 3). Maurer (1979), in a 2-year study of the unemployed, concluded that work continues to be a fundamental human need and provides not just a livelihood, but an essential passage into human community.

Fundamental to the profession of OT is the concept of work. As an occupational performance area, work encompasses vocational and educational activities, care of others, and home management. When individuals engage in work it is a productive activity, therefore, work is a medium and goal of OT (Jacobs, 1995). Work behaviors, skills, and physical capacities are performance components that constitute

important elements of work. Work skills refer to those skills that can be learned or perfected, such as typing, computer efficiency, or machine operation. Work behaviors include those behaviors necessary for successful participation in a job or to live independently, such as personal hygiene, accepting and following supervision, and getting along with others (Jacobs, 1995). Physical capacities are those abilities that allow an individual to perform work movements, such as sitting, standing, reaching, walking, stooping, bending, fingering, and handling.

Work skills, behaviors, and physical capacities are required to perform the tasks of an actual job. Problems experienced by workers related to cumulative trauma disorders, traumatic injuries, workplace accidents, or psychological distress affect work performance. OT intervention for the

Key Concepts

- Legislation and regulation: The implementation of laws, rules, and regulations that impact the practice of work.
- Job analysis: Structured analysis to identify the physical/functional aspects of work.
- Functional testing: An evaluation of an individual's physical abilities to perform work tasks.
- Goal setting related to return to work: Designing programs with goals that match the physical abilities of the worker to the functional requirements of the job.
- Treatment plan: A plan that identifies problems and interventions and determines goals for the purpose of returning the individual to the job.
- Work simulation: Actual or simulated work activity that matches the critical demands of the employee's job.
- Communication with work re-entry team: The process required to keep everyone focused on the return to work plan.

Essential Vocabulary

Cumulative trauma disorders: Work-related musculoskeletal/peripheral nerve disorders associated with highly repetitive tasks and/or forceful activity.

Ergonomics: Application of scientific information to the design of objects, systems, and environments for human use.

Functional capacity evaluation: Systematic evaluation of an individual's physical/functional capacities related to the performance of work movements.

Graded activities and work tasks: Activities/tasks that are increased in their duration, weights, heights, forces, and frequency as the worker's physical abilities increase.

Reasonable accommodations: Any change in the work environment to enable a qualified individual with a disability equal employment opportunity.

Work rehabilitation: Structured rehab, uses a graded program of exercise, education, aerobic conditioning, and actual or simulated work tasks to return persons to their jobs.

worker who is suffering from injury or illness addresses deficits related to work performance.

OT/OTA COLLABORATION

By developing a collaborative relationship, the OT and OTA use and combine their unique skills to deliver efficient, effective OT services (Glanz & Richman, 1997). The OT and OTA can have a positive impact on the individual who has had work interrupted by injury or illness. The OT focuses on problem identification, problem analysis, and the planning required for problem solution. The OTA focuses on delivery of direct services and documenting client response and progress. The OT/OTA team addresses both the physical and psychosocial issues affecting the worker's ability to function on the job. Each has a role that requires good communication between each other and with members of the work re-entry team (Glanz & Richman, 1997). The work re-entry team includes many individuals, the most important being the worker. Who will participate in a work re-entry team depends on the needs of the individual worker. Team members may include the following.

- Health care providers, including the physician, OT, and OTA
- Representatives of the employer, including human resources personnel, the occupational health nurse, safety manager, union representative, and department supervisor
- A rehabilitation consultant or case manager who may be representing the insurance company

In striving to achieve the best outcome for the client, the OT and OTA may also interact with engineers, ergonomists, architects, vocational specialists, and attorneys.

OCCUPATIONAL THERAPIST'S UNIQUE ROLE IN THE RETURN TO WORK PROCESS

The experienced OT practitioner possesses characteristics gained from his or her education and clinical experience, which make him or her uniquely suited for a major role in the rehabilitation of persons with industrial injuries (Ellexson, 1985). The OT practitioner's knowledge of injury and illness, understanding of psychosocial behavior, and knowledge of the rehabilitation system provides the basis for the application and use of clinical reasoning tools. These tools are used by the OT practitioner in recommending intervention programs to improve occupational performance (Moyers, 1999). In the case of

dealing with the industrial injury, clinical reasoning tools include the ability to analyze tasks and the ability to creatively adapt the physical environment (Ellexson, 1985). OT practitioners will also need the knowledge, skills, and abilities to deal with the administrative, regulatory, and cultural issues that affect the medium of work. The outcome of OT intervention should result in safe and functional return to work or identification of issues preventing work re-entry.

In providing services to the injured worker, the OT's and OTA's understanding of community is necessary to establish a working relationship with the client. The OT and OTA may come from different backgrounds and, as a result, can help one another gain insight into and mutually share their perceptions about the client's community, culture, values, work behaviors, and how these affect the treatment planning and goal setting process (Grady, 1995).

FRAMES OF REFERENCE

OT practitioners often find the biomechanical, human occupation, and compensatory frames of reference helpful in guiding treatment for the employee who is recovering from work-related illness or injury. The biomechanical frame of reference provides a basis for treating the musculoskeletal problem. The OT practitioner selects activities that are directed toward the individual's deficits, such as strength, ROM, and flexibility. Compensatory techniques in the form of job modifications may be necessary if the worker is unable to perform the critical job demands. Through the use of the human occupation frame of reference, the worker is guided in a direction that enhances self-esteem, supports worker behavior, and maintains worker identity. The employee, through this process of system organization, competency in social roles, and successful role performance, acquires the ability to put his or her efforts toward regaining the physical capacities necessary to return to work.

RETURN TO WORK PROCESS

OTs and OTAs address both prevention and intervention when dealing with injured workers. In the case of an injured worker who cannot go back to work following acute care, the OT may be asked to perform functional testing to determine work ability. The worker may have deficits in strength, ROM, flexibility, or endurance that prevent him or her from returning to the job. A return to work rehabilitation program may be necessary to address these deficits and prepare the worker for the transition to work. The return to work program could take place in a clinical setting, at the workplace, or a combination of both.

To determine actual job demands when designing a work rehabilitation program, a job site visit may be necessary. The COTA may go to the workplace to analyze the job. Combining information about the worker's abilities and deficits and information from the job site visit is important when designing a return to work program. This information can also assist the employer in determining job modifications or reasonable accommodations that may be necessary to allow the worker to return to the job.

The OTR and COTA communicate with the physician in providing information regarding a client's readiness for work. In most states, it is the physician who makes the final decision for release to work. The OTR and COTA, through planning, assessment, direct service, and evaluation, help maximize a safe and productive transition from rehabilitation to a work environment. If return to work is not realistic due to physical or psychological issues, the OTR and COTA provide the necessary information so care or intervention can be directed to the correct health care provider or vocational specialist.

Regulatory Considerations

To be effective in the treatment of the industrial worker, OT practitioners must be aware of laws and regulations affecting both workers and employers. The laws that have the greatest impact on OT practitioners providing services to injured workers and employers are the Americans with Disabilities Act (ADA), the Occupational Health and Safety Act (OSHA), and workers' compensation.

Americans with Disabilities Act

The ADA was passed in 1990. The ADA prohibits the exclusion of individuals with physical or mental disabilities from jobs, services, activities, or benefits (Kornblau & Ellexson, 1995). Employers are required to provide reasonable accommodations to those individuals protected by the ADA. Reasonable accommodation as defined by the ADA includes any change in the work environment or the way work is customarily performed that enables an individual with a disability to enjoy equal employment opportunity (Kornblau & Ellexson, 1995). The OTR and COTA may be involved in assisting the employer to design reasonable accommodations for individuals with disabilities.

Workers' Compensation

Workers' compensation laws are a product of the 20th century. The workers' compensation system protects the rights of workers with illnesses or injuries sustained on the job. Workers' compensation pays wage replacement and medical costs for the worker. Although each state workers' compensation law is different in its administration, interpretation, and benefit level, states do share some common principles (Ellexson, 1985).

Workers' compensation is a major cost to employers. The average employer pays 2% to 3% of payroll for workers' compensation insurance (Larson, 1995). The OT practitioner through timely, efficient, effective service can have a positive impact on reducing workers' compensation costs incurred by the employer.

Occupational Safety and Health Administration

In 1970, Congress established OSHA. As defined in legislation P. L. 91-596, the mission of the Occupational Safety and Health Act of 1970 is to ensure, so far as possible, every working man and woman in the nation has safe and healthful working conditions. It is up to the employer to enforce the standards set by OSHA. Refusal to do so can result in significant fines and reprimands. OTRs often work with employers on ergonomics and safety issues related to OSHA compliance.

Case Study 1

Background Information

John is a 42-year-old auto mechanic who has worked for the same employer for 14 years. John sustained a right shoulder injury when reaching overhead to remove a transmission from a car. John was seen by a physician and referred to a therapist for treatment of his shoulder. Following his acute therapy program, John continued to report pain and discomfort in his right shoulder.

Assessment

John was referred to the occupational rehabilitation department for a functional capacity evaluation (FCE) to determine his ability to perform work tasks related to his job as an auto mechanic. The OTR performed the FCE. The results of the FCE outlined John's current physical abilities and limitations. John showed no deficits in his ability to walk, stand, or sit. He was able to perform low positional activities, such as kneeling, crouching, and squatting. John showed decreased physical capacities in the following areas: floor to waist lift was limited to 30 pounds, working with the right arm overhead could only be done occasionally, and push and pull was limited to 30 pounds of force for 20 feet.

At the request of the OTR, the COTA visited the worksite to determine the physical job demands of the auto mechanic position. From her job analysis, the job demands were identified as follows:

- Lifting—Frequently. Lifts car, truck, and van tires 20 to 50 pounds, up to 125 pounds (rarely) from ground to chest level when removing or replacing tires on vehicles (assistance is available when lifting above 50 pounds).

- Push/pull—Occasionally. Moving tire racks about 25 feet, from inside garage to outside. Fifty pounds of force is required to push or pull the racks.
- Reaching/elevated work—Frequently. A 32-inch horizontal reach is required to work under hood of vehicles. A vertical overhead reach is required to work underneath vehicles that are positioned on the hoist.

Treatment Planning

Based on the results of the FCE and the job analysis, it was determined John would benefit from a work rehabilitation program. The OT developed the treatment plan from the results of the FCE and the job analysis information received from the OTA. The program would address John's deficits in right upper extremity strength and endurance and the functional work tasks of lift, push, pull, and overhead work.

The long-term goal of the program was return to work at his previous job in 3 to 4 weeks.

John would start in the clinic 5 days per week at 4 hours per day. After 3 weeks he would return to work full-time and alternate between modified duty and his regular job. A 1-week transition would be allowed to return to full-time on his previous job. The program goals included:

1. Education on safe lifting and body mechanics when handling tires, tools, and equipment and performing other auto mechanic job duties.
2. Cardiovascular conditioning, including exercise bike, upper body ergometer, and walking program, to increase endurance to perform job tasks for 8 hours.
3. Continuation of the graded exercise program started in acute therapy to increase strength and flexibility in the right shoulder.
4. Work simulation activities, including lifting tires from ground to chest level as when removing or replacing tires on vehicles, reaching overhead while using tools to simulate working on cars, and pushing and pulling carts to simulate moving the tire racks in and out of the building.

The OTA, under the supervision of the OT, carried out the treatment plan. The exercises, cardiovascular conditioning, and work simulation activities were graded to achieve the return to work goals in 3 weeks.

The OT re-evaluated John's physical status at the end of week 1 and adjusted the program based on his physical capacities and functional status. The OTA implemented the changes as directed by the OT. Based on John's progress, the OTA was able to increase the amount of time spent on work simulation tasks.

The employer was contacted by the OT to discuss ergonomic considerations related to the reaching and static postures required of the auto mechanics when working on vehicles on the overhead hoist. One of the changes made was to have longer sockets made for some of the wrenches. This would minimize the reaching distance when loosening or attaching nuts and bolts. A second change was to suspend the air hoses from the ceiling rather then having the mechanics hold them up while working on a vehicle. This minimized the static loading of the arms and shoulders while working in the overhead position.

Work Transition

Following week 3, the OT reassessed John's physical capacities. Based on his progress, John was released to return to work by his physician. Prior to actual return to the job, the OT, OTA, rehabilitation consultant, employer, and John met at the workplace to make sure the work transition plan was clearly understood by all parties. John would spend his first week at work alternating 4 hours of modified duty with 4 hours of regular duty. The modified duty included sweeping, cleaning tasks, and processing customer work orders. The regular duty included performing safety checks and maintenance on cars, light trucks, and vans. Prior to John returning to work, the employer had made the ergonomic changes discussed with the OT.

Program Discontinuation

The OTA made a job site visit the first week to monitor John's transition from modified duty to the regular job. The OTA made sure John was using the techniques he had learned and practiced in the work rehabilitation program to complete his work tasks. She also observed the ergonomic changes made by the employer. After 1 week of transition back at work, John was able to perform his previous job on a full-time basis. He returned to his regular job and was discharged from the occupational rehabilitation program.

Clinical Problem-Solving

Two weeks after John returned to work his employer called the OT. John was refusing to follow his return to work recommendations. John told the employer he did not think his return to work program was any good. The OT talked with the OTA to find out if John had raised any of these issues during his return to work program. The OTA stated John had not voiced any concerns. The OT arranged a meeting at the worksite with John, his employer, herself, and the OTA. John was given the opportunity to express his concerns. The OT did not dwell on why he did not bring up these concerns during the work rehabilitation program. The OT focused the interaction with John and his employer on concerns related to the work setting. While it was important for John to express his concerns, it was equally important for him to take responsibility for his part of the return to work plan. The discussion at the meeting was directed toward John's transition to work. In the future, if John identified areas of concern related to his recommendations, he would tell his employer. He and the employer would develop a plan to address the issue. If there were changes in the job tasks, equipment, or work methods, the employer would contact the OT to assess the changes and make sure John was working within his physical abilities using good ergonomic principles. What other factors might be involved with John's resistance and how could the OT/OTA team address these?

CASE STUDY 2

Background Information

Mary worked as a financial planner for a large brokerage firm. She had recently been diagnosed with multiple sclerosis. At about the time of Mary's diagnosis, her company was planning a project to remodel all employee offices. The human resources director was concerned that Mary's office be remodeled to accommodate the physical changes she might experience depending on the progression of her multiple sclerosis. The human resources director contacted an OT she had worked with in the past. The OT was asked to meet with the office design architect to discuss the office blueprints. The OT was also asked to meet with Mary to make sure both her current and future needs were considered with the workstation redesign. The OT met with the architect to review blueprints of the proposed workstation and made specific recommendations. The OTA interviewed Mary and reviewed work simplification and energy conservation techniques related to both the placement of office equipment and performance of specific work tasks. The OT and OTA then identified employee and worksite issues and made recommendations to the employer. Employee and worksite issues and recommendations include the following.

1. Proper sitting
   - Employee and worksite issues—The existing chair does not fit properly. The chair arms are too high, not adjustable, and require the employee to hike up her shoulders to use them. The lumbar support is fixed and does not allow individual adjustment.
   - Recommendations—When selecting a chair, consider the following chair characteristics:

   a. The ease with which the height can be adjusted.
   b. Whether the seated position can be changed easily.
   c. The type of support provided by the seat pan and back rest.
   d. The adjustability of the angle formed between the seat pan and backrest.
   e. The lumbar support of the chair.
   f. The base of support and if the chair swivels.
   g. Material and padding that makes up the chair.

2. Leg/chair clearance
   - Employee and worksite issues—Blueprints of the work counter were reviewed regarding leg clearance when using an office chair and allowing enough leg clearance for eventual wheelchair use.
   - Recommendations—The supports that hold up the counter will be designed to maximize leg clearance and movement both for office chairs and wheelchair use.

3. Computer work area
   - Employee and worksite issues—The computer will be positioned in a corner with an under-the-counter keyboard. According to the architect, the under-the-counter keyboard is adjustable and has an attached mouse holder.
   - Recommendations—Make sure adequate knee clearance exists with the under-the-counter keyboard and mouse holder. With this corner arrangement, enough space will exist that the work area could be modified in the future to allow Mary to rest her arms on the countertop to provide more upper arm, shoulder, and forearm support when using the keyboard.

4. Work area
   - Employee and worksite issues—The employee wanted the work area designed with enough space so work papers could be left on the desk.
   - Recommendations—The workstation will be designed in a U-shape to allow two corner work areas, one for the computer and keyboard and one for writing tasks and projects.

5. Lighting
   - Employee and worksite issues—The employee would like task lighting as well as overhead lighting.
   - Recommendations—The lighting set up will allow counter height switches to adjust the overhead lighting and space and wiring for individual desk lamps for task lighting.

6. Energy conservation/work simplification
    - Employee and worksite issues—The work area should be set up to minimize energy output to achieve work tasks. The employee stated she often gets fatigued walking out to the printer.
    - Recommendations—Counters will allow both writing and computer work without having to put away papers. Space for a printer will be factored into workstation design.

Upon completion of the report, the OT and OTA met with the human resources director and the employee to make sure there was a clear understanding of the recommendations. The meeting also validated the feasibility of the recommendations. The human resource director will stay in contact with the OT and told the employee to bring to her attention any issues she felt could be addressed by OT.

Clinical Problem-Solving

One week following the meeting, the OT received a call from the human resources director. The human resources director had just been informed of budget cuts in the dollars allocated for office remodeling. The OT was asked to prioritize Mary's needs since the project was being scaled back. The OTA and OT developed a plan and met with the human resources director and Mary. The following was determined as a result of the meeting.

- A new chair was an immediate priority, as the existing chair did not fit properly.
- The current work area needed temporary changes to allow space for both computer work and tasks requiring desk space. This would address issues related to energy conservation and work simplification.
- The above work areas would be temporary. At the suggestion of the OT, Mary's office was first on the remodeling schedule. If Mary's condition changed and it became necessary for her to use a wheelchair, remodeling would be done immediately.

The OTA would work with Mary on the fitting of a new office chair and assist with the temporary changes and accommodations to her workstation. What changes would be needed if Mary were pregnant or had arthritis?

REFERENCES

Bing, R. K. (1989). Work is a four-letter word! A historical perspective. In S. Hertfleder & C. Gwin (Eds.), *Work in progress: OT in work programs*. Rockville, MD: AOTA.

Ellexson, M. T. (1985). *The unique role of OT in industry. Work-related programs in OT*. Binghamton, NY: Haworth Press.

Glanz, C. H., & Richman, N. (1997). OTR-COTA collaboration in home health: Roles and supervisory issues. *Am J Occup Ther, 51*(6), 446-457.

Grady, A. P. (1995). Building inclusive community: A challenge for occupational therapy, 1994 Eleanor Clarke Slagle Lecture. *Am J Occup Ther, 49,* 300-310.

Jacobs, K. (1995). Preparing for return to work. In C. A. Trombly (Ed.), *OT for physical dysfunction* (4th ed.). Baltimore, MD: Williams & Wilkins.

Kornblau, B. L., & Ellexson, M. T. (1995). Reasonable accommodation and the Americans with Disabilities Act. In S. J. Isernhagen (Ed.), *The comprehensive guide to work injury management*. Gaithersburg, MD: Aspen.

Larson, B. L. (1995). Work rehabilitation. The importance of networking with the employer to achieve successful outcomes. In S. J. Isernhagen (Ed.), *The comprehensive guide to work injury management*. Gaithersburg, MD: Aspen.

Maurer, H. (1979). *Not working: An oral history of the unemployed*. New York, NY: Holt, Rinehart & Winston.

Moyers, P. A. (1999.) The guide to occupational therapy practice. *Am J Occup Ther, 53*(3), 247-322.

Management of Practice Issues

Documentation

Harriet Ann Backhaus, MA, COTA/L, ROH
Karen Sladyk, PhD, OTR/L, FAOTA

INTRODUCTION

It is important for the OTA to have a good understanding of the principles of documentation. While documentation policies and procedures vary considerably among facilities and often have unique aspects, certain principles apply to all methods of documentation.

The following components of documentation will be discussed:

- Purpose of documentation
- Review of the OT/OTA role responsibilities in the documentation of OT process
- Documentation for reimbursement
- Reporting OT services
- Examples of documentation

Confidentiality

According to the OT *Code of Ethics* Principle 2, confidentiality is to be considered at all times. Confidentiality means that the practitioner never allows information about the patient to be shared verbally or in writing with anyone the patient has not approved. Information about a patient can come from the patient or the written or computer-generated medical record. The OT practitioner must respect all patients' rights and work hard to make sure all staff respect privacy. Examples of breaking confidentiality include tossing old notes in the garbage, talking about patients at lunch or home, taking documentation home to finish notes, or approaching a former patient in the community before they approach you.

PURPOSE OF DOCUMENTATION

OT documentation is a legal document, protecting the rights of both the patient and the therapist (Perinchief, 1998). Documentation supports the treatment given in the care of the patient and the patient's response to that treatment (AOTA, 1995a). In addition, documentation ensures accurate communication for reimbursement from third party payers, such as insurance companies, Medicare, and Medicaid. The OT has the ultimate responsibility of the OT docu-

ESSENTIAL VOCABULARY

Assessment: Specific tools used in the evaluation process.

Discharge documentation: Summary of treatment progress at the discontinuation of services.

Evaluation: The process of gathering intake information.

Screening: Determines the need for evaluation.

Third-party payer: An insurance or HMO company paying for OT services.

Treatment plan: Legal document that outlines the map of treatment.

KEY CONCEPTS

- Confidentiality: Patient/client information is kept private.
- Documentation: Legal document used to communicate with other team members and record patient progress.
- Reimbursement process: Documentation required for OT services to be covered by a third-party payer.
- Prospective payment system: Medicare ruling designed to control treatment costs.

mentation, with the OTA contributing to the total plan (Early, 1996).

Each facility offering OT services has to adhere to the guidelines established by the particular accrediting agency for that facility. Examples of accrediting agencies that govern these facilities are:

- Joint Commission on Accreditation of Healthcare Organizations (JCAHO)
- Commission on the Accreditation of Rehabilitation Facilities (CARF)
- Comprehensive Outpatient Rehabilitation Facility (CORF)
- Federal and state agencies
- Individual state laws (Perinchief, 1998)

Facilities may adopt certain criteria for monitoring note-writing and ensuring the proper use of acceptable terminology and abbreviations. Documentation can also be used as part of quality assurance reviews for ensuring accountability in the organization or system (Perinchief, 1998). Since every provider strives for quality care, the documentation system must reflect that quality as well. It is important to realize that any part of the medical record, including OT documentation, can be used in legal proceedings. Co-signature of all OTA documentation is needed if required by law or the specific facility.

OTA Responsibility in the Occupational Therapy Process

The OTA is responsible for contributing to the OT process. The OT process includes screening, assessment and evaluation, treatment, re-evaluation, and discharge. The OTA responsibility is outlined in the OT Roles document prepared by the OT Task Force (AOTA, 1995b).

Screening

Screening is the process by which OT practitioners determine the need for evaluation and treatment. This includes chart review, interview, and observations to determine whether OT is needed. The OTA can, after establishing competency, perform parts of the screening component and report back to the OT. The AOTA document *Standards of Practice for OT* includes components of the OT process that can assist in developing competency (AOTA, 1995b). Competency is established when two people performing the same or equivalent procedure will obtain the same or equivalent results. Competency is determined by the supervising OT.

Initial Evaluation (Assessment)

Evaluation is the process of gathering a database and interpreting the findings for the development of a treat-

ment plan. The OTA can observe the OT perform the evaluation. After achieving competency, the OTA can, under the supervision of the OT, administer standardized tests, score test protocol, and complete data collection procedures, such as record reviews, interviews, general observations, and behavioral checklists. The OTA can also report the factual data orally, in writing, or both. Information from the assessment is then incorporated by the OT into an initial note. AOTA's *Elements for Clinical Documentation* (AOTA, 1995a) states that documentation should include the following elements:

- Patient's full name and case number on each page
- Date stated as month, day, and year
- Identification of type of documentation and department name
- Signature with a minimum of first name, last name, and professional designation
- Countersignature by an OT on documentation written by OTAs if required by law or the facility
- Acceptable terminology as defined by AOTA and/or the facility
- Facility-approved abbreviations

The initial note should contain information including:

- Referral source and when the referral was received
- Information obtained during the first session, which can include structured observation and formal evaluations
- Plans for further OT intervention, which include identification of problems, long- and short-term goals determined by the patient and therapist, methods to obtain those goals, the frequency of the treatment, and the anticipated outcome of the treatment (Early, 1996)

Reassessment

Reassessment is the process of gathering current information on the patient's functioning and using this information to decide whether to continue OT treatment, revise the treatment plan, or discontinue the treatment. Reassessment is an ongoing procedure. Tasks relevant to the screening and evaluation process apply to reassessment. The OTA can determine the need for reassessment and report any changes in the patient's performance that might indicate the need for reassessment. The OTA may also contribute to the reassessment by performing any tasks as requested by the OT.

Treatment Planning

Treatment planning involves preparation and implementation of the treatment plan. The OT is ultimately responsible for the outcome of the OT intervention and, as such, develops the OT goals for the patient based on establishing the problem list as identified by the assessment data and the goals of the patient. It is critically important to consider the goals of the patient (Hirama, 1996). The OT and OTA need to allow the patient to participate in the selection of meaningful goals and the methods to achieve those goals. The patient needs to feel that the goals are relevant to him or her. By asking the patient what is a concern for him or her, the OT or OTA can make a more informed decision as to the plan of treatment. The OTA contributes to the development of the goals and can assist the OT in developing the treatment plan. Goals need to reflect a patient action, a specific time frame, and a qualifier of the action. Components of goal writing can be referred to with the mnemonic RUMBA (Early, 1996; Perinchief, 1998):

- Relevant—The goal should reflect the patient's goal and be related to function.

- Understandable—Jargon should be avoided; stated so others can understand.

- Measurable—Stated in terms of frequency and duration.

- Behavioral—Behaviors that are observed and are measurable.

- Achievable—Goals that can be accomplished in a reasonable time.

Examples of goals using the RUMBA guidelines are:

- Within 3 days, the patient will be able to eat 50% of a light meal with an adaptive fork and no spillage of food in 20 minutes.

- After reviewing a bus schedule in the clinic and with no cues from the therapist or peers, the patient will be able to correctly identify the bus route and time of pick-up to get to work on time.

The treatment plan is carried out by the means of individual or group treatment using a variety of therapeutic media (Early, 1996). The documentation of the OT treatment plan and the patient's physical and verbal responses to it are written in the progress note. The OTA will be involved in the writing of progress notes, as it is the OTA who delivers a substantial amount of the OT intervention (Hirama, 1996).

Progress notes may be written daily, once a week, once a month, or as dictated by the individual facility or agency, and each facility may use different formats. Some settings require a daily notation in the patient's medical record that reflects the patient's response to treatment on that day. The OTA must be familiar with the time frame for documentation in the specific setting he or she is working.

Information included when writing progress notes are as follows (Early, 1996; Hirama, 1996):

- A description of the patient's response to the OT treatment. Examples include any remarks made by the patient during the treatment session that may indicate how the patient is tolerating treatment or if the patient sees any progress since treatment began.

- A summary of the patient's actual progress or lack of progress since the last note, stating what activities the patient has been participating in, and the frequency of the participation. The type of therapeutic exercise or activity used should also be noted (e.g., dressing training with compensatory techniques, participation in a cooking group, community mobility training, or participation in a self-ROM group).

- Any new information gathered through observation or evaluations since the last note is also documented. This information may include either positive or negative changes in physical or mental status, cooperation, and motivation. The current status of long- and short-term goals is reviewed and any changes that are indicated are documented. A goal may have been achieved or may no longer be appropriate.

The importance of the progress note is to document the patient's functional performance in order to justify continuation of OT services. The means by which the patient is working toward achieving the goals should be stated. In addition, it is important to include your justification for recommending that the OT treatment continues. If the plan or goals need changing, the OTA must collaborate with the OT.

Discontinuation of Intervention

When a person receiving OT services achieves the goal(s) established by the OT process, or if the goals were unable to be met, the service is discontinued.

The planning for discharge begins when the patient is first seen by OT. Important areas to be aware of throughout the intervention plan are:

- The patient's living arrangements after discharge.

- The activities and occupations the patient will assume.

- The need for additional assistance to carry out these activities of life.

- The services available to the patient (e.g, home health OT, adult day care, mental health services, rehabilitation centers, or possibly outpatient OT) (Early, 1996).

Discontinuation of OT services is documented in the discharge summary or discharge note. The OT is responsible for the discharge note, with the OTA determining the need for assessment of the discharge status. The discharge note is a summary of the course of the patient's treatment and includes:

- The number of sessions the patient attended.
- A report of the patient's progress, including the status of the goals.
- Changes in the patient's performance since initially treated.
- Any recommendations for further OT intervention or the need for other services.

REIMBURSEMENT FOR SERVICES

Payment for OT services comes from several sources (Bailey, 1998; Schwartz & Engle-Ramirez, 1996). These include federal, state, private and commercial insurers, grants, and self-pay sources. Funding usually comes from two kinds of payment systems: insurance and grant programs. Insurance programs include Medicare, Medicaid, workers' compensation, pre-paid health plans (HMOs, PPOs), and private insurance plans (Blue Cross, etc.). Some individuals pay for services themselves, and this is referred to as self-pay.

Medicare continues to be the largest funding agency for OT. The Prospective Payment System (PPS) became a part of the Medicare reimbursement system in 1983 (Bailey, 1998). This system affects most OT services under the Medicare guidelines. Skilled nursing facilities and home health services came under PPS guidelines in 1998 as a result of the Balanced Budget Act of 1997. Under PPS for skilled nursing facilities, fixed payments will be made for care including OT services. The Health Care Financing Administration (HCFA) has guidelines for reimbursement, which must be followed. For Medicare Part A, the minimum data set (MDS) is the basis for reimbursement. With Medicare Part B, International Classifications of Diseases (9th rev.) Clinical Modification (ICD-9-CM) codes are used in conjunction with the Health Care Financing Administration Common Procedure Coding system (CPT) codes (HCFA, 1999). AOTA has worked tirelessly to overcome some of the stifling rules developed under PPS (McCann, 2000). For example, students can bill for treatment again, the outpatient cap of $1,500 has been lifted for 2 years, and optometrists can refer to OT. This is just one reason it is important for all OTAs and OTs to be members of AOTA. Please note that many of these PPS codes are under constant revision and the most current sources should be consulted regarding this reimbursement issue, another benefit of AOTA membership.

Grant funding is also a large funding resource for OT and includes programs such as the Education for All Handicapped Children Act (P. L. 994-142), community mental health centers, the Older Americans Act, and Social Security Title XX-Social Services (Bailey, 1998). All of these sources can have OT as a part of their program for specific populations as outlined in the rules of the programs. Each funding source has specific documentation issues.

Documentation guidelines vary to the source of reimbursement. Insurance programs have more definite guidelines as to the services covered in specific settings. Some documentation systems have been streamlined in the form of critical pathways, which have daily treatment goals developed before the patient arrives. Grant programs allow for state or local regulations, which typically conform to broad national goals (Perinchief, 1998.)

UNIFORM TERMINOLOGY

Since sources of reimbursement review documentation to decide funding for those services OT provides (Bailey, 1998), patient performance should be documented by the use of uniform terminology, as outlined in the *Uniform Terminology for OT* (3rd ed.) (AOTA, 1994). Reimbursement will not occur unless documentation is complete and reports performance in functional terms, and uniform terminology provides the language to do so.

Uniform terminology defines the performance areas and performance components of OT services. The third edition updated the initial uniform terminology guides to reflect changes in theory and practice and added the performance context.

The occupational performance areas are:
1. ADLs
2. Work activities
3. Play or leisure

The occupational performance components are:
1. Sensorimotor components
2. Cognitive integration and cognitive components
3. Psychosocial skills and psychological components

Uniform Terminology (3rd ed.) (1994) further outlines the preferred terminology to be used when addressing these areas in OT documentation and should be referred to when writing notes.

It is evident that regardless of the note format used, certain areas should be consistently addressed, using the acceptable OT terminology and reflecting functional performance.

For example, if an OTA notices that a patient in a day treatment has improved in attendance, refused less often, has increased participation in group activities, and is now able to complete projects, this should be included in the progress note, and the OT should be updated. The documentation of these observations may enable the patient to continue in OT, since it shows that progress is being made.

Another example is that an OTA may observe through an ADL assessment that a patient with a left cerebrovascular accident has progressed from only being able to put on a shirt to putting on slacks and socks. Instead of stating that the patient has improved in ADLs, the OTA should specify which uniform terminology areas have improved compared to the last documentation. Changes in performance that represent a regression need to be noted also, and the OT should be informed to the change.

REPORTING OF OCCUPATIONAL THERAPY SERVICES

A facility may adapt its own note writing format based on specific populations and facility needs (Bailey, 1998). Whatever the format used, good documentation should always include a database, a problem list, and a treatment plan (Early, 1996), including long- and short-term goals. OT documentation must reflect the patient's functional performance in all areas of treatment.

One commonly used procedure to structure documentation is the problem-oriented medical record (POMR) (Hirama, 1996; Perinchief, 1998). The POMR consists of three sections, which include the database, the list of problems, and the plan for resolving the problems (Early, 1996). Notes adhering to the POMR system can be written in a narrative or paragraph form as long as the problems are clearly identified and the treatment or intervention plan and goals are clearly stated.

Many facilities use the POMR in the form of SOAP notes (Bailey, 1998). SOAP stands for subjective, objective, assessment, plan.

The subjective part of an initial or ongoing note done in the SOAP format refers to what the patient has to say, in addition to what the family or significant others have to report. At times, information from other disciplines may be included. Subjective information is based on report and is not measurable (Hirama, 1996; Perinchief, 1998). Reports from the patient or family can include the previous lifestyle or home situation, attitudes or feelings, complaints, and the patient's verbal response to treatment.

The objective part of the SOAP note refers to measurable and observable data obtained during the initial or ongoing evaluation (Hirama, 1996; Perinchief, 1998). Objective data comes from tests and measurements from structured evaluations such as the Purdue Pegboard, Kohlman Evaluation of Living Skills, and Allen's Cognitive Level Test. Data such as the results of ROM, muscle strength, sensory, or ADL performance can also be recorded here. In addition, the minutes of therapy or site of treatment can be reported in this section.

The assessment part of the note refers to the therapist's judgments as to how the limitations noted during the assessment data will affect the patient's functional performance (Perinchief, 1998). Additional data requiring interpretation from the practitioner is added to this section. For example, the patient's mood, affect, insight, or judgment is explained. Any problems discovered as a result of the objective data collected are listed here, for example, deficits in ADL status, decreased strength, or problem-solving difficulty. Problems are listed and numbered here. The problem list forms the basis for determining the goals.

The last part of the SOAP note is the plan. It is here that the long- and short-term goals are set (Hirama, 1996; Perinchief, 1998). In addition, the frequency and length of treatment is established. It is important to consider the patient's prior level of functioning, as this can help direct the plan of treatment. For example, if a patient lives in an assisted living facility and has meals provided, cooking may not be an important goal to include in the treatment plan. Treatment is always patient driven and should reflect what the patent will accomplish, not what the OT practitioners plan to do. For example, the plan section should always begin with "The patient will…" and should never just say "continue in present plan."

The SOAP format is convenient for both initial and progress notes. As mentioned earlier, progress notes reflect the recent treatment given. Progress notes are usually written weekly, unless the facility has other requirements. When writing a progress note using the SOAP format, the subjective part refers to what the patient reports about the treatment. The objective part of the note refers to the patient's current performance based on data found through specific evaluations, observations, and the use of therapeutic media. The assessment part of the progress note reflects the effectiveness of treatment and any changes needed, the status of the goals, and the justification for the need for continuing OT. Lastly, the plan includes any new goals, the treatment modalities to be used during the next treatment period, the frequency and duration of treatment, the need for further evaluations to be made, and recommendations (Hirama, 1996; Perinchief, 1998).

It is important to mention here that there are different methods of incorporating SOAP notes into the documentation process, and there may be slight differences in format depending on the type of facility and the patients who are treated. Some SOAP formats are more formal than others. The OTA must be familiar with the documentation format used in his or her specific facility (Bailey, 1998). If the SOAP note format is not being used in a setting, the OTA may still want to use the principles of the format to organize note writing.

While SOAP notes are commonly used in medical facilities, in the public school systems, documentation is referred to as the individual education plan (IEP). IEPs are required for all children receiving services under P. L.

94-142 of the Education for All Handicapped Children Act (Bailey, 1998).

IEPs must be established in writing before special education and related services can be provided (Case-Smith, Allen, & Pratt, 1996). The IEP is a collaborative effort by a team usually made up of a supervisory person, the child's parents, the child if appropriate, and others involved in the child's care, including the OT or OTA. The OTA provides the input based on the treatment sessions throughout the school year to the OT. The OT then completes the necessary documentation based on completing the end of the year evaluations.

Each school system has its own IEP outline, however, federal regulations specify that the following must be included in an IEP (Case-Smith, Allen, & Pratt, 1996):

- Present level of functioning.
- Goals and short-term objectives.
- Special education and related services to be provided.
- Dates for initiation and duration of services.
- Criteria for evaluation of the achievement of the goals and objectives.

Each discipline involved with the student contributes its plan of treatment, which is then incorporated in the master IEP.

CASE EXAMPLES

Figures 38-1 through 38-3 are examples of an initial evaluation, progress note, and discharge summary, respectively, based on the SOAP note format. Other styles of note writing include observation or narrative-style notes, which can be used in mental health settings. Observation notes give an accurate picture of what occurred during the treatment session.

SUMMARY

In summary, the OTA, under supervision of the OT, will use documentation to record the patient's status, develop a treatment plan, establish patient-directed goals, and record the actual progress in therapy (Early, 1996). Documentation will be specific to each setting, but as stated, good documentation includes reporting functional performance. This report is based on data collected from the assessment from which the treatment plan is developed. The treatment plan should reflect the choice of therapeutic media and patient-directed goals. *Uniform Terminology* (AOTA, 1994) should be used to ensure that the OT intervention program is being completely reported. In addition to the note samples given in this chapter, computerized documentation is being used in many settings. One type of computerized documentation is OT FACT (Perinchief, 1998). Also, many OT service providers, as well as other health care providers, have individualized computerized forms. Computerized documentation is helpful in time management, which is increasingly important as more demands are placed on OT practitioners.

Note: The term patient was used throughout this chapter as the person receiving OT services. Some settings will refer to this person as a client, student, resident, or member. Other settings may refer to the person by name or by another term specific to that setting.

A 72-year-old female with the diagnosis of status post right hip replacement with posterior approach secondary to degenerative joint disease, referred to OT by Dr. J. Smith on 2-17-00 for OT consult for ADLs. Surgery date: 2-15-00. Patient is toe-touch weightbearing. Patient treatment initiated on 2-18-00.

S. Patient complains of some hip pain. "It hurts but I can take it." Patient states that she lives in a one-story house with the laundry facilities in the basement. She reported she is a widow but has a daughter who assists with the shopping and heavy cleaning as needed. Patient states that she has had some difficulties with homemaking prior to the surgery but now reports she is pleased with the outcome of the surgery. She states she is hopeful to be able to resume the activities she had done in the past, "I can't wait to get back to my senior center groups."

O. Chart reviewed. Past medical history unremarkable except for history of degenerative arthritis. UE ROM: WNL. Sensation, coordination: No deficits noted. Functional transfers: Moderate assistance of one from bed to chair.

ADL status: Patient has limitations in hip range of motion in lower extremity secondary to precautions for total hip replacement and requires maximal physical assistance for lower extremity dressing. Patient reports she is independent in UE bathing and dressing but tires easily and needs to rest frequently.

A. Patient is cooperative and motivated to become as independent as possible. Patient showed good understanding of the hip precautions necessary for ADLs and later community mobility. Friends at the senior center seem to provide support and motivation. Patient understands the need for adaptive equipment and training in regard to the precautions.

Problem list:

1. Decreased performance in ADLs and leisure.

2. Decreased endurance for ADLs and leisure.

Rehabilitation potential: Good. Patient appears to be able to benefit from daily instruction in use of adaptive equipment, appropriate energy conservation techniques, and training in safe transfers. She was able to participate in this treatment planning and expressed her priorities.

P. Short-term goals: Patient will be able to:

1. Bathe and dress lower extremities with adaptive equipment and minimal physical assistance in 2 days.

2. Transfer to commode in room with minimal physical assistance in 1 week.

3. Verbalize energy conservation techniques as instructed for ADL tasks in 1 week.

Long-term goals: Patient will be able to:

1. Bathe and dress lower extremities independently with adaptive equipment by discharge.

2. Transfer to toilet in bathroom with appropriate safety equipment independently by discharge.

3. Will use energy conservation techniques and verbally report the benefits or concerns related to her leisure interests by discharge.

Treatment initiated for problem 1. Tolerance was good.

Jane Doe, OTR
2-18-00

Figure 38-1. OT initial note.

S. "I am using the adaptive equipment with the nurses."

O. Problem of decreased performance of ADLs:

Patient is able to don and doff slacks and socks with long-handled dressing equipment with occasional minimal assistance. Patient transfers to the commode with raised seat and rails with minimal assistance to maintain weight-bearing status. Patient instructed in energy conservation techniques and was given a handout.

A. Patient is limited by need for verbal cues at times to maintain toe-touch weightbearing status. She becomes frustrated when she forgets the weightbearing rules. Short-term goals achieved. Long-term goals reviewed and remain appropriate. Occupational therapy intervention continues to be needed to progress to independence in ADLs and leisure.

P. New short-term goal 4: Patient to bathe and dress lower extremities with verbal cues and long-handled sponge, dressing stick, sock aide in 3 days. As patient is able to tolerate present therapy schedule, the initial treatment plan remains appropriate with the above mentioned changes.

John Jones, COTA
2-25-00

Figure 38-2. Progress note (SOAP).

Initial visit: 2-18-00. Discharge visit: 3-1-00.

Patient with diagnosis of status post right hip replacement referred by Dr. J. Smith on 2-17-00 for ADL training, including mobility to pursue leisure interests.

S. Patient states she will have her daughter help her, but she states she can dress herself.

O. Problem of decreased performance in ADLs and leisure: Patient is independent in lower extremity bathing and dressing using adaptive equipment (reacher, long-handled sponge, sock aid, and dressing stick). Patient performs a sink-bath but has successfully demonstrated the use of a shower chair. Patient transfers to the toilet with raised seat and rails independently. Senior center was contacted by phone, and the bathroom there has the necessary equipment for patient's participation.

Problem of decreased endurance for ADLs and leisure: Patient was instructed in energy conservation techniques and is able to verbalize techniques appropriately. She reported that this has been most helpful in dressing and still having enough energy to go to the senior center. Patient will use the community disability transportation service for rides to the senior center until she is medically cleared to drive herself. Staff at the senior center have made arrangements for her first ride next week and will educate the patient on how to arrange the service.

A. Patient was independent in use of adaptive equipment, showed good judgment, and was able to follow posterior precautions.

Status of goals:

STG 1: Patient to bathe and dress lower extremities with adaptive equipment and minimal assistance in 2 days—Achieved.

STG 2: Patient to transfer to commode with minimal assistance in 1 week—Achieved.

STG 3: Patient to verbalize energy conservation techniques as instructed with 100% accuracy in 1 week—Achieved.

STG 4: Patient to bathe and dress lower extremities with verbal cues only in 3 days—Achieved.

LTG 1: Patient to bathe and dress lower extremities with adaptive equipment independently by discharge—Achieved.

LTG 2: Patient to transfer to toilet in bathroom with appropriate safety equipment independently by discharge—Achieved.

LTG 3: Patient will use energy conservation techniques and verbally report the benefits or concerns related to her leisure interests by discharge—Achieved.

P. Patient discontinued from OT secondary to discharge to home with daughter.

Recommendations: Continue to use recommended adaptive equipment for duration of precautions.

Follow-up: Home health OT.

Sally Smith, OTR
3-1-00

Figure 38-3. Discharge summary (SOAP).

REFERENCES

AOTA. (1994). Uniform terminology for occupational therapy (3rd ed.). *Am J Occup Ther, 48,* 1047-1054.

AOTA. (1995a). Elements of clinical documentation. *Am J Occup Ther, 49,* 1032-1035.

AOTA. (1995b). *COTA supervision information packet.* Bethesda, MD: Author.

Bailey, D. M. (1998). Legislative and reimbursement influences on occupational therapy: Changing opportunities. In M. E. Neistadt & E. B. Crepeau (Eds.), *Willard & Spackman's OT.* Philadelphia, PA: Lippincott.

Case-Smith, J., Allen, A., & Pratt, P. N. (Eds.). (1996). *OT for children.* St. Louis, MO: Mosby.

Early, M. B. (1996). *Mental health concepts and techniques for the OTA.* New York, NY: Raven.

HCFA. (1999). *Overview of medicare.* Www. medicare.gov.

Hirama, H. (1996). *The OT assistant.* Baltimore, MD: Chess.

McCann, K. (2000, January). The 2000 Medicare fee schedule. *OT Practice, 3.*

Perinchief, J. M. (1998). Management of occupational therapy. In M. E. Neistadt & E. B. Crepeau (Eds.), *Willard and Spackman's OT.* Philadelphia, PA: Lippincott.

Schwartz, K. B., & Engle-Ramirez, J. (1996). Occupational therapy and health care reform. In L. W. Pedretti (Ed.), *OT Practice Skills for Physical Dysfunction.* St. Louis, MO: Mosby.

OTA Supervision

Chapter 39

Sally E. Ryan, COTA, ROH, Retired
Karen Sladyk, PhD, OTR/L, FAOTA

INTRODUCTION

Throughout the history of the OTA, numerous questions have arisen regarding supervision issues. Questions continue about who supervises the OTA, under what circumstances, how frequently, and whether the supervision is close or general. Other questions concern who OTAs may supervise and the circumstances under which supervision may take place, as well as the experience necessary for assistants to provide supervision. This chapter discusses these issues and focuses on specific practice examples as well as guiding principles, patterns, and responsibilities of supervision. Utilization issues and related concerns will also be discussed. The importance of career enhancement opportunities is also emphasized.

Supervision may be defined as the process of providing guidance and direction to employees and others. It involves assuming responsibility for the actions of workers, students, volunteers, and others in carrying out the mission and goals of the unit, the department, or the system within a given organization. It also involves overseeing, managing, and pro-viding leadership. Individuals who assume supervisory roles must possess strong interpersonal, intraprofessional, and management skills. They must exhibit the ability to be role models, mentors, instructors, problem-solvers, arbitrators, and evaluators. Successful supervisors are comfortable in their roles and are often characterized by their supervisees as effective, caring, and involved. They are attuned to individual needs and are committed to helping individuals achieve their full potential, resulting in exemplary delivery of services and high job satisfaction. Moreover, they are effective team builders who have a keen understanding of the many ways that technical and professional staff members provide complementary skills, and they create an environment where collaboration is valued.

TERMINOLOGY

For the reader to have a good understanding of the many facets of supervision, it is important to know the meaning of the following terms and designations based on the official documents of AOTA (AOTA, 2000).

KEY CONCEPTS

- Supervision: Process of providing guidance and direction to others.
- Service competence: Consistently demonstrated skills equivalent to a professional.

- Entry-level practice: The OTA or registered OT who has less than 1 year of practice experience; the OTA is competent to deliver OT services, as stated in the AOTA entry-level role delineation, under the direction of an OT.

- Intermediate-level practice: The OTA or OT who has 1 to 3 years of practice experience and is competent to carry out entry-level tasks. The OTA exhibits skills to carry out a variety of ADLs in treatment and may be developing additional, more advanced skills in a special interest area.

- Advanced-level practice: The OTA or OT who has 3 or more years of practice experience and has achieved the intermediate level. The OTA has demonstrated advanced level skills that may be clinical, educational, or administrative.

- Close supervision: Direct, on-site, daily contact.

- General supervision: Frequent, face-to-face meetings at the worksite and regular communication between the OT and the OTA by telephone, written documents, or electronic conference. According to Medicare guidelines, general supervision is initial direction and periodic inspection of the actual activity; however, the supervisor need not always be physically present or on the premises when the assistant is performing services. AOTA recommends that general supervision of the OTA should be used only after service competencies have been demonstrated to the supervising therapist. These authors also emphasize that contact by the OT may be less than daily but should be a minimum of three to five direct contact hours per week for the full-time OTA. Supervision time is prorated for the part-time OTA.

- Service competence: Implies that the OT and OTA can perform the same or equivalent tasks and obtain the same results. This assurance is necessary whenever an OT delegates tasks to an OTA.

- OT aide: Designation given to individuals who perform routine tasks in the OT department. Through on-the-job training they learn skills in transporting patients, setting up treatment activities, maintaining supplies and equipment, and other related activities.

- Volunteer: Unpaid worker who assists with varying tasks in the department such as typing, filing, preparing bulletin boards, serving refreshments, maintaining the library, and shopping for patients (AOTA, 2000).

GUIDING PRINCIPLES AND PATTERNS

The AOTA has suggested supervision guidelines for OTAs (AOTA, 2000). These documents summarize supervision of OTAs in typical practice settings but does not present information about assistants who practice as activities directors, educators, or in other nontraditional roles where they do not provide OT treatment services. The following principles and patterns of supervision were drawn from these sources.

Supervision Levels of Personnel

1. Entry-level OTAs require close supervision from an OT or intermediate or advanced-level OTA for delivery of patient services. General supervision by an experienced OT or OTA is needed for management and administrative tasks. Entry-level OTAs should not have supervisory responsibilities.

2. Intermediate-level OTAs require general clinical supervision from an intermediate- or advanced-level OT. General supervision from an experienced OT or advanced-level OTA is needed for management and administration.

3. Intermediate-level OTAs may provide administrative supervision and clinical direction to entry-level OTAs and OTA Levels I and II fieldwork students. Intermediate-level OTAs may supervise aides and volunteers.

4. Advanced-level OTAs require general clinical supervision from an intermediate or advanced-level OT; general management supervision is provided by an experienced OT. Advanced-level OTAs provide administrative supervision and clinical direction to entry-level OTAs and OTA levels I and II fieldwork students, as well as supervise aides and volunteers (Schell, 1985).

Service Competency

1. It is the responsibility of the supervisor to establish the supervisee's level of service competency. A variety of methods, such as observation, videotaping, independent test-scoring, and co-treatment can be used.

2. Service competency is more easily established for frequently used procedures. Infrequently used procedures may require closer supervision.

3. It is suggested that the acceptable standard of agreement set by the OT to be met by the supervisees is three consecutive agreements before service competency has been established (AOTA, 2000).

Patient Condition

1. Regardless of the patient's condition, the OTA may not independently evaluate or initiate the treatment process prior to the OT's evaluation;

however, the OTA may contribute to the evaluation process.

2. More supervision is required for the OTA who is working with a person whose condition is rapidly changing due to the need for frequent evaluation, re-evaluation, and treatment modifications.

3. Treatment techniques that require simultaneous re-evaluation of the treatment response are more appropriately performed by an OT.

4. The OTA requires close supervision in implementing a treatment program for the acutely ill individual due to the complex problems and the degree of change frequently seen.

5. The OTA may carry out treatment with a greater degree of independence for patients who are stable or non-acute, or who have a controlled condition.

6. It is the OTA's responsibility to report all changes in patient performance and any other pertinent facts to the supervising therapist (AOTA, 2000).

Regulations and Standards

1. It is the responsibility of every supervisor and supervisee to know and adhere to the supervisory and related regulations set forth by Medicare, Medicaid, and other third party payers who provide reimbursement for OT services that the supervisor and supervisee carry out. For example, the Medicare guidelines for OT state that while the skills of a qualified OT are required to evaluate the patient's level of function and develop a plan of treatment, the implementation of the plan may also be carried out by a qualified OTA functioning under the general supervision of the qualified OT.

2. It is the responsibility of every supervisor and supervisee to know and adhere to the supervisory and related regulations set forth by Medicare, the Joint Commission on Accreditation of Healthcare Organizations (JCAHO), and the Commission for the Accreditation of Rehabilitation Facilities (CARF) when working for institutions that fall under their jurisdiction.

3. It is the responsibility of every supervisor and supervisee providing OT services in a state that has regulatory laws, such as licensure, registration, or certification, to know and adhere to the supervisory and related regulations required by that state.

4. It is the responsibility of every supervisor and supervisee to know and adhere to the *Standards of Practice* (Appendix B) and the *Principles of OT Ethics* (Appendix C) established by the AOTA (AOTA, 2000).

General Employment

Because supervision is a collaborative process between the supervisor and the supervisee, it is extremely important for each individual to have a clear understanding of his or her respective responsibilities (Cohn, 1998). Examples of these responsibilities are shown in Table 39-1.

UTILIZATION OF PERSONNEL

Some OTs serving as supervisors are recognizing the need to utilize OTAs more effectively due to increased demand for services, budget constraints, and limited availability of personnel (Brooks, 1982). The term "cost-effective" means producing the best results in relation to dollars spent. In an article on calculating cost-effectiveness of OTAs, Dennis (1988) presents convincing data that supports the cost-effective assumption. Linroth and Boulay (1988) also stress the need for employing more OTAs in terms of increased productivity and cost-containment. Over the past 30 years, concern has been voiced regarding the underutilization of assistants. The pattern of employment seen in many OT departments confirms the problem. Recent changes in Medicare funding have left many OT departments confused about services and billing by OTs and OTAs. Some departments have responded by hiring only OTs, while others have continued to support OTAs. An interesting contrast is seen in the field of engineering, where it is not unusual for one professional engineer to supervise six technicians. Despite great strides, the OT profession needs to increase its efforts to provide a better balance of technical and professional personnel in the delivery of patient services.

The Army Medical Specialist Corps provides an example of effective utilization of assistants, as the ratio of OTAs to OTs in the majority of their clinics in the United States is quite high. It is also significant to note that military workloads and levels of productivity are considerably higher than those found in the civilian sector (Swift, 1991). More utilization models and related patterns of supervision such as these are needed to allow the OT to provide more services to more patients.

Care must also be taken to ensure that OTAs are not overutilized. Failure to hire the proper level of personnel for the job requirements and to provide adequate supervision is unacceptable. OT services cannot be provided by an OTA who is not receiving OT supervision and must be discontinued (AOTA, 2000). Evert, in her 1992 Presidential address (Evert, 1993), provides a scenario that typifies the supervisory dilemmas faced by many OTAs when an OT is not available: the OTA must often refuse to treat the patient, even in the face of administrative pressure to do so.

Table 39-1

Examples of Supervisor and Supervisee Roles

Supervisor	*Supervisee*
Provide orientation to the facility and program	Participate in orientation activities
Assess periodically level of competency	Participate in competency assessment activities
Define and assign specific responsibilities	Carry out responsibilities effectively, seeking clarification if unsure
Establish criteria for performance evaluation and timelines	Discuss criteria and establish clear understanding of expectations
Schedule formal and informal meetings to identify problems, needs, and concerns and to solicit ideas	Participate regularly in meetings, openly and honestly discussing issues and providing feedback and ideas
Give feedback relative to areas of future growth and skill development, providing resources as needed	Seek new knowledge and skills and set professional goals
Develop and modify job descriptions	Recommend changes in job description

CAREER OPPORTUNITIES

A good supervisor must provide opportunities for challenge, growth, and advancement for supervisees as vehicles for career enhancement. Strickland (1988) describes a career development planning model adopted by a large medical facility for employees in the OT department. Career ladders have been established that provide a variety of options for both OTs and OTAs, including development of adaptive equipment and techniques, professional writing, educational presentations, and development of new programs and projects. Opportunities such as these can be a shared collegial experience among OTs and OTAs, which enhance day-to-day working relationships and, ultimately, job and career satisfaction.

SUPERVISION PARTNERSHIP

Supervision is often disliked by many people due to the unknowns that might come up in supervision meetings or negative experiences from the past. Students have likely had supervision from former jobs or faculty in OTA school and have likely had mixed results. A common problem is over-interrupting the supervision feedback and personalizing the information, causing hurt feelings between the supervisor and supervisee. Each supervisor has his or her own style. Ideally, the supervisor is open-minded and prepared for the task of guiding the OTA in his or her professional development. Ideally, the supervisee wants feedback to grow professionally by improving procedural, interactive, and conditional skills.

Depending on the needs of the OTA and the department, formal supervision meetings should be set in a regular schedule. A new graduate with a supervising OT in the same immediate treatment area as the new OTA may require less formal supervision than a new graduate working in different areas of a large facility. A new graduate needs daily face-to-face contact with his or her supervisor. In addition, a formal weekly 30- to 60-minute meeting should be arranged. These meetings should be documented by the OT as supervision meetings. These notes may be needed at a later date to show progress in the OTA's professional development. Accreditation agencies such as JCAHO expect supervision to be documented, and co-signing notes is not considered supervision.

The supervisee should come to meetings with a prepared list of questions based on his or her caseload. The supervision meeting should begin with a review of issues from former meetings and an update on those issues. The supervisor should then ask about current issues. Together the supervisor and supervisee should develop a plan of action for dealing with the current issues. A timeline for reporting back on the current issues should be developed. The supervisor should assist the OTA in problem-solving and clinical reasoning. The supervisee should be prepared to actively participate in this process. The supervision process becomes non-productive when the OTA simply asks, "What should I do?" with a problem, and the supervisor simply directs the answer. If appropriate, the supervisor may suggest helpful resources to further develop the OTA's professional development.

From time to time, there may be style differences between the supervisor and supervisee. This may develop when there is disagreement between different treatment approaches or disagreement on supervision approaches. Ideally, both parties can address the issues openly. The following are suggestions for dealing with problem supervision.

- The OTA's supervision needs are not being met— The OTA, using "I" statements, clarifies his or her needs. For example, "I need to meet with you at our regular scheduled time consistently because I feel uncomfortable with my current caseload. I understand we cannot meet today because of the important meeting, but I hope I can spend some time with you tomorrow morning." Notice how many "I" statements there are compared to "you" statements. "I" statements show that the OTA is taking personal responsibility and not insulting the supervisor with blame.

- The OTA's supervision is not being documented— Often the supervisor does not know that supervision must be documented. Remind the supervisor and if the problem does not resolve, ask if it is acceptable to document supervision yourself. These documentation notes are legal documents that can be requested by administration or outside agencies at any time. Ideally, supervision documentation will be used to document professional growth, including service competence, and be used for promotions and recommendations.

- The supervisor and supervisee have different styles—The OTA can ask that supervision styles be one of the topics of discussion for the next supervision meeting. If the supervisor's style is autocratic, the OTA can inform the supervisor that as a professional goal, she would like to participate in a supervision process that is more collaborative and reciprocal. If the OTA feels the supervisor's style is too open, that she cannot get the specific answers she needs, she can inform the supervisor that she would like to participate in professional conversations but to relieve her initial anxiety, she would like specific direction on this problem. Using "I" statements as discussed above are effective in dealing with different styles because they do not attack the style but only say, "I need something different."

CASE STUDY

Sue is a recent graduate of an accredited OTA program and has been working for 11 months in a large skilled nursing facility with 60 beds of subacute rehabilitation. Most of her clients are orthopedic cases but she is starting to see more people with stroke and head injury. Although she never thought she would miss school and all the homework, she has been recently thinking about furthering her education to learn more about the clients she currently sees.

The staff of the OT department where Sue works usually gathers for lunch in the ADL kitchen. The four OTs and the three other OTAs all have different opinions of what Sue should do. Two OTs feel she should return to college to become an OT. Two OTs feel she should return to college and major in kinesiology or biology. The other OTAs have varying opinions about what continuing education she should do but agree she should not go back to college. To complicate things further, her family also has different opinions.

At supervision, Sue brings up the issue of conflicting advice about returning to school. Her supervisor, Lori, asks a few probing questions to find out what Sue has been thinking to this point. Lori then asks about the opinions Sue has been offered, and they discuss the possible reasons each person had in offering their specific advice. Sue comes to see that each opinion offered is a reflection of the things that person values. Lori asks Sue about short- and long-term goals. Sue says that she is interested in learning more about her clients with neurological impairments for now, but would like to teach a lab at the local community college OTA program "some day." Lori is familiar with the community college that Sue is talking about and shares her information about teaching there. Lori asks Sue to think about her goals and come up with a list of educational options that best fits her professional development goals. Lori tells Sue about the resources the facility can offer her for professional development.

At the next supervision meeting, Sue says she would like to return to school with the eventual goal of completing her BS in psychology. Sue believes that this major would allow her to best understand her neurological clients from both a science and art perspective. She addressed her long-term goal with her family, who agreed they could be supportive of her part-time study. For now, Sue wanted to learn about head injury as quickly as possible. Sue wanted to know if Lori could help with this short-term goal. Lori reinforced Sue's decision-making process and supported her long-term goal. Together they developed a plan to reach her short-term goal. First, Sue would be partnered with an OT with expertise in head injury. They would co-treat for 2 hours per week while

Sue maintained her current caseload. Second, because Sue was a member of AOTA, she could participate in home-based, self-study material on cognition available to members. The facility would reimburse her costs if she presented an in-house inservice on what she learned as it related to her specific facility. This inservice would allow Sue to see if she liked the classroom teaching experience. If Sue was pleased with the inservice experience, the facility would offer the inservice free of charge to the community college students to give Sue further experience. Lastly, Sue would check the Internet for possible accredited college courses about head injury. Because the Internet is full of unreliable information, Sue and Lori agreed that the best approach for finding solid information about head injury treatment was to stick with an accredited college. Further, she may be able to transfer the Internet class as an elective in her BS program if the college offered regional accreditation.

Notice that Lori never gives Sue advice, but instead guides Sue to make her own choices and decisions.

SUMMARY

Supervision is a complex and dynamic process that involves a variety of skills and abilities. Ideally, it is a process of collaboration and reciprocation between the supervisor and the supervisee. It should be viewed as a partnership between professional and technical personnel.

Supervision is a process of providing guidance and direction to others. It involves assuming responsibility for workers and others in carrying out the mission and goals of the unit, the department, or the system within an organization. Knowledge of discipline-specific terminology and designations is necessary and provides a foundation for understanding OT supervision principles and patterns. These are delineated and discussed in terms of levels of personnel, service competency, patient conditions, regulations and standards, and general employment. Examples of supervisor and supervisee responsibilities are stressed. Models for increased utilization of technical personnel that demonstrate increased delivery of services in a cost-effective manner are needed. These models should also emphasize ways that technical and professional personnel can be challenged and achieve career growth through varied options. Career enhancement opportunities are necessary to build relationships with workers and increase job and career satisfaction.

REFERENCES

AOTA. (2000). *Official documents of the AOTA.* Bethesda, MD: Author.

Brooks, B. (1982). OTA issues: Yesterday, today, and tomorrow. *Am J Occup Ther, 36,* 567-568.

Cohn, E. S. (1998). Interdisciplinary communication and supervision of personnel. In M. Neistadt & E. B. Crepeau (Eds.), *Willard & Spackman's OT.* Philadelphia, PA: Lippincott.

Dennis, M. (1988). Calculating cost effectiveness with the OTA. In J. A. Johnson (Ed.), *OTAs—Opportunities and Challenges.* New York, NY: Haworth Press.

Evert, M. M. (1993). New president's address: Daily practice dilemmas. *Am J Occup Ther, 43,* 7-9.

Linroth, R., & Boulay, P. (1988). OTAs: Preparation for change. In J. A. Johnson (Ed.), *OTAs—Opportunities and Challenges.* New York, NY: Haworth Press.

Schell, B. (1985). Guide to classification of OT personnel. *Am J Occup Ther, 39,* 803-810.

Strickland L. R. (1988). Career ladder development for OTAs. In J. A. Johnson (Ed.). *OTAs—Opportunities and Challenges.* New York, NY: Haworth Press.

Swift, R. (1991). Chief, Army Medical Specialist Corps, personal correspondence.

The Role of the OTA as an Activities Director

Chapter 40

Sally E. Ryan, COTA, ROH, Retired

INTRODUCTION

The position of activities director, coordinator, or supervisor is one for which the OTA is well qualified. With an educational background in human development throughout the lifespan, disabling conditions, the teaching/learning process, group dynamics, and activity analysis, as well as an understanding of every individual's need for purposeful, meaningful activity, the OTA is able to carry out activities programs of exceptional quality.

Activities directors are employed in a variety of settings including community centers, large apartment and condominium complexes for the well and the disabled, group homes, halfway houses, institutions for people with mentally retarded or chronic mental illness, and long-term care settings for the elderly and others. Since a large number of OTAs are employed as activities directors in long-term care facilities, this chapter focuses on principles and applications for those settings. Although in many cases the majority of people residing in these facilities are elderly, a growing number of younger individuals are also residents. Whatever the site or the population, activity planning must meet the unique needs and interests of the consumer. Special measures must be taken to ensure that these individuals do not feel isolated due to age or residence. The activities director is often in a position to help develop these social partnerships.

DEFINITIONS

An activities program may be defined as an ongoing plan for providing meaningful activities, which is determined in relation to the individual needs and interests of those involved. Such programs are designed to provide a variety of opportunities for individuals to participate in activities, with the goal being to promote their physical, mental, and social well-being (National Association of Activity Professionals [NAAP], 1990; American Therapeutic Recreation Association [ATRA], 1987).

An activities director is employed by the facility and is directly responsible for planning, scheduling, implementing, documenting, managing, and evaluating an activities

KEY CONCEPTS

- Activities director: A person responsible for organizing and implementing a variety of activities designed to meet the needs of a specific population.
- Activity program: Meeting the needs of a resident's healthy activity level.
- Resident: The Medicare description of a person living in a long-term care facility.

program. The term *resident* is used in keeping with the terminology adopted in the current Medicare and Medicaid standards for long-term care facilities (Health Care Financing Administration [HCFA], 1999). The program is designed with the overall goal of meeting the individual resident's needs for healthy activity that will aid in maintaining optimum levels of functioning and quality of life.

An activities consultant is a qualified individual who is employed by the facility to provide guidance to the activities director about all aspects of the activities program (American Therapeutic Recreation Association [ATRA], 1998). This person may also provide consultation to other staff members and departments as requested by administration. OTs, experienced OTAs, therapeutic recreation specialists, and social workers often provide consultative services.

LEGISLATION AND REGULATIONS

The Department of Health and Human Services established the toughest requirements to date for Medicare and Medicaid programs in 1995 for long-term care facilities (HCFA, 1999), including specific regulations for activities departments and personnel. Complete copies of all regulations are available from state health/human services offices.

Many of the legislative improvements center around the Nursing Home Reform Amendments of the Omnibus Budged Reconciliation Act (OBRA) of 1987, which were designed to improve the standards of nursing homes "from the bottom up" and became law in 1990 (Saltz, 1990). Establishment of these amendments is an attempt to set minimum standards across the country for all nursing homes that receive federal aid. A database (HCFA, 1998) of the results of Medicare inspections of each nursing home in the United States is updated yearly on the Medicare website (www.medicare.gov). These standards address the following:

1. Rights and quality of life
2. Preadmission screening
3. Assessment and quality of care
4. Training of nurse's aides
5. Annual resident review
6. Facility survey and certification
7. Enforcement

Experts have noted that the standards for resident assessment are one of the most important provisions of the law. Resident rights are produced to free choice and freedom from chemical and physical restraints used for control, involuntary seclusion, discipline, or staff convenience (Saltz, 1990). Further, the new requirements mandate that individuals be assessed in terms of strengths as well as weaknesses, level of initiative and involvement, and personal preferences, with an emphasis on resident outcomes.

In addition to these federal regulations for skilled nursing facilities (SNFs) and intermediate care facilities (ICFs), most state health departments and licensing agencies have specific regulations for activities programs. The activities director must have a complete understanding of all of these regulations before initiating an activities program.

CAREER AND EDUCATIONAL INFORMATION

The ATRA shows the demand for activity staff to continue to grow in the new millennium (1998). Activity staff should have training in physical, biological, and behavioral sciences. The activity department should be designed similar to other therapeutic departments in the facility. The director and all employees of the department must have a job description that specifically outlines all responsibilities and expectations. The following items should be included:

1. Job title, supervisor, and supervisees.
2. Qualifications, including formal education and training and any specialized training that might be required, such as recommendation, reality orientation and reminiscence techniques, cardiopulmonary resuscitation (CPR), and first aid.
3. Licensure and/or certification requirements.
4. Skills such as effective written communication, verbal communication, and related public relations activities.
5. Required participation in continuing education and professional activities.
6. Specific activities responsibilities, such as assessing individual resident activities needs; planning, scheduling, implementing, documenting, and evaluating the activities program. Definitive time lines should be included (e.g., weekly, monthly, or quarterly).
7. Participation in the care planning process, including specific requirements for attending meetings and frequency.
8. Staff and volunteer recruitment, training, supervision, evaluation, and termination.
9. Inservice education training responsibilities for staff and volunteers.
10. Reports to be prepared and their frequency.
11. Procurement and maintenance of supplies and equipment.
12. Orientation activities for new employees and residents in the facility.
13. Other responsibilities, such as coordinating a barber, beautician, and voting appointments.

Table 40-1

Eight Activity Categories

Physical activities: These activities might include participation in exercise groups, sports, and games such as lawn bowling, shuffleboard, badminton, and daily walks.

Social access activities: Activities in this category include parties, picnics, meals at community restaurants, and tea time. The primary goal is to provide an opportunity for patients to interact socially. Family members should also be invited to some of these events.

Creative activities: Crafts, calligraphy, creative writing, and oil and watercolor painting are examples of creative activities. Such endeavors provide an outlet for creative expression, and although they often are presented in a group setting, socialization is not required.

Productive (work substitute) activities: Many people have a need to be engaged in a productive activity. Work on community service projects, such as flyer fundraising packets for the American Cancer Society or stuffing envelopes for a local charity, should be provided. Other work-related activities include writing and producing a daily newspaper, rolling bandages for the Red Cross, and baking items for a bazaar. Productive volunteer endeavors such as these allow the participants to continue to make a meaningful contribution to society.

Educational activities: Opportunities for lifelong learning are virtually endless. Photography clubs, music appreciation groups, and book review and discussion groups are examples. Individual activities, such as learning to speak a foreign language or to operate a computer, should also be included.

Leisure activities: Almost everyone needs time to read a good book, write letters, listen to the radio, or view a favorite television program. Quiet strolls in the park or just sitting on the patio observing and enjoying nature can be meaningful, refreshing pastimes.

Spiritual activities: Spiritual needs can be met in a variety of ways, such as participation in Bible study groups, a choir, or regularly scheduled religious services in the facility as well as the community. A missionary group often assists in fulfilling spiritual needs as well.

Democratic community activities: Living in a residential community affords members many opportunities to assume roles in determining the future of their community. These empowering activities include organizing forums for discussion and resolution of issues of mutual interest, forming a resident and state council to discuss problems and concerns and to establish policies, writing editorials for the facility newspaper, and organizing advice related to political and social issues that impact on the quality of life of the participants. Because they focus on opportunities for individuals to redevelop a sense of purpose in their lives, samples may be found under the categories of creative, productive, and democratic community activities, as well as others.

14. Methods and frequency of evaluation; conditions of probationary employment.

Job descriptions should be reviewed and modified as necessary, at least on an annual basis. Sample job descriptions for activities directors are often available from state health departments.

DEVELOPING AN ACTIVITIES PLAN

The first step in developing an activities plan is data collection about the likely participants. The medical record and the resident pre-admission history will provide information regarding the primary and secondary diagnosis, precautions and limitations, physician's approval for activities participation, the resident's birthday, nationality, social history, and the name of a family contact (ATRA, 1991).

Another step in the data collection process is to determine the interests of the residents. A structured questionnaire or interview may be used to seek information in specific areas of activities. One method is to divide potential activities into the following eight activity categories:

1. Physical
2. Social
3. Creative
4. Productive (work substitute)
5. Educational
6. Leisure
7. Spiritual
8. Democratic community activities

These are described further in Table 40-1.

Another method of categorizing activities is in terms of their potential to be supportive, provide maintenance, or provide empowerment. The following definitions are drawn from the *Standards of Practice* (1990) of the National Association of Activity Professionals (NAAP).

Supportive activities promote a comfortable environment while providing stimulation or solace to those individuals who cannot benefit from either maintenance or empowerment activities. Such activities are usually provided to those individuals who may be severely cognitively or physically impaired or those unable to participate in a group program. Examples include providing soft background music; placing plants, pictures, and other colorful objects in the resident's room; and providing sensory stimulation.

Maintenance activities provide the individual with opportunities to maintain physical, cognitive, social, spiritual, and emotional health. These areas are delineated under the eight activity categories discussed in Table 40-1.

Empowerment activities focus on the promotion of self-respect by providing opportunities for self-expression, choice, social responsibility, and personal responsibility. These activities differ from those designed to provide maintenance.

Whatever methods are used to categorize activities, it is important to ensure that every resident has an opportunity to participate in meaningful activities that are of interest and based on individual needs, strengths, and goals (ATRA, 1991). Activities that require decision-making should be emphasized as well, and resident collaboration should be a focus at every stage of treatment.

If potential participants fill out a questionnaire, an interview should also be arranged to verify and expand each resident's needs. If residents are reluctant to discuss items on a questionnaire, a more generalized approach may be used by asking open-ended questions such as:

- What activities did you enjoy before coming to the nursing home?
- What are some of the things you did during your spare time this week?
- If you were the activities director, what do you think would be an important activity to provide?

The interviewer should provide added cues as necessary to keep the responses to questions on target. Speaking with family members and other staff is also recommended to gain as much additional input as possible, especially if the resident is cognitively impaired or uncommunicative. Figure 40-1 provides an example of a form that may be used.

Once the data are gathered, the information must be tabulated and categorized and priorities established in terms of available staff, volunteers, space, existing supplies and equipment, community resources, and operating budget. For example, if the category of creative activities indicates that many residents are interested in arts and crafts, a general session should be scheduled daily.

Perhaps a small number are interested in knitting. While they could participate in the general group, they may also enjoy forming a knitting club that meets once a week to work on a special project, such as knitting hats and mittens for a children's home or homeless people in the community.

Initial activity planning can best be accomplished by setting up a general grid calendar with days on the left, including Saturday and Sunday, and the eight major categories of activities listed across the top. Enter the large group activities first—those in which residents indicated the greatest interest, such as crafts, movies, concerts, and games. Next, enter the small group activities, such as baking, gardening, and oil painting. Determine which of these activities the existing staff and volunteers can supervise, and identify additional needs. Be sure that necessary space, supplies, and equipment are available. Look for gaps in the plan and be creative about introducing new activities. It is also important to determine whether activities are primarily active or passive in terms of degree of participation. Every effort should be made to schedule out-of-building activities, such as picnics, shopping tours, and visits to zoos, so that residents maintain contact with the community. Some individuals will prefer not to join groups; therefore, time must be set aside for individual activity participation.

Activities needs cannot be totally met by a program that only schedules events Monday through Friday during the usual daytime working hours. Flexibility is necessary, and every effort should be made to provide some activities in the evenings and on weekends. Arrangements can usually be made for the assigned staff members to take compensatory time off during the regular workweek. The proposed activities plan should also be evaluated to ensure that at least some of the activities are held at a time when family members can participate, and efforts should be made to encourage them to do so.

Once the general grid plan is developed and staffing patterns are established, it is important to look at timing of the events. Consideration must be given to regularly scheduled activities such as meals, routine nursing care, physicians' rounds, occupational or physical therapy schedules, and visiting hours. These times are appropriate for the activity staff to document progress and complete department maintenance responsibilities.

Public Relations

Effective public relations are an important component of activity planning. When the final monthly plan is developed, it must be communicated as widely as possible. Copies should be provided to administration and all departments in the facility, as well as to each resident at least 7 days in advance. Large weekly posters should be made and posted in prominent locations throughout the

Name _____ Room_____ Admit Date _____

Date of Birth_____ Age _____ Hometown _____

Marital Status _____ Children_____ Grandchildren _____ Great Grandchildren ____

Siblings _____ Do any live nearby? _____

Ethnic/Cultural Background _____

Languages Spoken _____ Religion ___ _____

Education_____

Occupations _____

Work History _____

Registered Voter _____ Veteran_____ Branch of Service _____

Clubs and Organizations _____

Interests: (Code – S = small group; G = large group; I = individual)

Note: Interviewer should give examples in each category below.

- Physical activities _____

  _____

- Social access activities _____

  _____

- Creative activities _____

  _____

- Productive activities _____

  _____

- Educational activities_____

  _____

- Leisure activities_____

  _____

- Spiritual activities _____

  _____

- Democratic community activities _____

  _____

- Typical Day Profile_____

  _____

- Typical Week Profile _____

  _____

Life Goals_____

  _____

Previous Living Arrangement_____

Physician _____ Reason for Admission _____

Diagnosis _____ Functional Limitations/Strengths_____

Mobility _____ Vision_____

Hearing _____ Comprehension _____

Orientation_____ Behavior_____

Attention Span _____ Other _____

Contact Person _____ Phone_____

Address_____

Figure 40-1. Activity interest questionnaire, developed by S. E. Ryan, 1991. (Reprinted from Ryan, S. E. (1993). *Practice issues in OT: Intraprofessional team building.* Thorofare, NJ: SLACK Incorporated.)

Table 40-2
Activity Program Individualized Treatment Plan

Problem/need: Few social contacts; rarely participates in any group activities.
Capabilities/strengths: Articulate; knowledgeable about current events and sports.
Activity goal: Participation in one small group event.
Approach: Invite to current events group or sports group as a resource person; offer a choice and structure role to be as non-threatening as possible; stress that others are interested in the information that individual could share.

building. Individual posters should also be made to advertise special events, such as a concert or a bazaar. If a public address system is available, use it to make daily announcements of forthcoming events. Flyers can be mailed to family members when events are scheduled in which they may participate. The community should also be informed through providing local newspapers with press releases of activities of interest, such as a resident's 100th birthday or an announcement of the individuals who received ribbons for their entries in the county fair.

Related Planning Principles

Activities planning must always occur at least 1 month in advance. Failure to do so will produce undo stress for the director, staff, and volunteers and will result in unmet resident activities needs. Even the most thorough planning will not be flawless. The activities director must have alternative plans to draw upon when, for example, the high school band does not show up for a concert or a torrential rainstorm ruins picnic plans. Flexibility, adaptability, and resourcefulness are important attributes of the successful activities director.

Individual activity plans should be developed for every resident and be included in the total resident care plan. Problems and needs are identified and specific objectives are established along with methods for accomplishing the goals. Copies of both state and federal regulations should be obtained to be sure all required information is included. A brief example of a plan is provided in Table 40-2 (NAAP, 1990).

A confidential card system should be developed for each resident's individual activity plan. The resident's card should also have information on the primary and secondary diagnosis, limitations and precautions, physician's permission to participate in activities, birthdate, and other pertinent social history facts. Preferences should also be noted, such as small group vs. large group participation and afternoon activities vs. morning or evening activities. Locating the card system in a central but secure place, such as the activity department office, will allow all staff members convenient access to it. Additional infor-

mation on patient care planning and specific activity plans appears in the section on Records and Reports.

IMPLEMENTING THE ACTIVITIES PROGRAM

Once initial planning has been completed, the activities program is implemented, often gradually over several weeks. As activities take place, the activities director must carefully monitor all aspects to ensure that the programming is effective in helping to meet residents' goals. The following items are of particular importance:
1. General attendance and degree of participation.
2. Adequacy of staff and volunteer coverage.
3. Adequacy of space, furnishings, equipment, and supplies.
4. Adequacy of lighting, ventilation, temperature control, and general safety.
5. Effectiveness of communication with other departments.
6. Timing in relation to other activities taking place in the facility.
7. Specific ways to improve the activity and the degree of participation the next time it is presented.

Another helpful method is to break activities down into very specific activity components, particularly if they tend to take too much time or participation is less than expected. An example would be the weekly songfest. This activity is made up of at least 12 distinct parts:
1. Furniture arrangement.
2. Transportation for non-ambulatory participants.
3. Introduction of song leader and pianist.
4. Distribution of song sheets.
5. Use of an overhead projector with enlarged words to songs.
6. Use of clapping and marching activities.
7. Distribution and use of rhythm instruments.
8. Playing "Name that Tune" game.
9. Collecting and storing supplies and equipment.

10. Returning non-ambulatory residents to their units.
11. Rearranging furniture.
12. Documenting participation.

Keeping a clipboard close at hand is a good idea so that observations relative to the issue presented in the preceding sections may be recorded immediately. It is also important to seek critiques from participants, as well as staff members and volunteers. An activities planning committee should be established to review past events and make recommendations for future activities. Feedback should be incorporated into a regularly scheduled quality improvement plan.

Resident Motivation

A successful activity program involves much more than planning and carrying out a variety of activities. It must also include the creation of an atmosphere that is warm, friendly, caring, and as non-threatening as possible; an atmosphere that offers decision-making opportunities and promotes independence; and an atmosphere where residents are offered encouragement and support but are never coerced or forced to participate. These are very important motivational factors (Wlodkowski, 1990).

The main activity room should serve as a gathering spot for those who just want to get away from their room for a while. Space should be provided for people to observe the activities taking place, particularly new residents. Serving coffee and tea, within diet restrictions, is a method to comfortably include observers in the activities group. It encourages socialization and may increase motivation to become directly involved in the activity.

Motivation comes from within, but it can be enhanced by showing a genuine interest in the residents. Sometimes writing a short personal note to invite an individual to participate will be a motivating factor. Others will be motivated or drawn to activities because they can be assured of some degree of success and they feel "needed" by the other group members. For example, a person who is not interested in working on the mosaic mural in the dining room may be willing to spend hours sorting tile so that the others can work more efficiently.

RECORDS AND REPORTS

A system of regular documentation must be established in keeping with the requirements of federal, state, and facility regulations. The general categories of documentation include resident care plans, activity plans, activity notes, activity schedules, and participation records. The latter must be maintained for all group and one-to-one activities and should be a part of the resident's permanent record. Confidentiality must be maintained for all resident records and reports. Records should also be maintained for all staff members and volunteers, indicating hours worked as well as major responsibilities. Budget reports must be prepared regularly, and the administration of the facility may require monthly summary reports of the activities program, as well as an annual report. The activities director will also be responsible for developing and maintaining an activities policies and procedures manual. It is also advisable to keep records of supply needs and an inventory of equipment and furnishings.

Resident Care Plans

One of the main purposes of resident care planning is to assess needs and problems in a systematic way. Specific goals are established and methods are identified for accomplishing them. The resident care plan must be completed soon after admission and must include a comprehensive activity assessment. Comprehensive resident care plans promote a coordinated effort in providing medical as well as multidisciplinary services for the individual. Effective care planning must include the resident, the family, significant others, as well as the primary health care providers in the facility. Resident care plans must be reviewed and revised regularly. Medicare and Medicaid regulations require the use of a standardized assessment called the Resident Assessment System, which includes a minimum data set (MDS) to provide a framework for planning (AOTA, 1990). The activity assessment must reflect information from the MDS. After admission, the MDS is used as a means of updating the staff relative to the resident's status, particularly during times of change.

ACTIVITIES PLANS

Activities plans are developed, evaluated, and updated on a regular basis, usually monthly. They are a part of the resident's clinical record. The activities director must allocate specific blocks of time each week for this task to ensure that all plans are always up to date. To assist in this process, a system should be developed for staff and volunteers to share daily observations of individual residents. A notebook with a page for each resident is a simple way of collecting the information. A personal computer may also be used. An example of the way these observations might be written is shown in Figure 40-2. Whatever system is developed to share information, the activities director must be sure the documentation is secure and confidential.

In addition to contributing to the activity plan, observation notes such as these will also assist the activities director in evaluating each resident's degree of progress in attaining goals.

12/5/99. Task: Mosaic flowerpot. Participation: Initially slow to begin but worked for 1 hour. Said he was nervous about being the current event group leader next week.

S. Basket, Volunteer

12/7/99. Task: Mosaic project. Participation: Mr. J not pleased with final results, stated it looks too "girly." He was able to problem solve by suggesting he give it to the nurse for the day room. Expressed interest in wood puzzle.

B. Melling, Activity Aide

Figure 40-2. Sample of recorded observations.

3/21/00. During the past week, Mr. Johnson participated in 9.5 hours of scheduled therapeutic recreation events. Mr. Johnson actively participated in woodworking activities every weekday morning for 1 hour. He frequently takes a nap after lunch but participated in the weekly photography club and the current events group in the afternoon. He was the discussion leader of the current events group on two occasions this week. He initially appeared nervous about this role, but reported he was pleased with his skills after several members complimented him. He also visited the library twice this week and stated that "reading is one of my greatest pleasures." When asked to take a leadership role in a new book club for both residents and staff, he was excited and agreed to be on the planning committee meeting next Monday. He is maintaining the level of activity noted last month.

Jane Doe, COTA, Activities Director

Figure 40-3. Sample activities note.

Activities Notes

Activities notes (Figure 40-3) are included in the resident's clinical record and should be written by approved staff whenever change is noted or at least once a month. A good activity note should include a summary of the types of activities the person had been participating in, the frequency of participation, and the time involved. Notes should reflect maintenance, progress, or decline. Quotations may be used. All notes must be dated, written legibly in ink, and signed. Use of abbreviations should be avoided unless the facility has an approved list of abbreviations for use in records. Activity notes must be objective, accurate, and complete. They should relate directly to the activity plan and the total resident care plan.

Participation Records

Participation records should be maintained on a daily basis to provide an overall view of activity trends and fluctuations. Such records will reflect individual resident activity and inactivity. Further, these records are a barometer of interest in specific activities. Such records may also be used to provide justification for hiring additional staff members. Graph paper may be used to develop a simple participation recording form. The names of all residents are listed on the left-hand side and the different activities are listed across the top. To save space, use a coding system such as "C"=crafts, "B"=baking, and "G"=gardening. It is important to remember that if people come to the activity area and fall asleep, they have not participated and should not be listed on the participation record.

Activities Schedules

Activities schedules are generally the monthly calendar of events. These schedules should be filed, as they provide specific information on the variety of activities offered and when. The schedules may also be coded to indicate whether activities require active or passive participation and the number of staff members and volunteers that are needed for each activity. Review of past schedules is a great help in planning for future events.

Activities Reports

Summary reports of the activities program are written regularly as required by the administration and at least annually. A typical report might include information about the number of residents participating in the eight major activity areas (physical, social, creative, productive, educational, diversional, spiritual, and democratic community) with a breakdown of individual and group activities. New or unique events may be highlighted. Budget information should be included in the categories of income, expenditures, and cash on hand. The number of staff and volunteers should be noted as well as consultation services received. Inservice training programs for staff and volunteers should be briefly described.

Policy and Procedure Manual

The activities director is responsible for developing, reviewing, and revising the departmental policy and procedure manual. A policy may be defined as a statement that describes how basic program objectives can be met.

Subject: Birthday parties.

Policy: A monthly birthday party shall be held in the facility.

Purpose: To honor all residents who are celebrating a birthday during that month.

Responsibility: The activity director shall be responsible for planning and carrying out the party.

Procedures:

1. Written invitations will be sent to all residents celebrating a birthday during a given month. Invitations will also be sent to family members.

2. The date, time, and location of the party will be advertised at least two weeks in advance. All residents and staff are invited.

3. Corsages and boutonnieres will be provided for those being honored.

4. Cake, ice cream, and beverages must be ordered from the dietary department at least one week in advance of the event. Provisions for those on special diets must be accommodated.

5. Prizes may be awarded to the youngest and the oldest residents who are celebrating their birthday.

6. Musical entertainment will be provided.

Figure 40-4. Policy and procedures for a birthday party. (Reprinted from Ryan, S. E. (1993). *Practice issues in OT: Intraprofessional team building*. Thorofare, NJ: SLACK Incorporated.)

Policies are not subject to frequent change. Procedures are methods for carrying out the policy and are subject to modification as need arises. For example, the policy and procedures for conducting a birthday party might be written as shown in Figure 40-4.

STAFFING NEEDS

The literature yields little information on the topic of staffing requirements. This author believes that the employment of one full-time activities director for every 50 to 60 residents should be an absolute minimum in skilled and intermediate care facilities. Individual state regulations and licensing agencies may specify other minimums for activity personnel. It should be kept in mind that providing a minimum number of activities personnel may not allow maximum services to be provided in meeting the residents' individual activity needs and enhancing their quality of life.

As more individuals become actively involved in the activities program and increased needs are identified, it may be necessary to increase the staff size. Before hiring additional personnel, a specific job description must be developed that includes most of the items described in the beginning of this chapter. Administration must approve all new staff positions. Plans and procedures must also be developed for orienting and evaluating new employees and providing for their continuing education.

Volunteers

Although volunteers are a most important asset to any activities program, they should never take the place of paid staff under any circumstances. Rather, they should be used to enhance the program.

Before a volunteer program is initiated, legal and insurance issues must be considered to ensure that adequate liability safeguards are provided. Volunteers should be recruited, screened, and trained using a developed protocol, as needs arise to assist in increasing the effectiveness of the program. They can often provide some of the extra services that personalize the program, particularly in relation to individual needs. Volunteers can carry out a variety of tasks including letter writing, resident and departmental shopping, leading songfests, teaching creative activities, and word processing. Volunteers may be recruited through facility posters, more formal advertising in church and synagogue bulletins, high school/college newspapers, and general announcements at neighborhood events. All volunteers must have specific job descriptions and hours. Volunteers should participate in an orientation and training program. Records of service need to be maintained on each volunteer for service awards, letters of recommendation, or hours required to meet some other need, such as college applications or scouting awards. It is important to recognize volunteers for their contributions at least annually. Certificates or pins should be presented at a special gathering in their honor.

Program Management

As a departmental manager, the activities director must develop systems and approaches that will provide for the most effective and efficient delivery of activities services to meet the goals of the residents, the department, and the health care facility. Failure to do so may result in decreased motivation and interest on the part of workers and participants.

It is the responsibility of the supervisor to develop and utilize objective tools, such as job descriptions and evaluation forms to measure employee performance. The supervisor should also encourage the staff to participate in self-evaluation activities on a regular basis (ATRA, 1993). Individual job performance goal setting should be a collaborative process between the supervisor and the supervisees. When specific deficits in performance are noted, the supervisor should be constructive in the criticism given by providing guidance, resources, and opportunities that will assist the worker in skill improvement.

Above all, an effective supervisor must be caring, honest, objective, be willing to carry "a fair share" of the workload, and be open in relationships. A person who provides a strong role model and demonstrates a sincere interest in the well-being of those he or she supervises is indeed effective.

Interdisciplinary Role

Most health care facilities view the activities director as a department head and an integral member of the health care team. The activities director should participate in all department head meetings and patient care planning conferences, as the delivery of effective activity services depends on cooperation from and coordination with a number of other departments. Efforts should be made to develop both structured and informal communication channels that will ensure quality resident care and the achievement of goals.

Continuing Education

We live in an age where change occurs very rapidly, particularly in our health care delivery systems. The activities director, in collaboration with administration, staff, and volunteers, and with necessary outside consultation, must identify the continuing education needs and develop a plan to meet these needs (ATRA, 1993). Such a plan must include the required financial support. For example, many facilities require all staff members and volunteers to take a first aid course, and some require specialized training in cardiopulmonary resuscitation (CPR). As residents' needs change, staff members may also need to be trained in the techniques of reality orientation, remotivation, and reminiscence therapy. The activities director and everyone involved in the delivery of activities services must be given opportunities to participate in continuing education courses and workshops to ensure that existing skills are maintained and new ones acquired. Continuing education is important to provide necessary activities services, to enhance those services, and to be responsive to the changing needs of the residents.

Financial Planning Role

The activities director is responsible for financial planning for the department and must have skills in developing and managing a budget. The main categories that must be considered in budgeting are salaries, non-expendable equipment, expendable equipment and supplies, maintenance and repair, travel, and professional development. Projected income and cash-on-hand figures should also be included.

Salary

Salaries are generally the largest budget item. In planning, consideration must be given to actual salary amounts as well as post-probationary raises, merit and cost of living increases, overtime costs, and annual bonuses. Social security contributions, health care benefits, retirement plans, and life insurance costs must also be included. Consult with the human resource manager of the facility.

Non-Expendable Equipment

Purchases of major items, such as stereo systems, tables, and desks, are included in this category. Generally, this is equipment that is not "used up" and is expected to last 5 to 20 years. Before requesting new equipment, it is wise to check with other departments such as housekeeping to see if the needed items are in storage or available from another area of the facility.

Expendable Equipment and Supplies

This category of budget planning is likely to result in mistakes due to false assumptions or inaccurate information. The big problem lies in determining just exactly what is "expendable." Generally, any item that is "used up" over a short period of time is considered expendable. According to my own "Ryan Rule," "Anything smaller than a large bread box, that is not bolted down, kept under lock and key, or constant surveillance is eventually expendable." Table looms, radios, coffeepots, and hand tools are among the items that frequently disappear. Office supplies, crafts, food, and day-to-day supplies are all expendables.

Interdepartmental Activities

Another aspect that makes budget planning difficult is "who pays for what" when several departments participate in an activity. For example, when a picnic is held in the park, is the cost of food charged to the dietary department or the activities department? If a nurse's aide is designated to assist with the activity, are the hours worked charged against the nursing budget or the activity budget? Matters such as these must be resolved with administration prior to the event. Once these questions have been answered, more accurate planning can occur. One method is to keep track of actual expenses for 3 months, multiply that amount by four, and add at least 12% to cover inflation and margin of error.

Maintenance and Repair

Routine maintenance is required for sewing machines, powered woodworking tools, computers, and all audiovisual equipment. Departmental painting and redecorating may also be included in this category.

Travel

Expenses incurred for bus rentals for resident outings are generally the largest item in this category. If the facility has a vehicle for resident use, determine if any charges are made to your department. Reimbursement of employee and volunteer mileage for errands and shopping should also be covered in this budget category.

Professional Development

In light of the many rapid changes in health care policy, coupled with new research, legislation, and resulting changes in the provision of services, it is important for activities directors and activities personnel to have opportunities for professional development. Costs for continuing education courses and workshops, conventions, conferences, meetings, books, journals, related travel, and per diem costs are items that should be covered.

Income Sources

Cash donations, bazaar receipts, and bake sale proceeds are examples of income sources. The activities director must have a clear understanding of exactly what the administration expectations are for income-producing activities. Although some activities may be self-supporting in terms of revenue generated, it is an unreal expectation to believe an activity will generate enough income to cover expenses. Activities programs should never be forced to exploit resident endeavors to raise money.

Consultation

A consultant is a person who is employed by a facility on a contractual basis to provide indirect service. Consultants may be used to give information, assist in strategy development and problem resolution, to clarify issues, and to advise (AOTA, 1993). Typically, a consultant is employed by administration to provide services to a department or several departments in relation to specific concerns. Consultative services may be as short as a one-time visit or may extend over several months or years depending on the nature of the consultation required. It is important to understand that a consultant works "outside" the facility and brings expertise and an objective viewpoint to the facility.

The activities director might use a consultant to assist in providing information about and interpretation of federal and state regulations regarding activities programming. Other areas in which a consultant might offer assistance include continuing education and general community resources, activity suggestions for non-participating residents, establishing resident care planning goals, and suggesting ways to improve departmental management procedures. A consultant can also be a valuable resource for developing strategies for improved communication with another department or individual.

It is very important to note that when an OT is employed as a consultant it does not mean that OT services are being provided. Further clarification is found in the official position paper of the AOTA (1994) entitled *Position Paper: OT and Long-Term Services and Supports.*

Coordination of Occupational Therapy and Activities Services

In recent years, I have become increasingly concerned about the apparent "division" in some long-term care facilities that provide both activities and OT services. These services may not be coordinated and there may be little effort to reinforce the residents' goals from OT in the activity program. Informal observation and feedback from individuals working in the field present an interesting contrast in terms of "what is" and "what could be." A number of nursing homes and other long-term care facilities employ OTs and OTAs on a contractual basis to provide direct services under what is often viewed as a medical, rehabilitation model, frequently oriented primarily to physical dysfunction. The same facility may also employ OTAs to deliver activity services under a more holistic, humanistic, supportive, and maintenance model. Unfortunately, communication between the two services may be minimal. For example, a person with hemiparesis may be working on coordination activities in OT and an OTA in the activities department could reinforce treatment, but this coordination may not take place in many instances. It is imperative these efforts are coordinated and that the service providers critique their respective models and methods of service delivery to ensure maximum benefits to the recipients that are also cost-effective.

New Model for Long-Term Care

The Lazarus Project provides a model that should be considered as a possible solution to the problems in long-term care facilities that extend beyond those discussed previously. The model outlines the politics of empowerment based on a community model of democratic governance where residents, staff, and administration participate equally in creating an environment that is responsive to all member needs, thus improving the quality of life for those residing in these facilities (Kari & Michels, 1991). The OTA serving as an activities director or a direct OT service provider can have a marked influence in bringing about the necessary changes in 2000 and beyond, using the innovative principles stressed in this important work.

The Lazarus Vision

It seems fitting to leave the reader with a vision for the future in which the profession can play a vital role. While members of other age groups may be served by nursing homes, the needs of the frail elderly deserve particular attention. Therefore, the vision statement from the Lazarus project is shown in Figure 40-5 to provide a vehicle for study, reflection, and challenge, and a catalyst for implementing needed change (Kari & Michels, 1991).

Summary

The role of the OTA as an activities director offers many challenges and opportunities. Skills in assessing activities needs, planning, implementing, documenting, managing, and evaluating programs are essential. An activities director must also have strong interpersonal, leadership, supervision, and management abilities. The need for qualified activities personnel in long-term care facilities for the elderly and others is increasing, and the educational background of OTAs provides them with excellent preparation for such positions; however, employment of an OTA or OT consultant does not mean that OT direct services are being provided.

Recent federal legislation is emphasized and provides a foundation for following topics. Discussion of specific documentation needs and financial and other management tasks provides the reader with basic information. Interdisciplinary roles and consultation are a focus as well. The need for coordination between activities services and OT services is addressed and culminates with a brief dis-

cussion of a model for service delivery in the 2000s and beyond and in which OTAs can play a vital part, regardless of their specific roles in the provision of long-term care services.

Acknowledgments

Appreciation is extended to Nancy Kari, MPH, OTR, and Peg Michels, MA for sharing material from the Lazarus Project. Special thanks is also given to Shirley H. Carr, MA, OTR, FAOTA, for her critique and helpful comments and to Pamela Hayle, therapeutic activities programmer, for providing information and forms. Penny Boulet, COTA is also acknowledged for providing resources.

References

American Therapeutic Recreation Association. (1987). *Definition of therapeutic recreation.* Alexandria, VA: Author.

American Therapeutic Recreation Association. (1991). *Standards for the practice.* Alexandria, VA: Author.

American Therapeutic Recreation Association. (1993). *Standards for the practice of therapeutic recreation and self assessment guide.* Alexandria, VA: Author.

American Therapeutic Recreation Association. (1998). *Career information.* Alexandria, VA: Author.

AOTA. (1990). *Resident assessment system.* Rockville, MD: Author.

AOTA. (1993). Occupational therapy roles. *Am J Occup Ther, 47,* 1087-1099.

AOTA. (1994). Position paper: OT and long-term services and supports. *Am J Occup Ther, 48,* 1035-1036.

Healthcare Financing Administration. (1998). *Choosing a nursing home.* Washington, DC: Author. #HCFA-10121.

Healthcare Financing Administration. (1999). *HCFA fact sheet.* Washington, DC: HCFA Press Office.

Kari, N., & Michels, P. (1991). The Lazarus Project: A politics of empowerment. *Am J Occup Ther, 45,* 719-725.

National Association of Activity Professionals. (1990). *Standards of practice: Section A—Standards of care.* Washington, DC: Author.

Saltz, D. L. (1990). Celebration marks reform of nursing homes. *OT Week, 4*(41), 12-13.

Wlodkowski, R. J. (1990). *Enhancing adult motivation to learn.* San Francisco, CA: Jossey-Bass.

The Lazarus Project Vision

The Lazarus Project believes that frail elders can be contributing members to society. It is through contribution that individuals exercise power and are able to live a life of meaning and dignity. Empowerment happens when communities are created—communities which govern themselves by drawing on the diverse strengths of members to address common problems.

The Lazarus Project believes this kind of community can be created in nursing home environments. This requires a broad, holistic understanding of health. This concept of health includes the ability to have authority in one's life, to shape one's environment, and to extend influence within a broader public world.

Aging is a public issue; it is not simply an individual experience. When people become older and more frail, their ability to be contributing members to society changes. In a society that measures worth in terms of contributions and influence, the loss of physical and cognitive capacity quickly defines frail elders as "a problem." One of the ways the public has chosen to address this "problem" is to separate itself from chronically ill and disabled elders by "institutionalizing" the aging.

The authors of the Lazarus Project believe that the focus on the medical and service missions of long-term care institutions views residents as incapacitated rather than as contributors. When this assumption becomes embedded in the institution's governing system, it can lead to a loss of power for all involved—the residents, the staff, administrators, and families. This loss of influence constrains an institution's ability to effectively respond to the problems of aging.

Figure 40-5. The Lazarus Project vision. (Reprinted from Ryan, S. E. (1993). *Practice issues in OT: Intraprofessional team building.* Thorofare, NJ: SLACK Incorporated.)

Functional Ethics

S. Maggie Reitz, PhD, OTR/L, FAOTA

INTRODUCTION

The focus of the chapter is on you as a student gaining a working knowledge of functional ethics—the ability to apply knowledge of ethics to the day-to-day life of the OT student. This information will be especially helpful during your transition to the role of OT practitioner. However, additional training, ongoing reading, and self-study will be required for you to be an ethical, competent practitioner who is able to negotiate the complexities of today's practice arenas.

This chapter will help provide you with an initial understanding of ethics as it relates to the roles of the OT student and the future OT practitioner. A description of the *OT Code of Ethics* (AOTA, 2000) is provided. Professional and unethical behaviors are discussed. Problem behaviors not supported by the *OT Code of Ethics,* but sometimes exhibited by OT students, are identified. This section is followed by a brief discussion of dilemmas that practitioners may face. Finally, a practical method for analyzing and resolving ethical dilemmas is presented. Resources to assist

the student at arriving at an appropriate response to ethical issues are described.

LANGUAGE OF ETHICS

Some of the terminology in a discussion of ethics can initially be confusing and intimidating. After learning a few basic terms, however, "the richness and importance of ethics to the profession's ability to enact its values becomes readily apparent" (Reitz, 1997, p. 248).

Ethics

What are ethics? If you were to ask this question of beginning OT students or even random people on the street, you would receive a variety of responses. However, it would be easy to find common themes among the varied responses. These themes would probably include concepts involving values such as honesty, truthfulness, morals, and doing the "right" thing. Themes such as these are either represented or interwoven in the core values and attitudes identified by the profession of OT (AOTA, 1993). These core values and atti-

KEY CONCEPTS

- Ethics: Honesty, truthfulness, and morals.
- Code of ethics: A pledge of high values and principles for occupational therapy.

ESSENTIAL VOCABULARY

Beneficence: Prevent harm.

Duty: Meeting one's responsibilities.

Fidelity: Keep your word.

Nonmaleficence: First do no harm.

Veracity: Being truthful.

tudes are ideals that are essential to any discussion of OT ethics. They "are organized around seven basic concepts—altruism, equality, freedom, justice, dignity, truth, and prudence" (AOTA, 1993, p. 1085).

Mosey (1981) describes ethics as being the analysis of voluntary human behavior which impacts others, "the institutions of the society, or the physical, mental, or the moral development of the individual" (p. 20). In an AOTA publication, ethics are defined as "the pattern of values and norms which are assumed and taken for granted in a given cultural, professional, or institutional setting...Ways of determining right and wrong" (1998, p. 27). Ethics are the foundation of a culture and the broader society, as they provide guidance to its members regarding their relationships with others. The manner in which the ethical beliefs of a society are carried out is of special importance to those in the society who may be in danger of mistreatment due to age, illness, or other possible areas of discrimination.

Nonmaleficence and Beneficence

A glossary of other terms often found in discussions of ethics is available in the *1998 Reference Guide to the OT Code of Ethics* (AOTA, 1998). This glossary includes definitions for the terms beneficence and nonmaleficence. Reitz (1997, p. 248) also provides a brief discussion of these terms, which is included below.

During discussions of ethics in medicine and health, the terms nonmaleficence and beneficence are used. Nonmaleficence means, "above all [or first] do no harm" (Beauchamp & Childress, 1989, p. 120). On the other hand, beneficence means (besides not harming the patient), health care providers have a duty to remove or prevent harm, to provide a benefit or beneficial services to the patient, and to balance "benefits and harms." (Beauchamp & Childress, 1989, pp. 194, 195)

Duty, Veracity, and Fidelity

Although similar in meaning, these terms are not identical. "Duty is a broad term which includes the important behaviors of meeting one's responsibilities and performing one's work competently... this means completing the tasks required by your role as an OT student in a safe, ethical, and skilled manner" (Reitz, 1997, p. 248). Veracity simply means to be truthful, while fidelity means keeping your word (Beauchamp & Childress, 1989).

CODE OF ETHICS

Mosey (1981) describes the necessary criteria that distinguish a job from a profession. One of these criteria is a code of ethics. A profession and its code of ethics nor-

mally develop and evolve over time. In addition, forces of society shape both. Mosey views a code of ethics as a "contract" between a profession and the society it serves. The earliest written form of a code for OT practitioners was entitled the "Pledge and Creed for OTs" (Mosey, 1981). This document remained unchanged until 1977 (Mosey, 1981). In 1976, Wells published "an excellent critique of the 'Pledge and Creed' and a rationale for the major revisions" that were soon to be approved (Mosey, 1981, p. 65). Since 1977, the profession's code of ethics has continued to evolve and has been revised four times: in 1979, 1988, 1994, and 2000 (AOTA, 1998). This document is reviewed every 6 years.

The AOTA's *OT Code of Ethics* "is a public statement of the values and principles used to promote and maintain high standards of behavior in OT" (AOTA, 2000, p. 1). Seven principles are included in the current version of the code. These seven principles center on the well-being of those who receive our services, confidentiality, competence, complying with laws and policies, the provision of accurate truthful information, and the fair treatment of colleagues and other professionals (AOTA, 2000, pp. 1-4). The principles contained in the code help to clarify our core values and provide guidance by showing their connection to the daily life of an OT student or practitioner.

The latest version of the *OT Code of Ethics* is available via the Internet by selecting "About Us," then "Code of Ethics," and finally "Code of Ethics 2000" from the AOTA's homepage at the following address http://www.aota.org. This document can be easily accessed and should be periodically reviewed by OT students and practitioners.

When a student becomes a member of AOTA, he or she commits to following the Code of Ethics and its enforcement procedures (AOTA, 1998). The enforcement procedures also appear in the *1998 Reference Guide to the OT Code of Ethics* (AOTA, 1998). Although a student may not be a member of AOTA, the OT program in which he or she is enrolled may use this Code of Ethics as part of its OT student Code of Conduct. It is suggested that you determine which code or codes apply at your particular educational setting as well as those that may be specific to your state or geographical practice area. Although most state regulatory boards use AOTA's *OT Code of Ethics* as their standard of ethical behavior (Hansen, 1998b), it is wise to ensure that you understand and follow any and all applicable ethical codes.

PROFESSIONAL BEHAVIOR

A job becomes a profession once it has been recognized as such by a society (Mosey, 1981). The profession is then awarded certain privileges, such as status. In return, however, the profession has a responsibility to serve that society in a competent and respectful manner. Professional behavior is necessary for all students and practitioners of a profession to uphold its responsibility to society. Professional behavior encompasses a wide array of behaviors that are important for success in both the classroom and treatment environments. Examples of professional behavior that are important factors in students' academic and clinical success include punctuality, enthusiasm, cooperation, communicating appropriately—both verbally and nonverbally—the ability to accept criticism, and being nonjudgmental.

Many OT programs have developed feedback mechanisms to encourage the development of these crucial behaviors among students. Kasar, Clark, Watson, and Pfister developed a form at the University of Scranton, which includes 10 items that address such topics as communication skills, initiation, and clinical reasoning. This form appears as an appendix in a textbook on professional behaviors (Kasar & Clark, 2000).

It is important for students to receive frequent feedback regarding the skills and behaviors they have successfully mastered, as well as those requiring additional work. The presence of unprofessional behavior indicates an area in which feedback is needed. Some examples of unprofessional behaviors include missing class, failing to contribute your fair share to a group project, leaving trash in the classroom, and engaging in side conversations during class. Often students do not realize the impact of these behaviors on others. Many of the above mentioned unacceptable behaviors are distracting to teachers as well as to student peers. These behaviors are not tolerated during fieldwork placements or employment settings and should also not be tolerated in the academic setting.

Unethical Behavior

Acting in a manner counter to the principles detailed in any ethical code or student code of conduct that apply to you is unethical behavior. Some students, at times, engage in unethical behavior. When confronted about these behaviors, they often express dismay and confusion, not understanding that their behavior is unacceptable and bothersome to others. They are, after all, not "bad" people. They mean no harm, and therefore often fail to see the "wrong" in what they have done. Upon further questioning, however, students behaving unprofessionally or unethically often admit they simply had not thought clearly about their behavior and had allowed the stress of school or other important life roles to cloud their judgment.

Problem behaviors vary in seriousness. The resulting consequences usually vary in direct proportion to the seriousness of the problem behavior. Behaviors described above as being unprofessional, such as engaging in side

conversations during class, can be viewed as both unprofessional and unethical. They are viewed as unethical since the behavior is contrary to the core values of freedom and equality, because the behavior disturbs the educational process of their peers. Regardless of how disruptive this particular behavior is viewed on a continuum of problem behaviors, it is far less serious than, for example, plagiarism. Plagiarism and other serious unethical behaviors will be discussed below.

Problem Student Behaviors

It is important, as a preventive measure, to outline possible behaviors students may lapse into that can put them at risk for failure or expulsion from their OT program. This way you, as students, can monitor your own behavior and develop appropriate behaviors and skills that are needed to be a competent student and future practitioner. The development of positive professional habits is easier and more rewarding than the difficult challenge of changing poor habits once they are ingrained. In addition, you should be aware of unprofessional and unethical behaviors in others and develop skills to appropriately confront peers who engage in such behaviors. It is also important to remember that as a member of an institution or organization, you may be obligated to report breaches of student conduct codes or the OT Code of Ethics.

A variety of problem behaviors are described below. This list is by no means exhaustive but serves to illustrate inappropriate behaviors that are sometimes encountered by OT academic and clinical faculty. When a fellow student observes such behaviors, he or she should be aware that it is quite appropriate to confront the individual or individuals involved. This confrontation may not be easy. Help in analyzing the situation may be needed and is available from a number of sources identified later in this chapter. Although confronting unethical behavior is not easy, it ultimately benefits the individuals involved as well as the profession and society.

Some of the behaviors described below are blatantly unethical (e.g., plagiarism); these behaviors are on the very serious end of the continuum of unethical and unprofessional behaviors. Other behaviors, however, may be less obvious and could be argued as being non-issues by some individuals (e.g., misguided motivation to become an OT practitioner). These behaviors have been placed at the end of the list and are followed by a discussion of the associated ambiguity.

Confidentiality

As an OT student, you will have access to a variety of personal information about patients and their families.

Depending on the size of your community and your fieldwork placement, you may know these people either directly or indirectly. The temptation to gossip can be strong but must be avoided. In addition, telling "war stories" can help health professionals cope with the human suffering encountered during the process of assisting people in adapting to stressful circumstances. However, care must be exercised both in terms of to whom and where these stories are told. Be careful to maintain proper confidentiality and respect for patients.

Students should respect the confidentiality of information that is shared by peers and instructors in class. "Due to the nature of OT education, sometimes students and instructors have personal examples that are relevant to class discussions. This information should be respected and not used for gossip" (Reitz, 1997, p. 252). Confidentiality is required under principle 3E of the OT Code of Ethics, which states: "OT personnel shall protect all privileged, confidential forms of written, verbal, and electronic communication gained from educational, practice, research, and investigational activities unless otherwise mandated by local, state, or federal regulations" (AOTA, 2000, p. 2).

Sexual/Dating Relationships

It is inappropriate for students to date their instructors, supervisors, or patients. Most schools have policies that address this issue. Many professional ethical codes also prohibit this behavior either directly or indirectly. In some places, certain professions, such as psychologists, specify that such relationships are considered inappropriate even after the professional relationship has ended (State of Maryland, Title 10, 1992). Students should seek clarification of the prevailing code at their educational institution and within the regulatory body of their state or other applicable jurisdiction. Dating and maintaining a sexual relationship with a patient would be in violation of Principle 1 of the OT Code of Ethics as stated below:

OT personnel shall maintain relationships that do not exploit the recipient of services sexually, physically, emotionally, financially, socially, or in any other manner. (AOTA, 2000, p. 1)

In addition, students should be aware that engaging "in a sexual relationship with a minor or patient with mental impairments would be breaching Principle 1 which relates to beneficence (Kyler-Hutchison, 1998a, p. 47). "It is widely acknowledged that engaging in sexual relations with a minor is also committing a criminal act" (Kyler-Hutchison, 1998a, p. 47).

Lack of Commitment to the Educational Process

At times, students, for a variety of reasons, may be unaware of or lose sight of the importance of individual assignments and the purpose of those assignments relative to the goals of the overall curriculum. Sometimes this lack of awareness is of limited consequence. However, at other times it may lead students to dismiss assignments as "busy work" and cause them to use shortcuts that undermine the true goals of the assignments. These shortcuts often involve some sort of cheating. This cheating can take the form of reworking a friend's old paper and submitting it as original work, collaborating on an assignment that was supposed to be completed independently, making up data instead of collecting it, taking old papers or drafts of other students' work from the recycling bin or trashcan, or sharing answers during an exam. All of these behaviors are serious and may result in equally serious consequences as determined by your specific OT program. They also show a lack of understanding and respect for the curriculum. Assignments are carefully crafted to ensure that each student develops the skills he or she needs to be a competent practitioner. Cheating, therefore, can negatively impact the development of skills necessary to be a competent practitioner. It is also inconsistent with the core values of justice and truth and Principles 4 through 6 of the OT Code of Ethics. The end result is that cheating shortchanges the student and the profession, but, most sadly, it is likely to hurt the future patients of those engaging in this behavior.

Appropriate Collaboration vs. Cheating

The faculty in OT programs are responsible for assisting in the development of therapists through a variety of methods including individual and group work. The faculty is also responsible for evaluating the academic performance of each student to determine his or her level of skill, knowledge, clinical reasoning, and readiness for clinical placement. Each student's individual and group work must be examined to properly conduct this ongoing evaluation. Faculty members complete this task in order to ensure that you, as students, receive the feedback necessary to develop into competent and ethical OTs.

Group activities and assignments are meaningful learning tools. However, it is important to remember that your study partners will not necessarily be there beside you as you treat patients in your future careers. You must each be able to function independently as competent therapists. Even when working with other team members, you must be capable of providing competent and thorough patient care independent of the skills of your colleagues. However, this independence does not mean that as an OT practitioner you are prohibited from seeking additional supervision or mentoring when needed. In fact, it is encouraged by Principles 4D and 4G of the OT Code of Ethics.

Plagiarism

In general, plagiarism is considered "unauthorized use of works or ideas from others without permission or proper credit. Using the 'intellectual property' of others without permission or proper credit constitutes theft, as would improper acquisition of physical property" (Pigg, 1989, p. 103). Most OT schools and OT publications follow the recommended style described in the most current (1994) *Publication Manual of the American Psychological Association* (APA), which is often referred to as the APA Publication Manual. This manual states that "quotation marks [must] be used to indicate the exact words of another" (APA, 1994, p. 292). In addition, the APA Publication Manual indicates that when paraphrasing is used, proper citation must be provided. Students should also be aware that resources found on the Internet and other electronic media are also covered by rules of plagiarism.

Plagiarism is a form of cheating. Not only does it falsely represent a student's knowledge, but it also fails to provide well-deserved credit to individuals who have worked hard to add to the body of knowledge. Plagiarism can be the result of poor time management or lack of understanding about professional writing. However, neither of these reasons are a sufficient excuse for this behavior. Every OT student is responsible for knowing what plagiarism is and for taking steps to prevent it. Plagiarism is also inconsistent with the core values of justice and truth addressed in Principles 4 through 6 of the *OT Code of Ethics*.

Lack of Respect for Resources

There are probably few experiences that are more frustrating to students than to spend time identifying articles needed for a project and then find that the articles have been ripped out of the identified journals (Reitz, 1997). It is also frustrating for students planning to print a paper in a computer lab to find that they cannot do so because someone failed to correctly log off the computer or incorrectly reconfigured the printer cables. Students need to respect shared learning resources and take responsibility for learning to use technology correctly. Vandalism and theft of materials, which are more extreme examples of failure to respect shared resources, are a breach of Principle 54A of the *OT Code of Ethics*. This principle states that "OT personnel shall familiarize themselves with and shall seek to under stand and abide by applicable Association policies; local, state, and federal laws; and institutional rules" (AOTA, 2000, p. 2).

Faculty and Student Collaboration

Excellent research and program development can occur when students and faculty work together. To ensure that this relationship is positive, it is important to address a number of issues prior to the initiation of the project. These issues include "authorship, ownership of data, and subsequent use of data" (O'Rourke, 1989, p. 101). Students who work on a collaborative project with a faculty member and then write an article based on the project may be unaware of the need to share authorship or acknowledge the assistance of others. Depending upon the scope of the faculty member's contribution, it may be appropriate to share authorship or possibly use a form of joint authorship with the faculty member acknowledged as primary author. O'Rourke (1989) indicates that the following contributions merit joint authorship: idea generator, designer, implementer, data processor, data analyzer, editor or writer, or graduate assistant (p. 102).

The APA Publication Manual (1994) provides the following guidance:

> Authorship encompasses... those who have made substantial scientific contributions. Substantial professional contributions may include formulating the problem or hypothesis, structuring the experimental design, organizing and conducting statistical analysis, interpreting the results, or writing a major portion of the paper. (p. 294)

Assigning appropriate authorship is supported by Principle 7B, which states "OT practitioners shall accurately represent the qualifications, views, contributions, and findings of colleagues" (AOTA, 2000, p. 3).

As a student, you should be aware of any published policies or procedures in your program that pertain to student and faculty responsibilities associated with faculty projects. If you are planning to participate in a collaborative activity with a faculty member and your school does not have a policy, helpful resources can be found in the health education literature (Greenberg, Allen, & Noland, 1981) and the OT literature (Kyler-Hutchison, 1998b). In addition, other OT programs may be willing to share their research and publication ethics policies.

Limited/Specialized Interest

Some faculty members strongly believe that future OT practitioners should be committed to all humans and their quest to maximize their human potential. Students who wish to be OT practitioners but only work with a certain subset of patients are often viewed with concern by these OT faculty. They may question the appropriateness of admitting students who wish to work only with children, patients with hand injuries, or patients with physical disabilities.

These concerns are based on a number of factors. When students make premature decisions about areas of specialization they may close themselves to opportunities for learning and other future career possibilities. Student biases concern faculty, as they may indicate a lack of compassion for humanity as a whole, a lack of the ability to work with chronic patients, or a lack of desire to work with patients who are seen in some way as undesirable. With today's changing job market, there is no guarantee that future employment options will match the narrowly selected patient group desired by the student. Students need to be competent and willing to work with any and all individuals, families, and communities in need of OT services. The profession must uphold its responsibility to address the above concerns, as clearly supported by Principle 1A, which states that "OT personnel shall provide services in a fair and equitable manner. They shall recognize and appreciate the cultural components of economics, geography, race, ethnicity, religious and political factors, marital status, sexual orientation, and disability of all recipients of their services" (AOTA, 2000, p. 1).

Misguided Motivation to Become an OT Practitioner

In the past, potential OT practitioners were frequently attracted to the field by its creative, humanistic approach to health. Individuals who wished to make a difference in the health and welfare of society became OT practitioners. As the demand for OT services increased through the years, so did salaries. Some faculty members have voiced concern regarding the commitment of students who were primarily attracted to the profession by job security and financial rewards. The following questions are examples of this concern. What happens now that the job market has shifted and salaries have declined in some areas? Will these individuals remain committed to their patients and the profession? Will these individuals charge their patients fairly? Will they pay for necessary continuing education? Will financial concerns continue to be the primary factor in their decision-making?

The need to pose and answer questions similar to those above is supported by Principles 1A, 1C, and 4D. In addition to these principles, one can argue that an individual selecting the profession for misguided reasons is not being truthful or honest to the ideals as articulated in the Core Values and Attitudes of the profession (AOTA, 1993).

One may argue, however, that the values of a profession change as both society and the profession itself change. What if students are only partially attracted to the profession due to high salaries? Is the concern raised above still appropriate? An emphasis on financial compensation may not be "wrong" as long as practitioners are competent and uphold the *OT Code of Ethics*. What do you think?

The above example shows that ethics is often not clear-cut. There can sometimes be different interpretations of codes of ethics. In addition, a situation that may initially appear to be problematic may not truly be so once more information is gathered. It is important to avoid jumping to conclusions when confronted with a possible ethical dilemma. It is equally important to avoid rashly accusing someone of wrongdoing in the "heat" of the moment. The best way to approach a potential ethical issue is to systematically analyze the situation and follow one of the various models available to guide decision-making.

PRACTICE DILEMMAS

Many of the problem behaviors described above would be considered unethical if exhibited in a practice setting. For example, lack of respect for resources in the clinical environment is unethical in the case of practitioners using either computers or copying machines for personal reasons. Arriving late for team meetings or engaging in side conversations during meetings, family conferences, supervisory conferences, or patient rounds is unethical since it impacts negatively on colleagues and patient care. Thus, this type of behavior is contrary to the concept of beneficence described earlier in this chapter. Individuals encountering peers engaging in unethical workplace behaviors such as these are obligated to take appropriate action.

Some practice dilemmas involve issues of documentation, supervision, and billing. Documentation must be timely, accurate, and describe practice that is appropriate for the level of education and experience of the OT practitioner. This assertion is supported by Principle 4E, which states that "OT practitioners shall protect service recipients by ensuring that duties assumed or assigned to other OT personnel match credentials, qualifications, experience, and scope of practice" (AOTA, 2000, p. 2). It is also supported by Principles 4D and 5C.

One aspect of supervision is addressed in Principle 4E, as stated above. In addition, Principle 5A states that OT practitioners shall comply with local, state, and federal laws. This means that the OT practitioner is responsible for being familiar with laws that relate to OT practice, including those associated with supervision. Since laws and institutional rules—especially those pertaining to supervision—can vary, it is recommended that students and practitioners be aware of all laws that relate to their geographic and specialty areas. State regulatory boards can be helpful in obtaining this information.

All billing must be accurate and appropriate. It is the responsibility of OT practitioners to be aware of billing charges. Without this knowledge, it is difficult to fulfill Principle 1B, which states, "OT practitioners shall strive to ensure that fees are fair and reasonable and commensurate with services performed. When OT practitioners set fees, they shall set fees considering institutional. local, state, and federal requirements, and with due regard for the service recipient's ability to pay" (AOTA, 2000, p. 1).

ANALYZING ETHICAL DILEMMAS

There are several methods to use when analyzing an ethical situation (Aroskar, 1980; Hansen, Kamp, & Reitz, 1988; Kyler, 1998; Reitz & Kyler, 1998). These methods are similar in many ways. One method that embodies the essence of the various methods was developed by Hansen and Kyler-Hutchison and used by Kyler-Hutchison in her contribution to the text *Ethical and Legal Dilemmas in OT* (Bailey & Schwartzberg, 1995). This method includes finding the answers to the following four questions:

1. Who are the players in the dilemma?
2. What other facts or information are needed?
3. What actions may be taken?
4. What are the possible consequences of each action? (Bailey & Schwartzberg, 1995, p. vi)

After answering these four questions, you should have a better understanding of the situation and be able to select a course of action you are comfortable with and are able to defend.

PROFESSIONAL RESOURCES

A variety of human resources are available to assist you in analyzing an ethical dilemma and following through with your decision. These resources include your faculty advisor, faculty members, program director, and state association president. Other individuals include state regulatory board members, the Ethics Officer at AOTA, the Chairperson of AOTA's Commission on Standards and Ethics, and the Director of Regulatory Affairs at the National Board for Certification of Occupational Therapists (NBCOT).

Various documents that provide guidance are also available and should be referred to if you are thinking of reporting a breach of ethics. One of these documents, the *Enforcement Procedure for OT Code of Ethics—Revised*, is included in the *1998 Reference Guide to the OT Code of Ethics* (AOTA, 1998). Another useful document, *Disciplinary Action: Whose Responsibility* (Hansen, 1998a), is actually a useful chart that helps the student or practitioner determine the organization to which a report should be directed.

An article by Hansen (1998b), chairperson, Commission on Standards and Ethics from 1988 to 1994, further details the ethical jurisdiction and roles of three primary organizations that process complaints regarding breaches of ethics. These organizations include AOTA, NBCOT, and state regulatory boards. Additional articles in the *1998 Reference Guide to the OT Code of Ethics* (AOTA, 1998) cover such important topics as confidentiality and fieldwork, contractual agreements, preventing fraud and abuse, reporting a peer, and informed consent.

Additional literature exists that helps the OT student and practitioner to continue to study this important area of OT practice. Another AOTA publication, *Effective Documentation for OT* (Acquaviva, 1998), contains chapters that discuss fraud and ethical and legal issues surrounding OT documentation. The *OT Search* is an online bibliographic database that is accessible from the AOTA home page to individuals and institutions subscribing to this service. This database can assist the student in locating additional articles pertaining to ethics. The student is encouraged to use the reference list following this chapter to further his or her understanding of OT ethics.

SUMMARY

A profession must uphold its duty to society and do all that is reasonable to protect the public from unethical practitioners. It is the profession's duty and responsibility to educate and assist students and practitioners in developing and maintaining a high level of ethical practice. OT students must prepare to be fully competent, ethical practitioners. This preparation includes the development of a solid foundation in ethical behavior. This chapter has provided an introduction to ethics, the *OT Code of Ethics*, and a way to analyze ethical dilemmas. It has also provided information regarding resources for further study and assistance with ethical concerns. Students are strongly encouraged to use these resources. OT students and practitioners must consistently uphold the highest ethical standards. Failure to do so is a disservice to our patients, their families, and the society we serve.

ACKNOWLEDGMENTS

The author would like to express her appreciation for the assistance provided by the following individuals: Janie B. Scott, MS, OTR/L, FAOTA, for her review of content; Frederick D. Reitz, for his review of grammar and writing mechanics as well as providing coffee as needed; and Jessica Reitz, for shoveling snow so I would not be distracted and could make my deadline.

REFERENCES

Acquaviva, J. D. (1998). *Effective documentation for occupational therapy* (2nd ed.). Bethesda, MD: AOTA.

American Psychological Association. (1994). *Publication manual of the American Psychological Association* (4th ed.). Washington, DC: Author.

AOTA. (1993). Core values and attitudes of occupational therapy practice. *Am J Occup Ther, 47,* 1085-1086.

AOTA. (1994). OT Code of Ethics. *Am J Occup Ther, 48,* 1037-1038.

AOTA. (2000). OT Code of Ethics 2000 (online). Available http://www.aota.org/members/area2/links/LINK03.asp.

AOTA. Commission on Standards and Ethics. (1998). *1998 Reference guide to the OT code of ethics.* Bethesda, MD: Author.

Aroskar, M. (1980). Anatomy of an ethical dilemma: The practice (Part II). *American Journal of Nursing, 80,* 661-663.

Bailey, D. M., & Schwartzberg, S. L. (1995). *Ethical and legal dilemmas in OT.* Philadelphia, PA: F. A. Davis.

Beauchamp, T. L., & Childress, J. F. (1989). *Principles of biomedical ethics* (3rd ed.). New York, NY: Oxford University Press.

Greenberg, J., Allen, R., & Noland, M. (1981). Ethics and policy governing faculty and students. *Journal of the American College Health Association, 30,* 141-142.

Hansen, R. (1998a). Disciplinary action: Whose responsibility? In AOTA, Commission on Standards and Ethics. *1998 Reference guide to the OT Code of Ethics* (p. 38). Bethesda, MD: Author.

Hansen, R. (1998b). Ethical jurisdiction of occupational therapy: The role of AOTA, NBCOT, and state regulatory boards. In AOTA, Commission on Standards and Ethics. *1998 Reference guide to the OT Code of Ethics* (pp. 39-41). Bethesda, MD: Author.

Hansen, R. A., Kamp, L., & Reitz, S. (1988). Two practitioner's analyses of OT practice dilemmas. *Am J Occup Ther, 42,* 312-319.

Kasar, J., & Clark, E. N. (2000). *Developing professional behaviors.* Thorofare, NJ: SLACK incorporated.

Kyler, P. (1998). Framework for ethical decision making-revised. In AOTA, Commission on Standards and Ethics. *1998 Reference guide to the OT Code of Ethics* (p. 34). Bethesda, MD: Author.

Kyler-Hutchison, P. (1998a). Unethical and illegal: What's the difference? In AOTA, Commission on Standards and Ethics. *1998 Reference guide to the OT Code of Ethics* (p. 47). Bethesda, MD: Author.

Kyler-Hutchison, P. (1998b). Issues in ethics: Who's the author? Who's the owner? In AOTA, Commission on Standards and Ethics. *1998 Reference guide to the OT Code of Ethics* (pp. 51-52). Bethesda, MD: Author.

Mosey, A. C. (1981). *OT: Configuration of a profession.* New York, NY: Raven Press.

O'Rourke, T. W. (1989). The student-professor relationship. In N. K. Iammarino, T. W. O'Rorke, R. M. Pigg, & A. D. Weinberg (Eds.), Ethical issues in research and publication. *Journal of School Health, 59,* 101-102.

Pigg, R. M. (1989). Integrity in the publication process. In N. K. Iammarino, T. W. O'Rorke, R. M. Pigg, & A. D. Weinberg (Eds.), Ethical issues in research and publication. *Journal of School Health, 59,* 103-104.

Reitz, S. M. (1997). Ethics for students. In K. Sladyk (Ed.), *OT primer: A guide to college success* (pp. 245-255). Thorofare, NJ: SLACK Incorporated.

Reitz, S. M., & Kyler, P. (1998). Ethical issues in documentation. In J. D. Acquaviva (Ed.), *Effective documentation for OT.* (2nd ed., pp. 237-272). Bethesda, MD: AOTA.

State of Maryland, Title 10, Department of Health and Mental Hygiene. (1992). *Board of Examiners of Psychologists, Code of Ethics and Professional Conduct, p. 2.* [10.36.05]. Health Occupation Article.

Teamwork and Team Building

Ellen Berger Rainville, MS, OTR, FAOTA
Toné F. Blechert, MA, COTA, ROH
Marianne F. Christiansen, MA, OTR
Nancy Kari, MPH, OTR

INTRODUCTION

"...The idea of enhancing critical partnerships through the conscious pursuit of collaborative relationships may be one of the most valuable strengths and timely opportunities for OT in the 1990s and beyond" (Grady, 1990).

OT practice, like that of many other professions, has undergone tremendous change in recent years. One result is that OT practitioners, OTRs and OTAs, are increasingly likely to be asked to participate as members of teams—in education, in health care, on treatment units, in community settings, in management systems, etc.—the list is endless. The expectations inherent in these requests are as variable as the requests themselves. OT practitioners who do not fully understand team dynamics may unintentionally respond to these expectations inappropriately and then feel unsuccessful in their team-related work activities. Because teamwork is such an important part of today's world, OT practitioners need to be knowledgeable and competent in teamwork theory and practice in order to serve their consumers well.

Being an effective team member requires specialized knowledge and responsibility (Dunn et al., 1989). Team members must possess highly sensitive interpersonal communication skills (Navarra, Lipkowitz, & Navarra, 1990; Spencer, 1989), have knowledge and understanding of team development and dynamics (Blechert, Christiansen, & Kari, 1987; Gardner, 1988; Heming, 1988; Magrab et al., 1981), and demonstrate the ability to engage in collaborative work relationships (Grady, 1990; Guiffrida, 1991; Scheller, 1990). While team participation can be a challenging and sometimes even painful process (Dunn et al., 1989), its rewards include shared pride in goal achievement, increased confidence, and the satisfactions of high rapport (Gardner, 1988; Navarra, Lipkowitz, & Navarra, 1990; Scheller, 1990). The purpose of this chapter, therefore, will be to increase your knowledge and skill related to professional team process and function.

Becoming a respected and accepted member of the team is an important goal and a satisfying experience. There are many kinds of teams. We have all been on one

ESSENTIAL VOCABULARY

Interdisciplinary: Several disciplines collaborate in decision-making.

Intradisciplinary: Treatment within a discipline.

Mastery: Feeling control over one's environment.

Maturation: Goal renewal and improvement.

Ministration: Feeling closeness with co-workers.

Multidisciplinary: Several disciplines treat the person.

Transdisciplinary: An integrated team collaborates and often shares treatments.

KEY CONCEPTS

- Teamwork: Successful team dynamics working to the patient's benefit.
- Team building: Members feel ministration, mastery, and maturation.

type or another—sports, scouts, church or civic groups, charitable activities, and others. A team is defined as "a group of individuals who are committed to a shared purpose, to each other, and to working together to achieve common goals" (Briggs, 1997, p. xxi). Effective teamwork can contribute to the welfare of one's patients, create high morale among staff members, and foster a collaborative and an educational climate in the work setting (Beggs, 1962).

The term *effectiveness* is one of the "buzz words" of the millennium. Increased health care costs, productivity demands, and personnel shortages, coupled with maldistribution and attrition patterns, have produced problems in the effective delivery of OT services (AOTA, 1991). In geographic areas where there is an ample supply of both therapists and assistants, often only therapists are hired, or when assistants are hired, they are underutilized. The latter situation can engender decreased job satisfaction, lowered professional commitment, and attrition for OT personnel. With increased demands for cost-effective services, every effort must be made to reduce this attrition. Intra- and interprofessional team building are possible solutions. Some OT leaders feel that teamwork is "critically important to the vitality and expansion of the profession" (Blechert, Christiansen, & Kari, 1987).

An effective team is built on the character and competencies of its members. Team efforts are strengthened as members improve their professional and personal abilities. Satisfied, contributing team members are helpful to patients and to each other. These individuals demonstrate a basic personal security. They are confident of their knowledge and abilities and comfortable and honest about their limitations. Much has been written about the team process. This chapter will provide an overview of some key information about this important aspect of service delivery. Once you have begun to serve on a team, if not before, you will wish to pursue some of the additional information available. Some ideas for obtaining further information about teams are provided for you at the end of this chapter.

Types of Teams

Table 42-1 illustrates some important differences between groups and teams. As you can see, teams involve careful, intentional interactions aimed at facilitating achievement of the team's mission and goals. Service on a team offers opportunities for creative expression, for professional development and specialization, and for ongoing learning, along with great responsibility. Each team member shares responsibility for the actions of the group. For some, this is a supportive environment, for others, it can be intimidating. In any case, it can be a great adventure.

There are many types of teams. Teams are characterized by their purpose, such as educational team, rehabilitation

services team, management team, as well as by the ways in which they are organized and how their members interact. These interactions fall along a continuum from multidisciplinary to transdisciplinary, as illustrated in Table 42-2.

Qualities of Effective Teams

Team members need to have effective communication; they must listen to each other, assert their own points of view, and negotiate constructively in order to have the best outcomes (Henneman, Lee, & Cohen, 1995; Stewart, 1990). Teamwork is characterized by shared understandings, goals, values, visions, and responsibilities. These must occur in both word and deed (Brown, Thurman, & Pearl, 1993; Crepeau, 1991; Dunst, Trivette, & Deal, 1988).

In the early 1960s, Levinson and his colleagues conducted an important study of workers at a new company. They found that the employees were engaged in a process of fulfilling mutual needs and expectations. A climate of successful reciprocity (a mutual giving and receiving or exchange) was built and the following contributing behaviors were observed:

- Others are treated as individuals.
- Individual differences are appreciated.
- Relationships are established with those who are different.
- Flexibility is shown in stressful situations.
- Satisfaction is derived from a wide variety of sources.
- Strengths as well as limitations are accepted.
- Realistic self-concepts are exhibited.
- Activity and productivity are evident.

These behaviors and others are important to the success of teamwork and team building efforts (Blechert, Christiansen, & Kari, 1987; Levinson, 1962). The mutual trust and respect that characterize successful team collaborations are evident when the team demonstrates:

- Equitable access to information
- Equal opportunity
- Fair representation
- Reliable interactions
- Open, positive attitudes
- Frequent kudos
- Mutual recognition of competence and caring (Briggs, 1997; Stewart, 1990).

Factors that inhibit successful teamwork include:

- Problems with scheduling and time
- Differing values about team interaction, emanating either from the team members or from their organizations

Table 42-1

Groups Versus Teams

Groups	Teams
Members think they are grouped together for administrative purposes only. Individuals work independently; sometimes at cross purposes with others.	Members recognize their interdependence and understand both personal and team goals are best accomplished with mutual support. Time is not wasted struggling over "turf" or attempting personal gain at the expense of others.
Members tend to focus on themselves because they are not sufficiently involved in planning the unit's objectives. They approach their job simply as a hired hand.	Members feel a sense of ownership for their jobs and unit because they are committed to goals they helped establish.
Members are told what to do rather than being asked what the best approach would be. Suggestions are not encouraged.	Members contribute to the organization's success by applying their unique talent and knowledge to team objectives.
Members distrust the motives of colleagues because they do not understand the role of other members. Expressions of opinion or disagreement are considered divisive and non-supportive.	Members work in a climate of trust and are encouraged to openly express ideas, opinions, disagreements, and feelings. Questions are welcomed.
Members are so cautious about what they say that real understanding is not possible. Game playing may occur and communication traps may be set to catch the unwary.	Members practice open and honest communication. They make an effort to understand each other's point of view.
Members may receive good training but are limited in applying it to the job by the supervisor or other group members.	Members are encouraged to develop skills and apply what they learn on the job. They receive the support of the team.
Members find themselves in conflict situations which they do not know how to resolve. Their supervisor may put off intervention until serious damage is done.	Members recognize conflict is a normal aspect of human interaction, but they view such situations as an opportunity for new ideas and creativity. They work to resolve conflict quickly and constructively.
Members may or may not participate in decisions affecting the team. Conformity often appears to be more important than positive results.	Members participate in decisions affecting the team, but understand that their leaders must make a final ruling whenever the team cannot decide or an emergency exists. Positive results, not conformity, are the goal.

Table 42-2

Team Interaction Continuum

Intradisciplinary

One or more members of one discipline provide treatment to the individual. Generally, other disciplines are not involved. If other disciplines are involved, communication is limited.

Multidisciplinary

A number of professionals conduct assessments and interventions independent from one another. Some formal communications occur between involved professionals. Resources and responsibilities are individually allocated between disciplines.

Interdisciplinary

Several disciplines agree to collaborate for decision making. Evaluation and intervention are still conducted independently, within defined areas of each profession's expertise. Formal communications, such as treatment planning meetings, do occur to exchange information, prioritize needs, and allocate resources and responsibilities.

Transdisciplinary

An interdisciplinary team whose members are committed to ongoing communication, collaboration, and share decision making for the patient's benefit. Evaluations and interventions are planned cooperatively. Programs are often the responsibility of a primary interventionist, but treatments are often shared. Ongoing training, support supervision, cooperation, and consultation among disciplines is important to this model.

- Unacknowledged or unresolved differences among team members
- Inadequate resources
- Inadequate communication
- Poor management (Rosin et al., 1996)

Among the qualities of a successful OT practitioner, several are worthy of discussion as they relate to effective teamwork. These are cooperation, flexibility, and creativity.

Cooperation

Team members work together to achieve common goals. In this effort, each individual must pay attention to the details that make cooperation possible. The OTs and OTAs on the team must be well-informed about one another's activities. Cooperation allows the opportunity to teach and learn, to give and receive, and to increase the competence of all involved. A respectful attitude toward the other members of one's team is extremely important. As people work together more closely, they will learn a great deal of information about each other. Team members must be discrete and avoid petty gossip. Cooperation is easiest if trust is maintained.

Flexibility

A successful team member sees change as positive. New or changing approaches and methods are met with an open and accepting mind. This openness to change encourages all team members to think creatively and express ideas freely.

Creativity

OT personnel pride themselves on their creative abilities. Certainly one would hope for an atmosphere that encourages creativity among staff members. Teamwork demands an environment that is permissive enough to allow new ideas to develop, yet structured enough to provide order and direction for all members. The organizational environment can facilitate or inhibit team functioning. Therefore, the purpose and philosophy of the work setting and each team member's understanding of his or her own duties and the duties of other departmental members is very important. There are many management tools that support team members. One such tool is the job description, a list of the tasks that one is expected to perform at work. A written copy of one's job description as well as those of co-workers can increase team members' understanding of shared and individual responsibilities.

TEAM BUILDING

Napier and Gershenfeld (1983) define team building as a process that facilitates the development of a group of people with respect to their unique needs, their degree of readiness, and their past experience. They also point out the importance of team members having opportunities to experience each other in a wide variety of situations, as well as through activities that provide permission for a group to look at its own behavior and also to explore new ways of approaching problems in order to be more effective. Effective workplace team building is founded on the principle that teamwork meets specific needs of people in the areas of ministration, mastery, and maturation. When these needs are effectively met, the individual and the team grow and flourish. If these needs are not met, team dysfunction will occur (Blechert & Christiansen, 1986; Levinson, 1962).

Ministration

Ministration refers to our need to feel a sense of closeness with co-workers; to feel safe, guided, and supported; and to experience acceptance, trust, and respect. For example, think for a moment about how it feels to be a new OT staff member or student—everything seems so unfamiliar, or so it seems. Team members who provide extra orientation, anticipate questions, and indicate a willingness to listen to the students' fears and uncertainties help meet your ministration needs. When a team member tells you that it is okay to make a mistake and demonstrates an understanding that errors are an inherent part of the learning process, you feel a certain level of safety and support.

Some people may need a significant amount of support (ministration) in their work, whereas others may require very little. Some staff and students are uncomfortable telling their supervisor how much support they need in order to function effectively; however, some of us are fortunate to have a supervisor who can sense these needs without being told. It is important nonetheless for people to take responsibility and communicate any feelings of discomfort or lack of support, as well as appreciation for support given. If the supervisor is unable to provide the support needed, he or she should be prepared to offer other sources of gratification. The team experience often helps to fill this gap. When students' and staff members' needs for ministration are met, they are likely to perceive the workplace as "caring."

Mastery

The need for mastery is concerned with the desire to explore, understand, and, to some extent, control oneself and one's environment (Levinson, 1962). Mastery involves increasing proficiency in job activities. This occurs through role exploration, practice experience, reflection, and performance review. The need for mastery can be met in a variety of ways, such as developing a high level of expertise and an enhanced role in a particular area of therapeutic intervention. Also, taking advantage of opportunities to provide leadership to others through assuming supervisory and educational roles enhances mastery at many levels. Feedback on all professional activities should be actively sought from supervisors, peers, consumers, and other knowledgeable persons, and these ideas are incorporated into your practice.

A supervisor who is sensitive to the student's or staff person's need for mastery will provide an appropriate measure of control early in the fieldwork or employment experience. This control may take the form of offering choices in assignments for instance. Supervisors usually appreciate a student's or employee's interest in achieving independence; therefore, it is important to verbalize one's specific goals and needs. For the OT assistant, important competencies to be achieved must include more than those relevant to consumer care. For example, the ability to deal adequately with professionals from other departments, as well as other OT personnel, should be important goals.

Maturation

Maturation involves personal and professional goal renewal, risk-taking for goal achievement, and the empowerment of others. For example, the OTA who seeks out activities and programs that maintain as well as expand his or her professional roles is demonstrating a mature desire to be a lifelong learner. Seeking new responsibilities involving risks, such as developing a new program and becoming a mentor to another person are other ways that this need can be addressed. If maturation needs are met, a person unfolds; if they are not, the person stagnates (Levinson, 1962). Fieldwork provides reality testing opportunities for a student as concepts learned in school are applied in a real situation. This reality testing takes the form of feedback from supervisors and patients as a result of one's efforts. Feedback provides a student with the sense of growth necessary for some maturation to take place.

DEVELOPMENTAL TEAM BUILDING

The developmental team chart shown in Table 42-3 presents a team building process organized according to stages of team development, characteristics of the particular stage, supervisor tasks, team member tasks, and communication issues. The levels of ministration, mastery, and maturation are also delineated. When using this chart, it is important for the reader to consider the following:

- Developmental information may be used to assess current team functioning.
- Developmental factors that may enhance group functioning are important team builders.
- The stages listed are not absolute and may overlap.
- Teams are unique and their experiences may not always parallel the chart.
- Teams evolve according to their experiences along the developmental continuum (Blechert, Christiansen, & Kari, 1987; Bull, 1976; Corey, 1981; Hagberg, 1984).

TEAM MEMBERSHIP

The purpose of a health care, educational, or rehabilitative team is to provide the best possible service to the consumer through the sharing of information and expertise and the coordination of services. A professional member usually heads the team, although it is possible for the consumer to serve as team leader. It is most common for a representative of the organization(s) with professional responsibility for the implementation of services to serve in that role. The members of the team may include any number of people who provide services or assistance for the consumer. For example, in home health care, the team might include the consumer, physician, nurse, social worker, certified nurse assistant, homemaker, spouse, and OT practitioner(s). In the public school, it might include the special education administrator, classroom teacher, parent, child, and OT practitioner(s). Involvement of the consumer at every level of team decision-making and action is critical to outcome. It is important to assess for yourself how much teams value and respect the consumers of their care. Those who respect their consumers, even to the level of seeing them as equal participants on the team, are likely to have such respect for all team members. As stated earlier, such mutuality contributes to the success and satisfaction of a team. Table 42-4 provides brief definitions of the professionals with whom OT practitioners commonly interact.

As we work with professionals from other disciplines, it is useful to ask them about their professional fields. You will learn a great deal about their knowledge and skills by understanding their education, philosophy, goals, values, etc. You will enhance your professional services by drawing out the expertise of others and you in turn will enhance theirs.

Although the information on effective team building presented in this section can be applied to many professional team interactions, a critical focus is the intraprofes-sional relationship between OTs and OTAs. The relationship of teamwork to effective service delivery in OT has been identified as a major theme for our profession. If personnel within the same profession can work effectively as team players, it seems that teamwork that includes others will follow easily.

In summary, it is very helpful to understand the roles and responsibilities as well as the respective contributions of each team member. Teams that work well together are best able to accomplish such objectives as:

- Establishing a climate of mutual respect and effective working relationships.
- Appreciating the value of others' perspectives on assessment and intervention.
- Communicating effectively regarding the consumer's needs, including scheduling.
- Cooperating in planning and providing cost-efficient, considerate services.
- Evaluating the outcomes of services and the consumer's satisfaction with care.

TEAM ROLES AND FUNCTIONS

Table 42-5 illustrates the interrelationships of group, individual, and situational characteristics on the team process. Team members play multiple roles on the team, often quite different from those specific to their discipline. As the team develops, personality, education, values, and experience interact to influence team members toward different roles. Skilled team leaders can use this phenomenon to benefit their team, and team members learn to rely on each other through the sharing of roles and responsibilities. Table 42-6 lists typical roles of team members.

SUMMARY

Effective teamwork and team building are essential processes in the profession of OT. They contribute to quality service delivery and morale, and they can also have a significant influence on reducing OT and OTA attrition. Teamwork qualities include cooperation, flexibility, and creativity. OT practitioners work with many different people to share information, coordinate schedules, and provide the most effective overall services. The basic needs of ministration, mastery, and maturation provide a theme that carries over into the developmental team chart, which presents a team building process organized according to specific developmental stages of teams. The identification of team characteristics, supervisor and member tasks, and communication issues provides a matrix that can serve as an important tool for improved team building.

Table 42-3
Developmental Team Chart

Stage of Team Development	Characteristics	Supervisor's Tasks	Team Members' Issues	Communication
I. Initiation Stage Exploration and definition of member roles and responsibilities within the context of team and work settings.	Prior to and in the beginning phase of team formation, individuals may experience self-doubt, role ambiguity, and a degree of powerlessness in the work setting.	Promote atmosphere of acceptance and trust: state expectations openly, encourage discussion of members' expectations. Encourage commitment to learn building by helping members: identify skills, areas of strength and interest, increase self-esteem. Provide general definition and direction for newly formed team: define situation and resources available, define roles/responsibilities for members.	Learn and explore role expectations. Begin to share resources, identify own areas of expertise and interests.	Express anxieties and insecurities of new relationships. Verbalize support for team efforts. Demonstrate acceptance and begin to develop trust.
II. Transition Stage Adjustment and rearrangement of roles to create a team.	Team members experience increased anxieties, defensiveness, and struggles for control. Reclarification and adjustments of roles are evident. Group norms are forming. Relationship issues are important at this stage.	Provide encouragement. Manage conflict openly. Provide structures for team to make decisions, solve problems, and set priorities. Effectuate intervention strategies if needed. Reclarify roles, team goals.	Develop skills, gain confidence. Learn about the organizational structure. Commit self to teamwork.	Begin to identify and deal with conflicts openly. Verbalize group norms and values. Encourage team affiliation by engaging in community building activities.
III. Working Stage Tasks are identified and achieved.	Team members experience cohesion and productivity. Conflicts are dealt with openly and are effectively managed.	Refine leadership skills. Allow team members more autonomy and support development of their professional skills. Provide liaison functions with the external organization. Help team members find solutions to difficult problems; provide resources and support services. Assess and evaluate work done relative to the team's overall performance.	Participate in the planning, decision-making, and execution of tasks. Clarify personal goals. Ask for direction/support from supervisor. Participate in task evaluation. Develop sense of mastery.	Communicate support and challenge members through feedback. Discuss how methods of problem solving, decision making, and conflict management occur in the team.
IV. Interdependence Stage Team members are effective in their work; achieve interdependence in their working relationships.	Team members are mutually supportive, take pride in the team, value each other, and experience the team as interlocking roles.	Model collegial relationships. Become a mentor; empower others. Continue to develop personal and professional skills.	Reflect on self as a professional, reassess goals, offer peer evaluations. Form multiple points of view. Take risks; achieve greater competency.	Express valuing of team members and demonstrate support for each other's achievements.
Separation Team separation occurs at any stage; however, characteristics and tasks will be different depending on the maturity of the team.	Team members experience anxiety as they anticipate separation. There is an awareness of the successes and failures of the team.	Ensure opportunity for and assist members in summarizing, integrating, and interpreting the team experience. Provide a framework that will help members evaluate the team effort/individual roles. Allow time for members to resolve unfinished business and express feelings about the separation.	Summarize the team experience and the attainment of personal and professional goals. Evaluate personal and team performance. Define tasks for new members.	Express separation feelings. Avoid withdrawal/distancing of members. Give and receive feedback; discuss effect of current experiences on future teams.

(Reprinted with permission from Blechert, T. F., Christiansen, M. F., & Kari, N. [1987]. Intraprofessional team building. Am J Occup Ther, 41, 576-582)

Table 42-4

Professionals Who Often Serve on Teams with Occupational Therapy Personnel

Physician

A physician is a medical doctor who practices the science and art of preventing and curing disease and preserving health. In most states, physicians must prescribe medical treatments such as medication, surgery, and therapy. Occupational therapy personnel work with physicians who have varying specialty backgrounds. These specialists may include physiatrists (physical medicine and rehabilitation), psychiatrists (mental illness), neurologists (nervous system disease), orthopedists (musculoskeletal), ophthalmologists (vision), pediatricians (children), gerontologists (elders), and many more.

Psychologist

The psychologist is not a medical doctor, although he or she may have a doctoral (PhD or EdD) degree. A clinical psychologist functions in three areas: diagnosis, psychotherapy, and research. The psychologist administers diagnostic tests and conducts interviews in order to best understand the nature of the patient's problem. Psychological tests involve presentation of standardized challenges or situations. The varied reactions of different patients may then be observed and compared to typical responses. Many people are reluctant to reveal their thoughts in an interview, but may show a characteristic way of thinking in response to tests. Psychotherapy, a specialized type of counseling, may be performed with individual patients or patient groups, and families may be involved. Many psychologists have a background in statistics and research methods, and may be prepared to assist staff members who wish to do research by helping construct, design, and conduct clinical research projects and interpret results.

Nurse

The nurse is concerned with the health of the consumer as well as his or her comfort and care if ill. This involves evaluating and addressing the patient's physical, spiritual, and emotional needs through established nursing procedures and techniques. Nurses are responsible for a variety of therapeutic measures prescribed and delegated by the physician (such as administering medications) and must be able to observe and evaluate patient symptoms, reactions, and progress. Education, support, and anticipatory guidance for the consumer are important aspects of nursing practice.

Social Worker

The role of the social worker is to act as a liaison between the consumer and the community in order to make the best use of the resources available. Social workers may work in public or private hospitals, clinics, community settings, schools, agencies, correctional institutions, and home health. Individuals may be referred to a social worker for help with financial problems, nursing home or other specialized placement, or to access other needed services and benefits. Social workers are also skilled in individual counseling and group work as well as community organization. They may provide both direct services and consultation related to psychosocial issues.

Speech and Language Pathologist

Speech pathologists are concerned with an individual's ability to communicate. This includes attention to his or her understanding of language as well as his or her expression of ideas. Speech and language pathologists have background in learning and cognition, communication, and oral sensory and motor function. They may collaborate with occupational therapy personnel in any number of areas. Some typical speech and OT collaborations might include development of a nonverbal communication system, therapeutic feeding programs, and cognitive rehabilitative strategies. Speech pathologists are also concerned with auditory (hearing) ability and work closely with audiologists. The audiologist may also serve on the interdisciplinary team.

Physical Therapist

Physical therapists provide services for patients with disabilities resulting from disease or injury. Their focus is on mobility. Various modalities are used in physical therapy, including light therapy, which involves ultraviolet and infrared light; electrotherapy, which may involve diathermy and electrical stimulation; hydrotherapy, which includes equipment such as the Hubbard tank, whirlpool, and contrast baths; mechanical therapy, which involves massage, traction, and therapeutic exercise of various kinds; and thermotherapy, which involves heat such as paraffin baths and whirlpool. The purpose of physical therapy may be to relieve pain, to increase function of a

Table 42-4, continued

Professionals Who Often Serve on Teams with Occupational Therapy Personnel

body part by improving muscle strength and joint range of motion, to increase overall strength and endurance, or to improve mobility. Physical therapists assist people to be mobile with and without assistive devices. They are skilled in the use of wheelchairs, adaptive seating and positioning, walkers, crutches, canes, and other posture and mobility aides. They frequently collaborate with occupational therapy personnel.

Therapeutic Recreation Specialist

A therapeutic recreation specialist uses play, leisure, exercise, and other activities to meet individual needs. For example, for some people, group recreation may encourage positive relationships with others, improve body image, allow an outlet for emotional release, aid circulation and other body functions, and provide enjoyment and relaxation. Some activities used in therapeutic recreation are swimming, music, games and conduct dancing, dramatics, special events, and outings. Leisure counseling is also provided.

Vocational Rehabilitation Counselor

A person may need assistance in selecting appropriate and meaningful work or changing careers as a result of his or her illness or injury. For instance, a truck driver who has had a heart attack may need to find a job with less physical demands and stressors. A high school student may need help with career planning and with adaptations for college classes or job training programs. The vocational rehabilitation counselor may administer standardized tests, interest inventories, and aptitude tests as well as personal interviews in order to develop individualized plans for training and job placement. The OT and OTA may work with the vocational counselor in evaluating the work readiness, tolerance, coordination, and special skills.

Nutritionist/Dietician

The function of the nutritionist is to advise about (e.g., for people living on their own) or actually manage (e.g., in the hospital setting) the preparation and serving of food for consumers. This includes understanding complex nutritional needs and planning and preparing special diets. The nutritionist considers the caloric value, nutrient content, attractiveness, taste, and texture of foods and drinks. Occupational therapy personnel collaborate with nutrition staff in many ways—from the use of adaptive eating utensils and techniques to the preparation of nutritious meals and snacks to decisions about the texture of foods (so as to diminish risks such as swallowing problems or drooling).

Educator

The educator is concerned with the individual's learning. Educators are also known as teachers and have varied educational backgrounds. For example, some teachers are trained to work with children at certain ages and grade levels in schools; others are trained to work with young children and their families. Some educators have specialized knowledge in inclusion, reading, language, arts, music, etc. Their expertise and experience in creating environments and activities that promote learning and understanding is essential to the development of children and adults. Occupational therapy personnel often collaborate with educators on such areas as curriculum design, activity analysis, environmental modification, and special educational or instructional strategies.

Table 42-5

Team Dynamics

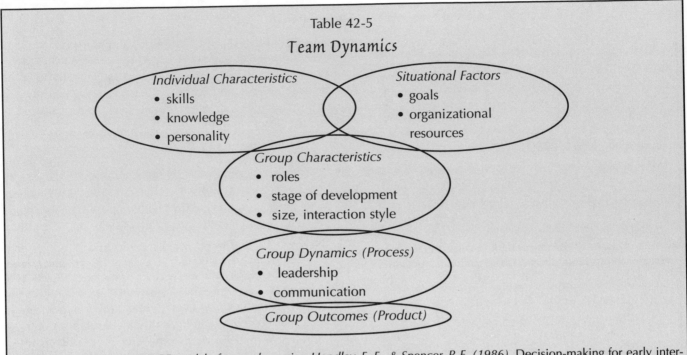

Individual Characteristics
- skills
- knowledge
- personality

Situational Factors
- goals
- organizational resources

Group Characteristics
- roles
- stage of development
- size, interaction style

Group Dynamics (Process)
- leadership
- communication

Group Outcomes (Product)

Adapted from Project BRIDGE model of team dynamics. Handley, E. E., & Spencer, P. E. (1986). Decision-making for early intervention services: A team approach. Elk Grove, IL: American Academy of Pediatrics.

Table 42-6

Roles of Team Members

Clarifier: Makes sure that the proposed plans are clear to everyone

Compromiser: Makes accommodations to others, especially in conflict situations

Consensus tester: Determines the team readiness to make decisions or take action

Elaborator: Makes sure that proposed plans are fully evaluated

Encourager: Praises others for their efforts and contributions

Energizer: Motivates the team into action

Gatekeeper: Makes certain that all team members have an opportunity to express their opinions

Harmonizer: Mediates conflicts on the team

Information gatherer: Collects information that is relevant to the issues

Initiator: Brings issues to the attention of the team

Observer: Provides constructive feedback on team dynamics and performance

Standard setter: Helps the team establish guidelines for the activities

Summarizer: Reviews all aspects of team issues and ideas

Tension reliever: Uses humor or changes in routine to reduce or avoid negative interactions

Acknowledgments

Ellen Rainville would like to gratefully acknowledge the important influence that her friend and colleague Joanne Miller has had on her understanding of collaboration between OTs and OTAs.

References

AOTA. (1991, June). Member data survey: Executive summary. *OT Week, 6.*

Beggs, D. (Ed.). (1962). *Team coaching: Bold new venture.* Indianapolis, IN: United College Press.

Blechert, T. F., & Christiansen, M. F. (1986). Intraprofessional relationships and socialization: The maturation process. In S. E. Ryan, (Ed.), *The COTA: Roles and responsibilities.* Thorofare, NJ: SLACK Incorporated.

Blechert, T. F., Christiansen, M. F., & Kari, N. (1987). Intraprofessional team building. *Am J Occup Ther, 41,* 576-582.

Briggs, M. H. (1997). *Building early intervention teams: Working together for children and families.* Gaithersburg, MD: Aspen.

Brown, W., Thurman, S. K., & Pearl, L. F. (1993). *Family centered early intervention with infants and toddlers: Innovative cross disciplinary approaches.* Baltimore, MD: Brookes.

Bull, N. (1976). *Teamwork: Working together in the human services.* New York, NY: J. B. Lippincott.

Corey, G. (1981). *Theory and practice of group counseling.* Monterey, CA: Brooks/Cole.

Crepeau, E. B. (1991). Achieving intersubjective understanding: Examples from an OT treatment session. *Am J Occup Ther, 45,* 1016-1025.

Dunn, W., Campbell, P., Oetter, P., Hall, S., Berger, E., & Stickland, L. R. (1989). *Guidelines for OT services in early intervention and preschool settings.* Rockville, MD: AOTA.

Dunst, C., Trivette, C., & Deal, A. (1988). *Enabling and empowering families: Principles and guidelines for practice.* Cambridge, MA: Brookline Books.

Gardner, H. G. (1988). *Helping others through teamwork.* Washington, DC: Child Welfare League of America.

Grady, A. P. (1990). Nationally speaking—Collaborative relationships: Opportunities for OT in the 1990's and beyond. *Am J Occup Ther, 44*(2), 105-108..

Guiffrida, C. (1991, December). Partnerships for change: Collaboration within and between professions. *Sensory Integration Special Interest Section Newsletter, 14*(4).

Hagberg, J. (1984). *Real power: Stages of personal power in organizations.* Minneapolis, MN: Winston Press.

Heming, D. (1988). The titanic triumvirate: Teams, teamwork and team building. *Canadian Journal of OT, 55*(1), 15-20.

Henneman, E. A., Lee, J. L., & Cohen, J. I. (1995). Collaboration: A concept analysis. *Journal of Advanced Nursing, 21,* 103-109.

Levinson, H. (1962). *Men, management and mental health.* Cambridge, MA: Harvard University Press.

Magrab, P., Elder, J., Kazuk, E., Pelosi, J., & Wiegerink, R. (1981). *Developing a community team.* Washington, DC: Georgetown University.

Napier, R. W., & Gershenfeld, M. K. (1983). *Making groups work.* Boston, MA: Houghton Mifflin Co.

Navarra, T., Lipkowitz, M. A., & Navarra, J. G. (1990). *Therapeutic communication: A guide to effective interpersonal skills for health care professionals.* Thorofare, NJ: SLACK Incorporated.

Rosin, P., Wjitehead, A. D., Tuchman, L. I., Jesien, G. S., Begun, A. l., & Irwin, L. (1996). *Partnerships in family centered care: A guide to collaborative early intervention.* Baltimore, MD: Paul Brookes.

Scheller, M. D. (1990). *Building partnerships in health care.* Palo Alto, CA: Bull Publishing.

Spencer, P. (1989). Team dynamics relative to exemplary early services. In B. E. Hanft (Ed.), *Family centered care* (pp. 4-43-4-50). Rockville, MD: AOTA.

Stewart, K. (1990). Collaborating with families: Reflections on empowerment. In B. E. Hanft (Ed.), *Family centered care.* Rockville, MD: AOTA.

Suggested Reading

Alpert, H. B., Goldman, L. D., Kilroy, C.M. & Pike, A.W. (1992). 7 Gryzmish: Toward an understanding of collaboration. *Nursing Clinics of North America., 27,* 47-59.

Fluegelman, A. (1976). *The new games book.* New York, NY: Doubleday.

Heerman, B. (1997). *Building team spirit: Activities for inspiring and energizing teams.* New York, NY: McGraw-Hill.

Rainville, E. B. (1997). Working with members of a treatment team. In K. Sladyk (Ed.), *OT student primer: A guide to college success* (pp. 159-170). Thorofare, NJ: SLACK Incorporated.

Scannel, E., & Newstrom, J. W. (1998). *The big book of team building games: Trust-building activities, team spirit exercises, and other fun things to do.* New York, NY: McGraw-Hill.

Management Issues and Models

Chapter 43

Christopher J. Leary, M.Div, MS, LPC, LADC

INTRODUCTION

The purpose of this chapter is to help the reader understand the multiple structures or models in which the OT practitioner will perform the duties of a human service professional in the practice of OT. Another word that we use to indicate a structure or model or context is paradigm.

Everything we do, whether in school, at work, or at home, is done within a specific context or paradigm. Life would be quite empty and meaningless if we did not have a specific paradigm or context in which we lived our daily lives and performed our daily tasks. In its simplest definition, paradigm can be defined as a model. Freud and Jung developed very specific theories to help understand the human psyche. These particular theories can be held up as paradigms or models in which we come to understand the human psyche from the point of view of each psychoanalyst. To carry this understanding of paradigm one step further, we could say that, in the Freudian paradigm, sexuality plays a significant role, while spirituality is more prominent in the Jungian paradigm. In addition, there can be multiple contexts or paradigms attached to a specific act or set of actions and behaviors.

When we define *service operations*, we are essentially defining the context or paradigm in which the practice of OT will take place. Therefore, we define service operations as the paradigm of OT practice that involves planning, structuring, organizing, and evaluating the practice of OT services within a specific environment. It must be noted that this paradigm has evolved dramatically over the past few years because of the demands of managed care companies who strive to reduce costs for insurance carriers by continually shifting the context in which they will pay for OT services. Many hospitals that have had fully staffed

KEY CONCEPTS

- Record keeping and data analysis: Used to document and evaluate program quality.
- Reimbursement procedures: Insurance companies, Medicare, and Medicaid are considered third party payers for services rendered by the OT practitioner.
- Accreditation: Verification by an independent organization who is qualified to verify that the health care facility and the OT department itself meet the minimum standard of care.
- Program evaluation and quality assurance: Maintaining quality programs.
- Continuing education: Ensuring that staff stays competent.
- Public relations: Developing community interrelationships.

ESSENTIAL VOCABULARY

Cost-effectiveness: Efficient utilization of goods, self, and personnel.

Fee-for-service: Paid according to face-to-face service rendered.

Indirect patient care activities: Scheduling, setting up, supervision, documentation, meetings, education, etc.

Inservice training: Educational services provided by the health care facility or independent organizations (public and private).

Malpractice: Performing tasks and/or duties in such a way that causes harm to the patient and/or others.

Negligence: Omitting tasks and/or duties that ought to have been performed.

Paradigm: Structure or model.

Risk management: Following established policy and procedure regarding risk in the work setting.

Science-based: Procedures utilized that have been proven effective via appropriate scientific research methodologies.

Service operations: Departmental/facility management.

OT departments in the past have been forced to combine departments and reduce staffing by merging many of the rehabilitation services under one department manager who may or may not be experienced in OT.

Managed care has had a major impact across all areas of health care. Hospitals, physicians, nurses, pharmacies, and all other health care providers are significantly affected by the decisions of managed care companies. It is vitally important to keep in mind the role that these managed care companies play as you continue to grow as a professional in your practice of OT.

This discussion of managed care is not intended to dishearten the reader. As you train to become a human service professional as an OT practitioner, you must seek ways to be innovative and adapt your skills and your art to health care in the new millennium.

SCHEDULING

Scheduling time for provision of OT services and for attendance at staff and departmental meetings as well as supervisory meetings is absolutely essential for the OT practitioner. Scheduling is often re-framed as "time management." Learning to manage your time in a demanding environment is what will ultimately define your success as a professional health care provider.

Many health care providers that were once paid according to a salaried structure are now paid according to a fee-for-service paradigm. In other words, they are paid only for the face-to-face time that they spend with the patient. All other administrative duties, paperwork, meetings, etc., are done on the provider's own time. Payment for services rendered is not given until the administrative paperwork is submitted to the health care facility.

RECORDING AND REPORTING

Documentation

We have a saying in the health care field, "If it isn't documented, it didn't happen." You can be the best OTA in the world but if you do not document your work accurately, your work does not exist to supervisory staff, administration, site reviewers, funding sources, and managed care companies. Your work becomes meaningless without appropriate documentation. As an OT practitioner, documentation is essential to the highest quality of care that you can provide for your patients. Indeed, all health care professionals ought to maintain accurate and complete records of treatment protocols with all assigned patients. All interactions with collateral service providers, whether verbal, written, or electronic, must be documented as well and kept as part of the medical record of the respective patient.

Evaluations, treatment plan with long- and short-term goals, objectives, methodology, progress notes, and a discharge summary are all appropriate forms of written documentation to be included in the patient's chart. Other documents to be included in the record are copies of written instructions given to the patient and/or the patient's family from OT services for implementation following discharge. Records of any equipment issued to the patient and the patient's family, along with instructions for use, must also be documented in the patient's medical record.

Treatment goals, whether long- or short-term, must be attainable and measurable. The objectives and the methodology indicate the structure for goal attainment. Because the treatment plan is structured in such a way, it becomes a dynamic document. It should continually be amended to reflect the progress that is made according to the established treatment protocol.

Technology has also advanced the practice of OT in areas of electronic documentation. Many health care facilities are converting from paper documentation to electronic. Bits of data are much easier to store than reams of paper in manila folders in large file cabinets. Traditional paper files were easier to protect under lock and key with respect to confidentiality. However, electronic data can be safeguarded against potential violations of confidentiality via appropriate use of passwords and secure data file storage. Many funding sources and managed care companies are requiring electronic submission of clinical data for quality assurance and reimbursement. Therefore, you as an OT practitioner would do well to familiarize yourself with current trends in computer clinical record keeping as well as the more traditional style of paper record keeping.

PREPARATION, MAINTENANCE, AND SAFETY OF THE WORK SETTING

The provision of OT, and indeed all health care, must take place in an environment that is clean and safe for the provision of such services. Health care facilities must adhere to strict codes of safety and hygiene in order to be licensed to operate by local and state authorities. In addition, the Americans with Disabilities Act requires that health care facilities provide optimum access for all people including those who require wheelchairs and other aids for mobility. Doorways, bathrooms, and offices must be able to accommodate the handicapped patient or staff person. In managing the environment of care, the health care facility should strive to provide a setting that is safe, effective, and accessible for all individuals who are served, all other staff members, and the public who have opportunity to enter the facility.

The Joint Commission on Accreditation of Healthcare Organizations (JCAHO) (1996) cites the following processes that are considered essential to managing the environment of care:

- Planning by organization leaders for the space, equipment, and resources needed to safely support the services provided. Planning and design are consistent with the organization's mission, vision, and values.
- Educating staff about the role of the environment in safely and effectively supporting care. The organization educates staff about physical characteristics and processes for environmental monitoring and reporting.
- Developing performance standards to measure staff and organization performance in managing the environment of care.
- Carrying out plans to create and manage the organization's environment of care. An information collection and evaluation system (ICES) is developed and used to continuously measure, assess, and improve the status of the environment of care.
- Reduce and control environmental hazards and risk.
- Prevent accidents and injuries.
- Maintain safe conditions for individuals served, visitors, and staff (JCAHO, 1996).

Environmental Considerations

It is the responsibility of the facility or hospital in which the OT department is situated to ensure that the environment for service is appropriate and safe. It is the responsibility of the individual OT practitioner to bring to the attention of supervisors and management any issues, circumstances, or situations that might compromise safety in any way for patients, staff, and the public in general. Safety is the responsibility of all employees of the organization.

Maintaining a safe environment requires that the health care professional be mindful of what types of things or behaviors compromise safety for patients, staff, and others. Such things as infection control procedures, universal precautions, storage of toxic chemicals and flammable substances, and knowledge of departmental and facility emergency and fire procedures are just some of the issues necessary to help maintain safety on the job for the OT.

The Department of Public Health and organizations for accreditation, such as JCAHO, require that health care facilities have a portion of the formal policy and procedure manual of the facility dedicated to risk management. In fact, it is ideal to identify a group of people who will

serve as the risk management committee for the organization. This committee has several responsibilities and tasks that fall within the scope of effective risk management. The first task is to set the policy regarding risk management for the facility. The board of directors must approve all policies for the facility. Once approved, the risk management policy must be distributed to all staff and patients. This can be done through posters, flyers, handouts, and formal orientation. All incidences of problems, regardless of how slight, must be documented and filed for review by the risk management committee. It is the risk management committee that makes recommendations to the administration for changes within the structure of the organization to help reduce risk of harm to any individual. The first rule of any health care professional is *primum non nocere,* that is, "First, do no harm." This rule extends and applies to the organizations that facilitate health care service as well. Risk management is the practical application of *primum non nocere* to the entire health care organization.

Emergency procedures must be clearly defined in departmental and facility policy and procedure manuals. In addition, emergency plans for evacuation in case of fire or other emergency must be clearly posted in every room of the facility. Directives for exiting the facility must be posted in all languages appropriate to the demographics of the facility. For example, if the facility is located in a city in which there is a high Latino population, then it is appropriate to have all signs and directives for emergency evacuation posted in both English and Spanish.

Since food preparation is sometimes part of the OT's treatment protocol, the proper storage and preparation of food becomes critical to preventing the growth and spread of bacteria. Therefore, infection control becomes an integral part of the OT practitioner's daily practice and agenda. One of the most effective means of preventing the spread of bacteria is through the washing of hands. Our hands are continually coming into contact with bacteria. For example, every time we touch a doorknob, money, table, chairs, or paper, our hands become reliable and efficient carriers in the spread of bacteria. It is a known fact that colds and viruses can be spread through the casual rubbing of one's eyes with unwashed hands. Use of hair nets, along with proper cooking and refrigeration of food, are essential to good infection control in the OT kitchen. In addition, some patients require strict infection control procedures because of compromised immune systems. Other patients may present a risk for infecting others because of the nature of their particular diseases. Some diseases that pose a threat to infecting others are hepatitis, herpes, AIDS, and urinary and respiratory infections.

MANAGING SUPPLIES

Escalating costs of health care and the decreasing responsibility and accountability of third party payers have resulted in large OT departments giving way to more compact services in smaller departments. In the current health care climate, it becomes imperative that OTs learn to manage supplies and inventory, as well as time, in the most cost-efficient manner. Although the responsibility for inventory management usually falls to some part of the administration, the OTA can participate in this very important part of departmental management. Input from direct care staff is very important in deciding which materials are absolutely essential for effective and efficient provision of OT services.

REIMBURSEMENT PROCEDURES

The budget for the OT department is usually closely managed by departmental administration. The budget is essentially a plan that analyzes the expected income for the department and/or facility as well as what expenses and costs might be incurred during a set period of time, usually the fiscal year. The budget is necessary to run the department and facility efficiently. Income generated by fees and monies that are given to the department by the facility are listed as revenues on the budget. Salaries, supplies, and other costs are listed under the expense side of the budget. The budget must balance and be approved by the appropriate authority prior to the onset of the fiscal year.

All businesses and health care facilities operate according to a budget. Accreditation organizations like to see input from staff in the development of the departmental or facility budget. Therefore, it is good to see documented in the departmental meeting notes that some time was set aside for budget development with staff. As a staff OT practitioner, you can provide input into the types of capital expenditures that need to be made in such areas as major pieces of equipment, departmental furniture, and training.

OT is considered a service that generates revenues for the facility. Because it is an income-generating service, it is critical that appropriate charges be accurate for the services rendered. In addition, the charges must agree with the documentation of the actual service. Many health care facilities have lost income because money had to be returned to a third party payer, such as Medicare, because the individual therapist was not clear in documentation as to what service was actually provided. The charge for the service was appropriate but the documentation did not support the charge. As stated previously, "If it isn't documented, it didn't happen."

Medicare and Medicaid are federally funded entitlements that provide medical insurance benefits under Title XVII and Title XIX of the Social Security Act. Medicare provides benefits primarily for the aged and the disabled, while Medicaid provides medical insurance benefits to those on welfare. Over the past few years, there has been an increasing trend in most states to move people off of the welfare rolls into gainful employment. Many states have set term limits to receive welfare benefits and will terminate needy people from the welfare program regardless of need if they have not secured gainful employment by the end of the term limit. Historically, Medicaid provided reimbursement to health care facilities but set the amounts that would be reimbursed. In contrast, Medicare would reimburse a health care facility at whatever it cost the facility to provide the service or services. Needless to say, many problems arose across the spectrum of health care related to Medicare reimbursement and fraud. Because of such abuses in the Medicare system, Medicare has tightened up on what services it considers reimbursable and Medicaid dollars have come under the fiscal authority of managed care companies in several different states resulting in fewer reimbursable services for the poorer segments of our society.

The Tax Equity and Fiscal Responsibility Act of 1982 and the Balanced Budget Act of 1997 brought about changes in how hospitals and other health care facilities were to be reimbursed by Medicare. Health care facilities were now subject to limits on reimbursement from Medicare. In addition, reimbursement is limited according to diagnostic-related groups. This resulted in a fixed cost to be reimbursed for an episode of illness, and the number of reimbursable treatments and/or treatment days in the health care facility would be limited.

Since these entitlements are coming more and more under the managed care umbrella, OT as well as other traditionally reimbursed services are not getting sufficient funds reimbursed for services rendered. The end result is that fewer medical benefits are given to those who have the most need, the elderly and the economically disadvantaged.

ACCREDITATION

Health care facilities are regulated and licensed according to local and state laws. In order to be licensed, the health care facility must adhere to the regulations for which the facility is licensed. In addition to governmental licensing and regulation, many health care facilities seek accreditation with a well-known certifying body. JCAHO is one such certifying body. JCAHO is a private, voluntary nonprofit organization that is made up of representatives from the American Hospital Association, the American College of Physicians, the American Medical Association, and the American College of Surgeons. A hospital, for example, that is preparing for a site visit from

JCAHO will hold multiple training sessions for all staff. The president and CEO, physicians, nurses, pharmacy staff, rehabilitation staff, including all occupation therapy staff, housekeeping staff, and food preparation staff are all targeted during a site visit. Every aspect of health care is monitored and scored. Once approved for certification, the hospital will proudly display a certificate that indicates certification by the joint commission.

In addition to JCAHO, the Commission on Accreditation of Rehabilitation Facilities (CARF) regulates the provision of rehabilitation services for disabled people. CARF is similar to JCAHO but differs in that it focuses primarily on rehabilitation services for the disabled.

PROGRAM EVALUATION

Program evaluation is the process of gathering data about a program by measuring clinical outcomes through formal surveys as well as other more traditional means of information retrieval. This process presents factual information for staff, administration, and the community about the quality and efficiency of the program. More and more funding sources in the nonprofit sector are demanding that outcomes studies be completed and results submitted to them on a regular basis. If the results slip below a statewide standard, then funding for such services may be reduced in the future.

MEETINGS

Official Documents of AOTA (AOTA, 2000) supports employee meetings of OT departmental staff members, both OT and OTA, for the following purposes:

1. Disseminating and receiving information.
2. Conveying information about the administrative policies of the institution or conditions of employment.
3. Discussing issues relevant to the management of the program.
4. Discussing issues relating to the development of the department or institution and its relationship to total health care.

All staff member have the responsibility to read, understand, and know the policies and procedures of the department and facility in which they are working. The employer has an obligation to introduce the individual staff member to the written policies and procedures, but it is the staff member's responsibility to learn them and know such policies and procedures. Accreditation organizations such as JCAHO or CARF want to see documented staff input into the development of departmental and facility policies and procedures. The staff meeting is an ideal place for this input to occur. Policies and procedures can be discussed and fine-tuned according to professional ethics and current treatment trends. Attendance at departmental and facility meetings is usually mandatory and is considered part of the professional responsibility of the individual staff person.

Supervision of the individual OTA by the OT may take place in a highly structured format or less structured. The need of the patients relative to the practice of the individual OTA will dictate the level of supervision to be utilized.

CONTINUING EDUCATION AND INSERVICE TRAINING

Continuing education and training for the OT are as essential to the professional life of the OT as food and water is to the biological life of the person. The practice of being a health care professional demands that each person maintains state-of-the-art knowledge about the theory and practice of OT. It is not sufficient that the accrediting organizations require a minimum number of hours of continuing education per year but you, as a professional person who cares for others, should require this of yourself. Reading the most current literature and journal articles can keep you tuned in to the latest trends in OT and its application. Inservice training is a wonderful opportunity to log in training hours at minimal cost to you personally. In addition, a training day presents opportunities for networking and marketing your department, facility, and yourself as a qualified OT health care professional in the community.

PUBLIC RELATIONS

Effective public relations for OT, as a health care discipline, is more important now than ever before. Over the past few years, managed care companies have consistently reduced the amount of money that they will reimburse health care facilities for OT services. This has resulted in many layoffs of qualified OT practitioners. Unfortunately, one of the most gripping realities of our current health care climate is that health care has become a commodity on the stock market. Regardless of how many times or in whatever creative ways they frame their existence, managed care companies do not manage care. They manage costs for care. They continually challenge the OT as well as all health care providers to come up with creative ways to provide the most effective treatment for the least amount of dollars so that the stockholders will continue to profit. Good public relations and effective marketing strategies are very important in this environment.

Despite some of the disagreeable issues that managed care companies have created for the provider of health care services, we should not overlook the good that has resulted from managed care. Unethical providers of care are now forced to adhere to rigid standards for provision of services. OT providers who have been faced with opportunities to find newer and more efficient ways of providing treatment in a cost-conscious environment have done so. Indeed, OT itself can be effectively integrated into a broader range of treatment settings and across other domains of health care than previously utilized (e.g., outpatient substance abuse and mental health treatment).

Research is a formalized investigation of activities for the purposes of improving the quality of OT patient care by means of recognized scientific methodologies and procedures. More and more governmental funding sources for nonprofit health care facilities are requiring hard data for quality assurance as well as research. Science-based programming is becoming the operative word in grant writing and public funding allocations. More and more weight is given to the programs that utilize science-based protocols and treatment practices. Historically, the average OT or OTA has not been oriented toward research and science-based treatment protocols. Charles Christiansen (1983), in an editorial written for the *OT Journal of Research* states that "…research continues to be viewed commonly as an activity foreign to our clients (patients) and irrelevant to our practice" (p. 195). He asserts that OTs will have difficulty in a competitive marketplace with dwindling resources if there is no research to validate the efficacy and value of the services provided.

Despite the fact that more intensive research skills are taught at the graduate level, it is imperative that all OTs and OTAs understand the basic skills associated with research and science-based treatment protocols.

SUMMARY

It is important for all OT practitioners to have an understanding of the structure and process involved in the administration and management of the department and facility in which they are working. Such skills as knowing how to manage time through effective scheduling of activities, maintaining appropriate documentation of records, and preparing and maintaining safety in the work area are essential and highly marketable skills for the OT. The OTA can be involved in such activities as quality assurance, program evaluation, and the process of accreditation via JCAHO or CARF.

Although service operations and management are functions reserved to the administration of the department and/or the facility as a whole, the process must be supported at the point of service delivery by direct care staff such as the OTs and OTAs. Care and pride in one's work at all levels of the institution affects every part of the health care facility and the care of patients.

REFERENCES

AOTA (2000). *Official documents of AOTA*. Bethesda, MD: Author.

Christiansen, C. (1983). An economic imperative. *OT Journal of Research, 37,* 195-198.

Joint Commission on Accreditation of Healthcare Organizations. (1996). *Comprehensive Accreditation Manual for Behavioral Health Care* (p. 401). Oakbrook Terrace, IL: Author.

Professional Development and Socialization

Chapter 44

Anne Birge James, MS, OTR
Marijke Kehrhahn, MA, PhD

INTRODUCTION

This chapter describes the processes by which the OTA develops and maintains competence, the combination of knowledge and skill necessary to provide excellent client care. *Professional socialization* is an interactive process that occurs through experiences. By developing learning relationships and engaging in learning activities, the OTA, whether a student or a specialist, continually enhances his or her knowledge and skills. Learning relationships and learning activities often present themselves in the process of solving clinical problems and expanding clinical knowledge into new areas.

As OTAs move through the phases of education, fieldwork, entry-level practice, job change, and specialization, they form relationships with educators, supervisors, mentors, fellow professionals, and clients with whom they will learn a great deal about the practice of OT. Continuing professional development activities, both formal and informal, will contribute to the OTA's competence and socialization. OTAs who have an open attitude toward learning are able to assess their skills and to plan for their ongoing development, which will successfully help them meet the learning challenges associated with becoming and remaining a competent practitioner.

COMPETENCE IN OCCUPATIONAL THERAPY PRACTICE

Mastering the knowledge and skills of OT practice is an important part of becoming a competent OTA. Gaining knowledge and skills is the focus of OT coursework and

---

KEY CONCEPTS

- Maintaining competence as a way of life: Adopting an attitude and a set of principles that give priority to the continual development of knowledge and skills.
- Supervision: A one-to-one process of goal setting, observation, coaching, and evaluation designed to promote professional competence.
- Learning relationships: Relationships with educators, supervisors, fellow professionals, and clients that provide opportunities for learning.
- Learning activity: Formal/informal activities that promote professional learning.
- Learning focus: The emphasis of learning at different phases of the professional socialization process.
- Professional development plan: A framework for individual assessment, goal setting, and planning for continuous professional development.
- Phases of professional socialization: The stages that the COTA goes through to become a fully competent professional.

ESSENTIAL VOCABULARY

Career breakpoint: A time of significant change in one's professional life.

Competence: Ability to apply knowledge and skills to perform successfully as an OT practitioner.

Continuing professional development: Planning, activities, and requirements to facilitate ongoing growth and development of OT professionals.

External adjustment: Changes in other professionals' knowledge, skills, or attitudes that result from a learning situation.

Internal adjustment: Changes in individual beliefs or behavior that result from a learning situation.

Mentor: A senior professional who acts as a role model to foster professional orientation and growth in a new professional.

Professional socialization: The personal development/social learning process by which a COTA develops into a fully competent professional.

Strategic compliance: A decision to comply with demands in the environment but retain different views concerning appropriate treatment strategies.

fieldwork. Competence, however, also involves skills beyond the body of knowledge of OT and includes professional behaviors such as interpersonal, organizational, and problem-solving skills (Fidler, 1996; May, et al., 1995; Youngstrom, 1998).

Competence can be defined as a complex interaction and integration of knowledge, judgment, higher-order reasoning, personal qualities, skills, values, and beliefs. Professional competence also embodies the ability to generalize competence or transfer and apply skills and knowledge from one situation and environment to another (Australian Association of OTs, 1994, p. 1).

The terms *interaction* and *integration* used in this definition emphasize the importance of combining knowledge and skills with professional behaviors so that the OTA can provide excellent client care.

Meeting the OT course requirements, successfully completing fieldwork, and passing the NBCOT certification examination are all methods of establishing initial competence. The profession of OT, however, is continually changing and evolving to meet the demands of the clients, the health care system, and society (Hinojosa & Blount, 1998). Expansion of technology and information occurs rapidly, constantly altering and improving the theories and techniques used by OT practitioners. Some areas of OT practice are becoming more specialized, requiring in-depth, complex knowledge and skills (Youngstrom, 1998). The constantly changing face of OT practice means that OT practitioners must frequently update their knowledge and skills to maintain competency after graduation. The following examples demonstrate just a few of the recent changes in OT practice.

- In 1977, there were five special interest sections in the AOTA. In 1998, that number had increased to 11 with two subsections (Youngstrom, 1998), supporting the notion that OT practice is becoming more specialized.

- Fifteen years ago, it would have been unusual to have a client with a personal computer. Now, it is important for the OTA to be familiar with computers as it is a common and important ADL for many clients.

- The World Wide Web was not readily available in 1994. Practitioners in the early 1990s did not require skills in accessing computer networks, which were of limited scope and typically not accessible from home. Now the Internet offers a tremendous range of potential services for people with disabilities, including shopping, communication, education, and social support. OT practitioners have a responsibility to be aware of the ways in which the Internet may be used to enhance function in the clients they serve.

- Practice settings have changed dramatically over the past 20 years. In the early 1980s, most OT practitioners worked in institutionalized settings, such as hospitals and nursing homes. Today, many work in community settings, including schools, outpatient clinics, and homes. The OTA in community practice is more likely to be treating clients without immediate access to an OT or other team member. Community practice requires more skill in independent problem-solving, decision-making, and collaboration with clients and family.

Competence, then, is not a place one arrives at when training is complete, but is, instead, a life-long process. Developing initial competency is typically a joint venture between academic and clinical educators and the student. The educators play a primary role in determining what should be learned and the student works hard to learn the knowledge and skills presented by the educator. The focus is on the basic skills needed to begin practicing as an OTA. Continued competency, however, cannot be so easily defined because it is not "generic." It must be determined based on the needs of the individual OTA, the clients served, the practice setting, and the profession as a whole. Maintaining competence, then, becomes the responsibility of the individual practitioner. Several documents written by the AOTA describe the practitioner as having a personal responsibility for maintaining competence (AOTA, 1993, 1994a, 1994b), suggesting that the OTA who does not participate in activities to maintain competence is not meeting the standards of professional practice. Fortunately, there are many ways to maintain clinical competence, many of which occur within the normal workday.

PROFESSIONAL SOCIALIZATION

The development and maintenance of competence occurs through a process called professional socialization. Schempp and Graber (1992) describe professional socialization as an interactive process that occurs through experiences (Figure 44-1). Experiences continually challenge our knowledge and assumptions or present us with a problem that cannot be solved with our current knowledge and skills. Finding a way to resolve these problems helps us to enhance our knowledge and skills, expanding our repertoire for future clinical practice. Learning relationships and learning activities can help us resolve the conflict or solve the problem.

The solution to the problem usually occurs in one of three ways (Schempp & Graber, 1992). The first approach is an *internal adjustment* in which the individual's beliefs or behaviors change based on what he or she has learned. The second approach occurs when the individual is able to bring new knowledge or skills to the sit-

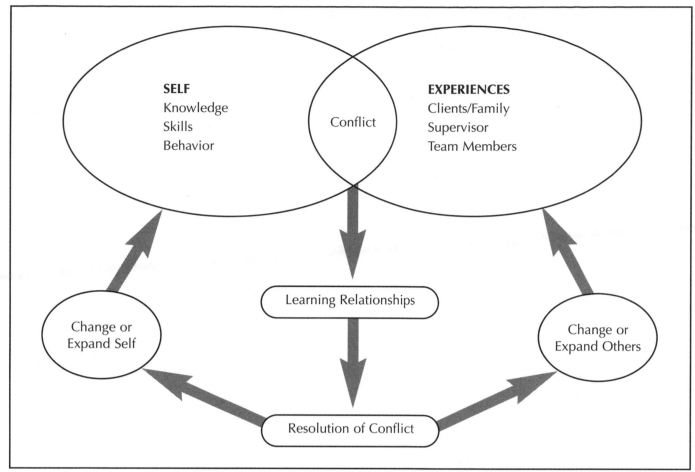

Figure 44-1. The process of professional socialization.

uation, resulting in an *external adjustment* (i.e., a change in others' knowledge, skills, or behavior). The third approach, *strategic compliance*, occurs when the individual complies with demands in the environment (i.e., changes his or her behavior) but continues to retain different views concerning appropriate treatment strategies. Because strategic compliance requires action that is in opposition with one's views and beliefs, it should not be considered as a long-term solution to a problem. It is, however, a useful strategy when the environment will change (e.g., the practitioner is leaving or a client or co-worker is leaving) or in a situation in which an external adjustment is possible, but will require time. In this case, it is better to comply with the recommended approach and work to make the changes necessary to apply a more effective approach in the future. The following is an example of the professional socialization process in action.

David was taught in school that a person with right-sided weakness from a stroke should use a stand-pivot transfer toward the left whenever possible because it is easier. During his clinical experience, however, he sees his clinical instructor transfer a client with right-sided weakness toward the right and she has the client squat rather

than stand. This transfer looks very different to him from what he was taught. It presents a *conflict* or problem for him to solve. Does he use the knowledge and skills he has or does he abandon them for this "new" way? He decides to investigate the problem with his clinical instructor. He describes to her what he learned about transfers in school and the differences he observed in the transfer approach she used. He has established a *learning relationship*. David's clinical instructor tells him that what he learned in school is one valid approach to transfers, but she is trying a different method with this patient based on an approach called neurodevelopmental treatment (NDT). She explains a little about the approach and gives David some handouts and articles to read that describe it further. She gives him a videotape about the transfer technique. These are examples of *learning activities*. David does his homework before his next fieldwork experience and comes to understand that there is more than one way to transfer someone with right-sided weakness. He has expanded his knowledge. He asks his clinical instructor to teach him how to do the NDT transfer, and this activity helps him to expand his skills. Now David has two transfer techniques to use. Further learning activities will help him to learn which technique to use under which circumstances. This is an example of professional socialization that led to an internal adjustment (i.e., a change in the person presented with the problem).

An example of professional socialization that results in external adjustment in others by continuing with the fieldwork experience is described in the first example. David is now skilled in NDT transfers and has been working with the client described above named Mr. Ortez. Mr. Ortez is progressing and now requires only minimal assistance using an NDT transfer. David is walking by Mr. Ortez's room one day and notices a nursing assistant helping him to transfer. She has him transferring to the left and is encouraging him to "stand up tall." Mr. Ortez appears confused and afraid. He is struggling to maintain his balance, and it is clear the nursing assistant is having to give much more than minimal assistance. David goes in to help with the transfer. When Mr. Ortez is safely in his chair, David finds himself faced with another conflict. He does not think that the nursing staff should transfer Mr. Ortez this way. In fact, it looked dangerous to both the client and the nursing assistant. But, he is not in charge of the nursing staff. He presents this problem to his clinical instructor (learning relationship). She tells David that the nursing department recently hired several new nursing assistants and that they were not taught NDT transfers as a part of their training. She asks David to help her prepare and present an inservice to new nursing staff (learning activity). This is completed and follow through with NDT transfers for clients who are using that approach improves. This is an example where the problem was used to encourage an external adjustment. The change occurred outside of the person who identified the conflict (David) through expanding the skills of others.

There are times when the solution to the problem does not occur in such a positive and easy way, and you may need to comply with a situation while personally disagreeing with the approach (strategic compliance). Jennifer is a student beginning level II fieldwork in a mental health setting. Her coursework and level I fieldwork supported the view that modifying the environment and task expectations is the most effective way to improve function for clients with clinical depression. Her first client on her level II fieldwork has a diagnosis of depression with significant functional limitations in home management skills. Jennifer presents her clinical instructor with a treatment plan that breaks meal preparation into sub-tasks that she feels the client can manage at this time. The focus of the plan is to support the client through these sub-tasks and gradually increase the complexity until she can cook a meal independently. Jennifer's clinical instructor reviews her treatment plan and asks her to try again. The clinical instructor explains that the philosophy of OT in the facility is to focus primarily on the

therapeutic relationship, as it is believed to be the most important component in enhancing a client's function. She believes that the tasks Jennifer has selected (cooking) leave inadequate time and opportunity for therapeutic use of self. She asks Jennifer to use treatment activities that are aimed at developing trust and provide opportunity for the client to discuss issues of importance to her. Jennifer also values the therapeutic relationship but continues to believe that a more direct functional approach is needed (conflict). She believes that her plan is more functionally relevant, yet still allows for development of the therapeutic relationship. She goes back to her textbooks and class notes (learning activity), e-mails her mental health instructor from school (learning relationship), and finds support for her views. She discusses the issue again with her clinical instructor, who is unwavering in her belief that treatment should be changed to focus more exclusively on the therapeutic relationship. Since Jennifer is a student and will be in this facility for only 8 weeks, the best choice for her is to go along with the clinical instructor (strategic compliance). Jennifer should approach this treatment with an open mind—she will likely learn some useful skills—but she can continue to maintain her belief in a treatment approach that views task adaptation as critical to effective treatment. Making a conscious decision to resolve a conflict through strategic compliance can in and of itself be a valuable learning experience. Jennifer has reaffirmed her beliefs by re-examining her knowledge in a critical way. If the strength of her conviction is maintained, she knows that she will need to find employment in a setting that is compatible with her views.

Professional socialization is a learning process based on learning relationships and learning activities. The following sections will describe more fully the myriad of relationships and activities that promote the professional development of OT practitioners.

Learning Relationships

Professional development literature in recent years has focused on the potential of social networks as sources of learning. In all that has been written on mentoring, clinical supervision, peer coaching, and team learning, the common element is the interaction between people for the purpose of promoting continued development. Working as a professional offers many ongoing opportunities for developing the knowledge and skills of an OTA. One of the greatest sources of learning is the OTA's relationship with others—in the classroom, in fieldwork sites, on the job, in continuing education courses, and through professional associations. The OTA will encounter many people in the health care field who have the capacity to help him or her learn and become a more proficient practitioner, such as teachers, fellow students, clients, supervisors, mentors, treatment team members, and colleagues.

The number of people who can serve as learning guides will expand as the OTA's career continues.

Sheckley and Keeton (1997) developed principles of professional development that highlight the importance of learning relationships. They pointed out that professionals who want to develop expertise must rely on a social network of fellow learners to challenge their thinking and share knowledge. Professional associates can promote reflection on experiences, add conceptual knowledge, develop applications of what has been learned to new situations, and assess the outcomes of interventions. They provide support, guidance, feedback, and input that will further professional learning. In this section, we will look at the relationships that will be part of the OTA's developing career and how those relationships promote ongoing professional socialization (Table 44-1).

Supervision

Supervision is an important component of education, training, and socialization of an OTA. Loganbill, Hardy, and Delworth (1984) define supervision as "an intensive, interpersonally focused, one-to-one relationship in which one person is designated to facilitate the development of therapeutic competence in the other person" (p. 4). The four primary functions of the supervisor are to:

1. Ensure the welfare of the client.
2. Enhance the growth of the supervisee.
3. Promote the supervisee's transition from one developmental stage to the next.
4. Evaluate the supervisee's performance.

To facilitate growth, the supervisor must find ways to promote the developing OTA's reflection on his or her clinical experiences, conceptualization of working knowledge, and application of newly acquired knowledge and skills. In addition, the supervisor encourages self-assessment and facilitates the development of new techniques and skills based on what is being learned through practice.

Supervisors use specific techniques, each serving an important function in the promotion of overall development. *Goal setting* and goal clarification are techniques that allow both the supervisor and the supervisee to state expectations and set a learning and performance agenda. Goal setting is important because it clarifies what the supervisee is to achieve and how the supervisor will judge his or her performance. *Observation* gives the supervisor a chance to see the OTA in action and to note his or her performance strengths and growth needs in light of expectations, standards of practice, and requirements. At times, supervisory observation will reveal opportunities for *instruction* or providing information, demonstration, or direction. Observation should also be coupled with *feedback*, "sharing knowledge of the results of an individual's performance with intent of changing that individual's behavior in a desirable direction" (Cohn, 1998, p.

795). Feedback is not judgmental of the person, but an assessment of the person's performance to clarify areas for specific improvement and examples of where to modify behavior.

Coaching is a process used by supervisors to help supervisees increase their sense of self-responsibility and ownership of their performance by promoting reflection and inquiry into their practices and professional activities. Good coaching from a supervisor will result in new awareness and new understanding that will ultimately have a positive effect on performance (MacLennan, 1995). Finally, *evaluation* is the systematic assessment of the OTA's performance to highlight areas of competence and specify areas that need improvement.

Perhaps the biggest challenge for both supervisor and supervisee is to work out a collaborative relationship that is inclusive of both the supervisor's style and the OTA's skills and needs. The OTA's collaborative behavior, maturity, level of expertise, and level of commitment will have an effect on how he or she is supervised and his or her overall experience of supervision (Glickman, Gordon, & Ross-Gordon, 1995). On a first fieldwork assignment, the student OTA will find that the supervisor will take more of the responsibility for supervisory activities, will observe and evaluate the OTA's performance closely, being more directive and explicit. As the OTA grows and develops as a professional, he or she will be expected to take on more of the responsibility for the supervisory relationship. Fully developed professionals are quite autonomous and become more a partner in the supervisory process. They bring questions, concerns, and clinical issues to their supervisors for feedback and bring successes to their supervisors' attention. Over time, the supervisor becomes less directive and more collaborative with the supervisee. The OTA's responsibility for growth increases as he or she develops into a full professional (Glickman, Gordon, & Ross-Gordon, 1995).

Supervision is truly a collaborative activity. The OTA and his or her supervisor must work together in the interest of growth and development. Bordin (1994) suggested that the working alliance between the supervisor and the supervisee helps make the relationship work. The development of a working alliance means agreeing on goals, agreeing on the ways to work together to reach those goals, and creating a positive bond or relationship. A good supervisor-supervisee relationship requires care, commitment, communication, respect, truthfulness, and trust (Bennett, 1997). Too many professionals ultimately stall their careers because they become defensive and unwilling to accept the feedback and advice of others. All professionals experience some barriers to being supervised. Personal barriers such as resistance to change, previous negative experiences, or attitudinal barriers, such as "I already know what I am doing" or "You're just picking on me," can really get in the way of benefiting from

---

Table 44-1

Day-to-Day Activities That Promote Ongoing Learning

- Reflection on clinical experiences
- Conceptualization of knowledge into working, applicable frames
- Deliberate practice in the use of new knowledge and skills
- Self-assessment
- Communication with other professionals
- Action-reflection: Implementing treatment plans, evaluating the outcomes, and revising plans and procedures
- Team meetings and case conferences

---

supervision. Sometimes organizational barriers, such as time pressures or limited opportunities for interaction with a supervisor, can stifle the learning relationship. Process barriers such as conflict or ineffective communication between the supervisor and the supervisee can also limit the value of supervisory feedback (MacLennan, 1995). Cohn (1998) stated that supervisees should be willing to try suggestions and evaluate barriers in an effort to overcome them. The OTA can enhance his or her own learning by being open to supervision, seeing supervision as a learning relationship, asking questions, listening thoughtfully, and taking advantage of the expertise that his or her supervisor has to offer (See Chapter 39).

Mentoring

Mentoring relationships are extremely helpful in promoting professional growth and development. A mentor is a senior professional who is selected by the developing professional or assigned by an employer to foster professional orientation and growth. Mentors often do not have supervisory responsibility for the OTA, but fill the OTA's need for a role model and a guide to how the system works and what is expected in the employing organization (MacLennan, 1995). A mentor may serve as an "inspirer," motivating and encouraging the new OTA to persist through difficult learning phases; "investor," devoting significant time and energy to the long-term future of the OTA; and "supporter," providing a listening ear and a gentle push (Butterworth, 1992). Many health care professionals look back over their careers and remember various colleagues who served as mentors during those times when their assumptions and knowledge were challenged through problems they could not solve.

Treatment Teams

The OT practitioner almost always works as part of a team of professionals who must work collaboratively to solve client-centered problems. Treatment teams provide collaborative opportunities for interprofessional learning, or learning among of group of professionals, often from different disciplines (Headrick, Wilcock, & Batalden, 1998). Sheckley and Keeton (1997) pointed out that adults learn best when they can tackle real problems, derive abstract concepts from their experiences, and test those concepts in new situations. The treatment team is an effective vehicle for continued learning because it offers opportunities for knowledge-sharing and problem-solving in a practical, relevant context.

Interprofessional learning does not occur when professionals are focused on rivalries, professional boundaries, and proprietary knowledge. Fortunately, as Headrick, Wilcock, and Batalden (1998) point out, most health care professionals have in common the personal desire to learn and the professional obligation to meet the needs of their patients or clients. The desire to learn and meet client needs often helps team members overcome the barriers to working and learning together.

Clients

There is no doubt that health care providers can and do learn from their clients. In the day-to-day work of the OTA, the information and feedback that clients give are a continuous source of knowledge and skill refinement. The process of assessing, identifying individual needs, and implementing individual treatment plans helps the OTA to develop an understanding of how theoretical and procedural knowledge applies to real-life situations. Working directly with a client gives a multitude of opportunities to learn what works, what does not, and why. It helps the OTA develop the skills for individualization, adaptation, and evaluation that are critical to providing quality services. Some clients may agree to serve as formal research subjects, allowing the OTA to develop an extensive description and case study from which to inform and develop practice. Other clients are natural teachers, providing the OTA with challenges, questions, and insights that lead to a higher level of understanding of individuals in need of OT, the conditions under which they live and work, and the value OT can have in supporting the client's goals. Almost any OT practitioner will be able to tell you stories about people they have served and how those people had a profound impact on their learning and growth as a professional.

Professional Relationships

Relationships with other OT practitioners will provide many opportunities for continued learning. For example, consider how much can be learned through conversations with fellow students. Some relationships developed in school will carry on into one's professional life, providing opportunities to share ideas, solve problems, give and get advice, and locate resources. Allen, Nelson, and Sheckley (1987) found that meeting with fellow professionals on a regular basis to discuss specific cases and general clinical issues was one of the two most highly valued and rewarding means of continuing professional development for psychologists. OTAs form relationships through work with fellow OT practitioners who offer ongoing opportunities for client- and content-focused dialogue that leads to continued competence.

Continued learning and professional development are the cornerstones of almost all professional organizations. Professional organizations offer many opportunities for members to get together and learn from each other. It is in the best interest of professional growth to join local, state, and national professional associations, such as AOTA, and to participate in them to form strong professional relationships.

The potential number of learning relationships continues to grow throughout the OTA's career. The OTA should seek out and build relationships that will not only support the development of continued competence but give opportunities to share knowledge with others.

Learning Activities

All professions value continuing professional development in order to maintain high standards within the profession and to build a rich body of professional knowledge. Continuing professional development is always expected and often required. Continuing education is required in many states to maintain licensure as an OTA. There are many reasons to pursue continuing professional development:

- To develop the technical expertise needed to best serve the client.
- To improve personal practice.
- To deepen one's understanding of critical topics and develop a specialty.
- To broaden the scope of knowledge.

- To remain current.
- To maintain certification or licensure.
- To develop the ability to work effectively in increasingly complex or unique clinical situations.

Continuing professional development is structured in both formal and informal ways to offer the OT practitioner literally hundreds of options for reaching and maintaining competence. This section will discuss a variety of options and offer a framework for creating a personal development plan.

Options for Continuing Professional Development

In order to meet the needs of a large and varied professional group, OT practitioners have created and organized a large number of formal activities for ongoing learning. Formal learning resources are developed and provided by technical schools, colleges and universities, professional associations, employment settings, and independent providers. Formal learning opportunities include:

- Continuing education classes—Similar to the classes that are taken in pursuit of a degree, continuing education classes are centered around a topic, meet a number of times, and are developed and led by one or more instructors.

- Seminars—Professional seminars are generally more interactive than classes because the participants are more actively engaged in developing the learning goals and contributing what they know to the learning process. Seminars may meet a number of times, like classes, which provides the advantage of getting to know other OT practitioners and sharing expertise with them.

- Workshops—Workshops are one-time learning events focused on a topic of interest, usually work-related skills or knowledge. Workshops are designed and conducted by a workshop leader and are often advertised through workplaces and professional publications.

- Inservice training—Many employers offer continuing professional development opportunities in the workplace. These presentations, workshops, and classes are called inservice training. Health care agencies often use inservice training to update professionals on agency policies and practices as well as relevant and necessary health care information that is required for accreditation or licensing.

- Conferences—Conferences offer a large number of learning opportunities at one time in one location. At a conference, you can access current materials, workshops, presentations, fellow OT practitioners, and product vendors. For example, AOTA sponsors a national conference annually that attracts thousands of OT practitioners. Conferences are a good way to find out about current issues and topics in your field. Many people find conferences fun and revitalizing.

- Publications—Magazines and journals offer another way to keep yourself up to date. Reading articles and research on current practices and issues in OT will give you a good sense of the current standards and expectations in the field, as well as a glimpse at what will be important in the near future. There are many publications written specifically for OT practitioners. The *American Journal of Occupational Therapy* is an excellent resource that comes as one of the many benefits for AOTA members. There are many other valuable journals. The Wilma L. West Library at the American Occupational Therapy Foundation (AOTF) has many resources and lists all available journals on its website (www.AOTF.org).

- On-line resources—The World Wide Web can be a valuable and convenient resource for continuing professional development because it provides access to specific websites, electronic conferences, and interpersonal communication with other professionals. Just a 15-minute search on "the web" can reveal hundreds of links to OT sites, including academic information, job information, research reports and opportunities, and current news.

- Audiovisual resources—There are an ever-increasing number of resources available—audiotapes, videotapes, and CD-ROMs—that are relevant to the OT field. Employing agencies, health care facilities, college and university libraries, and your local library may own or can help you locate and procure audiovisual materials.

As the OTA becomes socialized as an OT practitioner, he or she will encounter "in-practice" opportunities that hold tremendous educational potential. The in-practice learning activities include:

- Case conferences—Meetings to review specific cases and solve therapeutic problems surrounding cases provide opportunities to learn new information, see other practitioners in action, debate and resolve clinical issues, as well as develop problem-solving skills.

- Research—There are many forms of research that can yield new knowledge and skills. Conducting a literature review gives the researcher access to a tremendous amount of written information on a specific topic and requires that the researcher summarize and synthesize current knowledge. Participating in research on current practice provides the practitioner with opportunities to learn about how and why new treatment methods are effective.

- Writing and speaking—Writing an article, giving a talk, or teaching a class all offer the opportunity for the OT practitioner to reflect on and synthesize knowledge and experience and to share a unique viewpoint with others in the field.

- Volunteer participation on committees and commissions—Volunteering to serve on committees gives the learner a unique window into the field of OT, the current issues and concerns of the health care community and consumers, and available resources. Committees or commissions may be at the institutional level, such as a consumer support group; the regional level, such as a head injury advocacy group; or the national level, such as a certification policy task force. The opportunity to contribute one's expertise to resolve issues or develop new ways of thinking in the field is perhaps one of the most rewarding experiences available to competent professionals.

- Professional memberships and meetings—Joining and actively participating in professional associations, at the local, state, or national level, brings learners in contact with a wide variety of learning relationships and gives them opportunities to develop professional leadership skills. Professional organizations are run by volunteers who participate through activities such as organizing conferences, working with state licensure boards to ensure professional competency, or working with the legislature regarding health care reform.

Developing a Professional Development Plan

Just as clients benefit from the implementation of well thought out plans, the OTA will benefit from devising a plan for professional growth (Figure 44-2). In her article "Professional Reflection: Have You Looked in the Mirror Lately?", Marilyn Oermann (1998) suggests that health care practitioners should learn to identify competence needs and specific activities for meeting those needs on a continual basis. The first step in the personal planning process is to take a close look at the current working environment: What is the current environment demanding of me as a professional? What are the trends in the near future? What is going to be required of me over the next few years? (Epperheimer, 1997). The second step is a self-assessment. How am I prepared to meet the challenges? What skills and knowledge do I need to continue to be an effective practitioner? Oermann (1998) recommends that professionals assess their knowledge and skills for clinical practice, critical thinking, technological skills, professional values, communication and collaboration skills, leadership abilities, and attitudes about continued learning.

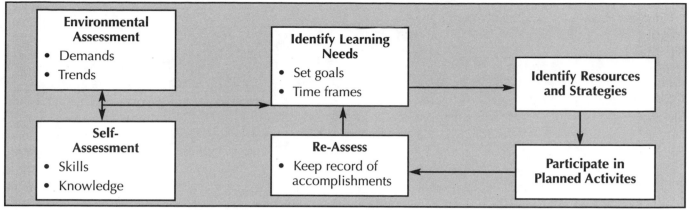

Figure 44-2. Planning for professional development.

Next, identify learning needs, set specific professional development goals, and identify the time frames within which the goals will be reached. Once development goals have been clarified, identify strategies and resources for meeting them. Seek resources through employers, professional colleagues, colleges and universities, and professional associations. These groups can give the best information about what continuing professional development activities and resources are available in your area and may also be able to help with financial assistance, such as tuition reimbursement or scholarships. Finally, keep a record of accomplishments and periodically assess progress toward professional development goals. Future job searches and marketability can be greatly enhanced by having a complete record of development activities.

Learning relationships and learning activities are crucial components of the professional socialization process. The process of professional socialization and the focus of the learning relationships and activities also tends to shift over time. Being aware of the typical phases of professional socialization can make the practitioner more sensitive to events in his or her career that offer unique opportunities of professional growth.

Phases of Professional Socialization

Professional socialization is a continuous process, however, the activities and the focus of professional socialization vary over time. The phases of professional socialization that follow were selected because they tend to be career "breakpoints" (i.e., a time when significant change occurs in one's professional life) (Schempp & Graber, 1992). Established relationships may be severed and new ones formed. Responsibilities may change significantly, requiring new skills or knowledge. Van Maanen (1977) stated that "breakpoints require the individual to discover or reformulate certain everyday assumptions about [his or her] working life" (p. 322). In other words, these breakpoints offer increased opportunity for the challenges—or conflicts—that facilitate learning and profes-

sional growth. The learning focus, learning relationships, and their relationship to the phases of socialization are summarized in Table 44-2.

Educational Setting

The professional socialization process begins within the required coursework for OTAs. Clearly, the learning focus at this stage is on the knowledge and skills needed for competent practice, with an emphasis on knowledge within the classroom setting. The "problems" stem more from a lack of knowledge than "conflicting" information. As described earlier, however, professional socialization requires an integration of knowledge and skills with professional behaviors. Educational programs are paying increased attention to professional behaviors and are making them a more explicit component of the curriculum by including them into course objectives and teaching students specific skills (Fidler, 1996; Raveh, 1995). Professional behaviors include abilities such as interpersonal and communication skills, management of time and resources, response to constructive feedback, problem-solving, critical thinking, professionalism, responsibility, commitment to learning, and stress management (May et al., 1995). Students may be presented with new ways of assessing and enhancing these behaviors that conflict with previously held beliefs and habits.

Fieldwork

Fieldwork offers continued opportunity for students to develop knowledge, but the learning focus shifts from knowledge to skills and professional behaviors. Students do not learn as many new things, but they learn how to apply what they know in a practical way. They are frequently presented with situations that do not "match" their expectations, presenting conflicts that become learning opportunities. For example, a student with an idea about what spasticity will look and feel like based on a description from a book may find that his or her "image" is very different from what he or she actually

Table 44-2

Phases of Socialization

Phase of Socialization	Content Focus	Learning Relationships	Process Directed By	Learning Activities
Educational	• General knowledge • Professional behaviors • (Basic skills)	• College faculty • (Clinical faculty)	• College faculty • Guidelines for accreditation	• Lectures • Case studies • Reading • Written assignments • Lab exercises • Role playing • Observation • Reflection
Fieldwork	• Skills • Professional behaviors • Knowledge	• Clinical instructor • Clients • (Other OT personnel) • (Team members) • (College faculty)	• Clinical instructor • (Student)	• Hands-on experience • Reflective dialogue notes • Team meetings • Reading/reviewing school
Entry-Level Practice	• Knowledge and skills that are setting specific • Professional behaviors with focus on independent self-management	• Clients • Supervisor • Other OT personnel • Team members • OT practitioners outside the institution	• OTA (self)—Supervisor collaboration • Institutional needs	• Hands-on experience • Reflective dialogue • Reading • In-services • Team meetings • Conferences • Workshops • Professional memberships
Job Changes	• Shift in knowledge and skills to meet needs of new setting • Refine professional behaviors in new relationships	• Clients • Supervisor • Other OT personnel • Team members • OT practitioners outside the institution (expanded since entry-level practice)	• OTA (self)-directed with supervisor input • Institutional needs	Renewed focus on: • Hands-on experience • Reflective dialogue • Reading • In-services • Team meetings • Conferences • Workshops • Revise prof. memberships (est. new affiliations) • Volunteer on committees
Specialization	• Focus on knowledge and skills specific to content area • Complexity of knowledge and ability to apply in varied situations is developed	• Clients • Supervisor • Team members • Specialists outside the institution • (Other OT personnel)	• OTA (self)-directed • Expert input (may or may not be OT) • Institutional needs	• Hands-on experience • Reflection • Reading • Writing • Assist with research • Presentations • Membership in specialty organizations • Volunteer on committees • Community service

sees and feels when he or she first works with a client with spasticity.

Entry-Level Practice

Significant changes in the professional socialization process occur at the breakpoint at which an OTA enters practice. The learning focus will shift to meet the demands of the setting. The new graduate will still be working on developing the skills and professional behaviors needed in clinical practice, but will be presented with new challenges that may not have occurred during fieldwork. Managing his or her own caseload rather than sharing a caseload, meeting productivity demands, learning about available resources, and learning the "politics" of an institution are all examples of new challenges for the entry-level OTA.

Now that the practitioner is an OTA and no longer a student, the process of professional socialization is directed by the individual. An OTA in an entry-level position should have ample opportunity for feedback and direction from the supervising OT, but the final decision about professional goals, learning relationships, and learning activities will be up to the OTA.

Job Changes

The professional socialization process continues even when the OTA stays with a single employer. A job change, however, often "recharges" growth and development of the employee by providing the OTA with new learning relationships and an environment that is less familiar and presents more challenges or "conflicts" to resolve. Enhancement of knowledge and skills often accelerates immediately following a job change as the OTA's learning focus shifts to refine and adapt the OTA's expertise to fit the needs of a different client group. A change in the practice setting can put new demands on professional behaviors, too, such as critical thinking, problem-solving, and communication skills.

Specialization

Not all OT practitioners choose to specialize in one practice area. Many practitioners enjoy the challenge of variety and opt to work in settings that require a breadth of skills. They may opt for varied practice settings when changing jobs in order to keep their skills "well-rounded." The process of professional socialization, however, in a specialized area of practice can offer the OTA unique experiences and opportunities. When the OTA specializes, the learning focus shifts to developing a depth of knowledge (i.e., learning a lot about one practice area). Examples of specialty areas in OT practice include pediatric mental health, hand injuries, industrial rehabilitation, geriatrics, neurologic rehabilitation, early intervention (birth to 3 years), and community mental health.

When entering a specialty field, the learning focus narrows, delving deep into the specialty content. The complexity of the knowledge base is enhanced.

SUMMARY

This chapter has described the process of professional socialization as it relates to developing and maintaining professional competence. Learning relationships and activities were included and the stages of professional socialization described.

Youngstrom (1998) described several traits and attitudes that can help the individual practitioner take responsibility for professional development and facilitate competency. These include:

- Have an open attitude toward learning. Learning should be seen as a continuous process that is facilitated by questioning one's own practice and conferring with others. The OTA with an open attitude for learning will always strive to find a better way.

- Be a self-evaluator. The OTA who assesses his or her own performance and seeks out feedback will open up many learning opportunities. Even though learning occurs naturally through experience, "without time given to self-evaluation and reflection, the practitioner cannot accurately assess the level of competence or target areas for development" (Youngstrom, 1998, p. 720).

- Make a professional development plan and make the time to carry it out. Without a plan that includes specific activities and dates, it is too easy to let time slip away and allow professional development slow.

REFERENCES

Allen, G. J., Nelson, W. J., & Sheckley, B. G. (1987). Continuing education activities of Connecticut psychologists. *Professional Psychology: Research and Practice, 18*(1), 78-80.

AOTA. (1993). OT roles. *Am J Occup Ther, 47,* 1087-1099.

AOTA. (1994a). OT code of ethics. *Am J Occup Ther, 48,* 1037-1038.

AOTA. (1994b). Standards of practice for OT. *Am J Occup Ther, 48,* 1039-1043.

Australian Association of OTs. (1994). *Australian competency standards for entry-level OTs: Final report.* Melbourne, Australia: Author.

Bennett, T. (1997). *Clinical supervision marriage: A matrimonial metaphor for understanding the supervisor-teacher relationship.* Paper presented at the Annual Meeting of the Southwest Educational Research Association, Austin, TX, January 23-25, 1997.

Bordin, E. S. (1994). Theory and research on the therapeutic working alliance. New directions. In A. O. Horvath & L. S. Greenberg (Eds.), *The working alliance: Theory, research, and practice*. New York, NY: John Wiley & Sons, Inc.

Butterworth, T. (1992). Clinical supervision as an emerging idea in nursing. In T. Butterworth & J. Faugier (Eds.), *Clinical supervision and mentorship in nursing*. New York, NY: Chapman & Hall.

Cohn, E. S. (1998). Interdisciplnary communication and supervision of personnel. In M. E. Neistadt & E. B. Crepeau (Eds.), *Willard & Spackman's OT* (9th ed.). Philadelphia, PA: Lippincott.

Epperheimer, J. (1997). Benchmarking career management. *HR Focus, 74*(11), 9.

Fidler, G. S. (1996). Developing a repertoire of professional behaviors. *Am J Occup Ther, 50*, 583-587.

Glickman, C. D., Gordon, S. P., & Ross-Gordon, J. M. (1995). *Supervision of instruction: A developmental approach*. Boston, MA: Allyn and Bacon.

Headrick, L. A., Wilcock, P. M., & Batalden, P. B. (1998). Interprofessional working and continuing medical education. *British Medical Journal, 316*, 771.

Hinojosa, J., & Blount, M. L. F. (1998). Nationally speaking: Professional competence. *Am J Occup Ther, 52*, 699-701.

Loganbill, C., Hardy, E., & Delworth, U. (1984). Supervision: A conceptual model. *The Counseling Psychologist, 10*(1), 3-41.

MacLennan, N. (1995). *Coaching and mentoring*. Brookfield, VT: Gower.

May, W. W., Morgan, B. J., Lemke, J. C., Karst, G. M., & Stone, H. L. (1995). Model for ability-based assessment in physical therapy education. *Journal of Physical Therapy Education, 9*, 3-6.

Oermann, M. H. (1998). Professional reflection: Have you looked in the mirror lately? *Orthopaedic Nursing, 17*(4), 22.

Raveh, M. (1995). Configuration of OT, professionalism and experiential learning—An integrated introductory course. *OT International, 2*, 65-78.

Schempp, P. G., & Graber, K. C. (1992). Teacher socialization from a dialectical perspective: Pretraining through induction. *Journal of Teaching in Physical Education, 11*, 329-348.

Sheckley, B. G., & Keeton, M. T. (1997). *Professional development: Perspectives from research and practice*. Chicago, IL: CAEL.

Van Maanan, J. (1977). *Organizational careers: Some new perspectives*. New York, NY: Wiley.

Youngstrom, M. J. (1998). Evolving competence in the practitioner role. *Am J Occup Ther, 52*, 716-720.

Human Developmental Chart

NEUROMOTOR DEVELOPMENT

Reflex Development

	Head/Trunk Control	Rolling/Crawling	Standing/Walking	Arm/Hand Function	Writing/Drawing
Prenatal Neonatal	Rooting Sucking Incurvation of spine Moro Extensor thrust ATNR STNR	Moro Asym. tonic m. Symm. tonic m. Tonic. labyr. Neon. neck r.	Plantar grasp Stepping Moro Placing Flexor withdrawal Extensor thrust Crossed extension	Palmar grasp Placing Traction Avoidance ATNR STNR	
2 mo. 6 mo.	Laby. righting Landau Prot. Extension	Neck/Body r. Laby. r-su Landau Tilt – pr/su Tilt – all 4s	Laby. r-pr. Pos. supporting Laby. righting Prot. Extension		
11 mo. 15 mo.	Tilting		Tilting/Hopping See-saw		

Voluntary Control

	Head/Trunk Control	Rolling/Crawling	Standing/Walking	Arm/Hand Function	Writing/Drawing
2 mo.	Lifts head when prone Head lag when pulled to sitting Falls forward in sitting position Back rounded				
3 mo.		Rolls back-to-side		Hands to midline Visual grasp Hands often open	
4 mo.	Had lag slight when pulled to sitting Lumbar curve only			Arms activate on sight of object Crude palm grasp Bilateral approach Holds 1 object	
5 mo.	Sits hyperflexed Head in line on pull-to-sit	Pivots in prone, arm propulsion movements			
6 mo.	Sits with support Begins to use supporting Reactions	Automatic rolling Assumes 4-point crawling posture		Unilateral approach begins Circuitous arm motion	

Age			
7 mo.	Sits alone momentarily	Sustains weight on extended legs / Bounces	
8 mo.	Belly crawling / Deliberate rolling	Holds 2 objects / Transfers object	
9 mo.	No longer uses arms for support in sitting / Assumes sitting independently / Leans forward, re-erects / 4-point crawl	Stands holding rail / Release beginning	
10 mo.	Sitting to prone	Pulls up to rail & lowers / Thumb & index tip prehension beginning	
11 mo.	Sits and pivots	Lifts foot at rail / Cruises	
12 mo. / 1 yr.			
15 mo.		Walks with one hand held / Assumes standing on own / Walks a few steps / Falls by collapse / Neat prehension / Places cube on cube / Casts object	Marks by banging or brushing / Marks rather than bangs
18 mo.	Seats self in small chair	Heel-toe progression in walking / Walks sideways (17m) / Walks backwards (17m) / Crude release (on contact with surface)	Holds crayon butt end / Scribbles off page / Whole arm movements / One color
21 mo.	Discards crawling	Squats in play / Down stairs hand held / Tries to stand on 6cm / Walking board / Kicks large ball / Tower 5-6 blocks	
24 mo. / 2 yrs.		Runs well / Walks with one foot on 6cm walking board (27cm) / Less handedness shift	Overhand grasp of crayon / Wrist action / Process rather than product
2½ yrs.		Jumps with both feet / Tries standing on one foot / Hops 1-3 steps on preferred foot / Attempts to step on walking board (33m) / Stands on 6cm walking / Board with both feet (38m) / Throws ball with poor direction about 5-7 feet / Throws bean bag into 12 in. hole from 3 feet	Holds crayon in fingers / Small marks / Imitates vertical/horizontal stroke

Age			
3 yrs.	Rides tricycle Alternates feet going up stairs Alternates feet part way on 6cm walking board (38m) Ascends small ladder alternating feet (38m)	Towers 10 blocks 10 pellets into bottle, 30 sec. Catches large ball with stiff arms Throws ball without losing balance, 6-7 feet Handedness	Copies circle Imitates cross Encloses space Simple figures Beginning designs Names drawing
3½ yrs.	Stands on 1 foot, 2 seconds Jumps from 8 in. elevation Leaps off floor with feet Together	Throws small ball	
4 yrs.	Propels and manipulates wagon Skips on 1 foot only Down stairs foot-to-step Balance on 1 foot, 4-8 Seconds Walk 6cm board part way Before stepping off Crouch for broad jump of 8-10 in. Hop on toes with both feet same time Carry cup of water without spilling Reciprocal arm motion in running pattern Ascends large ladder, alternating feet (47m)	Throws ball overhand Beginning adult stance throwing Catches large ball arms flexed but rigid	Pencil held like adult, wrist flexed Crude human figures "Suns" Copies cross
4½ yrs.	Hops on 1 foot, 4 to 6 steps Alternates feet full length of 6cm walking board (56m) Descends small ladder		More detailed human figures

5 yrs.	Roller skates, ice skates and rides small bicycle (5 or 6 yrs.) Skips alternating feet Stands indefinitely on 1 foot Hop a distance of 16 feet Walks long distance on tip toes Walks length of 6cm walking board in 6-9 sec. (60m) Running broad jump 28 to 35 in. Runs 11.5 feet per second Descends large ladder	Adult posture distance throwing Boys 24 feet Girls 15 feet Catches ball, hands more that arms, misses Bounces large ball	Buildings and houses Animals Idea before starting Copies triangle
6 yrs.	Stand on each foot alternately with eyes closed Walk a 4cm walking board in 9 seconds with one error Jump down from 12 in landing on toes only Standing broad jump of 38 in. Running broad jump of 40 to 45 in. Hop 50 feet in 9 seconds	Reach, grasp, release and body movement smooth Catch ball, 1 hand *Grip strength Boys 11.3 lbs. Girls 3.2 lbs.	Finger and wrist movement Copies diamond
7 yrs.	Motor performance continues to become more refined (running, jumping, balancing, etc.) Strength increases Learns to inhibit motor Activity	*Grip strength Boys 18.5 lbs. Girls 8.7 lbs.	
8 yrs.	Runs 5 yards per second Standing broad jump of 45 in.	*Grip strength Boys 26 lbs. Girls 14.4 lbs.	

*Dynamometer norms for dominant hand (average/mean) (unpublished) Scottish Rite Hospital for Crippled Children, Dallas, Texas.

3-dimensional geometric figures

Linear perspective

Distance throw
Boys 60 feet
Girls 35 feet

*Grip strength
Boys 45.2 lbs.
Girls 33.8 lbs.
Distance throw
Boys 95 feet
Girls 60 feet

*Grip strength
Boys 71.2 lbs.
Girls 46.2 lbs.

Boys distance throw
150 feet

Runs 6 yards per second
Standing broad jump of 60 in.

Boys standing broad jump 76 in.
Girls standing broad 63 in.

Boys run 6 yards, 8 in per second
Girls run 6 yards, 3 in per second

Boys run 7 yards per second

Boys standing broad jump 90 in.

Sensorimotor Development

Social and Play Development

Daily Living Skills

Body Scheme

Individual – mothering person most important

Other

Sensorimotor development (0-2 yrs.):
Tactile functions
Vestibular functions
Kinesthetic functions
Auditory functions
Olfactory functions
Gustatory functions

Vision

Rudimentary fixation
Reflexive tracking for brief periods

Sees light, dark, color and movement

Real convergence and Coordination

9 yrs.

10 yrs.
11 yrs.

14 yrs.

17 yrs.

Prenatal
Neonatal

2 mo.
6 mo.

11 mo.
15 mo.
2 mo.

Age	Visual / Perceptual	Sensory-Motor	Body Awareness	Social	Self-Help / Daily Living
3 mo.	Accommodation more flexible and eye coordinate smoothly				
4 mo.					
5 mo.	Size and shape consistency				
6 mo.	Depth perception / Visual tracking 90° / V and H planes / Color perception / Acuity / Discriminates strangers				
7 mo.				Stranger anxiety	
8 mo.					
9 mo.					
10 mo.					Holds bottle / Finger feeds
11 mo.					Drinks from cup (held)
12 mo. / 1 yr.		Integration of body sides (1-4 yrs.): / Gross motor planning / Form and space perception / Equilibrium response		Immediate family group important	Cooperates in dressing
15 mo.		Postural flexibility			Grasps spoon and into dish
18 mos.			"Tummy," legs, feet, arms, hand, face parts	Solitary or onlooker play	Feeds self, spills / Takes off hat, socks mittens / Unzips zippers / Toilet trained daytime / Handles cup well
21 mos.					Hold small glass 1 hand / Helps in getting dressed / Pulls on socks
24 mos. / 2 yrs.	Distinguishes vertical from horizontal lines	Strong tactile sense		Parallel play / Imitation	Pulls up pants / Removes shoes
2½ yrs.					Strings beads, snips with scissors, opens jar lid, turns door knob

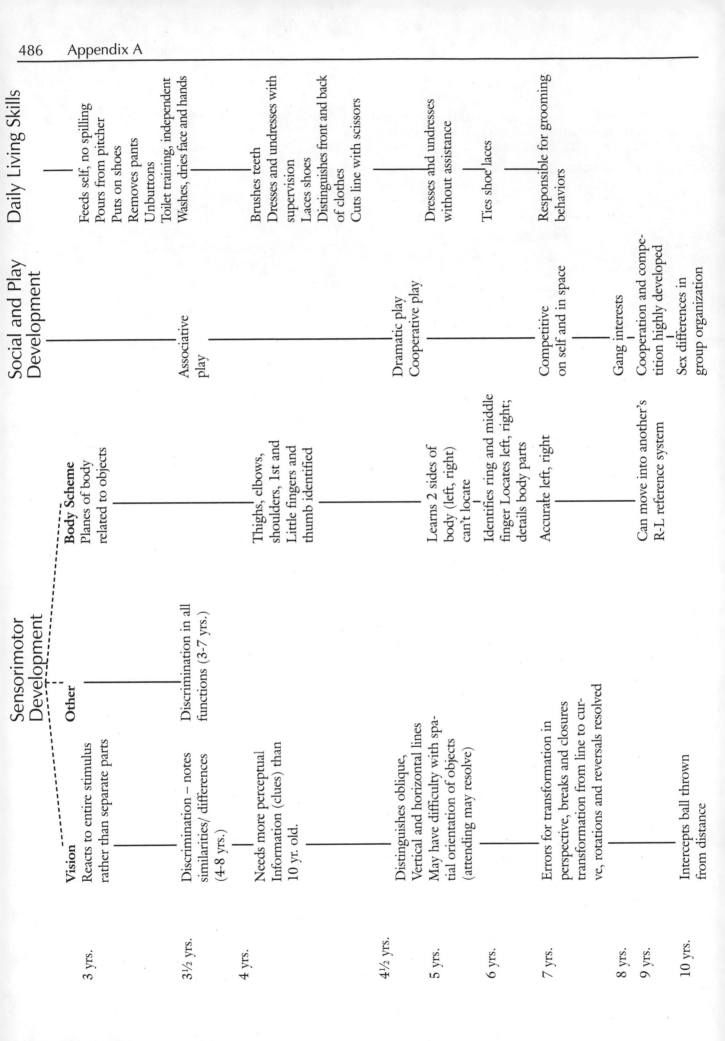

Age	Sensorimotor Development — Vision	Sensorimotor Development — Other	Sensorimotor Development — Body Scheme	Social and Play Development	Daily Living Skills
3 yrs.	Reacts to entire stimulus rather than separate parts		Planes of body related to objects		Feeds self, no spilling; Pours from pitcher; Puts on shoes; Removes pants; Unbuttons; Toilet training, independent; Washes, dries face and hands
3½ yrs.	Discrimination – notes similarities/differences (4-8 yrs.)	Discrimination in all functions (3-7 yrs.)		Associative play	
4 yrs.	Needs more perceptual Information (clues) than 10 yr. old.		Thighs, elbows, shoulders, 1st and Little fingers and thumb identified		Brushes teeth; Dresses and undresses with supervision; Laces shoes; Distinguishes front and back of clothes; Cuts line with scissors
4½ yrs.	Distinguishes oblique, Vertical and horizontal lines				
5 yrs.	May have difficulty with spatial orientation of objects (attending may resolve)		Learns 2 sides of body (left, right) can't locate	Dramatic play; Cooperative play	
6 yrs.			Identifies ring and middle finger Locates left, right; details body parts		Dresses and undresses without assistance
7 yrs.	Errors for transformation in perspective, breaks and closures transformation from line to curve, rotations and reversals resolved		Accurate left, right	Competitive on self and in space	Ties shoe laces
8 yrs.				Gang interests	Responsible for grooming behaviors
9 yrs.			Can move into another's R-L reference system	Cooperation and competition highly developed	
10 yrs.	Intercepts ball thrown from distance			Sex differences in group organization	

REFERENCES

Ayers. (1962). *Perceptual-motor training for children. Approaches to the treatment of patients with neuromuscular dysfunction.* Third International Congress WPOT.

Barsch. (1967). *Achieving Perceptual-Motor Efficiency.*

Cratty. (1970). *Perceptual and Motor Development in Infancy and Early Childhood.*

Gesell. (1940). *The First Five Years.*

Espenschade & Eckert. (1967). *Motor Development.*

Llorens. (1970). *Human development: The promise of occupational therapy.* Rockville, MD: AOTA

McGraw. (1945). *The Neuromuscular Maturation of the Human Infant.*

Mussen, Conger, & Kagan. (1963). *Child Development and Personality.* 3rd ed.

Peiper. (1963). *Cerebral Function in Infancy and Childhood.*

Appendix compiled by Mary K. Cowan, MA, OTR, FAOTA. (Reprinted with permission from Ryan, S. E. (1993). *The certified occupational therapy assistant: Principles, concepts, and techniques.* 2nd ed. Thorofare, NJ: SLACK Incorporated.)

Standards of Practice for Occupational Therapy

Linda Kohlman Thomson, MOT, OT(C), FAOTA,
Chairperson, Commission on Practice, AOTA

Permission was granted for the reproduction of this document by AOTA.

PREFACE

The Standards of Practice for OT are requirements for the OT practitioner (OTR and COTA) for the delivery of OT services that are client centered and interactive in nature (AOTA, 1995). The OTR supervises the COTA, and both work together in a collaborative manner to meet the needs of the client. However, the OTR is ultimately responsible and accountable for the delivery of OT services. This document identifies minimum standards for OT practice.

The minimum educational requirements for the OTR are described in the current *Essentials and Guidelines of an Accredited Educational Program for the OT* (AOTA, 1991a). The minimum educational requirements for the COTA are described in the current *Essentials and Guidelines of an Accredited Educational Program for the OTA* (AOTA, 1991b).

DEFINITIONS

- *Assessment:* Specific tools, instruments, or interactions used during the evaluation process. An assessment is a component part of the evaluation process (Hinojosa & Kramer, 1998).
- *Client:* A person, group, program, organization, or community for whom the OT practitioner is providing services (AOTA, 1995).
- *Evaluation:* The process of obtaining and interpreting data necessary for understanding the individual, system, or situation. This includes planning for and documenting the evaluation process, results, and recommendations, including the need for intervention and/or potential change in the intervention plan (Hinojosa & Kramer, 1998).
- *OT practitioner:* Any individual initially certified to practice as an OT or OTA or licensed or regulated by a state, district, commonwealth, or territory of the United States to practice as an OT or OTA (AOTA, 1997).
- *Performance areas:* Broad categories of human activity that are typically part of daily life. They are activities of daily living, work and productive activities, and play or leisure activities (AOTA, 1994c).
- *Performance components:* Elements of performance required for successful engagement in performance areas, including sensorimotor, cognitive, psychosocial, and psychological aspects (AOTA, 1994c).
- *Performance contexts:* Situations or factors that influence an individual's engagement in desired and/or required performance areas. Performance contexts consist of temporal aspects (chronological, developmental, life cycle, disability status) and environmental aspects (physical, social, political, cultural) (AOTA, 1994c).
- *Screening:* Obtaining and reviewing data relevant to a potential client to determine the need for further evaluation and intervention.
- *Transition:* Process involving actions coordinated to prepare for or facilitate change, such as from one functional level to another, from one life stage to another, from one program to another, or from one environment to another.

STANDARD I: PROFESSIONAL STANDING AND RESPONSIBILITY

1. An OT practitioner delivers OT services that reflect the philosophical base of OT (AOTA, 1979) and are consistent with the established principles and concepts of theory and practice.
2. An OT practitioner delivers OT services in accordance with AOTA's standards and policies. The nature and scope of OT services provided must be in accordance with laws and regulations.
3. An OT practitioner maintains current licensure, registration, or certification as required by laws or regulations.
4. An OT practitioner abides by AOTA's *OT Code of Ethics* (AOTA, 1994a).

5. An OT practitioner assures continued competency by establishing, maintaining, and updating professional performance, knowledge, and skills.

6. An OTR provides supervision for a COTA in a collaborative manner as defined by official AOTA documents and in accordance with laws or regulations.

7. A COTA seeks and follows supervision from a OTR in the delivery of OT services.

8. An OT practitioner is knowledgeable about AOTA's *Standards of Practice for OT*; the *Philosophical Base of OT* (AOTA, 1979); and other AOTA, state, and federal documents relevant to practice and service delivery.

9. An OT practitioner maintains current knowledge of legislative, political, social, cultural, and reimbursement issues that affect clients and the practice of OT.

10. An OTR is knowledgeable about research in the practitioner's areas of practice. An OTR applies timely research findings ethically and appropriately to evaluation and intervention processes and discusses applicable research findings with the COTA.

11. An OTR systematically assesses the efficiency and effectiveness of OT services and designs and implements processes to support quality service delivery.

12. A COTA collaborates with the OTR in assessing the efficiency and effectiveness of OT services and assists in designing and implementing processes to support quality service delivery.

STANDARD II: REFERRAL

1. An OTR accepts and responds to referrals in accordance with AOTA's *Statement of OT Referral* (AOTA, 1994b) and in compliance with laws or regulations.

2. An OTR accepts and responds to referrals for evaluation or evaluation with intervention in performance areas, performance components, or performance contexts when clients may have a functional limitation or disability or may be at risk for a disability or may be a risk for a disabling condition.

3. An OTR refers clients to appropriate resources when the needs of the client can best be served by the expertise of other professionals or services.

4. An OT practitioner educates current and potential referral sources about the scope of OT services and the process of initiating OT services.

STANDARD III: SCREENING

1. An OTR screens independently or as a member of a team in accordance with laws and regulations. A COTA may contribute to the screening process under the supervision of an OTR.

2. An OTR selects screening methods appropriate to the client's performance context.

3. An OTR communicates screening results and recommendations to the appropriate person, group, or organization. A COTA may contribute to this process under the supervision of an OTR.

STANDARD IV: EVALUATION

1. An OTR evaluates performance areas, performance components, and performance contexts. A COTA may contribute to the evaluation process under the supervision of an OTR.

2. An OT practitioner educates clients and appropriate others about the purposes and procedures of the OT evaluation.

3. An OTR selects assessments to evaluate the client's level of function related to performance areas, performance components, and performance contexts.

4. An OT practitioner follows defined protocols when standardized assessments are used.

5. An OTR analyzes, interprets, and summarizes assessment data to determine the client's current functional status and to develop an appropriate intervention plan. The COTA may contribute to this process under the supervision of an OTR.

6. An OTR completes and documents OT evaluation results within the time frames, formats, and standards established by practice settings, government agencies, external accreditation programs, and payers. A COTA may contribute to documentation of evaluation results under the supervision of an OTR and in accordance with laws or regulations.

7. An OTR communicates evaluation results, within the boundaries of client confidentiality, to the appropriate person, group, or organization. A COTA may contribute to this process under the supervision of an OTR.

8. An OTR recommends additional consultations when the results of the evaluation indicate that intervention by other professionals would be beneficial.

STANDARD V: INTERVENTION PLAN

1. An OTR develops and documents an intervention plan that is based on the results of the OT evaluation and the desires and expectations of the client and appropriate others about the outcome of service. A COTA may contribute to the intervention plan under the supervision of an OTR.

2. An OTR ensures that the intervention plan is documented within time frames, formats, and standards established by the practice settings, agencies, external accreditation programs, and payers.

3. An OTR includes in the intervention plan client-centered goals that are clear, measurable, behavioral, functional, contextually relevant, and appropriate to the client's needs, desires, and expected outcomes. A COTA may contribute to this process.

4. An OTR includes in the intervention plan the scope, frequency, duration of services, and the needs of the client.

5. An OTR reviews the intervention plan with the client and appropriate others. A COTA may contribute to this process.

STANDARD VI: INTERVENTION

1. An OTR implements the intervention plan through the use of specified purposeful activities or therapeutic methods that are meaningful to the client and are effective methods for enhancing occupational performance. A COTA may implement the intervention plan under the supervision of an OTR.

2. An OT practitioner informs clients and appropriate others regarding the relative benefits and risks of the intervention.

3. An OT practitioner maintains or seeks current information on resources relevant to the client's needs.

4. An OTR reevaluates during the intervention process and documents changes in the client's goals, performance, and needs. A COTA may contribute to the reevaluation process.

5. An OTR modifies the intervention process to reflect changes in client status, desires, and response to intervention. A COTA may identify the need for modifications and may contribute to the intervention modifications under the supervision of an OTR.

6. An OT practitioner documents the OT services provided within the time frames, formats, and standards established by the practice settings, agencies, external accreditation programs, and payers.

STANDARD VII: TRANSITION SERVICES

1. An OTR prepares a formal transition plan that is based on identified needs. A COTA may contribute to the preparation of a formal transition plan.

2. An OT practitioner facilitates the transition process in cooperation with the client, family members, significant others, team, and community resources and individuals, when appropriate.

STANDARD VIII: DISCONTINUATION

1. An OTR discontinues services when the client has achieved predetermined goals, has achieved maximum benefit from OT services, or does not desire to continue services. A COTA may recommend discontinuation of OT services to the supervising OTR.

2. An OTR prepares and implements a discontinuation plan that addresses appropriate follow-up resources. A COTA may contribute to the implementation of a discontinuation plan under the supervision of an OTR.

3. An OTR documents changes in the client's status between the initial evaluation and discontinuation of services. A COTA may contribute to the process under the supervision of an OTR.

4. An OTR documents recommendations for follow-up or reevaluation, when applicable.

REFERENCES

AOTA. (1979). The philosophical base of OT. *Am J Occup Ther, 33,* 785.

AOTA. (1991a). Essentials and guidelines of an accredited educational program for the OT. *Am J Occup Ther, 45,* 1077-1084.

AOTA. (1991b). Essentials and guidelines of an accredited educational program for the OTA. *Am J Occup Ther, 45,* 1085-1092.

AOTA. (1994a). OT code of ethics. *Am J Occup Ther, 48,* 1037-1038.

AOTA. (1994b). Statement of OT referral. *Am J Occup Ther, 48,* 1034.

AOTA. (1994c). Uniform terminology for OT (3rd ed.). *Am J Occup Ther, 49,* 1047-1054.

AOTA. (1995). Concept paper: Service delivery in OT. *Am J Occup Ther, 49,* 1029-1031.

AOTA. (1997). Bylaws. Article III, Section 1. Bethesda, MD: Author.

Hinojosa, J., & Kramer, P. (Eds.). (1998). OT evaluation of clients: Obtaining and interpreting data. Bethesda, MD: AOTA.

Adopted by the Representative Assembly 1998M15

Note: This document replaces the 1994 *Standards of Practice for OT.*

Occupational Therapy Code of Ethics — 2000

Ruth Hansen, PhD, OTR, FAOTA,
Chairperson, Commission on Standards and Ethics (SEC), AOTA

Permission was granted for the reproduction of this document by AOTA.

PREAMBLE

The AOTA's *Code of Ethics* is a public statement of the common set of values and principles used to promote and maintain high standards of behavior in OT. The AOTA and its members are committed to furthering the ability of individuals, groups, and systems to function within their total environment. To this end, OT personnel (including all staff and personnel who work and assist in providing OT services, (e.g., aides, orderlies, secretaries, technicians) have a responsibility to provide services to recipients in any stage of health and illness who are individuals, research participants, institutions and businesses, other professionals and colleagues, students, and to the general public.

The OT *Code of Ethics* is a set of principles that applies to OT personnel at all levels. These principles to which OTs and OTAs aspire are part of a lifelong effort to act in an ethical manner. The various roles of practitioner (OT and OTA), educator, fieldwork educator, clinical supervisor, manager, administrator, consultant, fieldwork coordinator, faculty program director, researcher/scholar, private practice owner, entrepreneur, and student are assumed.

Any action in violation of the spirit and purpose of this Code shall be considered unethical. To ensure compliance with the Code, the Commission on Standards and Ethics (SEC) establishes and maintains the enforcement procedures. Acceptance of membership in the AOTA commits members to adherence to the *Code of Ethics* and its enforcement procedures. The *Code of Ethics, Core Values and Attitudes of Occupational Therapy Practice* (AOTA, 1993), and the *Guidelines to the Occupational Therapy Code of Ethics* (AOTA, 1998) are aspirational documents designed to be used together to guide OT personnel.

Principle 1. OT personnel shall demonstrate a concern for the well-being of the recipients of their services (beneficence).

OT personnel shall provide services in a fair and equitable manner. They shall recognize and appreciate the cultural components of economics, geography, race, ethnicity, religious and political factors, marital status, sexual orientation, and disability of all recipients of their services.

OT practitioners shall strive to ensure that fees are fair and reasonable and commensurate with services performed. When OT practitioners set fees, they shall set fees considering institutional, local, state, and federal requirements, and with due regard for the service recipient's ability to pay.

OT personnel shall make every effort to advocate for recipients to obtain needed services through available means.

Principle 2. OT personnel shall take reasonable precautions to avoid imposing or inflicting harm upon the recipient of services or to his or her property (nonmaleficence).

OT personnel shall maintain relationships that do not exploit the recipient of services sexually, physically, emotionally, financially, socially, or in any other manner.

OT practitioners shall avoid relationships or activities that interfere with professional judgment and objectivity.

Principle 3. OT personnel shall respect the recipient and/or their surrogate(s) as well as the recipient's rights (autonomy, privacy, confidentiality).

OT practitioners shall collaborate with service recipients or their surrogate(s) in setting goals and priorities throughout the intervention process.

OT practitioners shall fully inform the service recipients of the nature, risks, and potential outcomes of any interventions.

OT practitioners shall obtain informed consent from participants involved in research activities and indicate that they have fully informed and advised the participants of potential risks and outcomes. OT practitioners shall endeavor to ensure that the participant(s) comprehend these risks and outcomes.

OT personnel shall respect the individual's right to refuse professional services or involvement in research or educational activities.

OT personnel shall protect all privileged confidential forms of written, verbal, and electronic communication gained from educational, practice, research, and investigational activities unless otherwise mandated by local, state, or federal regulations.

Principle 4. OT personnel shall achieve and continually maintain high standards of competence (duties).

OT practitioners shall hold the appropriate national and state credentials for the services they provide.

OT practitioners shall use procedures that conform to the standards of practice and other appropriate AOTA documents relevant to practice.

OT practitioners shall take responsibility for maintaining and documenting competence by participating in professional development and educational activities.

OT practitioners shall critically examine and keep current with emerging knowledge relevant to their practice so they may perform their duties on the basis of accurate information.

OT practitioners shall protect service recipients by ensuring that duties assumed by or assigned to other OT personnel match credentials, qualifications, experience, and scope of practice.

OT practitioners shall provide appropriate supervision to individuals for whom the practitioners have supervisory responsibility in accordance with Association policies, local, state and federal laws, and institutional values.

OT practitioners shall refer to or consult with other service providers whenever such a referral or consultation would be helpful to the care of the recipient of service. The referral or consultation process should be done in collaboration with the recipient of service.

Principle 5. OT personnel shall comply with laws and Association policies guiding the profession of OT (justice).

OT personnel shall familiarize themselves with and seek to understand and abide by applicable Association policies; local, state, and federal laws; and institutional rules.

OT practitioners shall remain abreast of revisions in those laws and Association policies that apply to the profession of OT and shall inform employers, employees, and colleagues of those changes.

OT practitioners shall require those they supervise in OT-related activities to adhere to the *Code of Ethics*.

OT practitioners shall take reasonable steps to ensure employers are aware of OT's ethical obligations, as set forth in this *Code of Ethics*, and of the implications of those obligations for OT practice, education, and research.

OT practitioners shall record and report in an accurate and timely manner all information related to professional activities.

Principle 6. OT personnel shall provide accurate information about OT services (veracity).

OT personnel shall accurately represent their credentials, qualifications, education, experience, training, and competence. This is of particular importance for those to whom OT personnel provide their services or with whom OT practitioners have a professional relationship.

OT personnel shall disclose any professional, personal, financial, business, or volunteer affiliations that may pose a conflict of interest to those with whom they may establish a professional, contractual, or other working relationship.

OT personnel shall refrain from using or participating in the use of any form of communication that contains false, fraudulent, deceptive, or unfair statements or claims.

OT practitioners shall accept the responsibility for their professional actions which reduce the public's trust in OT services and those that perform those services.

Principle 7. OT personnel shall treat colleagues and other professionals with fairness, discretion, and integrity (fidelity).

OT personnel shall preserve, respect, and safeguard confidential information about colleagues and staff, unless otherwise mandated by national, state, or local laws.

OT practitioners shall accurately represent the qualifications, views, contributions, and findings of colleagues.

OT personnel shall take adequate measures to discourage, prevent, expose, and correct any breaches of the and report any breaches of the *Code of Ethics* to the appropriate authority.

OT personnel shall familiarize themselves with established policies and procedures for handling concerns about this *Code of Ethics*, including familiarity with national, state, local, district, and territorial procedures for handling ethics complaints. These include policies and procedures created by the AOTA, licensing and regulatory bodies, employers, agencies, certification boards, and other organizations who have jurisdiction over OT practice.

REFERENCES

AOTA. (1993). Core values and attitudes of occupational therapy practice. *Am J Occup Ther, 47,* 1085-1086.

AOTA. (1998). Guidelines to the occupational therapy code of ethics. *Am J Occup Ther, 52,* 881-884.

AUTHORS

The Commission on Standards and Ethics (SEC):

Barbara L. Kornblau, JD, OTR, FAOTA, Chairperson
Melba Arnold, MS, OTR/L
Nancy Nashiro, PhD, OTR, FAOTA
Diane Hill, COTA/L, AP
Deborah Y. Slater, MS, OTR/L
John Morris, PhD
Linda Withers, CNHA, FACHCA
Penny Kyler, MA, OTR/L, FAOTA, Staff Liaison

Adopted by the Representative Assembly 2000M15

Note: This document replaces the 1994 document, OT *Code of Ethics* (*American Journal of Occupational Therapy, 48,* 1037–1038).

Prepared 4/7/2000

Internet Resources

Karen Sladyk, PhD, OTR, FAOTA

Trying to keep an Internet resource list current is like trying to hold water in your hands; but these sites are good places to start. Each site has been reviewed for accurate contact and has been judged as stable. The reader is cautioned to evaluate Internet information with extreme care. Because Internet information is not peer reviewed and the author is often unknown, the worth of Internet material is often of no scientific value. Internet information is fast but students are cautioned that the Internet does not replace scholarly inquiry.

To evaluate a web site, look for content accuracy first. Does the site publish information that you know is true from other reliable print forms such as journals? What seems to be the mission of the web site? To sell you something? Fundraise for their cause? Both sales and fundraising are acceptable Internet tools but does that seem to be the main purpose of a national organization's web site? Are author's names and peer-reviewed material available on the site?

Formats that are user friendly and assessable make a web site easier to use but do not be mislead by slick web sites that lack scientific content. Reliable sites usually have web masters that can accurately blend content and ease of use. The bottom line: Be careful of Internet information and make sure you confirm all content with non-Internet resources.

SITES THAT PROVIDE LINKS TO OTHER OCCUPATIONAL THERAPY SITES

The Health Professions Resource Center: www.THPRC.com

OT: www.occupationaltherapist.com

SITES OF INTEREST TO OCCUPATIONAL THERAPY ASSISTANTS

Administration on Aging: www.aoa.dhhs.gov

Advance for OT: www.merion.com/sitemap.html

Alzheimer's Association: www.alz.org

American Association of Retired Persons: www.aarp.org

American Cancer Society: www.cancer.org/frames.html

American Diabetes Association: www.diabetes.org/custom.asp

American Dietetic Association: www.eatright.org

American Occupational Therapy Foundation: www.aotf.org

AOTA: www.aota.org

Arthritis Foundation: www.arthritis.org

CBS Healthwatch: http://cbshealthwatch.health.aol.com

CINAHL: www.cinahl.com

CNN Food and Health: www.cnn.com

Discovery Channel: www.discovery.com

Elderhostel: www.elderhostel.org

Health Care Financing Administration: www.hcfa.gov

HealthFinder: www.healthfinder.gov

Health on the Net: www.hon.ch

HealthWeb: www.healthweb.org

Humor Matters: www.humormatters.com

ICIDH-2: www.who.int/icidh/

Juvenile Diabetes Foundation: www.jdfcure.org

Leisure and Aging Center: http://web.indstate.edu/nrpa-las/links.html

Medicare: www.medicare.gov

Muscle charts of the human body: www.ptcentral.com/muscles

Muscular Dystrophy Association: www.mdausa.org

National Cancer Institute: www.nci.nih.gov

National Council on the Aging: www.ncoa.org

National Eye Institute: www.nei.nih.gov

National Institute of Arthritis, Musculoskeletal, and Skin Diseases: www.nih.gov/niams

National Institute of Child Health and Human Development: www.nichd.nih.gov

National Institute of Diabetes, Digestive, and Kidney Diseases: www.niddk.nih.gov

National Institute of Health: www.nih.gov

National Institute of Mental Health: www.nimh.nih.gov

National Institute of Neurological Disorders and Stroke: www.ninds.nih.gov

National Institute on Aging: www.nih.gov/nia

National Institute on Alcohol Abuse and Alcoholism: www.niaaa.nih.gov

National Institute on Deafness and Other Communication Disorders: www.nih.gov/nidcd

National Institute on Drug Abuse: www.nida.nih.gov/NIDAHome1.html

National Library of Medicine: www.nlm.nih.gov/nlmhome.html

National Mental Health Association: www.nmha.org

National Osteoporosis Foundation: www.nof.org

National Parkinson Foundation: www.parkinson.org

National Rehabilitation Information Center: www.naric.com/naric

National Stroke Association: www.stroke.org

NBCOT: www.nbcot.org

Prevent Blindness: www.preventblindness.org

Public Broadcasting System: www.pbs.org

Sensory Integration International: http://home.earthlink.net/~sensoryint

Social Security: www.ssa.gov

US Government guidelines on evidence-based practice: www.ahrq.gov

Veterans' Administration: www.va.gov

World Federation of OTs: www.who.int/ina-ngo/ngo/ngo170.htm

World Health Organization: www.who.org

Index

BUILD *Your Library*

This book and many others on numerous different topics are available from SLACK Incorporated. For further information or a copy of our latest catalog, contact us at:

Professional Book Division
SLACK Incorporated
6900 Grove Road
Thorofare, NJ 08086 USA
Telephone: 1-856-848-1000
1-800-257-8290
Fax: 1-856-853-5991
E-mail: orders@slackinc.com
www.slackbooks.com

We accept most major credit cards and checks or money orders in US dollars drawn on a US bank. Most orders are shipped within 72 hours.

Contact us for information on recent releases, forthcoming titles, and bestsellers. If you have a comment about this title or see a need for a new book, direct your correspondence to the Editorial Director at the above address.

Thank you for your interest and we hope you found this work beneficial.